OTHER MONOGRAPHS IN THE SERIES
MAJOR PROBLEMS IN PATHOLOGY

Published

Evans and Cruickshank: *Epithelial Tumors of the Salivary Glands*

Mottet: *Histopathologic Spectrum of Regional Enteritis and Ulcerative Colitis*

Hughes: *Pathology of Muscle*

Thurlbeck: *Chronic Airflow Obstruction in Lung Disease*

Hughes: *Pathology of the Spinal Cord, 2nd ed.*

Fox: *Pathology of the Placenta*

Striker, Quadracci and Cutler: *Use and Interpretation of Renal Biopsy*

Asbury and Johnson: *Pathology of Peripheral Nerve*

Morson: *The Pathogenesis of Colorectal Cancer*

Azzopardi: *Problems in Breast Pathology*

Hendrickson and Kempson: *Surgical Pathology of the Uterine Corpus*

Katzenstein and Askin: *Surgical Pathology of Non-Neoplastic Lung Disease*

Frable: *Thin-Needle Aspiration Biopsy*

Wigglesworth: *Perinatal Pathology*

Whitehead: *Mucosal Biopsy of the Gastrointestinal Tract, 3rd ed.*

Jaffe: *Surgical Pathology of Lymph Nodes and Related Organs*

Wittels: *Surgical Pathology of Bone Marrow*

Forthcoming

Hughes: *Pathology of Muscle, 2nd ed.*

LiVolsi: *Pathology of the Thyroid*

Lukeman and Mackay: *Tumors of the Lung*

Mackay, Evans and Ayala: *Soft Tissue Tumors*

Mottet & Norris: *Histopathology of Inflammatory Bowel Disease, 2nd ed.*

Nash and Said: *Pathology of Acquired Immune Deficiency*

Neiman & Wolf: *Diseases of the Spleen*

Reagan and Fu: *Pathology of the Uterine Cervix, Vagina and Vulva*

Variakojis and Vardiman: *Pathology of the Myeloproliferative Disorders*

Clive Roy Taylor, MA., M.D., D.Phil., M.R.C.Path.

Professor and Chairman of Pathology
University of Southern California
Los Angeles, California

Immunomicroscopy: A Diagnostic Tool for the Surgical Pathologist

Volume 19 in the Series
MAJOR PROBLEMS IN PATHOLOGY

JAMES L. BENNINGTON, M.D., *Consulting Editor*

Chairman, Department of Pathology
Children's Hospital of San Francisco
San Francisco, California

1986

W. B. SAUNDERS COMPANY
PHILADELPHIA LONDON TORONTO MEXICO CITY
RIO DE JANEIRO SYDNEY TOKYO HONG KONG

W. B. Saunders Company: West Washington Square
Philadelphia, PA   19105

Library of Congress Cataloging-in-Publication Data

Taylor, C. R. (Clive Roy)
Immunomicroscopy: a diagnostic tool for the surgical pathologist.

(Major problems in pathology; v. 19)
Bibliography: p.
Includes index.

1. Pathology, Surgical. 2. Immunohistochemistry.
   3. Tumors—Diagnosis.   I. Title.   II. Series.
   [DNLM: 1. Histocytochemistry—methods. 2. Immunologic
   Technics. 3. Microscopy—methods. 4. Pathology—methods.
   W1 MA492X v. 19 / QZ 25 T239i]

RD57.T39 1986   617′.079   86–11824

ISBN 0–7216–8770–9

Editor: Suzanne Boyd

Designer: Terri Siegel

Production Manager: Pete Faber

Manuscript Editor: Lorraine Zawodny

Illustration Coordinator: Walt Verbitski

Page Layout Artist: Meg Jolly

Indexer: Dennis Dolan

Immunomicroscopy: A Diagnostic Tool for the Surgical Pathologist   ISBN 0–7216–8770–9

Last digit is the print number: 9   8   7   6   5   4   3   2

To my wife Susan for laughing, and not laughing, in the right places and to Emma, Ben, Jeremy, and Matt for avoidance of major physical and emotional trauma during this labor.

Contributors

CLIVE ROY TAYLOR, M.A., M.D., D.PHIL., M.R.C.PATH.,
Professor and Chairman of Pathology,
University of Southern California,
Los Angeles, California

with contributions by

ROY H. RHODES, M.D., PH.D.,
Neuropathologist, Assistant Professor of Pathology,
Cajal Laboratories, University of Southern California,
Los Angeles, California

ANDREW E. SHERROD, M.D.,
Pathologist, Assistant Professor of Clinical Pathology,
University of Southern California,
Los Angeles, California

BRUNANGELO FALINI, M.D.,
Universita di Perugia,
Perugia, Italy

Foreword

Progress in the field of anatomic pathology has been shaped in large part by the tools—gross examination, light microscopy, histochemistry, electron microscopy, and so forth—available to researchers at the time of their investigations.

Immunochemistry, which has its origins in the techniques of immunofluorescence, has relatively recently emerged as an important and powerful diagnostic tool following the development of immunoenzymatic, particularly immunoperoxidase, techniques and the demonstration that their use extended to routinely fixed, paraffin-embedded tissues. Dr. Clive Taylor, the author of this volume of the Major Problems in Pathology series, has played a major role in the development of this new field.

New discoveries are being made each day in the applications of immunocytochemistry to the diagnosis of neoplasms and infectious diseases. The immunoperoxidase technique has already proved an invaluable aid to the classification of neoplasms in terms of the cell of origin, direction of differentiation, and biologic activity. It holds great promise for further use in the characterization of a variety of tumors through elucidating unique immunophenotypic signatures.

In view of the extensive research on immunochemistry in pathology during the past few years, it is essential that the results of these studies be critically reviewed and summarized in a single reference source. Dr. Taylor provides in IMMUNOMICROSCOPY an authoritative review of the subject of immunochemistry that is encyclopedic and also is enjoyable reading. The monograph amply covers both the theoretical and practical aspects of the subject. It will be invaluable to pathologists, oncologists, surgeons, microbiologists and basic scientists.

James L. Bennington, M.D.

Preface

"Begin at the beginning, go on until you get to the end, then stop."

Advice from the King to Alice in her
Adventures in Wonderland.

LEWIS CARROLL (1832–1898)

This book sets out the basic theoretical and practical aspects of immuno-histology and immunocytochemistry. The content and format is designed for use primarily by the practicing surgical pathologist and histotechnologist, rather than for the research scientist or the avant garde investigator. Dedicated researchers already have a sufficiency, even a surfeit, of reading material in the recent literature, which includes some 1000 immunoperoxidase references in 1984 alone, not to mention countless reports describing the various scientific pursuits of the adepts of the immunofluorescence school. The majority of these papers are highly specialized in content, dealing with only one of many minutely focused research interests or with only one or another of the principal immunohistologic techniques. Such works, although fundamental to the advancement of knowledge and technique in immunohistology are, by their specialized nature, of limited value to the practicing surgical pathologist wishing to adopt and adapt these methods to more routine but clinically immediate purposes. This book is intended to provide a selected literature resource and a working text for the practicing pathologist, a text sound in theory and explicit in practical details, with ample discussion of interpretation and usage of immunohistologic techniques in diagnostic practice.

Of the basic immunohistologic techniques, immunofluorescence is the older (45th birthday this year) and the better established. Immunoperoxidase methods, although conceived more than 20 years ago, suffered a long gestation period and really only emerged into the light of day in 1974, with the demonstration of applicability of immunoperoxidase methods to routinely processed paraffin sections. This book seeks to present the basic principles of both the immunofluorescence and immunoperoxidase methods, with a marked emphasis on the latter. The similarities between these two techniques are greater than the differences, yet the differences may lead to a preference for one method over the other, according to the demands of the study in hand. These same differences have also resulted in long and acrimonious debates, which have borne little fruit in proportion to the time and energy consumed.

The author of this book has had experience with both immunofluorescence and immunoperoxidase methods, has been fortunate to work directly with several of the pioneers in this field, and has rubbed shoulders with many others.

This text is their creation as much as mine, and I acknowledge the debt, particularly to Drs. David Mason and Ian Burns (Oxford University), Dr. Stebbins Chandor (Marshall University, West Virginia), Dr. Robert Nakamura (Scripps Clinic, California), Drs. Mehrdad Nadji and Azorides Morales (University of Miami, Florida), and Drs. Florence Hofman, Paul Pattengale, Andy Sherrod, Alan Epstein and Sue Ellen Martin, with whom I am privileged to work at the University of Southern California. Dr. Brunangelo Falini (Perugia, Italy) made important contributions to the methods chapter while a fellow at USC; Dr. Andy Sherrod contributed greatly to the algorithm for anaplastic tumors described in Chapter 14; and Dr. Roy Rhodes (neuropathologist at USC) wrote the chapter on the central nervous system. Dr. Alan Epstein, who has recently joined our faculty, has also made major contributions with reference to the development and utilization of monoclonal antibodies. Many other fellows and visiting scientists have passed through, and in so doing have made their contribution; they include Dr. Jan van den Tweel (Heerlen, The Netherlands), Dr. Robert Maurer (Zurich, Switzerland), Dr. Tom Dura (Warsaw, Poland), Dr. Martii Aliviakko (Oulu, Finland), Dr. Lertikana Bhoopat (Chiang Mai, Thailand), Dr. Giuseppe Santeusanio (Rome, Italy), Dr. Olav Haugen (Trondheim, Norway), Dr. Dolores Lopez Vancel (Mexico City, Mexico), Dr. Demi Anagoustou (Athens, Greece), Dr. Gordana Stevanovic (Belgrade, Yugoslavia), Dr. David Ormerod (Currently at the Boston Eye Research Institute), Dr. Lena Krugliak (Israel), Dr. Wolfgang Friedmann (Berlin, West Germany), and a number of American fellows working with Dr. Robert Lukes, Dr. John Parker, or myself: Drs. Hank Williams, Doug Schneider, Richard Miller, Henry Slosser, Robert Modlin, Norman Levy, Michael Samoszuk, Eugene Yanagihara, and others who have played greater or lesser parts.

At different times we have separately championed one or other of the various immunohistologic techniques in mortal debate. Now in some areas we have agreement; in others, like gentlemen (and ladies), we agree to differ. This book is thus the result of a decade of healthy debate.

From this pool of knowledge, experience, and differing opinions, the goal is to provide a text that is useful to the surgical pathologist and clinical immunopathologist, both in describing the applications of immunohistology in general, and in guiding the choice as to the preferred method for particular purposes.

Immunohistology represents a relatively new area of pathology research and practice. Its potential usefulness is, I believe, very great. Widespread application of immunohistologic methods, by virtue of their great specificity, inevitably will transform histopathology from something resembling an art into something more closely resembling a science, with profound effects upon the way in which we recognize normal and abnormal cells by the microscope.

THE TEXT: ORGANIZATION AND BIBLIOGRAPHY

"It is much simpler to buy books than to read them, and easier to read them than absorb their contents."

WILLIAM OSLER
British Medical Journal
2:925, 1909

Chapter 1 deals with general principles, many of which apply both to immunoperoxidase and to immunofluorescence techniques, and include discussion of these methods in general terms. Subsequent chapters are divided into two groups; Chapters 2 and 3 describe technical aspects of fixation and the various immunoperoxidase techniques, and the remainder of the book is devoted to the practical applications of immunohistologic methods in diagnostic pathology. The rationale for selecting one method over another is given and discussed together with details of practical techniques and interpretation of the stained preparations. Certain key references are included within the text. However, most references are collected into tables covering particular topics; here the references are given by author and year with a brief commentary as to the relevance of the paper to the practicing surgical pathologist. This course has been adopted to achieve an uncluttered text from which the basic information pertaining to diagnosis may readily be extracted without wading through a morass of citations. The text presents a distillate of these tabulated references; access to the unadulterated original papers is given in a comprehensive bibliography at the end of the book. The appendices contain detailed staining protocols and information regarding commercial sources of the basic reagents and antibodies.

A HANDBOOK FOR EXPLORERS

Equipped with this book and a judicious selection of these wares, the pathologist may, without undue trepidation, venture forth into the still only partially explored world of immunohistochemistry. It will be something of an adventure. This is intended to be a guidebook; like all early guidebooks, it will be subject to repeated modification as the frontiers are defined and redefined. You, as co-adventurers are invited to share in this process.

CLIVE R. TAYLOR

Acknowledgements

The author is indebted to Betty Redmon, Cathleen Cooper, Jane Sindayen, and Elisa Arango for deciphering the manuscript in its various forms; to Barbara Felder, Betsy Yurth, Mary Drushella, Lillian Young, Brad Lyons, and Ray Russell for excellent technical support; and to Nick Douglas, who labored long over the production of the black and white prints included herein. Drs. Steb Chandor (Marshall University) and Bob Nakamura (Scripps Clinic, California) provided critical advice and crucial encouragement during the early stages of gestation.

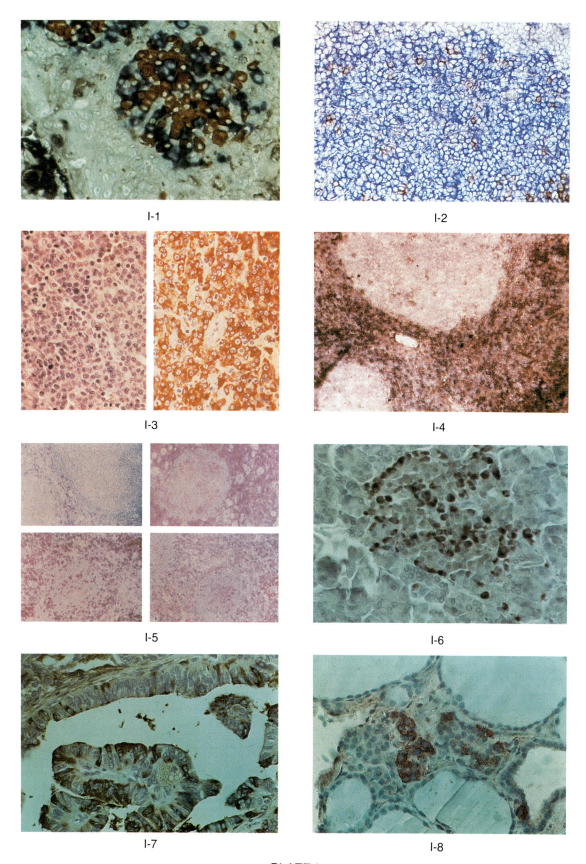

I-1

I-2

I-3

I-4

I-5

I-6

I-7

I-8

PLATE I

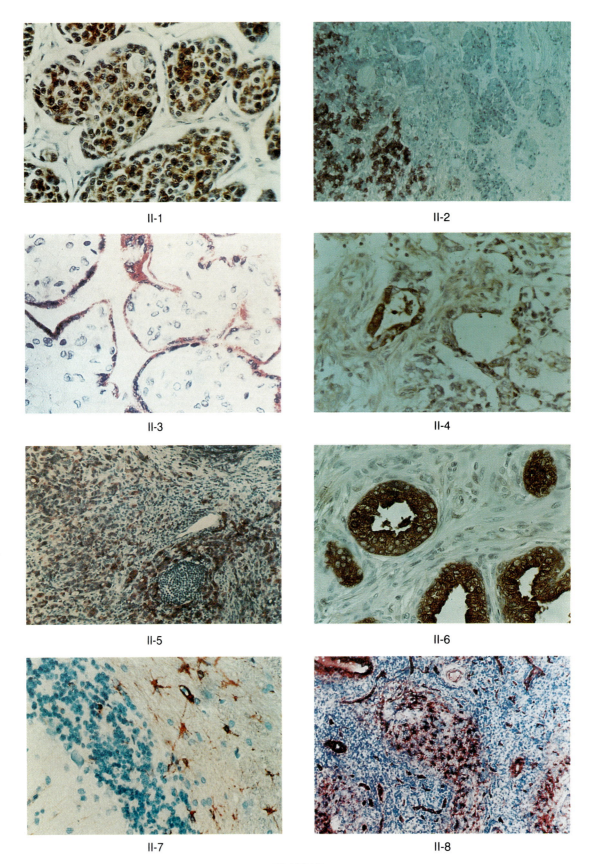

II-1

II-2

II-3

II-4

II-5

II-6

II-7

II-8

PLATE II

Contents

PRINCIPLES OF IMMUNOMICROSCOPY

"The pathologist with the highest CQ (credibility quotient) often carries the day."

TAYLOR AND KLEDZIK, 1981

HISTORICAL BACKGROUND

The Microscope in the Beginning

The history of medicine is in large part the history of advances in basic sciences and the translation of these advances into diagnostic or therapeutic practice.

In the beginning there were only "practitioners of the art," variously termed physicians or barber surgeons, according to their background and proclivities. Pathologists existed only to the extent that a practitioner piqued by curiosity or morbid interest might, when all else had failed, seek the final solution at the autopsy table. Indeed, by means of the meticulously detailed autopsy (Fig. 1–1A), with painstaking attention to abnormalities of gross anatomy, the "art" was advanced ever so slowly over a period of several thousand years from ancient to modern times.

In this context, at least with reference to pathology, the modern era commenced in the middle of the nineteenth century. It is easy to forget that Hodgkin's disease, a condition now diagnosed on the basis of minutely described microscopic characteristics, was first recognized 150 years ago (by Thomas Hodgkin, 1832) on the basis of detailed gross dissection of seven cases, without resort to microscopic examination. Indeed, it was not until a decade later, in 1842, that one of the first organized courses in histology was given, by John Hughes Bennett at the University of Edinburgh. Microscopes and microscopists certainly existed prior to this time, as evidenced by the extensive botanic illustrations of Robert Hooke (*Micrographia*, London, 1665); the zoologic, principally entymologic, drawings of Jan Swammardam (*Bybel der Na tuur*, Utrecht, 1669); and the 247 microscopes that Atonj van Leeuwenhoek (1632–1723) is

reputed to have possessed. Some have argued that the beginnings of histology date from the work of Marcello Malpighi (1628–1694), who delved into the microscopic world of embryology, portrayed the minute architecture of the spleen, and described red blood cells as "fat globules looking like a rosary of red coral," all this only a few years after Swammardam's first report of the existence of red corpuscles. However, these studies although startling in detail consisted only of accumulated sporadic observations and lacked the basis of an organized background of knowledge that Hughes Bennett was able to bring together for his histology course.

If Hughes Bennett deserves credit for his role in introducing histology into the curriculum and the minds of students of medicine, then Rudolf Virchow must be given credit for the first textbook of histopathology. Virchow's book, *Cellularpathologie*, was first published in 1856, with an English edition appearing in 1860 (Fig. 1–1B). It was based on a series of 20 lectures in which Virchow demonstrated, for the first time, that it was possible to establish the diagnosis and prognosis in many disease states by careful study, using the microscope, of cells and tissues. The concept that diseases resulted from imbalances of the body humors crumbled as physicians turned the pages of *Cellularpathologie* and were introduced to a new field of investigative and diagnostic medicine that was to form the foundation of histopathology.

The literature pertaining to microscopic anatomy and microscopic pathology grew rapidly as medical practitioners and researchers utilized the microscope to refine and redefine "old diseases" or to recognize and define hitherto undiscovered "new entities." Various staining techniques were developed

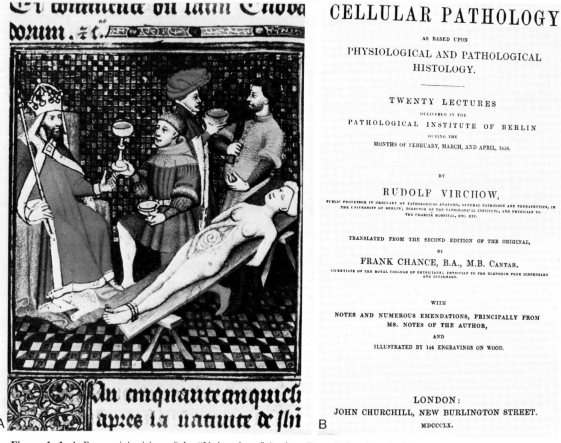

Figure 1–1. *A,* Boccaccio's vision of the "University of Ancient Rome" showing the Emperor Nero presiding at the autopsy of his mother Agrippina, whom he had put to death. (Original miniature in *Le Cas des Nobles et Femmes* [c1410]. Used with kind permission of Photographie Giraudon, Paris.) *B,* Title page for Cellular Pathology by Rudolf Virchow, English Language Edition, 1860. (Reproduced from a special edition issued by the Classics of Medicine Library, Birmingham, Alabama, 1978, by permission.)

to facilitate the study of tissue sections, staining cell nuclei, cytoplasm, or extracellular tissue components in a variety of contrasting colors. With each new report describing each new entity, the scope of histopathology was enlarged, with the result that within a few decades a major commitment of time and energy was required in order to become proficient in interpretation of the histologic appearances of normal and abnormal tissues. Thus the first pathologists emerged from the treacherous swamps of medieval medical practice onto the relatively firm ground that histopathology seemed to offer with respect to diagnosis of disease.

The practice of diagnostic histopathology, once established, changed little in principle during the succeeding 100 years. To be sure, numerous new morphologic criteria, some subtle to a degree, have been described, and many new entities have been established. Yet

the principles by which the histopathologist works and learns his trade have not changed significantly.

When first sitting at the microscope, the fledgling pathologist is faced with the problem of the recognition and nomenclature of each individual cell. What are the characteristic features that distinguish lymphocytes, erythroblasts, plasma cells, thyroid "parafollicular" C cells, and others?

Traditionally the pathologist has only two ways of seeking answers to these questions, only two ways of learning the art of "tissue diagnosis." First, he can show the slide to a more experienced colleague; the appropriate recognition criteria are then passed by word of mouth from pathologist to pathologist, from generation to generation. The second approach, at first sight more scientific in basis, involves a search of the textbooks or medical literature for a written description that corresponds to the cell in question, or even better, for a photomicrograph of a cell that upon comparison appears so similar to the cell visualized with the microscope as to justify applying to it the designation given in the textbook legend.

It is not too difficult to remind ourselves that criteria passed by word of mouth represent nothing more than an expression of the opinion of the experienced pathologist and that this opinion in turn paraphrases the opinion of his teachers. It is, however, rarely remembered that descriptions and illustrations in textbooks also are expressions of opinion and that these opinions, given additional weight and credibility by their appearance on the printed page, become tantamount to established facts. It is remarkable that histopathology, founded upon criteria derived from subjective opinions formed during the interpretation of cellular and subcellular patterns, has proven so successful and reliable over the years.

Nonetheless, experienced surgical pathologists recognize that many diagnoses are hedged with uncertainty as a direct consequence of the subjective nature of the judgments that pathologists must make.

Although knowledge of histopathology has advanced considerably, the basic principles of diagnosis based upon examination of a tissue section have not changed significantly since the time of Bennett and Virchow. However experienced the pathologist, the application and interpretation of morphologic criteria remain subjective. Diagnosis by examination of a tissue section is therefore often hedged with uncertainty, and opinions of experienced pathologists may differ critically with regard to the designation and import of any particular lesion. In such circumstances, when opinions differ, the diagnosis is usually resolved according to the consensus of opinions of several consulting pathologists, or in deference to the opinion of the most prestigious or the most forceful of those consulted. Thus the pathologist with the highest Credibility Quotient (CQ) (Fig. 1–2) often carries the day, and the diagnosis is considered final; there is no recourse to independent techniques for testing the rightness or wrongness of the prevailing opinion, upon which the ultimate diagnosis was based. Taylor & Kledzik, 1981.

The Need for Special Stains

Pathologists have long since recognized their fallibility, although they have not always publicized it (reviews, Taylor, 1978c, 1983a). They have therefore sought more certain means of validating morphologic judgments.

A variety of "special stains" were developed to facilitate cell recognition and diagnosis; most of these stains were based upon chemical reactions of cell and tissue components (histochemistry). In certain circumstances these histochemical strains proved to be of critical value in specific cell identification. More often they served merely to highlight or emphasize cellular or histological features that supported a particular interpretation without providing truly specific confirmation.

Immunohistology

The facility for performing a wide variety of truly specific special stains was available, at least in potential form, with the advent of a practical immunofluorescence technique (Coons et al, 1941). The immunofluorescence-labelled antibody method exploits the specific binding between antibody and antigen, utilizing antibody labelled with a visible marker (usually fluorescein isothiocyanate) as a visible probe for the presence of the corresponding antigen within tissue sections or cell preparations. The immunofluorescence

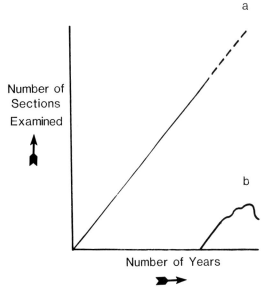

Figure 1–2. The workload accumulator graph (WAG) for calculating credibility quotient (CQ). WAG (a) shows a steady rise to infinity; the area under the line is a measure of the credibility quotient (CQ), which in this instance is awesome. WAG (b) represents a less impressive situation; the WAG has tailed off, the credibility quotient is correspondingly diminished, and the hedges of uncertainty loom tall in all directions. Type (b) WAGs stand to benefit most from immunohistologic methods; type (a) WAGs have the most to lose, particularly their aura of infallibility. It has been suggested that CQ and IQ show an inverse correlation.

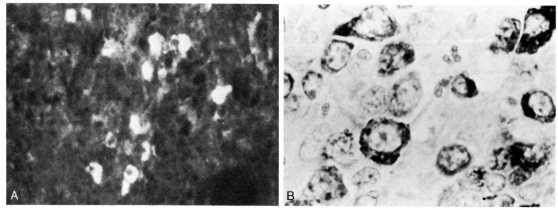

Figure 1–3. *A,* The immunofluorescent method on frozen sections; staining for IgG in plasma cells within a frozen section. Positive cells appear white. The morphologic features of positive and negative cells are not discernible. Frozen section, cold ethanol fixed (×320). *B,* The immunoperoxidase method on paraffin sections; portion of the same lymph node as in *A,* but fixed in formalin and embedded in paraffin. Staining for immunoglobulin is by the PAP method giving a positive black reaction in the cytoplasm. The chromogen is DAB (diaminobenzidine) the counterstain hematoxylin. The usual morphologic features upon which the pathologist relies for diagnosis are preserved. Note the diverse morphologic appearance of cells in the "plasma cell family," i.e., not many of the positive cells would be recognized as immunoglobulin-producing (plasma) cells by morphologic criteria alone (×900).

technique, popularized by the work of Coons (1941), Fagraeus (1948), and others, developed into a powerful research tool, generating an extensive literature. In time it provided the basis for the development of immunopathology as a flourishing, rapidly growing branch of investigative pathology. However, the immunofluorescence technique had little impact on diagnostic pathology as practiced by the surgical pathologist for reasons that relate principally to difficulties in applying the method to "routinely" processed paraffin-embedded materials.

Nonetheless, the success of immunofluorescence in pathology research created a pressing need for an alternative labelling system to avoid some of the disadvantages inherent in the immunofluorescent method, namely the need for specialized microscopy, application largely restricted to frozen sections and poor morphologic resolution (Taylor, 1983a) (Fig. 1–3A). Labels other than fluorescein isothiocyanate were sought. Of the many "labels" given trial, immunoenzyme techniques, linking antibody to an enzyme, in lieu of fluorescein isothiocyanate, proved most practical. Several enzymes were assessed in this system, including horseradish peroxidase, glucose oxidase, and alkaline phosphatase, together with a number of different substrate systems, for demonstration of the site of localization of enzyme-labelled antibody within tissue sections. Horseradish per-

oxidase in conjunction with diaminobenzidine and hydrogen peroxide as the substrate had advantages over other systems and became widely used.

The final critical step in making immunohistologic methods available to the surgical pathologist was taken in 1974, when it was shown that, using immunoperoxidase techniques, it was possible to demonstrate at least some antigens in routinely processed (formalin-paraffin) tissue (Fig. 1–3B). This discovery gave a new impetus to the use of immunohistologic methods. For the first time it was possible specifically to demonstrate a wide range of tissue components (antigens) in the types of tissues that the surgical pathologist has at his disposal when the need for special staining techniques becomes apparent in attempting to reach a diagnosis.

Only 10 years have passed since the feasibility of performing immunohistologic studies on routinely processed tissues was demonstrated with reference to the staining of immunoglobulin within plasma cells (Taylor, 1974; Taylor and Burns, 1974; Burns et al, 1974). In this decade, however, the range of antigens demonstrable in such tissues has increased enormously (Table 1–1); the literature contains reports of studies demonstrating more than 100 different antigens, many of which are relevant to the surgical pathologist as potential "special stains" with true specificity.

Table 1–1. Range of Antibodies That Have Been Successfully Employed for Demonstration of Antigens in Paraffin Sections

Hormones	Other Cellular Components *Continued*	Infectious Agents
ACTH	Ferritin	Herpes I & II
GH	Hemoglobin A	Hepatitis B surface Ag
LH	Hemoglobin F	Mouse mammary tumor virus Ag
LTH	Myoglobin	Rubella
FSH	Actin	Baboon endogenous virus
TSH	Myosin	Measles Ag
Parathormone	Keratin	Respiratory syncytial virus
Calcitonin	alpha$_1$-Antitrypsin	Buffalo pox
Thyroxine	alpha$_1$-Antichymotrypsin	*Legionella*
Thyroglobulin	alpha-Fetoprotein	*Kliebsiella*
hCG	Carcinoembryonic Ag	Group B streptococcus
beta-hCG	Mammary epithelial membrane Ag	Influenza
Testosterone	Hepatorenal Ag	Poliovirus
Estradiol	Pancreatic Ag	Varicella-zoster
Progesterone	Melanoma Ag	Cytomegalovirus (CMV)
Insulin	Prostatic acid phosphatase	Parainfluenza virus
Glucagon	Prostate specific Ag	Lymphocytic choriomeningitis virus
Somatostatin	Glial fibrillary acidic protein	Moloney virus
VIP	Tyrosine hydroxylase	Friend virus
Gastrin	Myelin basic protein	Shope fibroma virus
Secretin	Enkephalin (-like) Ag	SV 40
Motilin	Substance P	Human papilloma virus
Neurotensin	Enolases	Distemper virus
Cholecystokinin	Adenosine deaminase	Rotavirus
Renin	Terminal transferase	Polyoma virus
Vasopressin	Carbonic anhydrase	*Chlamydia*
Oxytocin	Cathepsin D	*Mycoplasma*
Neurophysin	Converting enzyme	*Trichomonas*
Bombesin	Factor VIII-related Ag	*Toxoplasma*
	Creatine kinase	*Trichophyton*
Receptors	Intestinal mucin Ags	Amebae
Transferrin receptor protein	HLA Ags	*Mycobacteria*
Estrogen receptor protein	Blood group Ags	*Leishmania*
	Surfactant apoprotein	*Fasciola*
Other Tissue Components	S100 Ag	HTLVI
Laminin	Neurofilament	
Fibrinectin	Vimentin	**Immunoglobulin Components**
Collagens	Desmin	Kappa, lambda light chains
Amyloid A protein	Mucin Ags	Gamma, alpha, mu, delta, epsilon
	Celomic Ags	heavy chains
Other Cellular Components	CALLA	J chain
Lysozyme (muramidase)	CLA	Secretory component
Lactoferrin	Endocrine granule Ags	C1, C2, C3, C4
Transferrin	Ia-like Ags	
	B cell Ags	
	Monocyte Ags	

Immunofluorescence vs Immunoperoxidase

This book is partly based upon a description of the theoretical principles and practical applications of immunohistologic techniques for the surgical pathologist and immunopathologist. For the surgical pathologist, the emphasis clearly is upon immunoperoxidase techniques, since these are most readily applied to routinely processed tissues. In diagnostic and investigative immunopathology, both immunofluorescence and immunoperoxidase techniques are applicable, and often immunofluorescence is preferred, particularly if morphology is not at a premium. Although the differences between immunofluorescence and immunoperoxidase techniques are given certain emphasis, particularly with regard to surgical pathology, it is important to stress that the principles underlying these two methods are identical up to the point that it is necessary to visualize the labelled moiety.

THE PRINCIPLES OF IMMUNOMICROSCOPY

"What is hidden from the eyes it is vain to conceive as though it were visible."

PARACELSUS, 1492–1546

A Specific Special Stain

This book is not an exercise in the esoteric; rather, it is an attempt to familiarize pathologists with relatively new techniques that are easily taught and readily learned, broad in application, simple in execution, but profound in implication for the future practice of pathology.

Clearly much progress has been made from the time that pathology texts devoted several pages to discussion of the importance of positioning the microscope at a north-facing window, the desirability of utilizing cloud-reflected light, the virtues of concave versus plano-concave mirrors, and the art of peering through the eyepiece with one eye, while the other eye, still open, focused on an infinity that the visual cortex must learn to ignore. Advances have occurred and knowledge has accumulated by meticulous application of time-honored morphologic principles with use of modifications of conventional histological techniques aided by a variety of histochemical stains. Immunohistologic methods promise to add a new dimension to the practice of histopathology, facilitating the specific demonstration of a wide range of cell and tissue components while conserving the ability to assess traditional morphologic criteria.

The aims of immunohistology are akin to those of histochemistry. Indeed, immunohistology builds upon the foundations of histochemistry; it does not replace histochemistry but rather serves as a valuable adjunct greatly extending the variety of tissue components that can be demonstrated specifically within tissue sections or other cell preparations. Charles Culling, author of one of the more popular histochemical texts (Culling, 1964), writes that an essay by Raspail, "Essai de Chimie Microscopique Appliqué à la Physiologie," is generally regarded as the "beginning of histochemistry." This dates from the same era in which Bennett was teaching his course in histology in Edinburgh and Virchow was assembling the material that would form the basis of his 20 lectures, "Cellular-pathologie"; to a large degree, these developments were interdependent, all reflecting the then current interest in microscopic anatomy.

Culling went on to state that "the object of staining tissue sections is to impart colour and therefore contrast to specific tissue constituents." Lillie (1965) has it that "the purpose of staining is to make more evident various tissue and cell constituents and extrinsic materials."

Most "routine" histopathologic stains utilize a range of dyes that bind differentially with tissue components by virtue of solution phenomena or various and largely ill-understood chemical reactions. The standard hematoxylin and eosin stain, the primary stain in surgical pathology today, falls within this category; the hematoxylin component preferentially stains nuclei, whereas the eosin dye preferentially colors the cell cytoplasm and extracellular components.

Histochemistry, to the degree that it is separable from "routine" histopathologic staining, seeks to exploit predictable chemical reactions between the constituents of a stain and the various molecules that are to be found in cell nuclei, in cell cytoplasm, or in intracellular or extracellular tissue components. Histochemical stains have the potential for specific demonstration of tissue components but often are limited in application because of complexities in the staining procedure or, more often, because of the fact that fixation and paraffin embedment so alter the structure of molecules within the cells as to obscure their otherwise characteristic chemical reaction. For example, many enzymes that otherwise might be demonstrated by addition of suitable colorogenic substrate systems are rendered inactive by conventional fixation and processing procedures. To some extent, therefore, many of the more specific histochemical stains for enzymes must be reserved for fresh unfixed cryostat sections, which often are not available when the pathologist realizes the need for a special staining technique.

Mann (1902) is reported to have said, "The object of all staining is to recognize microchemically the existence and distribution of substances which we have been made aware of macrochemically. It is not sufficient to content ourselves with using acid and basic dyes speculating on the acid or basic nature of the tissues, or to apply colour radicals with oxidizing or reducing properties. We should find staining reactions which will indicate the presence of certain elements such as iron, phosphorus, carbohydrates, nucleus and protamines and so on." Mann's incentives toward the development of specific histochemical methods apply even more to immunohistologic methods in which the potential exists to demonstrate an almost limitless range of tissue components, according to the presence of small three-dimensional "charge-shape" moieties that constitute antigenic determinants against which it is possible to prepare specific antibodies. These antibodies then can be used as specific probes to localize the corresponding antigenic determinants within tissue and cell preparations.

Antibodies as Specific Staining Reagents

An antibody is a molecule that has the property of combining specifically with a second molecule, termed the antigen. Further, the production of antibody by an animal is induced specifically by the presence of antigen; this forms part of the basic immune response.

Antibodies are immunoglobulin molecules consisting of two basic units: a pair of light chains—either a kappa or a lambda pair—and a pair of heavy chains—gamma, alpha, mu, delta, or epsilon—bound together by disulfide linkages. Light chains have a molecular weight in the region of 25,000, heavy chains a molecular weight of 50,000; thus the molecular weight of a whole immunoglobulin molecule such as IgG, consisting of a pair of kappa chains (or lambda chains) and a pair of gamma chains, is about 150,000.

The structure of an IgG immunoglobulin molecule is depicted in Figure 1–4A. IgG has two specific antibody (antigen-binding) sites,

Figure 1–4. *A,* Structure of an IgG molecule. In the text this structure is reduced diagrammatically to a bivalent molecule, different specifications being represented by different–shaped binding sites as in a, b, or c. *B,* Antigens and antigenic determinants. An antigenic molecule may be considered to consist of an immunologically "inert" carrier component and one or more antigenic determinants of like type (left) or diverse types (right).

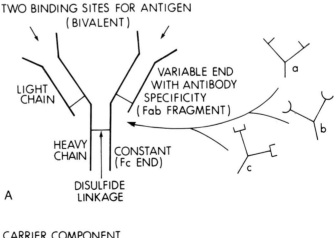

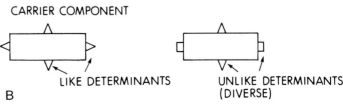

each able to bind specifically with one molecule of the inducing antigen. The binding sites are formed by the N-terminal ends of each light chain–heavy chain pairing, the specificity being determined by the exact amino acid sequences of the light and heavy chains. Thus different antibody molecules, having different specificities, display different amino acid sequences in the light and heavy chain components that comprise the binding site; these are termed the variable segments (idiotypes) of the light and heavy chains as opposed to the more constant sequences present at the opposite (Fc-constant) end of the molecule. For the purposes of depicting immunoglobulin molecules participating in the immunologic-immunohistochemical reactions described in this book, the organization of an immunoglobulin molecule may be further simplifed and represented as a bivalent molecule with two binding sites and a common linked portion corresponding to the constant segment (Fig. 1–4A).

An antigen may be any molecule that is sufficiently complex that it maintains a relatively rigid three-dimensional profile and is foreign to the animal into which it is introduced. Proteins and carbohydrates that are sufficiently complex to possess unique three-dimensional "charge-shape" profiles are good antigens; in fact, such molecules may bear more than one unique three-dimensional structure capable of inducing antibody formation (Fig. 1–4B); each of these individual sites on a molecule may be termed an antigenic determinant (or epitope), the determinant being the exact site on the molecule with which the antibody combines (Fig. 1–5).

An antibody, induced by a specific antigenic determinant, binds only to that determinant; theoretically the two binding sites of a bivalent antibody could bind to two separate determinants on the same or on separate molecules of antigen. In practice, in immunohistologic staining of antigens "fixed" within the rigid framework of a tissue section, it is probable that only one binding site of the antibody is bound. An antigen molecule bearing several determinants might theoretically bind several molecules of antibody, either antibodies of a single specificity (against a particular determinant present in

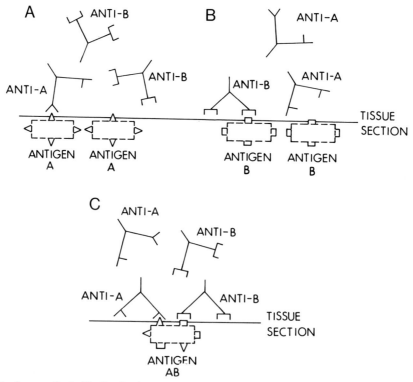

Figure 1–5. Antigen-antibody binding in tissue sections. Antigen-antibody binding is, in simplistic terms governed by matching of reciprocal "charge-shape" structures. In **A** anti-A antibody binds with the determinants in antigen A; anti-B does not bind. The reverse occurs in **B**. In **C** a molecule bears both determinants A and B, and both anti-A and anti-B bind.

multiple) or several antibodies of differing specificity (against two or more different determinants present in the same antigenic molecule) (Fig. 1–5). Again, in practice local steric interference may limit binding of multiple antibody molecules to sites that are spatially closely related.

Antibodies as Antigens

Immunoglobulin molecules are themselves sufficiently complex to contain several antigenic determinants; that is, an antibody molecule raised in one species may serve as an antigen when injected into a second species.

Any rigid part of the antibody molecule may serve as the antigenic determinant. Immunoglobulin molecules may thus possess several antigenic determinants, including determinants on both variable and constant parts of the molecule (Fig. 1–4A). In practice, antibodies are most easily produced against determinants present in the constant regions of the immunoglobulin molecule; such antibodies may particularly be used to distinguish the different light and heavy chains by immunologic means (eg, anti-kappa, anti-lambda, or anti-gamma, anti-alpha, anti-mu, and the like). The fact that immunoglobulin molecules can serve both as antibodies, binding specifically to tissue antigens, and as antigens, providing antigenic determinants to which secondary antibodies may be attached, is exploited in immunohistologic techniques; this binding forms the basis of the remarkable specificity and versatility that immunohistologic methods enjoy (Fig. 1–6).

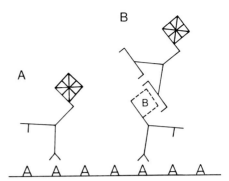

Figure 1–7. Antibodies as labels. For immunohistologic studies antibody molecules are made visible by the attachment of a flag, or label; the labelled antibody may be applied directly to the section (direct method, *A*) or may be used to detect binding of a nonlabelled primary antibody (indirect method, *B*).

Antibodies as Markers or Labels

Not only are antigen-antibody reactions specific, they also may be of such high affinity that once binding has occurred the antibody is dislodged only with difficulty. Thus specific antibodies can be used as probes to detect the localization of antigens within tissue sections or other forms of cell preparations. However, antibody molecules cannot be seen with the light microscope or even with the electron microscope unless they are labelled or flagged by some method that permits their visualization (Fig. 1–7). A variety of labels or flags have been employed, including fluorescent compounds and active enzymes that can be visualized by virtue of their property of inducing the formation of a colored reaction product from a suitable substrate system. Such methods have worked well in light microscopy and can, to some extent, be adapted to electron microscopy if the products are rendered electron-dense by suitable treatment. Alternatively, labels that are visible directly by electron microscopy may be used, such as gold, ferritin, or virus particles.

Immunofluorescence

Fluorescein isothiocyanate can be chemically linked to antibody, producing a fluorescent conjugate in which the antibody remains active. The sites of binding of such a conjugate in a tissue or cell preparation can be visualized by excitation with ultraviolet light, which causes the fluorescein to emit light in the visible wavelength (green; other labels give other colors, eg, rhodamine gives red).

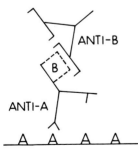

Figure 1–6. Antibodies as antigens. Anti-A antibody binds specifically to antigen A in the tissue section. Antigen B (B) is depicted as a second antigenic determinant that is part of the anti-A molecule; anti-B antibody, made in a second species, will bind to this determinant. Thus anti-B (the so-called secondary antibody) can be used to locate the site of binding of anti-A (the primary antibody) in a tissue section.

More recently other highly fluorescent substances have become available (eg, B-phycoerythrin).

Immunoperoxidase (Immunoenzyme) Methods

Immunoenzyme methods are based upon attachment of an active enzyme to a specific antibody, with utilization of the enzymatic activity of the enzyme to produce a visible color change in a substrate at the sites of localization of the antibody-enzyme complex within the tissue. The enzyme most commonly employed for this purpose is horseradish peroxidase; other enzymes that have been used include alkaline phosphatase and glucose oxidase.

The Different Methods of Immunostaining

Immunohistologic techniques have one principal aim in common—to attach the maximum amount of label at the site of localization of the antigen within the tissue with a minimum degree of nonspecific (background) binding of the labelled moiety. Considerable ingenuity has been exercised in achieving this, and a number of different techniques have been devised. The principles behind these techniques are described in this chapter, with discussion of some of the advantages and disadvantages of the different procedures. The more important techniques, which have found widespread application or are particularly useful under restricted circumstances, are described fully in subsequent chapters.

For the purposes of discussion in this chapter, the label utilized is horseradish peroxidase (as the prototype of the immunoenzyme method). Other enzyme systems such as glucose oxidase and alkaline phosphatase have been utilized successfully in some of these procedures, the direct and indirect conjugate methods, for example. Fluorescent labels such as fluorescein isothiocyanate have particularly been employed in the direct and indirect conjugate procedures (Fig. 1–7).

Peroxidase Antigen Method (Fig. 1–8). Horseradish peroxidase is a potent antigen, and when introduced into an experimental animal it induces a vigorous immune response with the formation of antibody against horseradish peroxidase. This sequence of

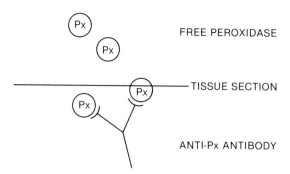

Figure 1–8. Peroxidase-antigen method. Following immunization with peroxidase (Px), the presence of nascent antiperoxidase antibody is detected by addition of free peroxidase.

events has been exploited in experimental animals as a means of demonstrating the sites of antibody production at light and electron microscopic levels.

An animal is immunized with horseradish peroxidase to induce an antibody response. Lymph nodes draining the site of antigen inoculation are resected at varying intervals following the final dose of antigen and processed for histologic examination. The sites of localization of the anti–horseradish peroxidase antibody within these tissue sections may then be demonstrated by the addition of free horseradish peroxidase, which will undergo specific binding to the nascent anti–horseradish peroxidase antibody formed within immunoglobulin-producing cells.

This method, which gives good results in cryostat sections and can be adapted for paraffin sections or for electron microscopic examination, has been particularly valuable for ultrastructural studies of the early sites of immunoglobulin production within immunoblasts and plasma cell precursors (Avrameas, 1975). The peroxidase antigen method, though extremely valuable in this particular experimental setting, is not useful in the investigation of human disease, requiring as it does immunization with horseradish peroxidase.

The Hybrid Antibody Method (Fig. 1–9). Not to be confused with hybridoma monoclonal antibodies, in which the antibodies are produced by hybridized cells, the hybrid antibody method is a technique by which two different antibodies, having distinct specificities, are split asunder chemically and then reconstituted so that two different specifici-

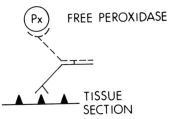

Figure 1–9. "Hybrid" antibody method. One specific site of the "hybrid" molecule binds to the tissue antigen (▲); the second site then serves to bind the free peroxidase label (Px).

ties come together within a single molecule, as illustrated in Figure 1–9 (see Sternberger, 1974). The hybridized molecule is depicted as having one specificity directed against the antigen in question (eg, rabbit anti-▲) and the second specificity directed against horseradish peroxidase (rabbit anti-Px). Hybridized antibody is added to the section, the anti-▲ specificity causing binding to the ▲ antigen within the tissues, leaving the antiperoxidase specificity to combine with horseradish peroxidase when this is added subsequently. The sites of localization of the horseradish peroxidase are then developed with a chromogenic substrate system, as for each of the other immunoperoxidase procedures. The method has the theoretical advantage of high specificity and is rapid. Disadvantages relate principally to the problems of preparing the hybrid antibody, particularly elimination of the nonhybridized antibody molecules from the final reagent. The sensitivity of the method is generally considered to be low, and it is not economical in terms of antibody usage; with the advent of monoclonal antibodies, these disadvantages may become less of a problem.

Direct Conjugate-Labelled Antibody Method (Figs. 1–10A and B). The method of attaching a label by chemical means to an antibody and then directly applying this la-

belled conjugate to tissue sections has been widely used in immunocytochemistry or immunohistology. As noted earlier, various labels have been employed, including a range of fluorescent substances (particularly fluorescein isothiocyanate and rhodamine), various enzymes (including horseradish peroxidase, alkaline phosphatase, and glucose oxidase) or certain electron-dense labels (such as ferritin). For the purposes of this chapter, we will deal only with fluorescein isothiocyanate and horseradish peroxidase as illustrative examples of the technique.

The process of chemical conjugation whereby the label is bound chemically to the antibody is described in more detail in Chapter 2. In preparing a labelled antibody conjugate, the aim is to attach the maximum number of molecules of label to each individual antibody molecule. It is desirable that 100 percent of antibody molecules should be labelled and that none should be rendered immunologically inactive by the labelling process. Similarly the labelling process must not inactivate the label (eg, quench the fluorescence or destroy the active site of the horseradish peroxidase enzyme). The final labelled reagent should not contain free molecules of label that might undergo nonspecific binding with the tissue section. Likewise, there should be no free molecules of unlabelled antibody, and similarly no molecules of antibody linked to inactivated label.

These are exacting requirements that are difficult to meet in the routine surgical pathology laboratory. However, conjugation methods have improved immensely in the past decade, and good, high-quality conjugates, both fluorescent and peroxidase, are available from a number of commercial sources (see Appendix 2).

The direct conjugate procedure has the advantages of rapidity and ease of performance. With this procedure the purity (ie, monospecificity) of the antiserum (antibody) is of critical importance, for if the antiserum contains a range of antibody molecules of varying specificities in addition to the antibody having the desired specificity, then all of these antibodies will be labelled during the conjugation procedure, and any or all may produce positive staining in tissue sections, leading to erroneous interpretation. The method, however, promises to be particularly suitable for use with monoclonal antibodies (vida infra) that are truly monospecific for an antigenic determinant and are not con-

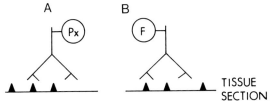

Figure 1–10. Direct conjugate method. The label, or flag, is attached directly to the antibody having specificity for the antigen under study. Px = peroxidase; F = fluorescein.

taminated with other antibodies having different specificities.

One practical disadvantage of the direct conjugate procedure is that for the detection of different antigens it is necessary to conjugate separately the appropriate primary antibodies. This can be time-consuming and, in addition, is a problem with reference to precious antibodies that may be available in limited amounts. Under such circumstances one is unwilling to risk a direct conjugation procedure involving some loss of the total amount of antibody. Finally, with regard to precious antibodies, the direct conjugate procedure usually demands that the primary antibody be utilized at a relatively high concentration in comparison with indirect and unlabelled antibody methods described subsequently; this circumstance can be an important factor in selecting the latter methods, for the precious primary antibody, used at a considerably higher dilution, lasts longer.

The Indirect, or Sandwich, Procedure (Figs. 11A and B). The indirect, or sandwich, conjugate procedure is a relatively simple modification of the direct conjugate method. It has the following advantages:

(1) Versatility is increased, in that a single conjugated antibody can be used with several different primary antibodies to detect several different antigens in different sections;

(2) the conjugation process is applied only to the secondary antibody, not to precious primary antibodies;

(3) the primary antibody can often be used at a higher working dilution (than in the direct method) to achieve successful staining;

(4) the secondary antibody, produced against immunoglobulin of the species from which the primary antibody is derived, is readily prepared with a high order of specificity and affinity; many commercial sources are available for conjugated secondary antibodies;

(5) the method lends itself to additional specificity controls compared with the direct conjugate procedure in that the primary specific antibody may be omitted, or another antibody of irrelevant specificity may be substituted, providing a valuable assessment of the validity of any staining pattern observed.

The indirect conjugate method is perhaps the most widely used immunofluorescence technique; initially, it was used extensively in immunoperoxidase studies but later was supplanted by unlabelled antibody methods.

All labelled antibody methods performed by the indirect procedure are strictly analogous in principle; the peroxidase and fluorescent indirect conjugate methods are illustrated in Figures 1–11A and B, respectively. The primary antibody, having specificity against the antigen in question (eg, rabbit anti-▲), is added to the section; the excess is washed off. The labelled secondary antibody, having specificity against an antigenic determinant present on the primary rabbit antibody (eg, swine antibody versus rabbit immunoglobulin), is then added; it serves to label the sites of tissue localization of the primary antibody, which in turn is bound to the antigen.

Unlabelled Antibody Methods—the Enzyme Bridge Technique (Fig. 1–12). The disadvantages of the chemical conjugation procedure—namely, the necessity for preparing a conjugate in which there is minimal denaturation of antibody and no inactivation of the label but in which there is 100 percent labelling of antibody with active label—may be avoided by devising techniques whereby the labelled moiety is linked to the antigen solely by immunologic binding. To achieve this end, Mason and colleagues (1969) developed a technique that has become known as the enzyme bridge method. This method is depicted in Figure 1–12. Three separate antibodies are employed, two from one species together with a bridge antibody derived from a second species. In the example shown in Figure 1–12, the primary antibody is rabbit antiserum against the ▲ antigen (rabbit anti-▲). The bridge antibody is a swine antiserum

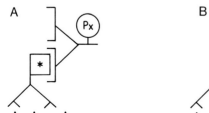 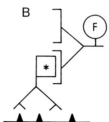

Figure 1–11. Indirect conjugate (sandwich) method. The primary antibody is unlabelled. The method utilizes a labelled secondary antibody, having specificity against the primary antibody. Boxed * = antigen determinant on primary antibody; Px = peroxidase label; F = fluorescein label.

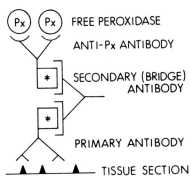

Figure 1–12. Enzyme bridge method. A second antibody is utilized to link (bridge) the primary antibody to an antiperoxidase antibody, which in turn binds to free peroxidase.

produced against rabbit immunoglobulin having specificity for the constant component of the primary rabbit antibody (ie, it is a swine antirabbit Ig). This bridging antibody is added in great excess so that, due to the intensity of competition, only one "valency" is bound to the antirabbit immunoglobulin; the second valency remains free, available for binding with any additional rabbit immunoglobulin added subsequently. Additional rabbit immunoglobulin is then added in the form of a rabbit antibody having specificity against horseradish peroxidase (rabbit anti-Px). This antibody attaches to the available

"antirabbit Ig" specificity sites of the bridge antibody, thus effectively linking the rabbit antiperoxidase antibody (anti-Px) to the primary anti-rabbit anti-▲ antibody, which in turn is bound specifically to the antigen under investigation (Fig. 1–12). The next step in this procedure is to add free horseradish peroxidase, which becomes attached to the antiperoxidase sites of the rabbit antiperoxidase antibody. Thus two molecules of the peroxidase label are effectively localized at the site of the ▲ antigen, using binding that is entirely immunologic in type.

Unlabelled Antibody Method—the PAP Method (Fig. 1–13). The PAP method is a second unlabelled antibody procedure that also avoids the problems inherent in chemical conjugation. First employed by Sternberger and colleagues for the detection of antitreponemal antibodies (referenced in Sternberger, 1974), the PAP system was reported to enjoy a sensitivity 100- to 1000-fold greater than comparable conjugate procedures. The principle of the PAP method is similar to that of the enzyme bridge method described in the preceding paragraphs. The acronym PAP denotes the peroxidase antiperoxidase (PAP) reagent that represents the third stage in this procedure.

The PAP reagent consists of antibody against horseradish peroxidase and horse-

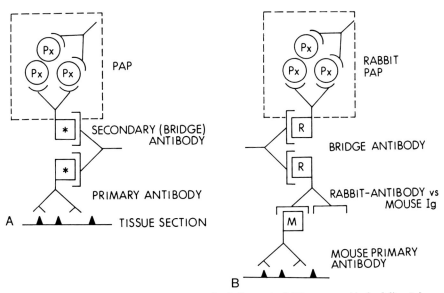

Figure 1–13. *A*, Peroxidase-antiperoxidase (PAP) method (3-stage). PAP reagent (dashed lines) is a preformed stable immune complex; it is linked to the primary antibody by a "bridging" antibody. *B*, PAP method (4-stage). PAP reagent (dashed line) is a preformed stable immune complex. Primary antibody in this example is murine (mouse Ig as in a monoclonal antibody); this antibody is followed by a rabbit antimouse Ig, a bridge antibody (e.g., swine antirabbit Ig) and rabbit PAP.

radish peroxidase antigen in the form of a small, stable, immune complex. Available evidence suggests that this immune complex typically consists of two antibody molecules and three horseradish peroxidase molecules in the configuration shown in Figure 1–13. The PAP reagent and the primary antibody must be from the same species (or from closely related species with common antigenic determinants), whereas the bridge antibody is derived from a second species and has specificity against the constant components of the primary antibody (eg, rabbit anti-▲) and the immunoglobulin incorporated into the PAP complex (eg, rabbit anti-Px). In the example depicted in Figure 1–13A, the primary anti-▲ antibody is made in rabbit; the bridge antibody is made in swine (ie, it is a swine antibody against rabbit IgG), whereas the PAP reagent is made from rabbit antibody against horseradish peroxidase (rabbit anti-Px) complexed with horseradish peroxidase antigen, utilizing a relatively straightforward procedure described by Sternberger and since modified by others. The bridge antibody serves as a "specific glue" to bind the PAP peroxidase-labelled moiety to the primary antibody that in turn is bound to the antigen under study. This method has become the most widely used variant of the immunoperoxidase technique for immunohistologic studies, particularly with reference to routinely processed paraffin sections. In part, its popularity is due to a reputation for a high degree of sensitivity coupled with the specificity and stability of the reagents.

One limitation of the PAP method has been that the antibody incorporated into the PAP reagent should be of the same species as the primary antibody. Most often this has been a "rabbit PAP" utilized with a primary antibody made in rabbit. Rabbit PAP cannot be used with a primary goat antibody or mouse antibody in a simple three-stage procedure, since a linking (or bridge) antibody cannot be prepared that will bind rabbit PAP to goat or mouse primary antisera. In order to utilize mouse or goat antibodies with rabbit PAP, one may adopt a four-stage procedure (Fig. 1–13B) with an additional primary stage: eg, mouse anti-▲ followed by a rabbit antibody against mouse immunoglobulin, bridge reagent, and then the rabbit PAP.

More recently PAP reagents have been prepared in goat and mouse, utilizing goat or mouse antiperoxidase antibodies (goat PAP, mouse PAP), facilitating the use of a three-stage PAP method with a goat or mouse primary antibody.

Similarly, if the primary antibody is of human origin, rabbit PAP is unsuitable, although PAP reagent made with chimpanzee immunoglobulin has sufficient cross-reactivity with the human immunoglobulin to permit use of a common bridge reagent. Similarly, cross reactivities with immunoglobulin of different species can be exploited successfully utilizing PAP made in one species with a primary antibody from another species. Such cross-species PAP techniques are, however, empirical and may be difficult to reproduce in other laboratories using antisera from other sources.

The growing desire to be able to use monoclonal antibodies (which are mostly mouse immunoglobulins) led to adaptation of the PAP method for use with murine primary antibodies. A four-stage technique can be used as described above, or the three-stage method using a mouse immunoglobulin PAP has proved successful and sensitive. The four-stage method may be more sensitive then the three-stage method with mouse PAP, though one pays the price of a more cumbersome procedure.

A recent and potentially useful variation of the PAP method utilizes immunoglobulin of the appropriate species (ie, same as primary antibody) chemically linked to horseradish peroxidase in lieu of a true PAP reagent (in which the peroxidase is linked immunologically by use of antiperoxidase antibody) (Such reagents are not commercially available; contact Dr. D. Y. Mason, John Radcliffe Hospital, Oxford, England).

The Biotin-Avidin Procedure (Fig. 1–14). The biotin-avidin procedure exploits the high affinity binding between biotin and avidin. Biotin can be linked chemically to the primary antibody (Fig. 1–14A), producing a biotinylated conjugate which, when added to the tissue section, localizes to the sites of antigen within the section. Subsequently avidin, chemically conjugated to horseradish peroxidase, is added; the avidin binds tightly to the biotinylated antibody, thus localizing the peroxidase moiety at the site of antigen in the tissue section. This method is rapid and has been used, particularly in an indirect procedure (Fig. 1–14B), to demonstrate tissue localization of monoclonal antibody; the secondary antibody could be, for example,

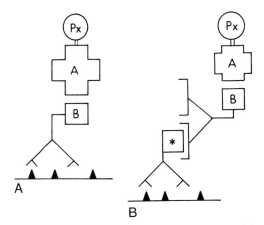

Figure 1–14. *A,* Direct biotin-avidin method. The primary antibody is linked to biotin (B); an avidin-peroxidase-conjugate (A-Px) is then added. *B,* Indirect biotin-avidin method. Used for monoclonal antibodies, the primary antibody is not conjugated; its localization is detected by a biotinylated secondary antibody.

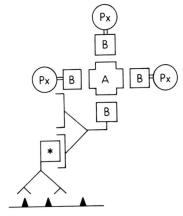

Figure 1–15. Avidin-biotin-conjugate (ABC) method. A biotinylated secondary antibody serves to link the primary antibody to a large preformed complex of avidin, biotin, and peroxidase. A = avidin, B = biotin, Px = peroxidase.

rabbit anti-mouse immunoglobulin conjugated with biotin. The method is apparently not as sensitive as the PAP method.

Two potential disadvantages exist. First, it has become apparent that different batches of biotin and different batches of avidin have differing affinities one for the other, and this affects quite drastically the sensitivity and reproducibility of the procedure in different laboratories. Second, some tissues contain significant amounts of endogenous biotin that may bind the avidin-peroxidase complex directly, thus producing nonspecific (false positive) staining. This can be combatted by suitable blocking techniques, at the expense of adding another step to the procedure (Chapter 2).

The Avidin-Biotin Conjugate (ABC) Procedure (Fig. 1–15). Hsu and colleagues (1981c,d) have developed a further modification of the biotin-avidin system that seems greatly to enhance its sensitivity to rival, or arguably to exceed, that of the basic three-stage PAP method. The method can be used either as a direct or an indirect technique. In the indirect technique (Fig. 1–15), the primary antibody is added, followed first by a biotinylated secondary antibody and next by the addition of preformed complexes of avidin and biotin horseradish peroxidase conjugate. This complex serves to localize several molecules of horseradish peroxidase at the site of the antigen within the section and apparently accounts for the enhanced sensitivity of the procedure. Again, one disadvantage is that different batches of biotin and

avidin have differing degrees of affinity, compromising the reproducibility of the system. However, by using matched batches of these reagents, these problems can be overcome; the method is then more widely applicable. Time for performance of the ABC conjugate procedure compares favorably with that of the PAP method. Binding to endogenous biotin remains a problem.

Protein A–Peroxidase Conjugate Method (Fig. 1–16). Protein A, derived from *Staphylococcus,* has the remarkable ability to bind with the constant (Fc) portion of immunoglobulin molecules from several different species. This binding capability may be exploited to develop a simple and rapid immunoperoxidase procedure. The only absolute requirement is that the primary antibody binds with protein A; most IgG molecules bind protein A, though affinity varies among

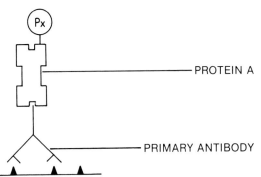

PROTEIN A

PRIMARY ANTIBODY

Figure 1–16. Protein A conjugate method. Protein A, labelled with peroxidase, binds to the Fc component of the primary antibody.

different IgG subclasses and in different species.

The method is depicted in Figure 1–16. The primary antibody, having specificity against the ▲ antigen is added to the section, followed by a protein A–peroxidase conjugate, which attaches specifically to the free Fc portion of the primary antibody. Binding of protein A to the Fc component is extremely rapid and of high affinity, such that the incubation period for the protein A–peroxidase conjugate stage can be as short as two or three minutes. One disadvantage is that in cryostat sections, the protein A–peroxidase conjugate will bind not only to the Fc component of any primary antibody that is added, but also to the Fc fragments of intrinsic immunoglobulins within the section. This does not appear to be a problem in the staining of paraffin sections, for the process of fixation and embedding so alters the Fc fragments that they are no longer capable of binding protein A. Clearly, the protein A–peroxidase (or fluorescein) conjugate method can be employed directly or as an indirect technique if the primary antibody that must be used will not bind protein A.

The Protein A–PAP Method (Fig. 1–17). The straightforward protein A–peroxidase conjugate procedure requires the chemical conjugation of horseradish peroxidase with protein A. To avoid the process of chemical conjugation, protein A may be used as the

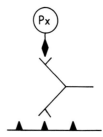

Figure 1–18. Labelled antigen method. The antibody is added in excess so that one valency is bound to the antigen in the section, leaving the second valency free to bind the labelled antigen that is added subsequently.

linking reagent in the PAP method, providing that both the primary antibody and the antibody incorporated within the PAP molecule are capable of binding with protein A. In practice this permits the use of primary antibodies from one species with PAP reagent derived from another species. It has the further advantage of being more rapid than the usual PAP method in that the protein A incubation and the subsequent PAP incubation may both be shortened to a matter of five minutes.

The Enzyme-Labelled Antigen Method (Fig. 1–18). The enzyme-labelled antigen method was devised as perhaps the ultimate in specificity among immunoperoxidase techniques. The principles of application of this method are illustrated in Figure 1–18. Only one antibody is employed; the method exploits the fact that antibody possesses two valencies, one of which may be bound to the antigen under study, with the second valency left free for binding with additional molecules of antigen added subsequently. The additional antigen is directly conjugated with horseradish peroxidase, thus this is an antigen–peroxidase conjugate (labelled antigen) procedure.

The method has some theoretical disadvantages in that high density of antigen in the section theoretically can cause both of the valencies of the antibody to bind to the section, leaving none free for bonding with the antigen-peroxidase conjugate; thus a false-negative result would be obtained. For this reason, the primary antibody is generally employed at a relatively high concentration. This method is therefore not economical in usage of the primary antibody and is best applied for the detection of antigens in which both antigen and antibody are in good supply. One major advantage is that the primary

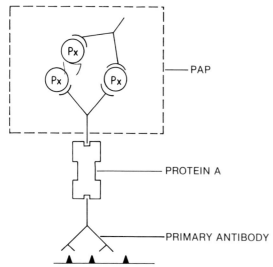

— PAP

— PROTEIN A

— PRIMARY ANTIBODY

Figure 1–17. Protein A-PAP method. The protein A is utilized to link the primary antibody (Fc) to the antibody (Fc) within the PAP complex.

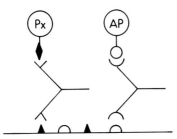

Figure 1–19. Labelled antigen double stain. Two different antibodies recognize their respective antigens in the tissue section, and subsequently bind only the corresponding labelled antigen (labelled with peroxidase [Px] or alkaline phosphatase [AP]).

antibody need not be particularly pure, as antibodies of irrelevant specificity will not be detected by this technique, even if they bind to the tissue section; lacking specificity for ▲ antigen, they will not bind the ▲ antigen–peroxidase conjugate and thus will not be visualized.

This method has proven particularly suitable for double-staining techniques whereby one seeks simultaneous staining of two antigens within the same section (Fig. 1–19). Using orthodox immunoperoxidase methods, one may encounter problems in cross-specificity in different reagents used, but with the double antigen method, the problems of cross-specific reactions are avoided owing to the fact that the label, linked to the antigen, will be taken up only by antibody that has specificity against that antigen.

For the purposes of double labelling, one may employ sequential immunoperoxidase stains, with different substrates, taking care to halt the reaction after the completion with the first substrate. Better, one may use the labelled antigen system (difficult, since investigators must first make the labelled reagents) or a peroxidase labelled antibody to locate one antigen and a glucose oxidase (or alkaline phosphatase)–labelled antibody for the second antigen. Double labelling is, of course, commonly employed in immunofluorescence systems, using fluorescein as one label (green) and rhodamine (red) as the other (see Chapter 2).

GENERAL APPLICATIONS: THE PARAFFIN SECTION

There are three limitations to the performance of immunoperoxidase techniques on "routinely" processed tissues:

(1) the experience and expertise of the investigator in performance of the technique and in interpretation of the results;

(2) The availability of specific antisera for detection of different antigens within the tissue;

(3) the degree to which the antigen in question survives the abuses of formalin fixation and paraffin embedment.

Of these, only the third is absolute, and even this appears not to be a major factor with reference to many different antigen systems.

Experience of the Investigator

The basic practical details of performing an immunoperoxidase stain have been set forth by many different investigators and are described again in this book. There is no definite "best" way, and different modifications may be adopted under different circumstances. The methods given in this book have given good service as basic laboratory procedures; performed in a routine fashion, they are consistently reproducible.

For those wishing to avoid the complexities of checkerboard titration studies, in order to establish the proper working dilutions of the various reagents, the use of immunoperoxidase "kits" is recommended. Such kits are available at present from several major commercial sources (Ortho, Dako, Biogenex, Miles, Lipshaw, Biomedia, and others). In using kits it is advisable for the user to follow strictly the producer's protocol (see Appendix 2).

As far as interpretation is concerned, this surely is a matter of experience. All pathologists are familiar with the diverse interpretations that may be placed upon a single histologic preparation when sent to different experts in different corners of the world, or even different "experts" in different corners of one department. Such vagaries of interpretation apply also to immunohistologic stains. It is important to emphasize that interpretation will always be suspect if performed in the absence of suitable controls—specifically, a negative control and, if possible, biological positive controls (see Chapter 2 for discussion of control procedures).

Availability of Specific Antisera

In the past the lack of availability of a wide range of antisera with a high degree of specificity for cellular and tissue antigens has constituted a serious limitation in extending the usefulness of immunohistologic techniques. However, in recent years with increasing interest in this method, the range of antisera available has increased considerably.

In part this is a result of the increased use of sophisticated techniques for the preparation of pure antigen preparations, permitting the production of high affinity conventional antibodies (antisera), which are then subjected to multiple absorption procedures to attain the degree of specificity necessary for immunohistologic techniques. It is important to emphasize that in assessment of such antisera, immunodiffusion assays for specificity may be inadequate, for they often will not detect "trace" antibody specificities that only become apparent when the antiserum is applied to tissue sections containing many different antigens. Again, this is discussed in the chapter concerning controls; the only adequate control system for assessing the suitability of a conventional antiserum for immunohistologic studies is a control system based upon immunohistologic assessment of specificity, using biologic "positive" and "negative" sections known to contain or lack the antigen in question.

Immunohistologic techniques have been

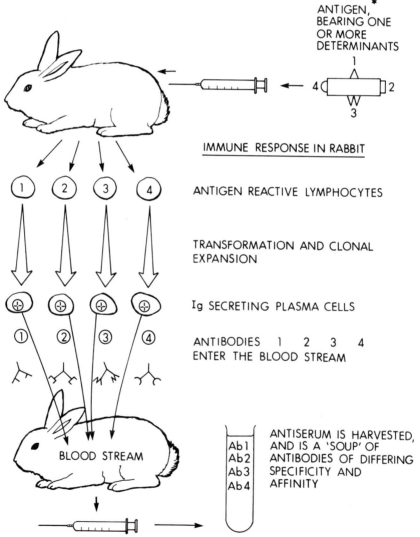

Figure 1–20. Production of conventional antibody. In practice a single molecule (antigen) induces the formation of several different antibodies, of differing specificity, affinity, and the like against the different determinants (or epitopes).

*Antigen shown bears four determinants—it elicits four different antibodies that constitute the antiserum.

given a further boost by the development of the monoclonal hybridoma antibody technique, a technique that has the potential for providing specific high–affinity monoclonal antibodies against an almost limitless range of antigens. The monocolonal antibody technique will be described only briefly here for the purpose of familiarizing the reader with the theoretical background necessary to assess the advantages and disadvantages of monoclonal antibodies. For details of practical technique, the reader is referred to the selected bibliography (the overall "monoclonal" literature is already so extensive that none of us has time to read more than a fraction of it).

In the production of a conventional antibody (Fig. 1–20), the different lymphocytes of the immunized animal have an opportunity to recognize and respond to the injected antigen (immunogen).

In practice even a single purified antigen bears several antigenic determinants, each of which elicits an immune response; even a single determinant can induce the formation of several antibodies of differing affinity and specificity. Only those lymphocytes having the appropriate receptors (recognizing an antigenic determinant of the immunogen) will react by proliferating to produce an immune response. The immune response is a complex series of cellular interactions involving macrophages, T lymphocytes, and B lymphocytes, and, even more specifically, particular subsets of these cells in different immune responses. The end result, with reference to antibody production, is that several clones of B lymphocytes, each clone possessing a receptor that serves as a recognition unit for the antigen, undergo proliferation. The products of B lymphocyte proliferation are plasma cells, which produce antibody with a specificity corresponding to that of the B lymphocyte initially stimulated by a particular antigenic determinant. The plasma cells secrete their (antibody) immunoglobulin into the serum; the combined production of the several stimulated clones into the serum of the immunized animal represents conventional "antiserum" that may be harvested and utilized in immunohistologic studies (Fig. 1–20).

Clearly such an antiserum contains several different molecular species of antibody having varying affinities and even varying specificities against the different antigens or antigenic determinants used to immunize the animal. (It is important to remember that antibodies may also be present to a whole range of antigens, including bacteria and viruses, that the immunized animal encountered in its existence prior to inclusion in your scientific endeavors as a source of antibody.) Thus in such a conventional antiserum, all these unwanted or potentially cross-reacting specificities must be removed by complicated absorption methods prior to use of the antibody in immunohistologic techniques, or alternatively, controls must be established to guard against misinterpretation.

On theoretical grounds there would be advantages to isolating a particular clone of B lymphocytes specifically responsive to the antigen in question and growing plasma cells derived from this clone alone in culture in order to harvest "pure antibody" from an in vitro system. In practical terms this cannot be achieved, for the B lymphocytes, like other normal cells, will grow only for a limited period of time "in vitro."

Malignant cells, however, have learned the trick of immortality, displaying the potential for unlimited growth in tissue culture, provided only that they are supplied with a suitable supportive medium and maintained under sterile conditions.

The hybridoma monoclonal antibody technique seeks to combine the potentialities of the B lymphocyte, which possesses the information to make specific antibody, with a malignant cell that "knows how to live forever" (Fig. 1–21). The hybridized product of these two cells might then be expected not only to produce the specific antibody but also to maintain production indefinitely in tissue culture.

The essence of this procedure is illustrated in Figure 1–21. A mouse is immunized with antigen; subsequently the immune-sensitized lymphocytes are harvested for fusion. The malignant cell population selected for fusion is usually a mouse myeloma line, particularly one that has undergone a mutational loss of its ability to secrete immunoglobulin. This mutational deficit is an advantage in that the myeloma cells will not produce their own intrinsic immunoglobulin, but following fusion they will produce only the immunoglobulin "ordered" by the B lymphocyte with which they are fused. Following suitable selection processes that, in fact, may be quite complicated and time-consuming, the various hybridoma clones, each producing a specific antibody in tissue culture, may be perpetu-

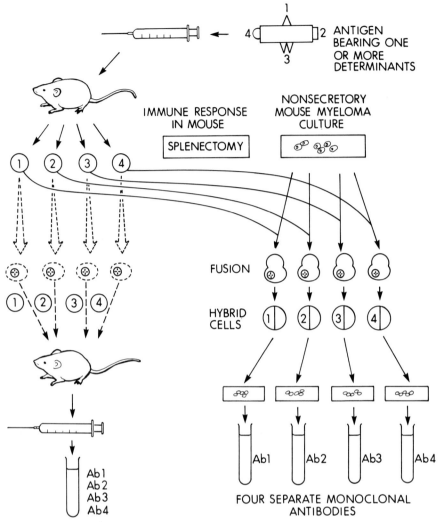

Figure 1–21. Production of hybridoma (monoclonal) antibody. On the left conventional mouse antiserum is produced, analogous to Figure 1–20. On the right four separate monoclonal antibodies result.

ated "in vitro." Pure monoclonal antibody of the desired specificity is then harvested and assayed for specificity, cytotoxicity, ability to fix complement, or suitability for immuno-histologic studies.

Limitations Due to Destruction of Antigen by Fixation

The combination of antigen with antibody depends upon the maintenance of the three-dimensional structural integrity of both antibody and antigen molecules. The specificity of antibody for a particular antigen and its ability to react with that antigen may only be preserved if that antigen maintains a particular three-dimensional configuration. Clearly

the processes of fixation and paraffin embedment may have deleterious effects upon antigenicity in terms of inducing alterations of three-dimensional "charge-shape" patterns (Fig. 1–22). Prior to the demonstration in 1974 (Taylor, 1974; Taylor and Burns, 1974) that immunohistologic techniques would serve to identify at least some antigens in paraffin sections, it was widely believed that "conventional means" of tissue processing (ie, formalin-paraffin) precluded the use of immunohistologic methods. Today it is recognized that the process of fixation does alter antigens; equally it is recognized that this process is not as catastrophic as once believed. A wide range of antigens is demonstrable in paraffin sections (Table 1–1), and this range increases daily. Much has yet to be learned

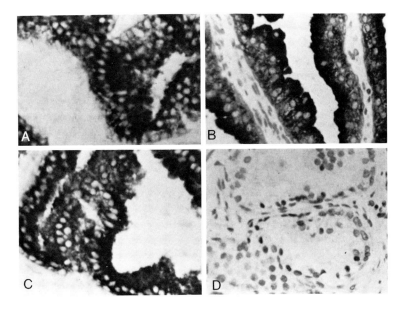

Figure 1–22. Four sections taken from a single prostate. *A* and *C* are frozen sections; *B* and *D* are paraffin sections. Of more than 70 monoclonal antibodies against prostatic acid phosphatase (from Hybritech), 9 stained both frozen and paraffin sections (*A* and *B*); the remainder stained only frozen sections (*C* and *D*), with no trace of reactivity in paraffin sections. This example underlines one possible disadvantage of monoclonal antibodies directed against a single epitope that may be destroyed in fixation, compared with conventional antiserum that contains several antibodies against different epitopes.

concerning the precise effects that different fixatives have upon different antigens. Table 1–2 summarizes the situation with regard to preserving the immunoreactivity of immunoglobulin under different conditions of fixation.

Information is accumulating slowly with regard to other fixation and processing techniques, but it is still not possible to formulate any general rule that will enable a surgical pathologist to predict whether a particular antigen will be detectable with a particular antibody following a particular fixation, processing, and embedding method. Indeed the only general rule remains an empirical one; the answer can only be derived by performing the experiment. Fixation is discussed at greater length in Chapter 3.

Table 1–2. Preservation of Immunoreactivity of Immunoglobulin in Plasma Cells Following Different Fixation Procedures*

Quality of Preservation	Fixation Procedure
Good	Precipitating, including Zenker's, Bouin's, and B-5
Intermediate	10% formalin†
Poor	Oxidizing: dichromates, permanganates

*Modified from Banks (1979).

†In our experience 10% FRESH buffered formalin also gives excellent results provided that fixation is not prolonged unnecessarily. As a general rule, FIXATION SHOULD BE FOR THE MINIMUM TIME CONSISTENT WITH GOOD MORPHOLOGY.

GENERAL APPLICATIONS—THE CRYOSTAT SECTION

Cryostat sections are employed preferentially whenever the stability of the antigen under investigation is in doubt. Cryostat sections may also be preferred when morphology is not at a premium or when the section serves merely as an "antigen source," and the prime interest is focused upon whether or not a particular serum added to the section contains antibody to an antigen present within the section (eg, testing for antinuclear antibody and so forth).

Immunofluorescence has traditionally served as the favored technique with cryostat sections. More recently immunoperoxidase procedures have been adopted by some investigators wishing to take advantage of improved morphologic resolution, ease of examination by light microscopy, or the permanence of immunoperoxidase-stained preparations.

Individual applications include

(1) detection of immunoglobulins and complement in renal biopsies;

(2) lymphocyte surface antigens in cryostat sections (in comparison with suspension-based assays);

(3) detection of "autoantibodies," antinuclear, antimitochondrial antibodies and others.

The principles of immunofluorescence methods are exactly those detailed for immunoperoxidase systems up to the point of visualizing the label. The direct and indirect methods are those most commonly applied (Figs. 1–10 and 1–11).

Throughout the text, reference is made to cryostat sections when these must be employed.

GENERAL APPLICATIONS— CYTOLOGIC PREPARATIONS

The recent shift in emphasis towards fine-needle aspirates has given new impetus to the utilization of immunocytochemical techniques for individual cell recognition in cytologic preparations from pleural or peritoneal effusions and in Pap smears as well as in needle aspirates. Since these types of cell preparations can be subjected to minimal or carefully controlled fixation, they are particularly suitable for demonstration of a wide range of antigens by immunocytochemical methods. Almost all of the immunostains that are effective in paraffin or frozen sections can be used with equal or greater facility in such cell preparations. Technical modifications are minor and are described in the text when appropriate.

2

THEORETICAL AND PRACTICAL ASPECTS OF THE DIFFERENT IMMUNOPEROXIDASE TECHNIQUES

"A grand hypothesis is not the usual path for advancement of medical knowledge. As a rule, first comes a new or improved method whose application to a variety of problems leads unexpectedly to greater understanding."

FRANK K. PADDOCK, 1841–1901

"All method is imperfect. Error is all about it, and at the least opportunity invades it."

BIOLOGIE DE L'INVENTION
CHARLES NICOLLE, 1866–1936

In this chapter the different techniques of immunoperoxidase staining, introduced in Chapter 1, are examined in greater detail. Practical and theoretical aspects that may lead to a preference for one technique over the others are given major emphasis. Some details of laboratory bench procedures are also given. It is recognized that the degree of detail given may be inappropriate for many readers experienced in utilizing these techniques; nonetheless, at the risk of causing minor offence, some of the minutiae are included, for successful immunohistologic staining depends upon the successful consummation of a series of interrelated individual steps. Although the rationale and technique for each step, when considered in isolation, may be painfully obvious, the implications and consequences of an imperfect technique at one step may be less obvious but still may condemn the whole staining procedure to failure.

The purpose of this chapter, therefore, is to provide the necessary information to assist the pathologist or investigator in the selection of an immunoenzyme technique that "fits the occasion," and further, to provide a sound practical basis for success in performance of whatever method is chosen.

Peroxidase vs Alkaline Phosphatase vs Glucose Oxidase

Discussion is centered upon immunoperoxidase methods in particular as the prototype of immunoenzyme methods in general. Techniques utilizing alkaline phosphatase or glucose oxidase as labels in lieu of horseradish peroxidase are analogous to the direct and indirect immunoperoxidase methods or to immunoperoxidase-avidin-biotin techniques; the theory and practice of these methods are interchangeable.

In the first chapter some of the advantages and disadvantages of these enzymatic labels, which may lead to an individual preference, were discussed. From the published literature

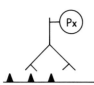

Figure 2–1. Direct conjugate method. The label, or flag, is attached directly to the antibody having specificity for the antigen under study. Px = peroxidase.

the overwhelming vote of most investigators is for use of immunoperoxidase as the primary technique, alkaline phosphatase and glucose oxidase methods being reserved for double staining or for specifically defined applications. This discussion, therefore, centers upon the immunoperoxidase technique, but the principles apply equally to other labels that may be employed (including other enzymes, immunogold, and so forth).

DIRECT IMMUNOPEROXIDASE METHOD

The direct immunoperoxidase method (Fig. 2–1) is similar to direct immunofluorescence (Chapter 1) but substitutes horseradish peroxidase for fluorescein isothiocyanate. This is the most simple method of immunoperoxidase staining, but it is less sensitive than the indirect and three-stage immunoperoxidase procedures and less economical in the use of primary antiserum (ie, requires the use of a greater concentration of a given

antibody). Furthermore, this method involves the need to label separately each primary antiserum with enzyme. This requirement may represent a problem if the specific antiserum is available only in minute quantities or if it is derived from some species, such as the mouse, from which the immunoglobulins are relatively more difficult to label with fluorochromes or enzymes, leading to poor-quality conjugates, with a lower degree of reactivity. In recent years methods for preparation of conjugates have improved dramatically (Table 2–1).

Peroxidase-labelled immunoglobulin (antibody) fragments (Fab or F[ab′]₂)* are mainly utilized for electron microscopic studies, in which optimal penetration of the conjugate (ie, small molecular size) is critical for detection of intracellular antigens, but these fragments are also finding increasing application in indirect techniques applied to frozen sections, for reasons that will be discussed subsequently (avoidance of Fc receptor binding).

In the direct technique the primary labelled antibody (peroxidase conjugate) is applied directly to the tissue section; following washing, the substrate is added, revealing the sites of localization of the peroxidase conjugate. This method can, therefore, be ex-

---

*A Fab reagent is part of an artificially split immunoglobulin molecule, effectively consisting only of the variable end-parts of the light chain–heavy chain pair; it contains a single antibody (antigen-binding) site. A F(ab′)₂ reagent is effectively two Fabs still attached together; it has two binding sites. Both Fab and F(ab′)₂ lack the Fc end of the molecule.

Table 2–1. Selected References–Materials and Reagents

Preparation and Utilization of Conjugates/PAP and Others	
Avrameas 1969	Glutaraldehyde conjugation
Boorsma & Streefkerk 1979	Relative merits of preparation of peroxidase conjugates, periodate versus glutaraldehyde
O'Sullivan et al 1979 Weston et al 1980	Dimaleimide method of conjugation
Nygren et al 1979	Glutaraldehyde conjugation
Nilsson et al 1981	Succinimidyl propionate conjugation
Bosman et al 1980a	Quick method for preparation of PAP reagent by precipitation, followed by resolubilization with excess peroxidase at low pH
Avrameas et al 1978	Conjugation of enzymes and antibodies
Slemmon et al 1980	Preparation of Fab-PAP (mw c.150,000; composition 2 Fab:1 HRP)
Yamase 1982	Shelf-life of PAP reagents
Sofroniew & Schrell 1982	Repeated use of diluted antisera in staining jars
Nusbickel 1980	Construction of incubator chamber
Paull & King 1983	Construction of incubator chamber
Automation/Quantitation	
Smith et al 1983b	Microdensitometry and PAP reagent
Dighiero et al 1982	Automated B and T cells using hemalog D system
Witorsch 1982	Densitometry, using electrophoresis densitometer
Peschke et al 1980	Image analysis of immunoperoxidase-stained paraplast sections

tremely rapid. In practical terms the principal difficulties relate to establishing controls for the specificity of the antibody applied to the tissue sections, to determining the appropriate titer for optimum staining, and to the conditions for incubation (time, temperature, buffer solutions, and the like).

Specificity

Under ideal circumstances you, the reader, are an immunochemist of some renown: you select and purify the antigen to a single molecular species; you immunize a rabbit from your own carefully monitored rabbit colony; you harvest the antiserum, separate the immunoglobulin, and subject it to final purification on an affinity column of pure antigen. Finally, you observe specific immunoprecipitation arcs that are totally abolished by preabsorption of antibody with antigen at equivalence.

However, if you were an immunochemist of renown, you would probably not be reading this book—except, of course, under ideal circumstances. For the purposes of this text, it is assumed that circumstances are less than ideal and that neither the author nor you are immunochemists of any renown whatsoever.

Are there any precautions that we should take regarding the specificity of our reagents, considering the less than ideal circumstances under which many of us labor? What should we aim for as specificity controls? What is the minimum control that is acceptable?

When a new primary antibody is acquired by your laboratory, whether prepared "in house," begged from a friend, or purchased from a commercial enterprise, reputable or otherwise, the onus of proof of specificity in your operating system is upon you, the investigator.

Traditionally the first step in establishing specificity has been to perform two-dimensional immunodiffusion precipitation (Ouchterlony) of antibody against antigen, the presence of a single arc indicating specificity. Such an assumption may not be justified, because the immunodiffusion method depends not only upon the purity and concentration of the antibody under test but also upon the purity and quality of the antigen against which diffusion occurs. The presence of a single arc is not a reliable indication that the antibody will display only a single specificity when applied to tissues; the immunodiffusion method usually employs a purified

antigen preparation (eg, some form of extract of the antigen from tissue) which by definition excludes the possibility of detection of the numerous other antigens that are not in the extract but may be encountered in tissue fluids, in cell cytoplasm, or upon cell membranes.

For example, this type of problem is commonly encountered in relation to antisera against viral antigens. An animal is immunized with virus grown in tissue culture; antiserum is harvested and shown to react with purified antigens from virus A, but not with antigens from virus B, C, or D (all grown and purified from tissue culture). The antibody may thus be claimed to be specific for virus A. Such a claim should not be confused with "monospecificity," for such an antiserum may contain a range of antibodies against tissue culture cell antigens and growth support media (animal serum proteins); any of the antibodies may cross-react with human cell antigens or with tissue fluid components, such as immunoglobulins or albumin. Thus any staining observed with this antiserum might include viral antigens, but to assume that all observed staining represents virus antigen would be rash and would not enhance one's reputation as a scientist, or even as a pathologist.

Also, it appears that immunodiffusion is not sufficiently sensitive to detect low levels of contaminating antibodies by the formation of arcs, although antibodies present in low titer are quite able to produce detectable staining of the corresponding antigens in tissue sections, particularly when the more sensitive immunoperoxidase methods are utilized. Thus, if immunodiffusion is to be the yardstick, assessment of specificity should include not only testing of antibody against purified antigen but also testing against human serum components, and possibly against tissue homogenates, for the presence of reactivity against any of the antigens therein (particularly immunoglobulins and albumin).

Finally, the above results should be regarded as preliminary; further assessment of specificity will need to be made directly on tissue sections; indeed the latter may be the only means of specificity control available. This operation involves the use of "biologic" controls, or "positive" and "negative" controls. The author recognizes that the use of this form of "jargonese" often is acutely painful for the pure immunochemist; indeed, reviews of papers submitted to reputable journals in which the reviewer's critique consists chiefly of long diatribes against the use of the terms "positive" control or "negative" control have been received. Nonetheless, these terms are used here, for they serve an invaluable purpose in the growing "routine use" of immunohistochemistry, ensuring or reminding that some form of specificity and technique control is essential. As a concession to the pedantic, the following digression gives these terms some formal definition.

Tissue Section Controls (So-Called Biologic Controls). In the context of immunoperoxidase staining of tissue sections, a "positive control" is a tissue selected for the purpose of obtaining a definite positive reaction. For a positive control there should be evidence based upon independent information that the antigen in question is present in large amounts in the tissue and that the integrity of the antigen is preserved in the tissue section available for study (see Figs. 12–1 and 14–25).

A "negative control" section is the reverse of this condition—namely, a section from a tissue known to lack totally the antigen under study. In many instances the presence or absence of antigen is presumed upon the basis of knowledge of the microanatomy, physiology, and biology of the tissue under study; hence the use of the term "biologic control."

For example, plasma cells may be presumed to contain immunoglobulin of kappa or lambda light chain type. Thus in staining an unknown tumor, for the purpose of detecting whether or not it contains kappa or lambda light chains, a section containing normal plasma cells, presumed to contain kappa or lambda light chains, would be the logical choice for a positive control. A section containing brain cells, adrenal cells, or other nonimmunoglobulin-containing cells, might be selected to serve as a negative control. It should be noted that in practice most tissue sections selected as positive controls (for example, sections of reactive tonsils chosen as controls for staining of kappa and lambda light chains—plasma cells positive) also include numerous cells that do not contain the antigen in question (eg, in the tonsil, cells other than plasma cells do not contain kappa or lambda light chains; indeed, plasma cells that contain kappa chain may serve as controls for lambda, and vice versa); these serve as negative control cells, directly alongside the positively stained cells. With experience

it is usually possible and is always wise to search for "positive and negative" control cells within the section under analysis. For example, in examining an unknown tumor for the presence of immunoglobulin, any normal plasma cells present at the periphery of the tumor may be utilized as "in-built" positive controls, whereas endothelial cells may serve as negative controls.

There is also a matter of philosophy to be addressed with reference to selection of control tissues. It is recognized that some antigens may be denatured by fixation and processing and rendered nondetectable. It is arguable whether the "positive control" section should be from tissue processed in an ideal way, so that antigenicity is likely to be preserved, or whether the positive control section should be from tissue processed in a manner identical to the tissue under study, in which it may not be known whether fixation or processing has adversely affected the antigen.

The former control (ie, optimizing preservation of antigen, exemplified by a frozen section) would serve as a positive control for the specificity of the antibody and for the successful performance of all of the steps of the immunostaining procedure but would give no information as to whether or not the fixation-processing method utilized for the tissue under study permits demonstration of the antigen. To answer this question, the second type of control would have to be employed; ie, a section from tissue processed in an identical manner and known to contain, at least prior to processing, the antigen under question. Under these circumstances a positive result in the positive control and a negative result in the tumor (both processed identically) would permit a statement that the tumor does not contain detectable amounts of the antigen; a negative result in both would indicate that processing has destroyed the antigen or, alternatively, that the staining technique itself is at fault or that the antibody lacks useful specificity for the antigen under study.

In practice, when setting up immunoperoxidase techniques within a laboratory, it is generally best to select an "in-house" control, processed in the standard manner, in which the antigen is presumed upon biologic grounds to be present. Only if the technique consistently fails to produce successful results on "in-house" tissue is it necessary to resort to the staining of frozen sections, or carefully

Table 2–2. Representative Dilution Titration to Determine Optimal Titer of Antibody for Use in Direct Conjugate Method

Intensity of Staining[1] of:	Serial Dilutions of Primary Antibody →					
	1/5	1/20	1/80	1/320	1/1280	1/2560
(a) Unwanted background[2]	+ +	+	±	±	±	±
(b) Specific antigens[3]	+ + +	+ + + +	+ + + +	+ + +	+ +	+

[1]Intensity of staining scored on a semiquantitative scale 0 to + + + +; ± indicates faint positivity of uncertain significance.

[2]Unwanted background staining may result from several different mechanisms (see text).

[3]Intensity of staining of specific antigen (eg, with titration of anti-kappa antibody–specific staining would be present in plasma cells).

processed tissues subject to optimal fixation, in order to establish that the negative findings are due to destruction of antigen by the fixation or tissue processing rather than to some failure in the labelled antibody technique itself.

In selection of controls for a particular antigen-antibody system, one, of course, may be guided by the literature or by the manufacturer of the reagents; however, such guidance is not a substitute for proving the efficacy of staining with "in-house" controls.

Optimal Dilution

The optimal dilution for use of an antibody in immunohistology is defined as that dilution at which the greatest contrast is achieved between the desired (specific) positive staining and any unwanted (nonspecific) background staining. Selection is subjective and is based not simply on the greatest intensity but rather on the greatest useful contrast (Table 2–2).

Serial dilution titration for determining the working dilution of an antibody is often referred to as checkerboard (or chessboard) titration; in the strict sense, a true checkerboard titration involves titration of two variables simultaneously (see indirect technique on following pages). The optimal titration in the example in Table 2–2 would be 1/80, for at that dilution the contrast (specific stain minus unwanted background) is greatest.

INDIRECT METHOD (Fig. 2–2)

The staining procedure is analogous to that for indirect immunofluorescence (Chapter 1), involving incubation of the sections with the specific "primary" antiserum, washing, then addition of the "secondary" peroxidase-labelled antiserum having specificity against

the primary antibody. The indirect method has a wider range of application than the direct method, for with only one labelled antibody (ie, the secondary antibody—eg, swine antirabbit immunoglobulin) it is possible to demonstrate, in serial sections, the sites of tissue binding of a range of primary antibodies (made in the rabbit in this example), against a range of different antigens. In addition, the indirect method is particularly useful when the specific antibody is available in too small an amount to be processed for conjugation or when the primary antiserum has a low antibody content.

Specificity Control

The indirect technique utilizes two antibodies: the primary antibody, having specificity against the antigen under study, and the secondary labelled antibody, having specificity against an antigenic determinant present on the primary antibody. For successful immunostaining, controls must be included to assess the specificity of both of these antibodies. In addition, both antibodies must be used at the optimal titer.

The specificity of the primary antibody

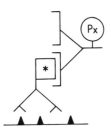

Figure 2–2. Indirect conjugate (sandwich) method. The primary antibody is unlabelled. The method utilizes a labelled secondary antibody having specificity against the primary antibody. Boxed * = antigen determinant on primary antibody; Px = peroxidase label.

against the antigen in question may be investigated by immunodiffusion precipitation methods described in the previous section or by the use of biologic controls. However, in the indirect technique the specificity of the secondary antibody must also be assured. It is essential that the secondary antibody does not, of itself, react with any antigens present in the tissue sections under study; otherwise, staining will be observed as a consequence of direct binding of the secondary antibody to these antigens. This unwanted (and unexpected) staining may then be confused with the specific staining that results from binding of the secondary antibody to the primary antibody, which in turn is bound to the specific antigen under investigation.

Negative Controls. In the indirect method and in unlabelled antibody methods to be described subsequently, a panel of negative controls (see Table 2–3) may be utilized to evaluate tissue specificity of the primary antibody and the secondary labelling reagents. This panel may include all or any of the following:

(1) "Negative antibody control" (saline): section is treated with phosphate-buffered saline in lieu of primary antibody; the addition of secondary antibody and all other steps are followed unchanged.

(2) "Negative antibody control" (normal serum): section is treated with normal serum from same species as the primary antibody in lieu of primary antibody; the addition of secondary antibody and all other steps are followed unchanged.

(3) "Negative antibody control" (irrelevant antibody): section is treated with immune serum (ie, antibody of irrelevant specificity) from the same species as the primary antibody; the addition of secondary antibody and all other steps are followed unchanged (see Fig. 12–1).

(4) "Negative antibody control" (pre-immune serum): section is treated with pre-immune serum from the animal that subsequently was immunized to provide the specific antibody; the addition of secondary antibody and all other steps are followed unchanged.

(5) "Negative antibody control" (absorbed antibody): section is treated with absorbed primary antibody (ie, primary antibody following absorption with an excess of specific antigen); the addition of secondary antibody and all other steps are followed unchanged.

(6) "Blocking antibody control": prior to addition of the primary antibody, an additional antibody with the same specificity, but from a different species, is added; the addition of secondary antibody and all other steps are followed unchanged.

(7) "Negative substrate control": section is stained, omitting both primary and secondary antibodies; addition of substrate and other steps are followed unchanged.

(8) "Biologic negative control": the primary and secondary antibodies and substrate all are added following the normal procedure, but the section utilized is specifically selected because it is believed to lack the antigen under study.

Sections used in negative controls 1–7 should be parallel sections taken in series with the

Table 2–3. Control Procedures

	Preliminary Stage	First Stage	Second Stage	
1. "Saline" control	0	PBS	2° antibody[2]	substrate
2. "Normal serum" control	0	normal serum[1]	2° antibody	substrate
3. "Irrelevant antibody" control	0	irrelevant antibody[1]	2° antibody	substrate
4. "Pre-immune serum" control	0	pre-immune serum[1]	2° antibody	substrate
5. "Absorbed antibody" control	0	1° antibody specifically absorbed[1]	2° antibody	substrate
6. "Blocking" control	specific antibody from species B[3]	1° antibody[1]	2° antibody	substrate
7. Substrate control	0	0	0	substrate
8. Biologic negative control	0	1° antibody[1]	2° antibody	substrate
9. TEST SECTION	0	1° antibody[1]	2° antibody	substrate
10. Biologic positive control	0	1° antibody[1]	2° antibody	substrate

[1]All these reagents at same dilution (equivalent protein concentration)—all from species A, including 1° (primary) antibody.
[2]2° (secondary) antibody with specificity versus 1° antibody (ie, anti–species A immunoglobulin).
[3]Specificity identical to 1° antibody but made in a different species.

test section that is stained for the antigen under study.

In all of the negative controls, the anticipated result, indeed the desired result, is lack of specific staining. However, the presence or absence of staining is of differing import in these different controls, and the conclusions that may be drawn from each are limited, as discussed following.

Negative control number 1 (saline) demonstrates that the secondary antibody alone shows no detectable binding to components within tissue sections under test; thus any staining observed in the test section, to which the primary antibody has been added, may reasonably be attributed to the effects of the primary antibody.

The use of a normal serum negative control (2) is based upon the observation that "normal" sera from different species may bind to various components within human tissue sections. The use of this negative control permits assessment of this possibility. However, it may be argued that the concentration of immunoglobulin in normal sera is considerably less than that in the primary antibody, which is an immune serum, and that for the comparison to be valid, equivalent amounts of immunoglobulin must be applied to the section. This had led some investigators to utilize the third form of negative control (3—the irrelevant antibody), in which sections are treated with an immune serum from the same species as the primary antibody but with an irrelevant specificity (ie, a serum raised against an antigen that is not expected to be present within the section under test); lack of staining in this control then gives a general indication that antisera from this species do not cross-react with human tissue components. This conclusion is not absolute, for it does not constitute proof that the individual animal from which the primary antibody was derived, did not possess cross-reactive components within its serum prior to immunization. This possibility can only be excluded by the performance of the fourth control (4—the pre-immune serum), in which two parallel sections are treated side by side, the first with the primary antibody and the second with pre-immune serum derived from that same animal prior to immunization. This control, however, is generally not available, unless the antibodies being used have been prepared personally by the investigator; certainly pre-immune serum

is rarely available for antisera that are purchased commercially.

Again, some immunochemists would argue that in applying normal serum or nonimmune serum as a negative control for the primary antibody it is important to add identical amounts of immunoglobulin; indeed, some authors have stressed the importance of application of equal microgram amounts of immunoglobulin. This preoccupation is, however, no more than a delusion of scientific exactitude, since in a conventional antiserum the specific antibody constitutes an unknown proportion of the total immunoglobulin, the remainder representing a variety of antibodies of irrelevant specificity. Only with affinity-purified antibodies, or more particularly with monoclonal antibodies, should one consider going to the length of applying equal amounts of nonspecific immunoglobulin versus specific antibody as determined by weight.

Treatment of a section with primary antibody following preabsorption with excess antigen (control number 5) provides one of the most satisfying negative controls, for if a loss of staining is observed following absorption of antibody with specific antigen, then it may be assumed that the staining observed with the nonabsorbed antibody is attributable to the presence of the antigen within the tissue section. However, even in this instance, there are some potential pitfalls that often are overlooked. The validity of this control depends upon the purity of the antigen used for absorption. For example, in attempting to make anti-A antibody, if the material used for immunization (the immunogen—ie, antigen A) contains, unsuspected, a small amount of a contaminant (antigen B), then the antiserum developed would contain antibodies against both antigen A and antigen B. Absorption of this antiserum with the immunizing material (ie, the immunogen containing antigen A and the unsuspected contaminant, antigen B) would lead to a loss of positive staining and then to a false conclusion—namely, that the antiserum is specific for antigen A. In fact, all of the staining observed in a tissue section might have been due to the presence of antibody against the unsuspected contaminant, antigen B.

In practice, usually only one of these five "negative antibody controls" is employed; preference would be for use of specifically absorbed control antiserum if available (control number 5); or failing this, an immune antiserum of irrelevant specificity, but from the same species, should be employed (control number 3). Pre-immune serum from the immunized animal, the source of the specific antiserum, should be used if available (control number 4).

Negative control number 7 is designed to test, not the specificity of the antibodies, but whether the substrate alone is affected by any of the surviving enzymes within the tissue section. Specifically, in the immunoperoxidase system this control is a test of whether or not endogenous peroxidase is present, for the presence of active endogenous peroxidase will induce formation of a colored reaction product that may be confused with the product of the immunoperoxidase reaction. Strategies for avoiding this particular problem are discussed later.

The "biologic negative control" (8) is a control section specifically selected to lack the antigen under study. This section is not a control in a strict scientific sense, but it may serve as a general warning, in that a positive reaction following treatment with primary and secondary antibodies and substrate indicates that the immunostaining system is staining cells known to lack the antigen; thus the specificity of the system must be examined more closely.

It is, of course, obvious that in most instances of staining of a tissue section for the presence of an antigen (eg, immunoglobulin), some cells in the section will contain the antigen (positive—eg, plasma cells), whereas other cell types making up the tissue contain no antigen; these latter cells (eg, fibroblasts, endothelial cells, and the like) should not stain, and their nonreactivity serves as an intrinsic negative control.

One other negative control has been advocated by some investigators, and this is the "blocking (negative) antibody control." In this form of control, the section is treated with specific antibody (against the antigen in question) derived from one species (eg, goat anti-kappa chain), followed by "primary" antibody of the same specificity but made in a different species (eg, rabbit anti-kappa chain); in theory, binding of the primary rabbit antibody to the antigen is impeded by the presence of the goat antibody that already is linked to the antigen. Thus the final stained product, after addition of the labelling reagents (eg, swine antirabbit immunoglobulin-peroxidase or conjugate) is expected to be reduced. On the basis that one specific antibody interferes with binding of a second specific antibody, this control serves as a further indication of the specificity of the system. One difficulty with this type of control is that the "blocking" is reversible, and if the primary antibody is of high affinity (as hopefully it is), it may simply displace by competition the blocking antibody, and the final staining reaction may not noticeably be reduced.

These control procedures are summarized in Table 2–3.

Optimal Dilution (Checkerboard) Titration

As with the direct conjugate procedure so with all other labelled antibody methods, it is imperative that antibodies are applied at the optimal dilution: the one at which greatest useful contrast is achieved. In two- and three-layer methods, exemplified by the indirect conjugate and PAP (vide infra) methods, respectively, each of the separate immune reagents must be applied at optimal dilution. In addition, the dilutions of the primary and secondary (and tertiary) antibodies are interdependent in terms of contrast developed by the procedure as a whole. This fact necessitates comparison of results obtained using several dilutions of the labelling reagent (secondary antibody) with several different dilutions of the primary antibody; comparison is achieved by checkerboard or chessboard titration (Table 2–4).

NONCONJUGATE PROCEDURES—SO-CALLED NONLABELLED ANTIBODY METHODS

Hybrid Antibody Method (Fig. 2–3)

The use of hybrid antibody has been well reviewed by Sternberger (1979a), who describes the preparation of antibodies with double specificity by the recombination of univalent fractions obtained following pepsin treatment of two antibodies of different specificity. The extension of this concept to immunocytochemical procedures involves hybridization of one antibody, specific to the antigen in question, with a second antibody, directed against the label (eg, ferritin or peroxidase). In this technique the antibody raised against the antigen under study is

Table 2–4. Determination of Optimal Titers for Indirect Immunoperoxidase Method—Checkerboard Titration

		\multicolumn{6}{c}{Dilutions of Primary Antibody →}
		1/5	1/20	1/80	1/320	1/1280	Negative Control[1]
	1/10	slide 1 + + + (+ +)	slide 2 + + + (+ +)	slide 3 + + + (+ +)	slide 4 + + (+ +)	slide 5 + (+ +)	slide 16 ± (+ +)
Dilutions of Secondary Antibody (Conjugate) ↓	1/40	slide 6 + + + (+)	slide 7 + + + (+)	slide 8 + + + + (+)	slide 9 + + + + (±)	slide 10 + + (±)	slide 17 − (±)
	1/160	slide 11 + + (+)	slide 12 + + (±)	slide 13 + (±)	slide 14 ± (−)	slide 15 ± (−)	slide 18 − (−)

EXAMPLE OF AN 18-SLIDE TITRATION

[1]Negative control (omit primary antibody, replace with pre-immune serum, or serum with irrelevant specificity; see negative controls).

[2]Intensity of specific staining is indicated on a scale of 0 to + + + +; nonspecific background is given in the same scale in brackets $\left\{ \begin{matrix} 0 \text{ to } + + + + ; \text{ eg, } + + + \\ (+) \end{matrix} \right\}$ indicates strong specific staining (+ + +) with moderate background (+).

Note: In this example optimal result is achieved with slide 9.

cleaved enzymatically (usually with pepsin) and reconstituted with similarly split antibody derived from the same species but directed against horseradish peroxidase. Following reconstitution a variable percentage of the antibody molecules have a double, or dual, specificity (one antibody site for the given antigen and the other for the enzyme label).

A significant disadvantage of this method is that the hybrid antibody preparations generally contain some nonhybridized antibody molecules (ie, antibodies with two identical binding sites), and these reduce the sensitivity of the method by competitive binding with tissue antigen. "Pure" hybrid antibody may be obtained by successive solid phase adsorption and elution on columns of each of the two antigens (the "given" antigen and peroxidase). However, this is time-consuming and wasteful of antibody; added to which

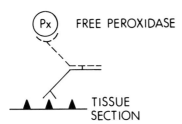

Figure 2–3. "Hybrid" antibody method. One specific site of the "hybrid" molecule binds to the tissue antigen (▲); the second specific site then serves to bind the free peroxidase label (Px).

elution of the high-affinity antibody, of greatest value in immunostaining, is difficult. For these reasons this method has not been used extensively. For details of the method and its application, the reader is referred to Sternberger's excellent monograph (1979a).

With the advent of the hybridoma method and the capacity for inexpensive production of large amounts of antibody, this method may find new favor as an alternative to conjugation techniques. It should be noted, of course, that for hybridoma or monoclonal antibodies the term *hybridoma* refers to the antibody-producing cells (which are fused hybrids—see Chapter 1), not to the antibody molecules, which are normal monospecific bivalent immunoglobulins.

Unlabelled Antibody Enzyme Method (Enzyme Bridge Method) (Fig. 2–4)

The unlabelled antibody enzyme method was introduced by T. E. Mason and colleagues in 1969. It is not widely used today, finding its main application as a second technique in double-labelling methods. However, the principles developed in the enzyme bridge method apply also to the PAP method devised shortly thereafter by Sternberger and collaborators: in the PAP method the third and fourth steps of the enzyme bridge procedure are effectively combined, as subsequently described.

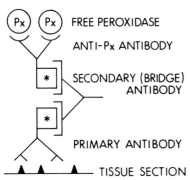

Figure 2–4. Enzyme bridge method. A secondary antibody is utilized to link (bridge) the primary antibody to an antiperoxidase antibody, which in turn binds to free peroxidase.

Four components are applied sequentially in the enzyme bridge method: primary antibody, secondary antibody, antibody against horseradish peroxidase, and horseradish peroxidase (Fig. 2–5). The first and third components of this immunostaining sequence must be prepared from the same species, or must show immunologic cross-reactivity. The system depends on utilizing the functional bivalent binding of the bridge, or linking, antibody so that binding to specific primary antiserum (eg, rabbit antiserum versus kappa chain) is primarily by one valency (site), leaving the second valency (site) free to bind with any additional rabbit immunoglobulin that is added subsequently (eg, the rabbit antiperoxidase antibody) (Fig. 2–5). In theory and to a large extent in practice, this is achieved by adding the bridge antibody in great excess, so competition for binding to the antigen sites on the primary antiserum is high, with only one of the two possible binding sites finding attachment in most instances.

This method does not require chemical conjugation between peroxidase and antibody and therefore avoids the risk of loss of antibody reactivity or enzyme catalytic activity that may occur in the conjugation procedure. The PAP method also shares this advantage but effectively combines the last two steps of the "bridge" method and is apparently more sensitive.

The PAP Method

The PAP method was first utilized for the demonstration of binding of rabbit anti-treponemal antibody to *Treponema pallidum* in smear preparations (Sternberger et al, 1970).

Positive staining was detectable at a dilution of anti-treponemal antibody of one in one million, a dilution one hundred to one thousand times higher than the greatest dilution giving detectable staining by indirect immunofluorescence techniques. This observation gave rise to the popular conception that the PAP method is exquisitely sensitive.

This apparently high degree of sensitivity proved seductive for pathologists and other investigators bent upon the detection of small amounts of antigen in tissue sections, particularly small amounts of antigen that might have survived fixation and processing in "routine" paraffin sections. Several groups of investigators working with different systems and different goals independently discovered that it was possible to demonstrate at least some antigens in fixed paraffin sections (immunoglobulins—Taylor, 1974; Taylor and Burns, 1974; pituitary hormones—Halmi et al, 1975; viral antigens—DiStefano et al, 1973); the PAP method, probably because of its great sensitivity, appeared to be particularly useful for this purpose.

The principles of the PAP method are illustrated in Fig. 2–6. The primary antibody is added to the tissue section at a dilution determined by checkerboard titration (vide infra), giving optimal contrast between positive staining and any nonspecific background reaction. Following washing, the secondary antibody is added in large molecular excess, so there is great competition for binding to the primary antibody already in place upon the section. Under these conditions binding of the secondary antibody by only one of its two valencies (antigen-binding sites) will be favored, leaving the second valency free, potentially able to bind specifically with more immunoglobulin from the same species as the primary antibody. Additional immunoglobulin from the same species (as the primary antibody) is then added in the form of a stable immune complex, consisting of antibody against horseradish peroxidase and horseradish peroxidase antigen (the PAP—peroxidase-antiperoxidase reagent). This immune complex is taken up specifically by the free binding sites of the bivalent linking antibody, which thus serves to link the primary antibody and the PAP reagent—provided, of course, that both the primary antibody and the PAP reagent are derived from the same species or share a high degree of immunologic cross-reactivity for the linking antibody. The principles are

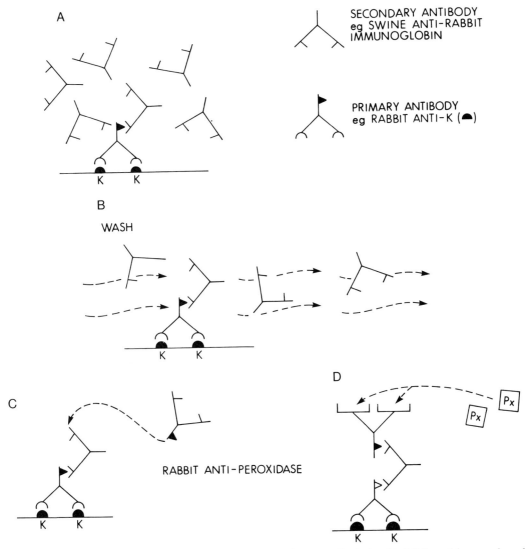

Figure 2–5. Enzyme bridge method, sequential steps. ***A,*** Primary antibody is added followed by a wash and the addition of secondary antibody in excess. ***B,*** Excess unbound secondary antibody is washed away. ***C,*** This leaves one free valency of swine anti-rabbit immunoglobulin antibody available to react with rabbit antiperoxidase added subsequently. ***D,*** The free peroxidase added as the final stage is bound by the antiperoxidase specificity of the rabbit-anti-peroxidase antibody. The chromogen is then added, producing a colored reaction product.

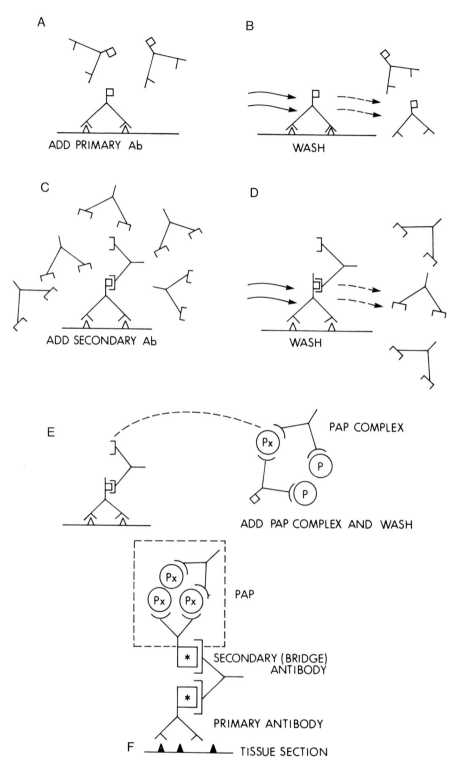

Figure 2–6, *A–E.* PAP method, sequential steps.

directly comparable with the enzyme bridge method, and the potential difficulties of chemical conjugation of peroxidase to the specific antibody are likewise avoided.

We do not imagine that you, not being immunochemists, wish to prepare your own PAP reagent, although the details on how to do so are clearly given by Sternberger and others (Sternberger, 1979a). In practical terms PAP reagents are relatively stable in dilution solution and are available from a number of commercial suppliers (see Appendix #2).

Structure of PAP Reagent

The structure of the PAP complex has been well defined by Sternberger and colleagues. PAP consists of three molecules of peroxidase and two molecules of antibody against horseradish peroxidase in a stable pentameric form, as illustrated in Figure 2–6.

From the point of view of the user, the major features of importance are that the activity of the enzyme is preserved, that the complex is stable even in high dilution (there appears to be some variability in the stability of PAP reagents prepared in different species, and by different manufacturers), and that the complex contains immunoglobulin characteristic of the species in which the anti-horseradish peroxidase antibody was prepared.

The antibody component of the PAP complex has specificity against the peroxidase components, the whole complex being bound to the secondary (linking) antibody by the specificity of that antibody, not by the specificity of the antibody within the PAP complex. This circumstance is of critical importance, worthy of emphasis, since this means that PAP raised in one species can generally only be utilized if the primary antibody is from the same species and if the linking antibody is a functionally bivalent antibody with specificity against immunoglobulin of that species.

This specificity to some extent limits the utility of a particular PAP reagent, for a rabbit primary antibody must be linked with rabbit PAP, and goat primary antibody with goat PAP, and so forth. The only exception to this rule, mentioned earlier, is when significant cross-reactivity is demonstrable between primary antibody from one species and PAP made in another (usually closely related) species (eg, human primary antibody—chimp PAP).

Titration of PAP Reagent

Given the availability of a PAP reagent, it is necessary to titrate the reagent to determine the dilution giving optimal staining in a system in which the other reagents have also been optimized (Table 2–5).

Ideally, all titrations should be in terms of micrograms of active reagent; in practice, this desired goal is rarely achieved, and we must content ourselves with expression of dilutions, meaning, of course, that the dilutions

Table 2–5. Checkerboard Titration for PAP Method*

Primary Antibody Dilution (eg, Rabbit Anti-Insulin)	Secondary Antibody Dilution (eg, Swine Antirabbit IgG)	PAP Dilution (Rabbit PAP)		
		1/20	1/80	1/160
		(Slide Numbers)		
1/80	1/10	1	2	3
	1/40	4	5	6
	1/160	7	8	9
1/320	1/10	10	11	12
	1/40	13	14	15
	1/160	16	17	18
1/1280	1/10	19	20	21
	1/40	22	23	24
	1/160	25	26	27
Control (omit primary antibody)	1/10	28	29	30
	1/40	31	32	33
	1/160	34	35	36

*A 36-slide checkerboard is shown; optimal dilutions of reagents are selected on the basis of that slide giving greatest useful contrast. With experience it may be possible to reduce the complexity of this titration, omitting some of the dilutions that experience (ie, previous use of similar reagents from the same source) has shown are unlikely to be optimal.

used in one laboratory (and reported in one paper) with a particular set of reagents cannot be transferred automatically for use in a second laboratory unless all reagents are identical.

Once optimal dilutions have been determined, the stock of undiluted reagent should be divided into convenient aliquots, for preparation of working dilutions immediately prior to use. Generally speaking, it is not wise to store reagents in a highly dilute form, unless additional protein or stabilizers are added to conserve activity, since reactivity may decline unpredictably. That stability of highly diluted reagents can be achieved is evidenced by the availability of commercial immunostaining kits (eg, from Ortho, formerly Immulok) that do contain prediluted reagents and have a shelf life of one year or more.

A principal reason for use of freshly prepared reagents from aliquots is avoidance of repeated sampling of a single reagent tube (or bottle), as by a Pasteur pipette, since this practice almost invariably results in bacterial contamination and loss of reactivity that is both unpredictable and aggravating. Here the "pure" scientists might learn a lesson from their often maligned cousins in the commercial sector, who have to a large extent overcome the contamination problem by providing diluted reagents in sealed dropper bottles whereby the reagent is directly dropped from the reagent bottle.

We have unashamedly borrowed this technique in our laboratory, and whenever we make up new dilutions of reagents for use over a period of several days we utilize these same small plastic dropper bottles.

Accelerated Staining, Overnight Staining, Humidity Chambers

It is convenient at this point to discuss variations in incubation time.

Standard incubation in most procedures is 30 minutes at room temperature. With multistage methods, such as the PAP method, successive incubation and washings result in a lengthy overall procedure. Some attempt has been made to shorten the procedure by incubation at 37°C in a hotplate humidity chamber; incubation for each step may then be 10 minutes or less. This approach, introduced by Ortho, who markets a hotplate, has been adopted by other investigators, some of whom utilize humidity chambers placed in

an oven at 37°C. This method is perhaps less effective than the hotplate owing to the longer time taken for reagents to reach a temperature of 37°C.

Incubation of slides in a humidity chamber is essential at 37°C and is advisable at room temperature, particularly in more arid climates. In practice, if a slide treated with antibody is permitted to dry, excessive nonspecific background staining invariably occurs. Even when total drying does not occur, evaporation of the antibody solution on the slide may result in an effective increase in antibody concentration, again producing unwanted background staining. Humidity chambers containing level slide racks may be purchased, or may be made rather easily from glass rods and plexiglass or glass plates glued together with water-resistant bonds. Staining racks upon which slides rest while incubating should be level to avoid drainage of antibody off the section to other areas of the slide.

Overnight (or extended time) incubation may also be employed in certain circumstances; here again a humidity chamber partly filled with water is essential. We have employed overnight staining to permit use of primary antibody at a high dilution; it is possible to achieve good staining, with reduced nonspecific background staining, by taking an antibody that gives reasonable results when incubated for 30 minutes, diluting it 10- or even 100-fold, and then incubating it for 12 to 14 hours. This method conserves precious antibody, reduces background staining due to nonspecific attachment of antibody (the antibody is present at a much lower concentration, favoring binding by high-affinity immunologic reactions), and may also be used to increase the intensity of staining from an antibody that produces only a weak positive reaction with normal incubation. In this method only the primary antibody is given prolonged incubation; other reagents are used normally.

Applications of PAP Procedure

Beyond the general discussion here, there are many reported variations in application of the PAP method. A selection of the pertinent literature is given in Table 2–6, including comparison with immunofluorescence methods and with conjugate and ABC procedures, reviews of utilization in paraffin sections, cell smears, and postembedment

Table 2–6. Selected References—General Methodology and PAP Method

Pinkus 1982 Wilkerson and Wilkerson 1982 Heyderman 1979, 1980 Bosman et al 1979 Nadji 1980 Hsu et al 1981b, c Montero 1981 Heitz 1982 Straus 1981	General review on paraffin-embedded tissues
Bergroth et al 1980	Used paraffin sections and cytocentrifuge preparations; compared indirect, bridge, and PAP methods; indirect method least sensitive
Clausen 1980	Compared indirect peroxidase, fluorescence, and PAP; PAP preferred
Sternberger 1979a	PAP method
Tougard et al 1979	PAP versus indirect conjugate for thin araldite sections
Zakharova et al 1979	Immunoperoxidase simpler than immunofluorescence and PAP method more sensitive
Wachsmuth 1982	PAP more sensitive than fluorescence in detection of amino-peptidase (frozen sections)
DiPersio et al 1982	PAP in paraffin, fluorescence in frozen and RIA; of equivalent sensitivity in detection of beta$_2$-microglobulin
Tinelli et al 1979	Study of human auto-antibodies, compared fluorescence versus peroxidase, alkaline phosphatase, and glucose oxidase conjugates; concluded peroxidase best
Banks 1979	Focus on hematopathology, but includes good discussion of controls and fixation
Laurent et al 1980	Comparison of conjugate versus PAP (for immunoglobulin)
Grube 1980	Semi-thin sections peroxidase/DAB, examined by light microscopy, then exposed to UV light gave specific yellow fluorescence with much increased sensitivity
Hsu & Ree 1980	Multiple "self-sandwich method," utilizing repeated applications of primary antibody and the specific antigen prior to bridge antiserum and PAP. Claimed a 50% increase in sensitivity without compromising specificity. Possible method for demonstrating some SIg in paraffin sections.
Naritoku & Taylor 1982	Evaluation of different immunohistologic methods for use with (mouse) monoclonal antibodies
Naiem et al 1982	Value of immunohistochemical methods in specificity screening of hybridoma supernatants
Laurent et al 1982	Surface Ig in smears; stained either as cell suspensions and then smeared, or stained directly as smears
Tubbs et al 1980c Vernon & Lewin 1980	Comparison of peroxidase versus fluorescence in lymph nodes
Jäger & Dörmer 1981	Cytophotometric method for quantitating immunoperoxidase staining of individual cells
Millar & Williams 1982	Preparation of a standard antigen slide for immunoperoxidase positive control
Dighiero et al 1980	Method for individual cell quantitation of immunoperoxidase staining (in mouse ontogeny and in human CLL)
Zafrani et al 1983	PAP most sensitive, but Fab conjugates penetrate best
Smith et al 1983b	PAP method and microdensitometry
Falini & Taylor 1983	Review of 10 immunoperoxidase methods

staining for electron microscopy. The reader should refer directly to these papers for details.

Protein A in Immunoenzymatic Techniques

Protein A is a protein covalently linked to the peptidoglycan part of the cell wall of most *Staphylococcus aureus* strains, one of the best producers being strain Cowan I (about 80,000 molecules of protein A per organism). An important property of protein A is its ability to bind to IgG immunoglobulins from several mammalian species, including man, rabbit, goat, and mouse. There are at least two sites in the intact molecule of protein A accessible for linking IgG, binding occurring through the Fc domain of the IgG molecule, close to the C1 binding site.

Table 2–7. Selected References—Protein A

Trost et al 1980a, b, c	Three papers describing use of protein A: *(a)* demonstration of ANA in SLE; *(b)* good description of use in light microscopy; *(c)* use at EM, with reference to pemphigus and pemphigoid and tissue-bound IgG
Notani et al 1979	Protein A in unlabelled antibody method
Falini et al 1980	Comparison of protein A with other methods, including PAP
Watts & Leathem 1980	Protein A–PAP method
Mandache et al 1980	Preparation of a "hybrid" reagent with dual specificity, using protein A to link two antibodies of different specificities

The affinity of protein A for IgG immunoglobulins varies from one species to another. For example, in the case of human immunoglobulin, the ability to interact with protein A is largely confined to the IgG1, IgG2, and IgG4 subclasses; whereas in that of mouse the IgG2a, IgG2b, and IgG3 subclasses are strongly reactive, but IgG1 is less so. Recently, however, it has been shown that IgG1 mouse myeloma immunoglobulin may bind staphylococcal protein A, although with considerably less avidity than it binds IgG2 proteins; it now appears that the differences in mouse IgG subclass binding to protein A are more quantitative than qualitative, probably reflecting the presence of several binding sites in IgG2 molecules, but only a few in IgG1 molecules. In addition, partial reactivity with protein A has been reported for monoclonal immunoglobulins other than IgG, both human and murine.

Protein A consists of a single peptide chain of approximately 42,000 molecular weight with high stability for heat and other denaturing agents. About 50 percent of the molecule appears to have an alpha-helical configuration. Coupling of protein A to other substances such as fluorescein, peroxidase, alkaline phosphatase, ferritin, and ^{25}I does not adversely affect the biologic properties of the native protein (IgG binding). Consequently protein A is currently used as immunologic reagent in a number of applications, including immunofluorescence, immunoperoxidase, immunoelectron microscopy, and radioimmunoassay techniques. Table 2–7 gives access to selected literature concerning the utilization of protein A methods.

Figure 2–7 depicts two protein A immunoperoxidase methods. In the two-stage conjugate method, a primary specific antibody is first applied, followed by the protein A–peroxidase conjugate; protein A–alkaline

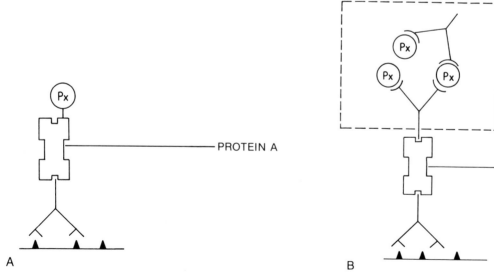

Figure 2–7. *A*, Protein A conjugate method. *B*, Protein A-PAP method.

phosphatase may also be employed. The three-stage technique uses unlabelled protein A as the bridging reagent between the primary antibody and the PAP immune complexes.

Protein A–peroxidase itself can also be utilized (without primary antiserum) as a labelling probe to detect tissue-bound IgG autoantibodies by virtue of their Fc components. The success of this method depends entirely on the ability of protein A conjugate to bind tissue immunoglobulins through Fc receptors. This goal is better achieved in frozen sections in which the Fc portions of IgG molecules appear to be preserved. In contrast, incubation of paraffin sections of IgG myelomas with protein A–peroxidase conjugate does not produce any labelling of the neoplastic myeloma cells, most probably owing to the denaturing effect of routine fixation and embedding procedures upon the Fc portion of cytoplasmic immunoglobulins.

It should be noted that the ability of protein A to bind Fc components of endogenous immunoglobulin in frozen sections is a significant disadvantage if the protein A method is used for detection of monoclonal antibody binding in frozen sections.

Blocking and titration studies indicate that the sensitivity of the indirect method employing protein A–peroxidase conjugate is similar to that of labelled antibody techniques.

Protein A–peroxidase appears to have, however, several advantageous properties with respect to the peroxidase-labelled conjugates in indirect methods in paraffin sections.

First, the specificity of the immunolabelling is enhanced with protein A–peroxidase, since the background activity is minor compared with that observed with peroxidase-labelled antibody, unless affinity-purified antibody is used; in the indirect conjugated antibody technique, the background staining may be attributed at least in part to the presence in the secondary antibody preparation of labelled nonspecific components, which can interact with unknown tissue constituents. In fact, when the primary antiserum is omitted (negative control), there is minimal binding of protein A to the tissue sections. Another factor that may contribute to the low background is the use of protein A–peroxidase at a high dilution (up to a ratio of 1:8000 protein A to primary antibody), taking advantage of the great affinity of protein A for the Fc portion of the IgG molecule.

When present, nonspecific staining can be completely eliminated by incubating the sections with 3 percent H_2O_2/10 percent egg albumin or by use of protein A diluted in a buffer containing mannose, glucose, galactose, and bovine serum albumin. The use of normal nonimmune serum for "blocking" (as in PAP methods) is not recommended, owing to possible cross-reactivity between protein A and the Fc portion of these nonspecific immunoglobulins.

Second, the use of protein A–peroxidase results in a significant reduction in processing time, since the binding of protein A to Fc portion of antibody reagent is very rapid.

Third, the protein A is able to react with immunoglobulins from several mammalian species, and, consequently, its use is not limited with respect to the species of origin of the primary antibody. It should, however, be remembered that IgG3 immunoglobulins in man and IgG1 immunoglobulins in mouse show a weak reactivity with protein A, resulting in decreased sensitivity when these IgG subclasses are part of the immunostaining sequence. In order to overcome this problem, protein A may be used in a three-step procedure, following incubation of primary mouse antibody with rabbit antimouse immunoglobulins that show high affinity for protein A.

Finally, the low molecular weight of protein A–peroxidase (80,000) as compared with that of peroxidase-labelled antibody (200,000) may be exploited for immunoelectron microscopic detection of intracellular antigens. Ultrastructural demonstration of fibronectin, viral particles, and IgG antibodies has been obtained by using direct or indirect protein A procedures. The anticipated molecular weight of a monomeric protein A–peroxidase conjugate is approximately 80,000; however, the protein A–peroxidase conjugation products obtained by the periodate method are high–molecular weight polypeptic aggregates, most suitable for light microscopy visualization. By using benzoquinone or glutaraldehyde as the cross-linking reagents in a two-step procedure, lower molecular weight protein A–peroxidase conjugates may be obtained. The recent introduction of new bifunctional reagents such as N-succinimidyl 3-(2-pyridyldithio)-propionate should further increase the ability to obtain monomeric protein A conjugates with better tissue-penetrating properties.

The three-stage protein A–PAP technique

is a modification of the classic PAP method. Because of its affinity for IgG immunoglobulins from various species, protein A may efficiently act as a bridge reagent between rabbit PAP and a primary antibody from species other than rabbit, provided the antibody has good affinity for protein A (heterologous PAP system). This method clearly has advantages for the detection of human or mouse immunoglobulins for which homologous PAP may not be available and is, in addition, much more rapid than the conventional PAP method, owing to the rapidity of protein A–Fc binding.

The Biotin-Avidin Systems

Avidin is a basic glycoprotein with a molecular weight of 68,000 and four high-affinity binding sites for biotin, a vitamin with a molecular weight of 244. The coupling of substances such as fluorescein, enzymes, and ferritin to either biotin or avidin does not inhibit the formation of biotin-avidin complexes; these two reagents are, therefore, often used in immunofluorescence and immunoperoxidase studies.

A comprehensive review of the utility of biotin-avidin systems in both ELISA and immunoperoxidase techniques has recently been published by Guesdon et al (1979). The techniques are illustrated in Figure 2–8, and access to selected pertinent literature is given in Table 2–8. Briefly, the tissue sections are incubated with the biotinylated primary antibody and then with avidin-peroxidase conjugate or unlabelled avidin and biotinylated horseradish peroxidase. Warnke and Levy (1980) have used a three-stage "indirect" system in which unlabelled primary antibody is followed by a biotinylated secondary antibody and finally by an avidin conjugate of horseradish peroxidase (Fig. 2–8).

All these methods have, however, the disadvantage of relatively low sensitivity, a problem when the antigen to be identified is present in the tissues only in extremely small amounts; for example, surface differentiation antigens defined by monoclonal antibodies. Berman and Basch (1980) succeeded in increasing the sensitivity of the two-step method threefold by adding another fluoresceinated antibody against biotin after the primary antibody and fluoresceinated biotin.

The avidin-biotin-peroxidase complex (ABC) method, recently developed by Hsu et al (1981c, d), is more sensitive than the basic biotin-avidin method. The ABC method may be utilized in a direct (with a biotinylated primary antibody) or indirect procedure, most commonly the latter. In the ABC technique, a biotinylated secondary antibody acts as a bridge reagent between the unlabelled primary antibody and the avidin-biotin-peroxidase complex (Fig. 2–8). The most intense staining reaction with the lowest background stain is generally obtained using ABC conjugates with avidin to biotin-peroxidase ratio of 4:1 (optimal concentration, 10 µg/ml avidin to 2.5 µg/ml biotin-peroxidase conjugate).

Because the intensity of staining of the immunoperoxidase reaction is a function of peroxidase activity, it has been suggested that the greater sensitivity of the ABC method may be related to the fact that the avidin-biotin-peroxidase complex is a lattice structure containing several peroxidase molecules. Claims for superior sensitivity of the ABC method, compared with PAP methods, have not been borne out in our laboratories using both rabbit PAP and mouse PAP reagents with the appropriate primary antibodies (vide infra). In our experience exploitation of the full range of sensitivity of the ABC method is often hampered by nonimmunologic binding reactions in many tissues.

The occurrence of nonspecific staining in biotin-avidin detection systems is attributable to one of several factors. First, nonspecific attachment of free avidin or labelled avidin to cellular components occurs to a variable degree, probably because of electrostatic interactions. Second, avidin preparations may show binding to endogenous biotin present at high concentration in many mammalian tissues, especially liver, adipose tissue, mammary gland, and kidney. The endogenous avidin-binding activity resulting from these mechanisms can be suppressed by preincubating the sections with free avidin (concentrations ranging from 0.1 to 0.01 percent) for 20 minutes and then, after a brief five-minute washing in PBS, with free biotin (concentrations ranging from 0.01 to 0.001 percent) for a further 20 minutes, as described by Wood and Warnke (1981). The rationale for this approach is that all four binding sites present in each added avidin molecule will be completely saturated by both the endogenous biotin and the free biotin added to the sections. Since each biotin molecule can link to only one avidin molecule, the final result is that none of these blocking reagents can bind to the free or labelled avidin or the

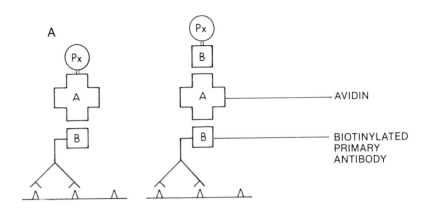

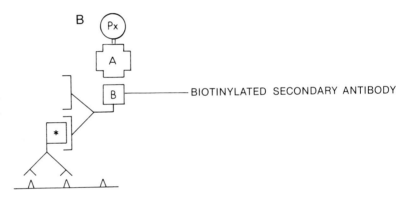

Figure 2–8. *A*, Direct biotin-avidin methods. *B*, Indirect biotin-avidin method. *C*, Avidin-biotin-conjugate (ABC) method (used as an indirect method).

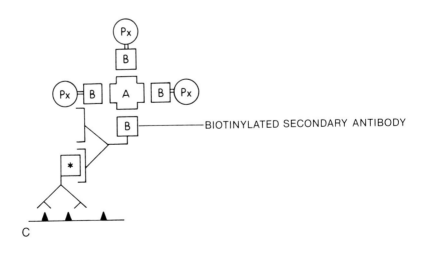

Table 2–8. Selected References—Avidin-Biotin Methods

Guesdon et al 1979	Authoritative use of various avidin-biotin methods; good technical paper
Yasuda et al 1981	Peroxidase-avidin conjugate
Hsu et al 1981a, b, c	Three essentially similar papers describing the ABC technique in detail
Heggeness & Ash 1977	Avidin-biotin and immunofluorescence staining for actin
Tolson et al 1981	Avidin-colloidal gold method
Warnke et al 1980	Use with monoclonal antibodies to leukocyte antigens in frozen sections
Wood & Warnke 1981	Endogenous avidin-binding activity
Banerjee & Pettit 1984	Endogenous avidin-binding activity

biotin in the subsequent stages of the immunostaining sequence. This blocking procedure is somewhat tedious but should be performed, at least as a control, in all stains of tissue sections in which the intrinsic biotin content and its distribution is unknown.

The ABC method has proved particularly valuable when used as an indirect technique for immunostaining with mouse monoclonal antibodies, by virtue of its sensitivity (eg, ABC with a biotinylated horse antimouse antibody).

3

FIXATION, PROCESSING, SPECIAL APPLICATIONS

"Though this be madness, yet there is method in't."

POLONIUS, in *Hamlet*, ACT II, SCENE 2

Immunohistologic techniques (immunofluorescence and immunoperoxidase) permit correlation of traditional histologic criteria with an independent system for cell recognition; namely, the visualization and localization of specific cell or tissue antigens or both. For optimal results both antigenic reactivity and morphologic detail must be preserved when the tissues are prepared for immunohistologic examination. Two methods are commonly used. The first method, that of the traditional morphologist, incorporates some form of "fixation," followed by dehydration and embedding in paraffin wax to provide a rigid matrix for sectioning. The second method involves minimal fixation and relies upon freezing to provide rigidity to the tissue for sectioning (cryostat or frozen section technique). More recently, fine-needle aspiration methods for producing cell smears have increased in popularity; these specimens, subject to brief fixation, are well suited to immunocytochemical techniques.

It is obvious that many factors may influence the ability to perform successful immunostaining: the form of fixation, the method of processing, the nature of the antigen, its concentration in the tissue specimen, and its distribution (intracellular, membrane-related, or extracellular).

In general, antigens present in relatively high concentration within the cytoplasm are preserved during fixation. Surface antigens, by contrast, are frequently denatured or "masked" by routine fixing and embedding procedures and are better analyzed by immunologic techniques in cell suspensions or frozen sections. For these reasons, many contemporary laboratories, recognizing the growing need for a variety of immunohisto-

logic studies, have adopted the policy of collecting and storing a small portion of each specimen in liquid nitrogen, thereby allowing staining of frozen sections if subsequent need becomes apparent. This procedure is in addition to fixing and processing material for paraffin embedding, which allows testing for many antigens, albeit some are destroyed. Touch imprints, fine-needle aspirates, cell suspensions, and cytocentrifuge preparations from small tissue samples provide additional alternatives to the paraffin section method (later in the chapter).

PARAFFIN-EMBEDDED SECTIONS

Fixation

Tissues that are to be embedded in paraffin wax are first "fixed" in order to optimize preservation of cell morphology; the choice of fixative profoundly affects the morphologic and immunohistologic results.

The ideal fixative for immunohistologic studies should not only be readily available, it should also be in widespread use in order to maximize the range and number of samples available for immunohistologic studies. The fixative should preserve antigenic integrity and should limit extraction, diffusion, or displacement of antigen during subsequent processing. Also, it obviously should give good preservation of morphologic details after embedment in a support medium (eg, paraffin). In addition, the fixative should allow adequate penetration of tissue by the immunochemical reagents, and it must not interfere with subsequent antibody-antigen reactions intrinsic to the immunostaining

Table 3–1. Selected General References: Fixation

Arnold et al 1974, 1975	Comparative study of processing and fixation methods
Boenisch 1980	General review and bibliography
Bosman et al 1977 Bosman & Nieuwen- huijzen Kruseman 1979	General review
Curran & Gregory 1980	Fixation and processing with reference to immunoglobulins
DeLellis et al 1979	Review of workshop
Mason & Biberfeld 1980	Review of problems, anomalous staining, etc.
Taylor 1978b	Practical and theoretical aspects
Banks 1979	Various fixatives
Pearse 1968	Excellent text; general histochemistry
Culling 1974	Text: histopathologic techniques
Lillie 1975	Text: histopathologic techniques

procedure. These are requirements in addition to the usual needs for low toxicity, stability on storage, and economy of use that apply to all routine fixation methods. Unfortunately, in everyday practice the more faithfully the morphologic detail is preserved by the fixative, the greater is the damage to the immunologic properties of the tissue components, so at the moment the separate demands of histology and immunohistology cannot be completely reconciled. Current techniques represent a working compromise (Tables 3–1 and 3–2).

Formaldehyde

Formaldehyde, a highly water-soluble, somewhat volatile gas, is marketed as formalin in a 37% to 40% solution. At this concentration formaldehyde is mainly present in the polymeric form and is not suitable for fixation purposes. For routine histopathologic diagnosis, tissue samples are usually fixed in 10% dilution of concentrated formalin (i.e., 4% formaldehyde), which is then neutralized with sodium acetate or buffered to pH 7.0 by a combination of monobasic and dibasic sodium phosphate. This fixative is known as 10% neutral formalin. At neutral pH, formaldehyde exists almost entirely in monomeric hydrated form (methylene glycol, $CH_2[OH]_2$) with a low molecular weight. In consequence, it penetrates the tissues rapidly.

Formaldehyde develops its fixative properties mainly by reacting with proteins. In general, it attacks any side group containing an active hydrogen. The active hydroxymethyl groups formed by this reaction may undergo condensation reactions with other nearby active hydrogen leading to methylene-type linkages between polypeptide chains that are the basis of fixation. Formaldehyde may also reduce disulfide linkage to two sulfhydryl groups that in turn may react with formaldehyde and take part in the methylene linkages.

For histochemical procedures the recom-

Table 3–2. Selected References: Fixatives

Dixon & Eng 1982	Fixatives for myelin basic protein: formalin good, mercuric chloride bad
Clausen 1980	Fixatives for alpha$_2$-antitrypsin: formalin good, Bouin's poor; prolonged fixation, adverse effect
Curran & Gregory 1980	For immunoglobulins formal acetate is best, mercuric chloride good; formalin requires trypsinization
Leathem & Atkins 1980 Banks et al 1979	Review of several fixatives for immunochemistry
Jacobsen et al 1980	Review of several fixatives and loss of staining with time
Mason et al 1980a	Advantages of mercury-based fixatives
Käyhkö 1980	Staining of J chain following Bouin's fixative
Konttinen & Reitamo 1979	Different fixatives in smears and sections, with special reference to lactoferrin
Bergroth et al 1982	Fixation–dependent false-positive staining
Reitamo et al 1980b	Baker's fixative (formol-calcium) good for cell smears
Sassen & Vander Plaetse 1980	Progressive loss of antigens in unfixed air-dried smears
Matthews 1981	Effect of clearing agents
Sainte-Marie 1962	The cold alcohol method
Brandtzaeg 1974 Brandtzaeg 1981	Cold alcohol (Sainte-Marie) method
Robinson & Dawson 1979	Formalin and neuroendocrine cells
Piris & Thomas 1980 Heyworth 1980 Bosman et al 1977	Fixation and staining of plasma cells
Bowling 1979	Processing of lymph nodes, ideal technique
Taylor 1980 a,b	Problems encountered

mended fixation time in 10% formalin is usually between 12 and 18 hours. Clearly, optimum fixation time is dependent upon rate of penetration and thus the size of the tissue blocks. In order to achieve good morphologic detail, fixation must exceed a certain minimum period (eg, 4 to 6 hours for 10mm × 10mm × 3mm blocks), but there is practically no upper limit to the time of fixation (ie, morphologic detail is still good after fixation for 96 hours or more). However, it is now recognized that antigenicity is lost progressively during the fixation process; the longer the period of fixation the less antigen remains intact as determined by specific reactivity with appropriate antibody. Thus for immunohistologic studies, fixation should be for the briefest period consistent with satisfactory morphology (eg, 4 to 6 hours).

The successful immunohistologic detection of many antigens in formalin-fixed paraffin sections is probably due to the fact that although some molecules are altered structurally so as not to react with antibody, they are present in sufficiently high concentration within the cytoplasm for a proportion to remain relatively intact. It should, however, be noted that in cases of faint or "negative" staining, the immunologic reactivity of some intracytoplasmic antigens may be increased (or restored) by incubating the paraffin sections with proteolytic enzymes, particularly trypsin (Table 3–3). Incubation of fresh formalin-fixed tissues with 30% saccharose solution has also been reported to restore some of the antigenicity lost during fixation. Such findings suggest that the denaturation caused by the formalin is probably reversible and that the antigens are only "masked" (ie, the antigenic determinants are rendered partially inaccessible by overlying methylene linkages that may be dissociated by incubation with trypsin, saccharose, or other substances, thus revealing again the antigenic sites). Comparative studies carried out on various fixatives indicate that solutions containing mercury or picric acid, compared with formalin, give the best preservation of intracytoplasmic antigens and that acidic fixatives may alter the antigens more than neutral ones.

A fixative containing periodate-lysine and paraformaldehyde does permit the utilization of several monoclonal antibodies in paraffin sections: Janossy's group (Collings et al, 1984) showed that 22 out of 27 monoclonals to membrane-related antigens were effective under these conditions.

Table 3–3. Selected References: Unmasking of Antigen by Trypsinization, Etc.

Mepham et al 1979	Proteolysis to improve staining for immunoglobulin
Deng & Beutner 1974	Formaldehyde, sucrose, preservation of antigenicity
Hautzer et al 1980	Trypsin for immunoglobulins
Radaszkiewicz et al 1979	Protease for HbsAg (hepatitis B surface antigen)
Pileri et al 1980b	Pronase enhances immunoglobulin staining
Eishi et al 1981	Optimal conditions for trypsinization
Jacobsen et al 1980	Loss of 15% of stainable Ig for each 24 hours in formalin
Curran & Gregory 1980	Various fixatives and trypsinization; comprehensive paper
Mason & Biberfeld 1980	Good review of problems and solutions

Mercuric Chloride–Containing Fixatives

Tissues fixed in mercuric fixatives usually show a greater number of positive cells and a more intense positive reaction within each individual cell than observed in formalin-fixed specimens, at least with regard to staining for intracellular immunoglobulins (Mason et al, 1980b; Curran and Gregory, 1980). Because of the good preservation of antigenicity with B5 and other mercuric chloride–containing fixatives, trypsinization becomes unnecessary; even if performed, there is no enhancement of staining. Moreover, the histologic details, particularly those of the nucleus in H&E stained sections, are considerably improved with this form of fixation.

Mercuric chloride is a good fixative but does not penetrate tissues well and may cause marked shrinkage. Therefore, it is usually combined with other fixatives. Formol sublimate, B5 fixative (a formalin–mercuric chloride mixture, neutralized with sodium acetate), Zenker's fluid, and Sousa's fluid are all examples of mercuric chloride–containing fixatives. These fixatives act more rapidly than formalin (blocks of lymph node 3mm thick are adequately fixed in B5 within 2 to 4 hours). They give an improved sectioning quality and preserve the morphologic detail better than formalin. However, tissues fixed with mercury-containing fixatives frequently show the presence of black mercuric precipitates. Although at immunoperoxidase staining such deposits are easily distinguishable from the diaminobenzidine reaction product, it is preferable to remove the mercuric deposits by incubating the sections with 0.5% iodine solution in 0.5% ethanol for 5 minutes, briefly rinsing in tap water, and then reincubating in 5% sodium thiosulfate for 5 minutes. This step may be performed prior to immunostaining or immediately prior to addition of the chromogen.

Many intracytoplasmic antigens, particularly immunoglobulins, can be demonstrated with mercuric fixatives; indeed, it has been demonstrated that formol sublimate and B5 are superior to formalin for preserving intracellular immunoglobulin antigenicity (see Table 3–2). The better preservation of antigen may stem in part from the reduced fixation time compared with formalin.

Picric Acid–Containing Fixatives

Bouin's and Zamboni's fluids are the two most commonly used picric acid–containing fixatives. Picric acid reacts with histones and basic proteins, which leads to the formation of crystalline picrates with amino acids. The process causes yellowing of the tissue specimens, which can easily be removed by treating with a saturated solution of lithium carbonate in 70% ethanol for 2 minutes. The tissue antigen reactivity is relatively unaffected by this technique. Comparative studies show that Bouin's fluid may be preferable to formalin and alcohol fixatives (eg, Carnoy's fluid) for the demonstration of intracellular immunoglobulins and J chain in paraffin sections (Käyhkö, 1980).

Immunoperoxidase staining for hepatitis B surface antigens (HbsAg) has been carried out successfully on sections of Bouin's fixed, paraffin-embedded liver specimens (Busachi et al, 1978). Studies have identified numerous neuronal proteins, defined by 18 different clones of monoclonal antibodies, after fixation of leech ganglions in Bouin's fluid for 4 hours at room temperature (Zipser and McKay, 1981). In contrast, two other neuronal antigens could be detected in tissue fixed in 4% paraformaldehyde but not in those fixed in Bouin's.

Alcoholic Fixatives

When immunohistochemistry was in its infancy, alcohol (ethanol) was a widely used fixative (eg, the Sainte-Marie cold ethanol method). The assumption that the antigenic structure of certain tissue antigens is preserved by fixation in cold alcohol was the basis of the Sainte-Marie method. Unfortunately, however, tissues fixed in alcohol alone undergo marked shrinkage and distortion with resultant poor morphology.

Following the discovery that many of the previously mentioned fixatives (eg, formalin, B5, Bouin's, and others) do permit some preservation of antigenicity, absolute alcohol alone is now rarely employed for immunohistologic studies. When used as a fixative, alcohol is usually combined with other substances (eg, formalin and acetic acid), as in Carnoy's fluid. As alcohol diffuses rather rapidly, 1 to 2 hours in Carnoy's fluid is sufficient to fix completely; the fixed tissue is then transferred directly to absolute alcohol.

Carnoy's fixative is the first choice for the immunohistologic demonstration of lactoferrin in paraffin-embedded sections (Konttinen and Reitamo, 1979). Absolute alcohol and acetone are also claimed to preserve the antigenicity of lactoferrin, but in tissues fixed with these alone, the lactoferrin leaks to the surrounding medium. Unfixed frozen tissue sections are usually adopted for the detection of leukocyte surface antigens, including common leukocyte antigen, with certain monoclonal antibodies, for the antigenicity of many of these surface antigens is altered by various fixatives; however, the antigenicity of common leukocyte antigen appears to be better preserved after fixation in Carnoy's than in other fixatives (Pizzolo et al, 1980). By contrast, Carnoy's has a detrimental effect on several other antigens, such as lysozyme, that are well preserved following formalin fixation.

Conclusion

As can be seen from the preceding discussion, there is no general rule. The critical issues are the same for all fixatives: penetration should be as rapid as possible; care should be taken to avoid the obvious pitfalls that preclude good histologic preparations, and fixation time should be the minimum consistent with good morphology. If several different antigens are sought, it is advisable to use more than one type of fixation procedure, preferably including some type of frozen technique for the very labile cell surface antigens.

For each new investigative study, it is wise to conduct preliminary experiments to determine the ideal fixation-processing method for the antigen(s) in question. Faced with the need to utilize previously fixed tissue, it is equally important to conduct a study to determine the extent of survival of the critical antigens in the tissue available.

In a "routine" laboratory it is advisable to establish a standard optimal fixation routine, with particular attention to standard block size, standard fixation time, and avoidance of prolonged exposure to alcohol, xylol (xylene), or host paraffin baths. Once this is standardized, experience will reveal which antigens can be reliably demonstrated. It is wise, whenever possible, to take a small sample of each specimen and "snap-freeze" it in liquid nitrogen for use should it be necessary to stain for some antigen that does not survive the "routine" method.

Fixation Time

Biopsy specimens of delicate tissues, such as lymph nodes, should be handled gently during surgical removal and should be fixed immediately (see Bowling, Table 3–2, for a good protocol). The development of anoxia, due to delays between removal and fixation or to delay during surgery concurrent with the use of clamps and ligatures, damages the cell membranes and consequently may render some cells permeable, permitting diffusion of cell products out of cells or entry of serum proteins into cells. This may account for anomalous immunoperoxidase staining patterns that have been observed, particularly the unexpected presence of serum proteins (including immunoglobulins) in a variety of cell types (see Mason and Biberfeld, 1980).

In addition, drying of the outer part of a biopsy specimen may occur, in part caused by the common practice of wrapping tissues in dry gauze for transmission to the pathologist. These problems may be compounded in autopsy materials and may lead to irregular loss of antigencity and irregular zones of nonspecific staining of cells with a variety of different antibodies. It has been suggested that during terminal cellular anoxia, a decrease in intracellular pH causes denaturation of tertiary and quaternary protein structures and, in consequence, a loss of antigenicity. Such loss of antigenicity may be exacerbated by diffusion of soluble antigens during phases of autolysis and by the deleterious effect of some fixatives upon some antigens; the net result is an incremental loss of staining with poor localization. It should be stressed that not all antigens are equally susceptible to anoxic degradation or diffusion, just as not all antigens are equally affected by fixation.

Once the specimen has been placed in the fixative, the optimal fixation time will depend on the diffusion rate of the fixative, the size of the tissue block, and the nature of the tissue (lung is readily penetrated; liver, less so). It is obvious that the outside of a tissue block becomes fixed before the inner part and that the larger the block, the longer the fixative will take to penetrate to the center. Therefore, if the block is too thick, overfixation of the outer portion of the tissue will occur; this circumstance may result in poor antibody penetration or in denaturation of antigens, even though the morphology may be satisfactory. Under these circumstances the immunoperoxidase staining may often be positive and specific in the center of the section, but not at the periphery. If the tissue is fixed for too short a time or if the block is too large, the reverse may occur, inadequate fixation and poor morphology in the center of the tissue and optimal immunostaining at the periphery (Fig. 3–1); all of these possibilities are persuasive evidence for the use of thin (3 to 5 mm) blocks for fixation. The optimal fixation time is, of course, also dependent upon the concentration of the fixative; both concentration of fixative and time of fixation of small blocks should be defined for immunohistologic studies. With reference to concentration, it should be remembered that the critical feature is the concentration of "active fixative" at the time of use, not the concentration as initially prepared some weeks or months previously when delivered to the clinic or operating suite. Fresh fixatives are important.

Fixative pH

In general, the most satisfactory morphologic and antigenic preservation is obtained using fixatives near neutral pH. In acid environment the antigenicity of the molecules may be lost, probably as a result of the destruction of the tertiary and quaternary structures of the proteins (Reitamo, 1978). The risk of antigenic denaturation is particularly high in fixatives containing acid substances (most commonly acetic acid) but may

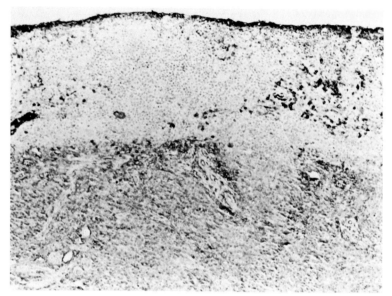

Figure 3–1. Fixation—the two-edged sword. Paraffin secretion shows spleen stained for immunoglobulin (Ig). The spleen was fixed by dropping it whole into a bucket of formalin, a sad practice with dire effects for the immunopathologist. The formalin penetrates only the outer few millimeters (upper part of figure); here the cytoplasmic Ig is preserved and the plasma cells can be stained (black dots). Serum Ig can be stained in small vessels (left), but surface Ig is rendered nondetectable. The deeper parts of the spleen remain partially fixed (lower part of figure); here autolysis occurs and immunostaining is fruitless.

be minimized by appropriate adjustment of pH to physiologic range.

An important often overlooked cause of low pH is the aging of some formalin solutions; the traditional approach of storing formalin over marble chips is probably not an adequate precaution.

Acid decalcifying agents, such as acetic acid, especially if used for a long time, may lead to the destruction of the antigenicity of many molecules in bone marrow biopsies (Banks, 1979).

Temperature

Within quite wide limits, the fixation temperature is probably not critical. Jacobsen et al (1980) have, however, reported that the sensitivity of the PAP method for the detection of intracellular immunoglobulin is increased after fixation at 4°C. It should be remembered that in the subsequent steps of tissue processing, paraffin infiltration of the blocks at temperatures over 60°C may cause marked antigenic denaturation in addition to loss of morphologic (nuclear) detail. Specific data are not available as to the relative antigenic loss at different temperatures during the embedding procedures; nonetheless, experience strongly suggests that paraffin impregnation should be carried out at less than 60°C, with the use of low melting–point paraffins, for the minimum time necessary to complete the process in small tissue blocks. In this respect, we probably still have something to learn from the work of Sainte-Marie

(1962), who twenty years ago showed that "cold alcohol–cold embedding" procedures provided improved capability for demonstrating tissue antigens by immunofluorescence.

Tissue Processing

In contrast with the fixation and embedding procedures, the remaining steps in the processing of tissues seem to have less influence on the results of the immunohistologic investigations. Matthews (1981) found, however, that the number of immunoglobulin-containing plasma cells and the intensity of the staining of every individual plasma cell was enhanced if either chloroform or Inhibisol was used instead of xylol as the clearing agent. B5-fixed tissues processed through chloroform or Inhibisol also showed less background staining. For unknown reasons, these differences were abolished by pretreatment of the sections with trypsin. In our experience the substitution of chloroform for xylol has not produced noticeable differences.

Embedding Media

Most of the reported studies of immunohistochemical techniques have employed either cryostat sections or "routinely" processed tissues, in which the embedding medium was "paraffin" (not otherwise specified).

There are many different commercial paraffins, including some with additional ingredients. Detailed data on the suitability of these for immunohistochemical staining for particular antigens are sketchy.

In practice the usual requirement in a laboratory about to develop the capability for immunohistochemical staining is that the method adopted works on the "in-house" material, both current cases and those on file as paraffin blocks. This is a limitation that precludes not only selection of the ideal fixative but also selection of the ideal processing method and embedding medium. In reality very few service laboratories have shown a willingness to overhaul or radically change their fixation, processing, and embedding techniques to achieve good immunohistochemical results; rather, every effort is made to adapt the immunostaining method to the material on hand. The difficulties intrinsic in this practice have been discussed. It must be emphasized that immunohistochemical methods, however good, cannot be expected to achieve reliable results in the face of poor fixation or embedding methods. If the "in-house method" cannot be changed radically, it should at least be overhauled with regular fresh reagents and minimal controlled fixation times. Dehydration and rehydration similarly should be standardized to the minimum time with small blocks and the lowest melting–point paraffins consistent with ambient temperature in the laboratory should be selected.

For those adventurous spirits contemplating more radical changes or for those embarking upon prospective studies in which immunohistochemical stains are essential, some of the source literature is given in Table 3–4.

FROZEN SECTIONS

Until recently only a limited number of antisera (anti-Ig, anti-J chain, anti-lysozyme, anti-hormone antibodies, and the like) were available, and in consequence relatively few molecular constituents could be detected in either normal or pathologic tissues. As described earlier, the integrity of the cytoplasmic antigens recognized by many of these antisera appear to be at least partially preserved in paraffin sections.

To a large extent, the newly introduced monoclonal antibodies, particularly those

Table 3–4. Selected References: Processing and Embedding

Stein et al 1984 Nemes et al 1982	Freeze-dried paraffin sections; excellent preservation of antigens
Dudek et al 1982	Quick freeze/freeze-drying for ultrastructural studies
Giddings et al 1982a	Immunoglobulin in araldite-embedded kidney
Peschke et al 1980	Use of paraplast
Takamiya et al 1979	Plastic semi-thin sections and protease
Judd 1980	Modified paraffin for thin sections
Beckstead et al 1981	Semi-thin plastic method for marrow
Rodning et al 1980 a,b	Epoxy resin method with removal of resin

with specificity for cell surface antigens, have overcome earlier limitations in terms of the range of different antibodies available and have made possible many new immunohistologic investigations. However, coupled with this unquestioned advance, an old problem has been aggravated—namely, the adverse effects of "routine" fixation and paraffin-embedding upon the immunologic reactivity of many of the membrane-related antigens (eg, surface immunoglobulins, Ia-like antigens, T–cell differentiation antigens, and so forth). There is a general consensus that most surface antigens are better preserved in frozen sections (Fig. 3–2) cut by cryostat from snap-frozen blocks than in paraffin sections, providing a real incentive to collect frozen blocks as well as formalin-paraffin tissues in all instances where immunohistologic studies may be contemplated.

Snap-Freezing Methods

Tissue must be as fresh as possible and should be snap-frozen with minimum delay by one of the following techniques (Johnson et al, 1978).

1. Solid CO_2–Alcohol Mixture. This is the method of choice for collection of large numbers of blocks from a specimen. Pieces of solid CO_2 are added, slowly to avoid "boiling over," to alcohol in a wide-mouth thermos until the temperature of the alcohol drops below $-20°C$. Small blocks of tissue, not more than 5mm thick, are then snap-frozen by placing them on the inner side wall of a hard-glass boiling tube to which they are self-adherent. The tube containing the specimen is then plunged into the freezing mixture until the tissue sample is below the level of

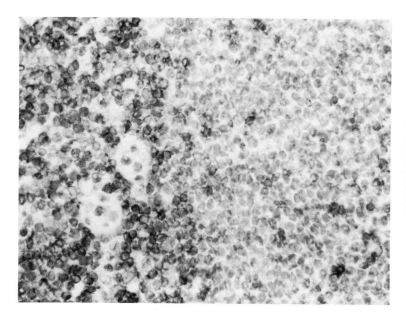

Figure 3–2. Lymph node treated with OKT11 (E rosette receptor) antibody; positively stained T cells appear as small black donuts. Frozen section, 3-amino 9-ethyl carbazole (AEC) with hematoxylin counterstain (×320). Many monoclonal antibodies are effective only in frozen sections.

the outer liquid. Great care must be taken to prevent the alcohol from entering the top of the tube, as this will hamper freezing and soften the block, making cutting difficult; it may also interfere with antigenicity. The tissues, which freeze quite rapidly (approximately 10 minutes), are then pried off the glass, placed in polyethylene bags, sealed, and stored at a temperature of −20°C or −70°C.

2. Liquid Nitrogen–Isopentane Mixture (Maxwell et al, 1966). This is the method of choice for small tissue specimens.

In order to freeze minute specimens (bone marrow, liver, kidney biopsies, and the like), the tissue sample may be placed in the bottom of a small cup (1cm × 1cm), which can easily be made by twisting tin foil around the end of a pencil. The cup is then filled with an inert embedding material (eg, Ames OCT compound) and immersed in either liquid nitrogen or isopentane–liquid nitrogen mixture for freezing. Another method of dealing with small tissue fragments is to sandwich them between larger fragments of another tissue (eg, mouse liver) and then to snap-freeze the "sandwich."

Because isopentane has a high thermal conductivity, the tissues freeze rapidly in this medium, and the irregular freezing caused by direct immersion in liquid nitrogen, which vaporizes when it comes into contact with the tissue, is avoided.

When freezing is rapid, the ice crystals formed are small (subcellular) and, in consequence, the morphologic artifacts encoun-

tered with large ice crystals are minimized. For these reasons some investigators prefer to use isopentane instead of liquid nitrogen as cooling agent, although in routine practice, freezing in liquid nitrogen itself usually produces satisfactory morphologic definition.

If isopentane is used, it should be precooled in liquid nitrogen to the point at which it forms opaque droplets (these droplets indicate that the isopentane is approaching its own freezing point of −160°C). The foil cup containing the biopsy specimen is held with forceps and immersed in the isopentane; the specimen may be dunked in and out a few times to reduce cracking that may be caused by uneven cooling. Precooled forceps are used for transferring the frozen specimen from isopentane to liquid nitrogen or to a −70°C freezer. Also, relatively simple freezing systems have recently become available commercially (eg, from Neslab, Inc., Portsmouth, New Hampshire).

Storage of Specimens

Thawing and refreezing damages the morphologic architecture of the tissue and creates a high level of background at immunohistologic staining, which is usually attributed to irregular diffusion and partial denaturation of antigens. Thus, once snap-frozen by one of the preceding methods, the tissue samples must be stored in the frozen state. Tissue hydration and antigenicity remain good for a period of up to 2 years when specimens are stored in individual sealed containers in liquid nitrogen. Because of the limited space inside liquid-nitrogen containers, some investigators prefer to transfer the snap-frozen specimens to small polyethylene bags and to store them in a freezer cabinet at −20°C or −70°C. Unfortunately, however, due to the dehydration of the specimen when stored at this temperature, sectioning becomes increasingly difficult on prolonged storage, and the risk of background staining is increased. For example, tissues conserved in a cryostat cabinet at −15°C only remain hydrated for 2 weeks. Miller and Hogg (1980) suggest snap-freezing in an excess of water to avoid dehydration. To do this, they place the tissue specimen with cut surface down in a conical universal polystyrene container to which 4ml OCT compound embedding medium has been added; then after snap-freezing in liquid nitrogen, the container is removed from the liquid nitrogen and is immediately three–quarters-filled with physiologic saline solution. The container is then tightly capped and again snap-frozen in liquid nitrogen for storage in a cryostat cabinet at −20°C until use. Hydration of the specimens handled in this way is maintained up to 1 year at −20°C.

Preparation of Frozen Sections

Sections from unfixed tissues snap-frozen in one of the above ways are obtained by cutting in a cryostat (eg, in a microtome that is housed in a refrigerated cabinet with a regulated temperature between zero and −30°C).

Morphologic detail is better preserved in paraffin-embedded tissues than in cryostat section (see Fig. 1–3). Nonetheless, assiduous attention to the technical aspects of freezing and sectioning can produce surprisingly good results so that, when counterstained with hematoxylin, sufficient morphologic detail is apparent for the identification of most cell types with reasonable confidence (Fig. 3–2).

Certain tissues containing little intrinsic support (eg, undecalcified bone marrow biopsies) are particularly difficult to cut on a cryostat. However, Rijntjes et al (1979) obtained satisfactory results by using a cryomicrotome originally designed for autoradiography sections. Another solution is to cut snap-frozen concentrated bone marrow particles (Falini, unpublished data; see also section on bone marrow in this chapter).

Tissues are usually sectioned at about −20°C by applying a minute amount of water or saline to the base of the frozen tissue block, so that it adheres to the chuck. Blocks may also be frozen on small cork mats to facilitate attachment to and removal from the chuck. Sections should be cut at 6 to 10 microns, or, in practice, as thin as possible consistent with the production of intact sections without tears, rents, or irregularities of thickness due to intermittent compression; these latter aspects of sectioning are largely matters of the quality of the cryostat and the expertise and devotion of the histology technician. The sections are then removed from the cryostat on glass slides and dried under an electric fan or simply at room temperature for two hours. Insufficient drying results in the sections becoming detached during the staining procedure or produces difficulties if subsequent fixation in acetone is attempted, owing to the immiscibility of acetone and water.

Several different techniques may be adopted for counterstaining frozen sections; some investigators prefer methylene blue, others hematoxylin and eosin. Roberts's modified celestine blue–eosin procedure has been proposed for improving nuclear detail (Roberts, 1966); briefly, the frozen sections are fixed in a complex-mixture fixative containing 10ml formalin, 56ml absolute alcohol, 5ml glacial acetic acid, 0.18g sodium chloride, 0.15g picric acid, and 30ml of distilled water. After fixation in this mixture for 3 minutes, the sections are rinsed in 70% alcohol and then stained for another 3 minutes in celestine blue–eosin mixture.

Some investigators prefer to use unstained frozen sections for immunohistologic investigations, achieving better contrast for the product of staining but at the cost of a major decrease in ability to categorize cell types morphologically.

The techniques utilizing freeze drying (to avoid orthodox dehydration) and subsequent paraffin embedment offer a valuable alternative permitting staining of leukocyte surface antigens with good morphology (see Nemes et al, 1982; Stein et al, 1984; Table 3–4).

FROZEN VERSUS PARAFFIN SECTIONS

A unique problem is created in frozen sections by the fact that soluble antigens may migrate from their original sites during the freezing process and in consequence may be falsely located at immunostaining or may be entirely lost. The heat generated by compression due to passage of the knife blade during cutting in the cryostat increases this problem. This phenomenon is particularly evident with low molecular weight intracytoplasmic and intranuclear antigens, like peptide hormones, terminal transferase, and so forth. Cytoplasmic hydrolytic enzymes also have been reported to diffuse in frozen sections within 30 seconds after sectioning, regardless of whether the frozen sections were fixed in acetone or not (Wachsmuth, 1976). Janossy et al (1980e) have noted that terminal deoxynucleotidyl transferase (TDT) tends to migrate from the nuclei in frozen sections but not in paraffin sections.

Fortunately, the antigens that are better preserved in frozen sections are mainly those located on the cell membrane (surface). These antigens are probably immobilized in the cellular membrane macromolecular network, which limits their diffusion. If the sections are fixed in acetone for a short time (usually 5 to 10 minutes) before being subjected to the immunostaining procedure, diffusion will be minimized, and the antigens will react in situ with the specific primary antibody. In addition, fixing sections in cold acetone tends to prevent detachment from the slide and adequately preserves morphologic detail.

Some investigators are, however, reluctant to fix frozen sections because of the risk of denaturing the antigens under study. Curran and Gregory (1980), for example, noted that if the frozen sections were fixed in formaldehyde before incubation with primary anti-Ig antibody, the surface immunoglobulins did not stain. Therefore, some researchers prefer to use unfixed frozen sections or to fix them only after the primary antibody of the immunostaining sequence has been applied. Difficulty may however be experienced in demonstrating antigens with differing diffusion rates (eg, intranuclear TDT) and membrane-related antigens such as Ia, common ALL, and human thymus-leukemia antigen (HuTLA) in frozen sections. Prefreezing fixation of the tissues would probably block the diffusion of the intranuclear TDT antigen but at the same time might cause denaturation of the cell surface antigens.

Although the enhanced preservation of antigenicity in frozen sections, compared with paraffin ones, may be considered a major advantage for the immunohistologic detection of certain surface antigens, it may of itself cause some technical problems.

First, unlike paraffin sections, in frozen sections the Fc receptors appear to be at least partially preserved (eg, Itoh et al, 1977) and may be the cause of false-positive reactions due to binding of labelled antibodies (consisting of whole molecules of IgG) via the Fc portion of the immunoglobulin molecule. $F(ab')_2$ reagents have been utilized in order to circumvent this problem; all the antibodies and the PAP complexes used in multilayer methods must be F(ab) or $F(ab')_2$ reagents in order to obtain real advantage. Contradictory results have been reported by other authors who have failed to observe nonspecific binding of immunologic reagents to Fc receptors in frozen sections. The low affinity of Fc receptors for nonaggregated immunoglobulins may, in part, explain these conflicting findings; whole monomeric peroxidase-labelled antibody molecules and mouse monoclonal PAP (Mason et al, 1982) (maximum antibody:peroxidase ratio, 1:2) may, in practice, be suitable for immunohistologic studies in frozen sections, owing to a preference of Fc receptors for larger aggregates.

Second, although the attainment of excellent preservation of antigenicity in frozen tissue is a critical condition for the success of immunologic investigations, the presence in the sections of excessively large amounts of the antigen may of itself cause some technical problems during the immunostaining procedures. For example, Bigbee et al (1977) found that the dilution of the primary antiserum adopted for the identification of a specific antigen in frozen sections using the PAP method may not be the optimal one for the detection of the same antigen in paraffin sections. In fact, using the primary antibody at identical dilutions, it appears that more antiserum may be bound in frozen sections than in paraffin sections, for in the latter the amount of intact antigen may be greatly reduced as a result of fixation or embedding procedures or both. Consequently the primary antiserum (antibody) often must be used at lower concentration in frozen than in paraffin sections, otherwise excessive binding of primary antibody to the tissue sections may paradoxically result in a negative stain, possibly by binding both valencies of the bridge or linking antibody, as suggested by Bigbee.

Finally, in utilizing frozen sections, the possibility of encountering endogenous enzymes with activities identical to (or similar to) those of the enzymatic label must be considered and combatted. As described later, endogenous peroxidase is a problem in paraffin and frozen sections alike; however, endogenous alkaline phosphatase is inactivated in routine fixation and processing, thus presenting difficulties only in frozen sections.

THIN SECTIONS AND ELECTRON MICROSCOPY

This book does not seek to address the subject of immunoelectron microscopy. Although the principles of immunostaining at electron microscopic levels are similar to those discussed here, there are major differences in terms of fixation and processing that necessitate consideration of radically different approaches to the staining of paraffin sections. Sternberger (1970a) has given an excellent review of ultrastructural immunocytochemistry to which the interested reader is referred.

Rather, this book seeks to reduce the need for electron microscopy by the dissemination of special staining techniques for cell identification that obviate the need for time-consuming ultrastructural studies in support of a histologic diagnosis.

One area of significant overlap between electron microscopy and light microscopy is the provision of "thin" sections; long used as a preliminary to electron microscopic examination of a tissue block, thin sections have recently found a place in the light microscopic examination of certain tissues, including liver, lymph node, and kidney. In many instances the preparation of thin sections requires the use of more rigid embedding media, identical or akin to those used in electron microscopy. Adoption of such media brings with it the attendant problems familar to immunoelectron microscopists. Table 3–5 provides a source literature to pre- and post-embedding staining methods applicable to immunohistologic staining of thin sections for light microscopy.

Such techniques are usually not available to the surgical pathologist and will therefore not be considered further here.

CELL SMEARS AND IMPRINTS

For a number of years after its introduction, the immunoperoxidase technique was

Table 3–5. Selected References: Immunoperoxidase in Thin Sections and Electron Microscopy

Sternberger 1979a	Excellent immunocytochemistry text
Tougard et al 1979	Araldite, PAP, conjugate methods
Dura & Gladkowska-Dura 1980	Transmission electron microscopy (EM) method for Ig
Nakane & Hartman 1980	Scanning EM
Gourdin et al 1979	Surface antigens by EM
Pelletier et al 1981	Pituitary hormones in plastic-embedded tissues
Gamliel & Polliack 1979	Review of scanning EM markers, including latex, viruses, gold, ferritin, and peroxidase
Takamiya et al 1980	Postembedding staining of plastic sections for immunoglobulin
Heyderman & Monaghan 1979	Resin-embedded sections; review
Rodning et al 1980 a,b	Immunoglobulins in resin-embedded sections
Giddings et al 1982a	Araldite, immunoglobulins, and complement
Smart & Millard 1983	Alpha$_1$-Antitrypsin in glutaraldehyde–fixed resin-embedded sections
Judd 1980	One-micron sections from modified paraffin procedure
Kuhlmann & Peshke 1982	Review; various fixatives, removal of resin for postembedding staining

mainly utilized for detecting antigens in tissue sections. However, like immunofluorescence techniques immunoperoxidase and other forms of immunoenzyme staining can be carried out on cell smears, cell imprints, and on cells in suspension; these preparations can then be examined by light or electron microscopy. Further details are also given in relation to study of "smears" of leukemias and lymphomas (Chapter 4).

Living cells, in suspension, exclude penetration of whole antibodies into the cytoplasm, thus only surface antigens are revealed with the live cell supension method (Fig. 3–3). By contrast, in imprints or smears, both cell surface and cytoplasmic antigens are accessible for reaction with the antibody, as the cell membrane is rendered permeable by drying or fixation.

The use of immunoperoxidase methods on live cell suspensions has a number of inherent technical disadvantages.

1. The removal of excess reagents by multiple washing and centrifugation is time-con-

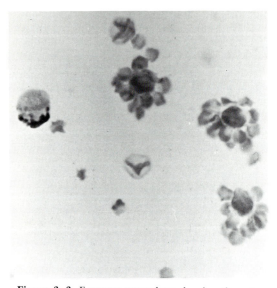

Figure 3–3. E rosette procedure showing three "rosetting" T cells; a single B cell is identified by a black cap of SIg using the immunoperoxidase method. The primary anti-Ig antibody was added to live cells in suspension at 37°C. The cells were washed and "rosetted," then smeared, fixed briefly in acetone, and stained by the PAP method. Counterstain hematoxylin and eosin (H&E) (×650).

suming, particularly in multistage immunocytochemical procedures like the PAP method, and may result in an unacceptably high loss of cells. For this reason many investigators prefer direct immunofluorescence or direct immunoperoxidase techniques for detecting surface antigens in cell suspensions. Only a single wash sequence is then necessary, but the sensitivity may be less than in multiple-layer methods.

2. As with fluoresceinated reagents, peroxidase-labelled whole antibodies and PAP complexes may bind nonspecifically to the cell surface via Fc receptors. The use of $F(ab')_2$-labelled antibody fragments resolves this problem, but all reagents must be $F(ab')_2$ in a multiple-layer method.

3. The Fc receptor–positive cells that do not synthesize their own surface immunoglobulin may adsorb serum immunoglobulins, thus resulting in false-positive results when immunocytochemical studies for the detection of surface immunoglobulin are performed. This problem can be overcome by incubating the cells for 30 minutes at 37°C to promote shedding of the adsorbed surface immunoglobulin. The principles are analogous to immunofluorescence and have been described elsewhere (Taylor and Parker, 1981—review paper).

Surface Antigen Staining of Live Cells

Rather than staining cells in suspension, some investigators prefer to effect the immunostaining of surface antigens by using viable cells attached to slides or wells coated with poly-L-lysine; since the cells are not fixed there is reduced risk of denaturation of surface antigens. This system has been successfully employed for

1. screening of monoclonal antibodies directed against cell surface antigens; for many antigens the cells can be "fixed" with low concentration of glutaraldehyde (0.025%) without detectable loss of antigenicity;

2. detecting HLA histocompatibility antigens and terminal transferase;

3. demonstrating platelet autoantibodies in patients with immune thrombocytopenia.

Table 3–6. Selected References: Specific Applications

Brown et al 1979	HLA antigens
Collings et al 1984	T and B cell antigens in paraffin sections using periodate-lysin–paraformaldehyde fixative
Druguet & Pepys 1977	Alkaline phosphatase method for whole blood lymphocytes
Eross et al 1978	Surface antigens (including HLA) by PAP method
Greenberger et al 1977	Lysozyme in blood cells
Hecht et al 1981	Staining for TdT
Judd & Britten 1982	Excellent review of different fixation/processing methods for demonstration of surface antigens; includes freeze-drying methods
Knowles et al 1977	Comparison of techniques for surface and cytoplasmic antigens
Lansdorp et al 1980	Quantitative method; staining of surface antigens in cell monolayers
Laurent et al 1980	Comparison of conjugate, PAP method
MacPherson & Kottmeyer 1977	Detection of antilymphocyte antibodies
Mason et al 1980b	Surface and cytoplasmic immunoglobulin
Nadji 1980	Review of immunoperoxidase technique for cytology
Reitamo et al 1980b	Immunoglobulin in cell smears
Schmidt et al 1980	Detection of antiplatelet antibodies
Tate et al 1980	Detection of antiplatelet antibodies in idiopathic thrombocytopenic purpura (ITP)

Certain technical requirements must be observed in order to avoid background staining in this procedure. First, the slides or wells should be pretreated with gelatin buffer in order to block free charges of poly-L-lysine which otherwise may nonspecifically bind antibodies by electrostatic interactions. Second, the cells should be fresh, in that stored "frozen" lymphocytes tend either not to adhere to the slide or to detach too easily. Third, as with paraffin or frozen sections, endogenous peroxidase activity must be inactivated, for low levels of surface staining may be obscured by intense cytoplasmic staining that could be due to endogenous peroxidase.

Surface Antigen Staining in Cell Smears, Imprints, or Cytocentrifuge Preparations (Table 3–6)

Another approach is to smear cells directly on slides and perform the immunostaining after air drying or short-term fixation. This gives good preservation of morphologic detail with minimal denaturation of membrane-related antigens, at least when suitable fixatives (vide infra) are used at low concentration for a brief period of time. In this method adherence of the cells to the slides is usually good, and the nonspecific binding of antibodies due to Fc receptors is minimal if brief fixation is employed. Also, this method permits the detection of both surface and intracellular antigens, in that air drying and routine fixation techniques render surface membranes permeable to antibodies (Hofman et al, 1982). Initial studies using this approach demonstrated that antigenicity of immunoglobulins (Fig. 3–4), lysozyme, lactoferrin, and ferritin was adequately preserved after 30-second fixation in buffered formol acetone at room temperature (Mason et al, 1975). This method has since been used successfully by researchers for the identification of a number of antigens such as immunoglobulins, lysozyme, acid phosphatase, gastrin, beta subunit of human chorionic gonadotropin, carcinoembryonic antigen (CEA), and alpha-fetoprotein. The most widely used fixatives are cold acetone, buffered formol-acetone or ethanol. For staining of lymphocyte surface antigens in frozen sections, cold acetone (reagent grade) is commonly used for periods of 30 seconds up to 10 minutes (Hofman et al, 1983). (Note that some antigens may be lost with prolonged fixation.)

Clearly, the introduction of a chemical fixation stage, prior to the primary antibody, introduces the possibility of denaturation of different antigens to varying and unknown degrees. For example, the antigenicity of lactoferrin, with a positive reaction confined to the neutrophil granules, is well-preserved after buffered formol-acetone fixation; but when the cells are fixed in Carnoy's fluid for 30 minutes, both the cytoplasm and the nucleus of neutrophils show a positive reaction. Such a reaction is difficult to explain, but it has been suggested that fixation in Carnoy's fluid may destroy the integrity of the secondary neutrophil granules, thereby allowing

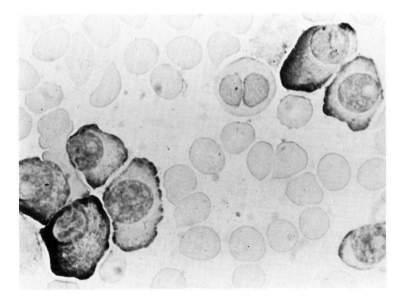

Figure 3–4. Peripheral blood smear showing light chain within a plasma cell leukemia (disseminated myeloma). Smear fixed in buffered formol acetone, DAB with hematoxylin counterstain (× 900).

the lactoferrin to migrate to other sites, such as the nucleus, in which anions may link to the cationic lactoferrin. In other studies immunoglobulin antigenicity was better preserved by fixing cell smears in Baker's formol calcium for 2 to 4 minutes (Reitamo et al, 1980b) than by the technique just described. In this manner extremely small amounts of intracellular immunoglobulin have been detected in pokeweed mitogen–stimulated lymphocytes. Thymic serum factor and similar antigens have been revealed by fixing thymic prints in 10% neutralized formalin for 10 minutes (Monier et al, 1980).

Another way to carry out the immunoperoxidase staining of smears, imprints, or cytocentrifuge preparations is to incubate the cells with the primary unlabelled antibody in suspension (Basten et al, 1978), followed by washing, smearing and fixation prior to application of the bridge antibody and the PAP complexes (Fig. 3–3). This approach avoids any denaturation of antigens caused by smearing, air drying, or fixation, and has given good results when applied for the study of cell membrane–related antigens detected by murine monoclonal antibodies. With this technique it is also possible to show the "capping" phenomenon otherwise not detectable in fixed cell preparations.

These approaches for revealing surface and intracellular antigens in cell smears have produced good results using the direct or indirect immunoperoxidase techniques. The ABC and PAP procedures tend, however, to be more sensitive; affinity-purified primary antibodies should be used for these methods, otherwise contaminant antibodies of unwanted specificity (that may be present in the primary antiserum) may give detectable positive reactions because of the high sensitivity of these techniques.

The use of alkaline phosphatase-labelled reagents for the detection of surface immunoglobulins in cell suspensions has been advocated because it allows the positive Ig-bearing lymphocytes to be easily distinguished from the endogenous peroxidase-containing cells, such as monocytes. This method may be applied for the enumeration of B lymphocytes in whole blood preparations, rather than in Ficoll-separated lymphocytes, thus circumventing false scores resulting from unavoidable and variable loss of cells during separation procedures. The ABC method has been widely employed for this purpose in double staining. Alkaline phosphatase–anti-alkaline phosphatase complexes

have also been used to demonstrate Fc and C3b receptors on the surface of peripheral blood cells (Pepys and Pepys, 1980).

Applications

Immunocytochemistry applied to cell smears has a number of immediate applications in clinical pathology. For example, it is possible to demonstrate monoclonality or monotypia (ie, the presence of a single light chain on the surface of a population of neoplastic cells) in cell smears of patients with lymphoproliferative disorders. In agreement with immunofluorescence studies, strong surface labelling has been observed in prolymphocytic and hairy cell leukemias, whereas cells of CLL, with a lower density of surface immunoglobulins, show a weaker staining reaction. When all of the immunoperoxidase staining steps (including addition of primary antibody) were performed on fixed cell smears, a diffuse staining pattern over the entire cell surface was observed. If, however, the cells were incubated in suspension with the primary antibody and subsequently smeared and fixed prior to the addition of the secondary antibody, the positive reaction appeared to be restricted to one pole of the cell ("capping phenomenon") (Fig. 3–3). Variations of this technique are suitable for T and B cell counting using monoclonal antibodies, for demonstration of Ia-like antigens, for identification of HLA antigens, and for detection of TDT and many viral and microbial antigens. This method is also amenable to double staining, demonstrating two antigens simultaneously.

ASPIRATION CYTOLOGY

All that has been written for cell smears also applies directly to smeared preparations made from fine-needle biopsy–aspiration, of lymph nodes or tumor masses. This technique has long been used in parts of Europe but has not found general favor among histologists, who feel that it is unwise to jettison the tissue recognition aspect of diagnosis for total reliance upon cytologic features. The more recent application of immunocytochemical techniques to fine-needle aspirates may change the philosophy by providing a more certain means of cell recognition. Also, aspiration smears, subject to minimal or no fixation, lend themselves well to immunologic staining methods.

Immunocytochemical techniques are applicable to Papanicolaou cervicovaginal smears and are being used increasingly for direct diagnosis of infectious disease. For example, Lozano de Arce et al (1985) examined PAP smears from 60 women with herpes simplex virus (HSV): approximately 50 percent had cytologic features suggestive of herpes, whereas 95 percent showed positive immunoperoxidase staining with HSV2 antibody. Eighteen controls were nonreactive. Such rapid and precise diagnosis clearly offers advantages over orthodox viral culture. These aspects are further discussed in relation to cervical and uterine cancer and human papilloma virus infection (Chapters 12 and 15). In addition, Pap smears can also be stained for CEA, various cytokeratins, and celomic and other "tissue specific" antigens to facilitate recognition of cervical and endometrial neoplasia (Chapter 14).

The use of immunocytochemical procedures with fine-needle aspiration biopsy is exemplified by the study of Katz and colleagues (1985), the staining prostatic material for prostate–specific epithelial antigen and prostatic acid phosphatase. They showed close correspondence between immunocytochemical staining of histologic sections and Papanicolaou smears obtained by fine-needle aspiration; it should be noted that successful immunostains were performed on previously stained Papanicolaou smears, by removing cover slips with xylene then rehydrating through the alcohols. This procedure clearly provides a method of last resort for immunocytochemical staining; the ideal method is to reserve fresh smears from aspiration needle biopsies for direct immunocytochemical staining should the need arise.

Readers wishing to familiarize themselves with the technique of fine–needle aspiration biopsy are referred to the book by Miller and colleagues (Miller and Kini, 1983), which deals principally with thyroid but includes a general technique, or the book by Frable, *Thin Needle Aspiration Biopsy* (Frable, 1984). A ready literature resource is provided by the new journal *Diagnostic Cytopathology* (Igaku-Shoin, New York/Tokyo, 1985).

BONE MARROW EXAMINATION

Preparation of both bone marrow smears and histologic sections is critical for a complete morphologic and immunologic evalua-tion of bone marrow. Immature cells may be more easily recognizable by morphology in bone marrow smears than in histologic sections. However, the assessment of overall cellularity and the proportions and distribution of abnormal cells is better achieved in sections. Both immunofluorescence and immunoperoxidase techniques have been employed to detect surface or cytoplasmic antigens in bone marrow cell suspensions and smears, as an adjunct to diagnosis. Sometimes, however, smears from bone marrow aspirates are unsatisfactory, because they are hypocellular or poorly representative of the total marrow cell population. This is a known problem in myelofibrosis, metastatic tumors, Hodgkin's disease, the non-Hodgkin lymphomas, and some leukemias. In addition, detailed morphologic and immunologic investigations of certain cell types may not be possible in bone marrow suspensions owing to naturally occurring low numbers. The same kind of difficulty is also encountered when one attempts to assess neoplastic cell populations in bone marrow aspirates taken after intensive chemotherapy.

In these circumstances, the study of the bone marrow structure and the distribution of the cells in situ becomes critical. The histologic examination of a bone marrow section allows study of the topographic relationship of the different cell types with the stromal, fatty, and osseous components, and the proportions of the different cell types may be more accurately assessed. The mode of infiltration of the bone marrow (ie, paratrabecular involvement) is also particularly important for the diagnosis of certain types of non-Hodgkin lymphomas (small cleaved follicular center cell lymphoma) and some acute leukemias (myelomonocytic type).

Certainly there are several techniques

Table 3–7. Selected References: Bone Marrow

Brynes et al 1978	Review
Rijntjes et al 1979	Frozen section method
Block 1976	Comparison smear, biopsy, section
Lukes & Tindle 1972	A method for particle section
Falini et al 1984	Frozen section, immunoalkaline phosphatase method
Moir et al 1983 Erber et al 1984	Method for both smears, applicable also to marrow

available for preparation of good histological sections of the bone marrow (Table 3–7). The most common are

1. aspiration with subsequent sections of concentrated bone marrow particles;

2. bone marrow biopsy of the posterior or anterior iliac crest followed by decalcification and paraffin-embedding, or embedment in methacrylate without prior decalcification.

Some authors prefer the particle-concentrating method for preparing histologic sections for morphologic and immunohistologic evaluation of the bone marrow (Lukes and Tindle, 1972). This procedure avoids the risk of antigenic denaturation related to the decalcifying agents, such as acids or EDTA. Several intracellular antigens, such as immunoglobulins, ferritin, lysozyme, and hemoglobin A and F have been successfully detected in B5-fixed bone marrow particle sections using this approach. In addition, with this method, immunohistologic identification of membrane-related antigens is possible in frozen sections of bone marrow, thereby avoiding the difficulties inherent in obtaining adequate 4-micron cryostat sections from undecalcified bone marrow biopsy.

The greatest drawback to relying on particle sections alone for histologic and immunohistologic evaluation is that the osseous abnormalities and the relationship of the hematopoietic cells with bony trabeculae cannot be adequately assessed. As noted above, the paratrabecular localization of lymphomatous cells is an important morphologic diagnostic criterion in certain lymphoproliferative disorders. Also, in situations with "dry tap," the relatively much larger sample size of a bone marrow biopsy may be a critical advantage.

For these reasons many investigators prefer to prepare histologic sections directly from decalcified paraffin-embedded bone marrow biopsies. Good preservation of some intracellular antigens has been observed after fixation and decalcification for 15 to 24 hours in a mixture of Zenker's fluid and acetic acid in a 20:1 volumetric ratio. The antigenicity of immunoglobulins is retained, at least partially, after fixation of trephine bone marrow biopsies for 3 hours in formol sublimate, followed by 48 hours fixation-decalcification in 10% acetic acid-formol saline. Others, however, have encountered less favorable results, and certainly the antigenicity of many molecules may be severely compromised by the decalcification procedures. Ethylenediaminetetra-acetic acid (EDTA) is considered a more bland decalcifying agent than low-pH methods.

Membrane-related antigens may be effectively demonstrated in cryostat sections of undecalcified bone marrow (difficult to cut), or in sections of marrow particles physically separated from bone fragments (difficult to separate), or, better, in sections of a snap-frozen concentrate of a marrow aspirate preparation that contains no bone. Falini and colleagues (1984) from Dr. Mason's laboratory provide an excellent approach that utilizes frozen sections of nondecalcified bone marrow biopsies with an immunoalkaline phosphatase label to avoid the problems of endogenous peroxidase activity in the numerous myeloid cell components.

SPECIAL APPLICATIONS OF IMMUNOPEROXIDASE METHODS

Human Antibody As a Primary Antibody

The classic PAP procedure cannot readily be applied to the study of antigen recognized by human antibodies since this would require a human PAP reagent, and the preparation of a human antiperoxidase antibody is clearly unethical. Two-stage conjugate and four-stage PAP immunoperoxidase techniques and the heterologous PAP method using chimp or baboon PAP have been employed to circumvent this problem. However, many of these methods suffer some loss of specificity contingent upon the use of additional antibodies with an associated increase in the risk of unrecognized cross-reactivity. Protein A methods have been shown to give a higher specific-staining:background-staining ratio than the above methods and may be preferred for demonstration of "human" antibodies.

For example, Biberfeld et al (1975) used protein A labelled with fluorescein in a two-stage technique to reveal human autoantibodies on frozen sections. A similar system was employed by McCallister et al (1979) to detect human IgG autoantibodies in cell suspensions from patients with immune neutropenias. More recently, Tate et al (1980) identified platelet-associated IgG in patients with different types of immune thrombocytopenias by using labelled protein A as a bridge reagent between human IgG autoantibodies and rabbit PAP on cytocentrifuged platelet preparations. It was claimed that this method proved more sensitive and more specific than the indirect immunoperoxidase technique. Trost et al (1980c) employed an indirect protein A technique for the demonstration and titration of antinuclear antibodies in SLE sera using mouse liver sections. These investigators also were able to use protein A–peroxidase as a labelling probe in immunoelectron microscopy for revealing autoantibodies in the skin tissue of patients affected by pemphigus and bullous pemphigoid. A "labelled antigen" method employing normal human IgG covalently coupled to peroxidase as an alternative to human PAP reagent represents yet another possible variation of the protein A method.

Thus for the detection of binding of human immunoglobulin, the following choices are available (among others):

1. Indirect conjugate: eg, using a peroxidase-conjugated antibody such as goat versus human Ig (all classes)

2. Direct protein A conjugate: eg, using protein A conjugated with peroxidase to detect presence of human IgG (by virtue of Fc linkage to protein A for IgG$_1$, IgG$_2$, and IgG$_4$ subclasses)

3. Four-stage PAP (rabbit): eg, goat anti-human Ig; rabbit antigoat Ig; swine antirabbit Ig (link antibody); rabbit PAP

4. Protein A-PAP (rabbit): eg, using protein A followed by rabbit PAP (linkage of Fc components of same human IgG (vide supra) to Fc of rabbit IgG in PAP complex)

5. Three-stage PAP (chimp): eg, rabbit antihuman Ig followed by chimp PAP

6. Human IgG-peroxidase complex: eg, rabbit antihuman Ig followed by human Ig covalently linked to peroxidase, a labelled antigen method.

Given a choice, one is, of course, presented with the burden of choosing. Differing circumstances and requirements dictate the choice.

In frozen sections the use of protein A methods may be contraindicated by presence of endogenous immunoglobulin of IgG class that may directly bind the protein A (independently of any human IgG added). This caveat applies to human tissues (containing human IgG) or to any animal tissues containing animal IgG subclasses that bind protein A. This is less of a problem in fixed tissues (particularly paraffin sections) because processing appears to so alter the structure of endogenous Fc components that they no

longer react with protein A. If this system is attempted, the use of negative controls (omitting addition of the primary human IgG antibody) is essential to determine the degree of endogenous protein A binding.

With this restriction any of the above methods may be utilized for detection of binding of human antibody to sections of nonhuman tissues. This is well exemplified by the typical test for antinuclear antibody (ANA) in which human (patient) serum is added to frozen sections of rat liver in an attempt to detect specific binding to liver cell nuclei. The procedure is commonly carried out by indirect immunofluorescence methods; in my view indirect immunoperoxidase methods will do the same job, but will do it better since a permanent preparation is produced that can be examined by ordinary light microscopy by one or more individuals to make the necessary reading and interpretation.

A similar rationale applies to detection of other human "autoantibodies" using frozen sections of animal tissues (anti–basement membrane, antimitochondrial, etc.).

In searching for binding of human antibodies in human sections, there is a potential problem—distinguishing endogenous immunoglobulins (present in serum, tissue fluids and inflammatory exudates) from any human immunoglobulin added to the section. In tissues containing only low levels of tissue fluid immunoglobulin or in those in which the presence of Ig is sought at a location where it normally is totally absent (eg, "prickle zones" in epidermis in pemphigus), the problem can usually be resolved by judicious interpretations, based upon experience, and by titration of the sensitivity of the system (ie, selection of the dilution of labelling reagents so that the traces of endogenous immunoglobulin are seen only faintly, permitting achievement of good contrast with the locally high concentration of immunoglobulin deposited in the basement membrane). It must be admitted that this approach offends the "pure" scientific instinct; certainly such maneuvers have been known greatly to arouse molecular biologists who accidentally stumble upon them. However, the establishment of a level of "sensitivity" for a laboratory test, that "ignores" normal levels, is a common occurrence in clinical immunology where low titers (1:2, 1:4, 1:8, and so forth) are routinely and deliberately ignored in serologic testing for the presence of serum antibodies (eg, VDRL, monospot, and others). In my view, as long as controls are included and the pathologist is aware of what he is doing (ie, looking for above-normal levels or abnormal distributions), this approach is practically defensible; it works best, of course, with experience.

It should not be forgotten that there also will be some differences between frozen sections and fixed tissue sections with respect to endogenous antigens such as immunoglobulin. In frozen sections (especially if unfixed until after sectioning) there may be extensive diffusion of free tissue fluid antigens and loss from the section. This may paradoxically be an advantage in detecting precipitated Ig or immune complexes that presumably do not diffuse, the detection of which is therefore enhanced by virtue of removal of "background" Ig.

In fixed tissues this fortuitous result is precluded, since fixation presumably locks all antigens in situ; a separate problem here is our lack of ability to predict the extent by which fixation may denature antigens. This has been discussed previously in this chapter.

In conclusion, for detection of antigens in human tissue sections utilizing "human" antibody, the use of fixed paraffin sections is preferable 1. because some endogenous Ig may have been denatured, reducing the background, 2. because Fc receptor activity is largely destroyed, 3. but ONLY if the antigen in question survives fixation and processing. Otherwise, frozen sections must be employed with the attendant difficulties described above.

For detection of in vivo–bound Ig (eg anti–basement membrane antibody) or immune complexes deposited in human tissues, the frozen section method is usually preferred, utilizing either fluorescent or peroxidase labelling methods (for example, see MacIver and Mepham (1980) for detection of Ig in paraffin sections of kidney).

Mouse Antibody As Primary Antibody: Immunohistologic Studies Using Monoclonal Antibodies

Note that however excellent the technique, however great the sensitivity, it will only be possible to detect antigen if it is present; many of the antigens recognized by currently available monoclonal antibodies are very susceptible to the adverse effects of fixation-processing (earlier in this Chapter). Thus

frozen sections are generally preferred for studies using monoclonal antibodies UNLESS IT IS KNOWN (or the investigator directly demonstrates) THAT THE ANTIGEN UNDER STUDY SURVIVES FIXATION AND PARAFFIN EMBEDMENT. When using frozen sections, the possibility of significant nonspecific binding of reagents to Fc receptors becomes a significant problem (whereas in paraffin sections Fc receptors appear to be effectively destroyed).

In the remainder of this chapter, it is assumed unless otherwise stated that frozen sections are to be employed; the possibilities of Fc receptor binding of the primary mouse antibody and of all of the labelling reagents must be weighed for all systems. In theory, nonaggregated, nonantigen–complexed Ig (the ideal antibody preparation contains neither aggregates or complexes) should not bind significantly to Fc receptors. Many conjugated antibodies contain complexes that will bind, and some authorities advocate the use of Fab or F(ab')$_2$ conjugates. Theoretically, success demands this requirement of all antibodies used, including the primary. In practice, we only occasionally have found evidence of significant binding of nonconjugated mouse monoclonal antibodies that could be attributed to Fc receptor binding; whereas apparent Fc binding of whole Ig conjugates has been encountered many times but is not invariable.

PAP complexes theoretically present a much greater problem since they are complexes, and as such are much more prone to Fc receptor binding. It is our experience that for different PAP reagents available commercially, Fc receptor binding varies widely both by source and species of Ig in the PAP. Controls should be employed to test for Fc binding prior to use.

Mouse monoclonal antibodies have some distinct advantages over conventional antisera preparations:

1. Theoretically they are "monospecific" and do not require extensive adsorption procedures.

2. They can be produced in large amounts from selected hybrid cell clones.

3. Their high specificity may reduce background staining caused by the nonspecific tissue binding of the unwanted contaminant antibodies always present in conventional primary antisera.

4. Results from different laboratories using monoclonal antibody from the same

source (ie, exactly the same reagent) can be compared.

The choice of a specific and sensitive immunologic detection system for use with monoclonal antibodies is critical for immunohistologic studies. Various immunoperoxidase techniques have been employed for detecting the binding of mouse monoclonal antibodies to tissue sections; these include: the two–stage conjugate method, the four–stage PAP procedure, the three–stage protein A technique, variations of the biotin-avidin system, and the three–stage PAP method using conventional or monoclonal mouse PAP.

Some of the multilayer methods give a high degree of nonspecific staining; in addition, they are time consuming. Although protein A has been successfully employed as a bridging reagent between mouse monoclonal antibodies and rabbit PAP, it has a relatively low affinity for the Fc fragment of some mouse immunoglobulins, especially IgG$_1$, and is thus inappropriate for use with some subclasses of monoclonal antibodies.

Variations of the biotin-avidin method found initial favor for use with monoclonal antibodies. Warnke and colleagues (1980) showed that satisfactory specificity and sensitivity may be achieved using an indirect biotin-avidin method. The sensitivity can be further enhanced by using the biotin-avidin-peroxidase complexes (ABC method). For optimum staining, all reagents should be titered independently. Controls should be included to monitor for binding to endogenous biotin and for nonspecific attachment to the section.

Mouse PAP Method

Conventional and monoclonal mouse PAP reagents have recently become available for immunohistologic labelling of monoclonal antibodies both in paraffin and frozen sections. Mouse monoclonal PAP complexes appear to have a lower molecular weight than the rabbit PAP complexes, probably due to the fact that mouse monoclonal antiperoxidase antibody, unlike rabbit antiperoxidase antiserum, recognizes only one antigenic determinant on the individual enzyme molecule and consequently can only form single complexes. The physiochemical characteristics of these monoclonal PAP reagents could be responsible for the high specific labelling obtained in frozen sections (ie, the relatively

low Fc receptor binding), because the linkage of PAP complexes to Fc receptors is more frequently observed with high molecular weight aggregates.

"In House" Experience of Techniques and Reagents

Avidin-biotin conjugate, ABC, protein A, monoclonal and conventional mouse PAP methods, four-stage method with rabbit PAP, and indirect conjugate methods have all been used extensively in our laboratories for the demonstration of a wide variety of antigens using monoclonal antibodies in frozen and in paraffin sections.

In our hands greatest sensitivity (ie, ability to use primary monoclonal antibody at a high dilution) was achieved with the ABC method, the mouse PAP (using a monoclonal mouse PAP) method, and the four-stage method using rabbit PAP (ie, mouse monoclonal—rabbit antimouse IgG–swine antirabbit IgG—rabbit PAP); of these the four–stage PAP method was most sensitive, but also the most time consuming. The ABC and the mouse PAP methods appeared to show comparable order of sensitivity, depending on the quality of the differing reagents. Of several different conventional (polyclonal) and monoclonal mouse (and rat) PAP reagents (conventional from Sternberger Immunocytochemicals and from Ortho, monoclonals from Ortho), the monoclonal PAP reagents gave the best results in terms of sensitivity; in addition, background staining was less.

ABC reagents (from Vector) showed considerable variation from lot to lot and sometimes gave higher levels of background staining when used to achieve comparable levels of sensitivity. Recently, more standardized reagents have become available and give excellent results.

Indirect conjugate methods gave good results with low levels of background (using goat antimouse IgG–peroxidase conjugate [whole or F(ab')$_2$, from Tago], although the sensitivity was less than with mouse monoclonal PAP (Ortho), necessitating use of the primary antibodies at higher concentrations (eg, with the conjugate method, Leu 4 at 1:40; with mouse PAP,.at 1:400 or more).

In essence, recommendations for use of mouse monoclonals are as follows:

1. First, try an indirect procedure using a whole Ig conjugate with specificity versus the Ig class of the monoclonal used as the pri-

mary. It seems obvious, but a goat antimouse IgG (gamma–chain specific) reagent will not (or certainly should not) give good results if the primary antibody is mouse Ig of mu class; although obvious, the "class" of the monoclonal is often overlooked in setting up new stains.

2. If the above approach produces too much nonspecific background (in the controls) that might be attributed to Fc binding of the conjugate, try using an F(ab')$_2$ conjugate (it will be considerably more expensive).

3. If the above approach produces only weak staining or demands use of the primary monoclonal antibody at a high concentration unacceptable for financial or other reasons, then try a monoclonal mouse PAP system or the ABC system. In our experience PAP is the most widely useful and applicable system but is more time consuming that the two preceding choices.

4. If all of these methods fail, take counsel with your colleagues and your conscience (recheck your controls; recheck the specificity of your labelling reagents—call the suppliers if necessary).

5. At this point remember that the ABC system may give good results when all else fails. Again be sure that the specificity of the reagents you obtain is appropriate for the primary antibody you wish to utilize.

DOUBLE IMMUNOENZYMATIC TECHNIQUES

Simultaneous staining of two antigens in the same section traditionally has been carried out by double immunofluorescence techniques that utilize the contrasting fluorescence of fluorescein and rhodamine conjugates.

The identification of two antigens in fixed paraffin-embedded tissues has been accomplished by immunoperoxidase staining of serial sections. Unfortunately, it may be very difficult to identify with certainty the same cell or cells in adjacent sections, especially if the cells under study are small. The use of ultrathin methacrylate sections has been advocated for this purpose, but the fixation and embedding procedures frequently cause denaturation or masking of antigens accompanied by failure of the immunoperoxidase staining procedure.

More recently, double immunoenzymatic techniques have been developed, permitting

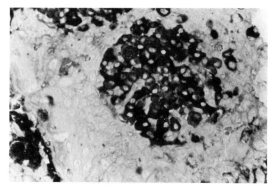

Figure 3–5. Medullary cords of chronically reactive lymph node showing double staining of plasma cells. Lambda chain is stained blue (deep black) using alkaline phosphatase and fast blue (BBN); kappa chain is stained brown (gray) using peroxidase and diaminobenzidine tetrahydrochloride (DAB). This is the double-labelled antigen method (Chapter 3); there is no counterstain. Paraffin section (× 320). See color plate I–1.

the demonstration of two antigens concurrently within a single section. These procedures offer several advantages over double immunofluorescence staining, including the fact that the two labels are visualized simultaneously (rather than sequentially, as is the case when using immunofluorescence). Furthermore, the morphologic details are better preserved in the immunoenzyme methods, and the colored reaction products are permanent, so stained preparations can be examined and re-examined at leisure (Fig. 3–5).

Double immunoenzymatic techniques have been adapted both for the peroxidase–conjugate antibody method and unlabelled antibody methods (selected references, Table 3–8). In these procedures the first sequence of antibodies staining one antigen may or may not be dissociated following the development of the peroxidase reaction with 3-3'-diaminobenzidine (DAB) as substrate. Staining for the second antigen is then carried out with a primary antibody of different specificity and a second, different substrate system for the peroxidase enzyme, usually 4-chloro-1-naphthol; this produces a contrasting blue-colored reaction product.

Various methods have been proposed for efficiently eluting antibodies from the sections without causing denaturation of the antigenic structures. Most of these methods are based on the incubation of the sections with acid solutions (usually glycine-hydrochloric acid buffer at pH 2.2 or 1N hydrochloric acid for 1 hour), which are known to produce dissociation of antigen-antibody

Table 3–8. Selected References: Double Staining

Joseph & Sternberger 1979 Sternberger, 1979b Sternberger & Joseph 1979	PAP sequential double staining without removal of primary antibody (used pituitary)
Gu et al 1981	Sequential double staining using PAP and immuno-gold
Valnes & Brandtzaeg 1982	Sequential double staining, using first DAB as first chromogen (blocks both first enzyme and first antibody site) followed by chloro-naphthol in the second stain sequence
Van Rooijen 1980	Excellent but brief listing of six different methods for double staining
Lechago et al 1979	Double immunoperoxidase-immunofluorescence method
Valnes & Brandtzaeg 1981	Double PAP-fluorescence method
Sofroniew & Schrell 1982	Double staining with novel reutilizable antibody method, involving immersion of whole slide in staining jar of antibodies
Schrell & Sofroniew 1982	Staining of adjacent thin sections to achieve "double" staining of individual cells (for cells large enough to be cut in two sections in parallel)
Malik & Daymon 1982	Alkaline phosphatase-horseradish peroxidase double staining
Falini et al 1982a	Double staining using labelled antigen method
Mason & Sammons 1978	Double staining—alkaline phosphatase-peroxidase
Hofman et al 1982	Double staining of cytocentrifuge preparations
Valnes & Brandtzaeg 1984	Sequential double staining without removing first set of reagents
Mason et al 1983	Double staining technique for monoclonal antibodies; immunoperoxidase/alkaline phosphatase
Moir et al 1983 Erber et al 1984	Cell cytocentrifuge method and double staining
Falini & Taylor 1983	Review of methodology, including double stains

H_2SO_4 in 140V of distilled water at pH 1.8) and subsequent reduction with 1% $NaSO_4$ for one minute.

In order to avoid the problem of antigen denaturation and partial removal of high affinity antibodies that may be observed with elution techniques, it has been proposed that the double staining procedure may be performed leaving in place the first set of reagents. Some authors have suggested blocking the Fc portion of the first sequence of reagents with protein A from *Staphylococcus aureus*; others believe this treatment unnecessary. Sternberger and colleagues (Table 3–8), for example, were able to demonstrate two antigens simultaneously without elution of the first set of reagents, in spite of the fact that the second primary antibody was of the same species as that used for the first antigen, while the same PAP labelling reagents were used for both; the success of this system may be due to the polymerized product of DAB oxidation (used for the first antigen–PAP method) blocking the catalytic site of peroxidase in the PAP complexes while also obscuring the antigenic reactivity of the first sequence of antibodies, thereby preventing the interactions with the second sequence antibodies and the second substrate system.

The possibility of nonspecific mixed staining reactions due to cross-reaction of the second sequence of antibodies with the first sequence may be minimized by use of a double immunoenzymatic method in which two specific primary antibodies, produced in two different species, are used in combination with two separate species-specific secondary antibodies coupled to different enzymes (eg, peroxidase and glucose oxidase). However, the staining of antigens by this method must be carried out sequentially and is time consuming. Mason and Sammons (1978) described a double immunostaining procedure in which two different antigens in one section are detected by the simultaneous application of the classical PAP procedure and the enzyme bridge method, with alkaline phosphatase as the second enzyme label. The double-labelled antigen method (Falini et al, 1982a) represents still another order of improvement; it is very rapid and reduces the possibility of cross-reactivity to a minimum. Briefly, the sections are incubated with a mixture of antisera against the two antigens to be investigated (eg, kappa and lambda light chains), followed by a mixture of kappa light chain labelled with peroxidase and

bonds. When using these systems, it is usually better to stain first with DAB, because the polymeric reaction product is insoluble under conditions when antibodies are removed from the section. Some investigators claimed successful antibody elution following 1 minute incubation of the sections with an oxidizing solution (0.15mol $KMnO_4$ and 0.01N

lambda light chain labelled with alkaline phosphatase (Fig. 1–19, Chapter 1). The peroxidase and alkaline phosphatase–labelled antigen tissue sites are then revealed using the appropriate chromogenic substrate for the two sections (ie, DAB/H_2O_2 for peroxidase (brown) and naphthol AS phosphate–fast blue BBN (clear blue) for alkaline phosphatase. The double antigen–staining technique allows a number of selected combinations of different antigens labelled with different enzymes to be used, the only limitation being the availability of an antigen in sufficient amount and purity for coupling to the enzyme label.

Application of Double Staining Methods

With the production of monoclonal antibodies, leading to the detection of an ever-increasing variety of antigenic molecules in human tissues, it is becoming progressively more important to be able to visualize selected pairs of antigens simultaneously in tissue sections; this is particularly evident in attempting to define the patterns of cellular specificity of the numerous monoclonal antibodies against leucocyte surface antigens. However, there are technical obstacles to double immunoenzymatic staining of monoclonal antibodies, arising from the fact that monoclonal antibodies are normally raised in the same species (eg, mouse or rat). As a result, the secondary antibody (eg, antimouse or antirat Ig), in the three-stage or indirect techniques, cannot distinguish between the two primary (mouse) antibodies. In order to circumvent this problem, Janossy et al (1980e), in attempting double–indirect immunofluorescence studies using OKT4 (helper phenotype) and OKT8 (suppressor phenotype) monoclonal antibodies, were forced to substitute one of the two monoclonal antibodies (OKT8) with a T cell–specific conventional horse antiserum (TH2) recognizing the same (or a closely similar) subpopulation of cytotoxic and suppressor T cells as OKT8.

The double–labelled antigen method does not have the cross-reactivity problem inherent in the indirect techniques, but unfortunately it is not suitable for double labelling using monoclonal antibodies in lymphoid tissues, for most of the differentiation antigens recognized by these antibodies are not, at least at present, available for direct labelling.

Two monoclonal antibodies, both directly labelled with different fluorochromes or enzymes, could theoretically be used in double-labelling experiments, but direct immunostaining procedures have a low sensitivity, and mouse antibodies have proved more difficult to label with fluorochromes than antibodies of most other species. Double labelling with monoclonal antibodies can be achieved by use of monoclonal antibodies of different IgG subclasses, together with subclass-specific secondary antibodies conjugated with contrasting labels; alternately, the appropriate subclasses of purified mouse myeloma proteins linked to different fluorochromes or enzyme labels could be used in a labelled antigen method. The recent introduction of microscale periodate conjugation methods (Ramanarayanan, 1981) permits labelling of small amounts of antigen with peroxidase, and renders the labelled antigen method more widely useful; labelled antigens reported include kappa and lambda light chains, IgG, IgA and IgM, complement C1q and C3, lysozyme, fibrinogen, albumin, prolactin, and luteinizing hormone.

Sequential Immunoenzymatic Staining

When one utilizes double immunoenzymatic staining, it is sometimes difficult to recognize double staining of individual cells, for the colored reaction product of one label may overwhelm the other. In these circumstances a sequential immunoenzymatic staining technique may prove useful. In this approach one antigen is stained; the sections are examined and photographed, and then the second antigen is stained in contrasting color. Sections are then re-examined, and identical fields are rephotographed for comparison.

A Practical Approach to Double Staining with Monoclonal Antibodies

A satisfactory double-staining method using monoclonal antibodies has been in "routine" use in our laboratory for some time (Hofman et al, 1982). The method is applicable both to frozen sections and to cytocentrifuge preparations.

Briefly, the procedure involves sequential application of two different staining systems, the first an indirect ABC peroxidase procedure using biotinylated horse antimouse IgG and linked to ABC peroxidase with AEC as

Figure 3–6. Follicular center cell lymphoma, small cleaved, diffuse pattern. This is a low level IgM producer, stained here both with a monoclonal antibody versus the idiotype (using an alkaline phosphatase conjugate method—blue) and anti-mu chain-specific antibody (using immunoperoxidase and AEC—red). In this instance almost all of the cells bearing SIgM (mu chain) belong to a single idiotype and give double staining (purple: red plus blue—appears black). Scattered cells bearing IgM but not reacting with the anti-idiotype reagent appear red (gray); these may be normal residual IgM-positive B cells, or they may be members of the neoplastic IgM clone that have lost this particular idiotype. In some instances two or more idiotypes, implying two or more clonal variants, have been detected within a single lymphoma. In immunohistology we still normally content ourselves with light and heavy chain typing, but staining for idiotypes is important if the use of anti-idiotype antibodies is contemplated for therapy. Frozen section (×320). (Anti-idiotype prepared by Dr. I. Royston.) See color plate I–2.

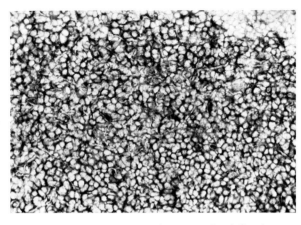

the substrate; the second an indirect conjugate method using goat antimouse IgG linked with alkaline phosphatase and fast blue BBN as substrate. Controls reveal that there is no detectable binding of the second labelling system (goat antimouse Ig/alkaline phosphatase) to the first monoclonal antibody in spite of common specificity; this circumstance presumably is due to steric interference. Mounting is in buffered glycerol jelly, in deference to the use of AEC, which is alcohol soluble, as one of the chromogens (Fig. 3–6).

*Some Immediate Applications of Double-Labelling Methods**

1. Assessment of plasma cell populations: myeloma versus reactive plasmacytosis (Fig. 3–5)

2. Assessment of other immunoglobulin-producing B cells (Fig. 3–6): lymphoma versus reactive proliferation, particularly useful for identifying focal monoclonality, as in the early stages of evolution of B-immunoblastic sarcoma in angioimmunoblastic lymphadenopathy

3. Recognition of the development of myelomonocytic or erythroblastic leukemia in a background of advanced myeloma

4. Double staining of pituitary hormones in assessment of hyperplasia and adenoma

5. Assessment of possible cross-reactive staining patterns of monoclonal antibodies versus cytoplasmic or cell surface antigens or both

————————

*Staining of adjacent serial sections may, of course, meet these needs if it is not possible to perform simultaneous double staining; in our experience, double staining of single sections is more easily interpreted. These applications are discussed more fully at appropriate locations in the text.

ENZYMES, SUBSTRATES, CHROMOGENS

Endogenous Enzyme Activity

The degree of susceptibility of an enzyme to denaturation and inactivation by a fixative varies. Some, like peroxidase, are preserved in both paraffin and frozen sections (Sternberger, 1979; Straus, 1971); others, like alkaline phosphatase, are completely inactivated by routine fixation and paraffin-embedding procedures (Falini et al, 1982a; Mason and Sammons, 1978) but retain their enzymatic activity in cell smears (Druguet and Pepys, 1977; Pepys and Pepys, 1980), in cryostat sections (Ponder and Wilkinson, 1981), and in tissues embedded in methacrylate at low temperature (Western and Bainton, 1981). Any residual activity of these endogenous enzymes must be abolished during immunohistologic studies in order to avoid false-positive reactions when utilizing the same, or similar, enzymes as labels.

Alternatively, one may use enzyme markers, such as glucose oxidase, that are not present and cannot be induced in human tissues, thereby circumventing problems of endogenous enzyme activity (Suffin et al, 1979).

Endogenous Peroxidase Activity Inhibition

Peroxidase and peroxidaselike activity (catalase and cytochrome oxidase) is present in a number of normal and neoplastic cells, including erythrocytes, granulocytes, eosinophils and hepatocytes. Furthermore, high endogenous peroxidase activity has been found in certain other tissues (eg, normal and neoplastic estrogen-sensitive tissues in rats—Andersen et al, 1975). Thus there is an ever-present risk of false-positive results when immunoperoxidase techniques are utilized for the study of tissues rich in blood cells, like bone marrow, or for the detection of estrogen receptors (Ghosh et al, 1978), necessitating almost "routine" use of a "peroxidase-blocking" step in the staining procedure coupled with a "substrate control" (ie, a section treated only with the hydrogen peroxidase–chromogen mixture to visualize the extent of endogenous peroxidase activity).

Various approaches have been devised for the inhibition of peroxidase activity. Streefkerk (1972) suggested incubating the sections with a mixture of methanol/H_2O_2 prior to the immunostaining procedure. Burns (1975) increased the H_2O_2 concentration in stepwise fashion to about 10%, with the additional purpose of also bleaching hematin, without achieving success under all circumstances.

Other "blocking techniques" have been proposed. Weir et al (1974) succeeded in neutralizing endogenous peroxidase activity and obtained good preservation of immunoglobulin antigenicity by incubating sections with 0.075% hydrochloric acid in ethanol at room temperature for 15 minutes before immunostaining.

In most situations we have obtained satisfactory results with methanol/H_2O_2. Some investigators (McMillan et al, 1981; Strauss, 1972) state that this is too drastic and may cause some denaturation of antigen. For example, McMillan observed that both methanol/H_2O_2 and hydrochloric acid mixtures had adverse effects upon some T cell antigens in frozen sections; under these circumstances it is preferable to use alternative methods for blocking endogenous peroxidase or to utilize the blocking step subsequent to incubation with the primary antibody (vide infra). In our experience this certainly is true for some of the lymphocyte surface markers detectable by use of monoclonal antibodies, although it is without adverse effect on most cytoplasmic antigens. When high quantities of an antigen are present—for example, intracytoplasmic immunoglobulins in mature plasma cells—the destructive power of methanol may not be particularly critical; however, it may become so when only tiny quantities are present, as is the case with membrane-related antigens.

Strauss (1972, 1976) advocated the use of phenylhydrazine, which appears to preserve the antigenicity of many molecules but suffers from the disadvantage that it does not completely inhibit the endogenous peroxidase activity of eosinophils. Robinson and Dawson (1975), in their study of gastrin, found that in their system the best way to avoid antigenic denaturation was to reveal endogenous peroxidase differentially: ie, first develop the endogenous peroxidase using 4-chloro-1-naphthol (giving a blue-gray color); next perform the immunohistologic stain, developing the peroxidase label with diaminobenzidine (giving a contrasting brown reaction product). A similar approach was in fact used by the author in the initial reports describing the feasibility of demonstrating immunoglobulin antigens in paraffin sections; alpha-naphthol pyronin was used for endogenous peroxidase (pink), followed by diaminobenzidine (brown) for the horseradish peroxidase label (Taylor and Burns, 1974; Taylor, 1974).

More recently, Fink et al (1979) attempted to solve the problem of antigen denaturation by incubating the sections with methanol/H_2O_2 after the addition of primary antibody, in order that the immunologic reaction with the tissue antigen would occur prior to any denaturation produced by the methanol. Clearly, the methanol/H_2O_2 mixture must be applied to the sections before the peroxidase-labelled antibody, or the PAP complexes, because not only animal endogenous peroxidase, but also the plant peroxidase (including horseradish peroxidase, the form most commonly used for preparation of conjugates and PAP complexes) is inactivated by methanol/H_2O_2 treatment.

Heyderman and colleagues (Heyderman, 1979; Heyderman and Neville, 1977; Heyderman et al, 1979) introduced a procedure in which sections are first incubated with 7.5% H_2O_2 in distilled water to inhibit the acid hematin and then in 2.28% periodic acid in distilled water to block endogenous peroxidase. Unlike methanol/H_2O_2, periodic acid can also neutralize the endogenous peroxidase activity of the endothelial cells. Because the aldehyde groups formed during periodic acid treatment may lead to nonspecific staining phenomena, the sections should be incubated with 0.02% sodium borohydride (Lillie and Pizzolato, 1976) in distilled water prior to addition of the antibodies. This method has given good immunostaining of CEA and epithelial cell membrane antigens. However, the authors pointed out that it may not be ideal for detecting antigens that contain a carbohydrate determinant (eg, blood group antigens), because periodic acid oxidizes sugar molecules, opening the ring structure between hydroxyl groups and producing loss of carbohydrate-related antigenicity.

Endogenous Alkaline Phosphatase Activity Inhibition

The growing use of alkaline phosphatase as an enzyme label in both single and double immunoenzymatic techniques has resulted in an urgent need for a satisfactory means of blocking the activity of endogenous alkaline phosphatase in fresh or frozen tissue. The enzyme is totally destroyed by routine fixation and embedding procedures but not in frozen sections (Mason et al, 1981), or cell smears (Pepys and Pepys, 1980).

The isoenzymes of alkaline phosphatase are widely distributed throughout human tissue (Fishman, 1974). However, high concentrations of alkaline phosphatase are often associated with absorptive cells, especially in the brush borders of the interstitial mucosa and the proximal tubules of the kidney. Alkaline phosphatase is also present wherever calcification occurs, particularly in osteoblasts. In addition, alkaline phosphatase activity is detectable histochemically on the surface of arterial and capillary endothelial cells, in stromal reticulum cells, in neutrophils, and in primary follicle and mantle zone lymphocytes in frozen sections of normal lymph nodes, spleen, and tonsils; alkaline phosphatase–positive lymphomas, mantle zone lymphomas (Namba et al, 1968) may originate from these alkaline phosphatase–positive lymphocytes.

For these reasons endogenous alkaline phosphatase activity must be blocked in frozen sections in order that immunohistologic staining patterns are not misinterpreted. There are various methods of inhibiting the activity of this enzyme (depending on the isoenzyme involved and its tissue location). A useful method is that described by Borges (1973) in which levamisole is added to the enzyme substrate solution at a final concentration of 0.1 mol, prior to its addition to the section at the end of the immunostaining process. The rationale of this approach is that levamisole easily suppresses the endogenous alkaline phosphatase activity present in most human tissue, but has no effect on calf intestine alkaline phosphatase, the form of enzyme most commonly used for preparation of antibody conjugates for labelled antigen methods and for the induction of conventional or monoclonal anti–alkaline phosphatase antibodies in "bridge" methods.

Immunoenzyme techniques using alkaline phosphatase as enzyme markers are not only useful for double immunoenzymatic studies but may also represent a valuable alternative to immunoperoxidase staining in the following situations:

1. Detection of antigens in tissues particularly rich in endogenous peroxidase (such as bone marrow)

2. Better preservation of antigenic structures following incubation of frozen sections with levamisole instead of with methanol/H_2O_2 mixture

Glucose oxidase has also been employed as enzyme marker for immunohistologic studies (Avrameas, 1969; Campbell and Bhatnagar, 1976; Suffin et al, 1979). Since this microbial enzyme is not present or inducible in normal mammalian tissue, it may be extremely useful in those situations in which other techniques produce high levels of endogenous staining that interfere with interpretation. Dr. James Robb at Scripps has developed a highly sensitive multilayer avidin-biotin variation of this technique, the so-called super-GAB method (glucose oxidase-avidin-biotin), involving repeated application of the glucose-oxidase-avidin-biotin reagents (Robb, 1981).

CHROMOGENS

For the different enzyme labels several different chromogens are available (Table 3–9).

With horseradish peroxidase, diaminobenzidine (DAB) may be preferred, since the brown reaction product is alcohol-fast and thus suitable for a wide range of counterstains and mountants. Amino-ethyl carbazole (AEC), giving a red color, has become more widely used recently. Although it is alcohol soluble, unlike DAB it is not on the FDA list of laboratory carcinogens and thus has been favored by commercial supplies of immunohistologic reagents.

Key references to different chromogens are given in Table 3–9.

For general purposes we routinely employ AEC (amino-ethyl carbazole). It also is the chromogen provided with most commercial kits; its use should be strictly according to the manufacturer's instructions.

AEC produces a crisp red color that contrasts well with a hematoxylin counterstain

Table 3–9. Selected References: Chromogens for Enzyme Labels

Marcollet et al 1980	Diaminobenzidine versus phenylenediamine plus pyrocatechol (Hanker-Yates reagent, a noncarcinogen)	Tubbs et al 1979	Comparison DAB versus aminoethyl carbazole (hCG staining)
Rathlev et al 1981	Glucose oxidase technique	Sheibani et al 1981	DAB versus phenylenediamine and pyrocatechol (Hanker-Yates)
Bulman & Heyderman 1981	Alkaline phosphatase technique; stress need to completely inhibit endogenous enzyme using Bouin's solution or periodic acid and potassium borohydride	Porstmann et al 1981	Comparison of phenylenediamine, dianisidine, aminoantipyrine and azino-di (3-ethylbenzothiazoline sulphuric acid-6)
Pelliniemi et al 1980	Storage of DAB as a frozen solution	Trojanowski et al 1983	Eight different chromogens reviewed
Vacca et al 1978	Low pH suppresses red cell pseudoperoxidase but not horseradish peroxidase (in PAP reagent) or neutrophil peroxidase	Hanker et al 1977	An alternative noncarcinogenic chromogen—blue/black
		Tinelli et al 1979	Glucose oxidase versus alkaline phosphatase versus peroxidase
Van Bogaert et al 1980	Good discussion of methods for blocking endogenous peroxidase	Sheibani et al 1980 Tubbs et al 1981 a,b Tubbs & Sheibani 1982	Review and practical application of the major chromogens for peroxidase

(NB: a "progressive" nonalcoholic hematoxylin should be used—eg, Mayer's, not Harris's). Secions must be mounted in an aqueous medium (eg, 80% glycerol—Aquamount contains small amounts of organic solvent and may cause slow diffusion or loss of stain), and dehydration through alcohol must be avoided since the red AEC product is alcohol-soluble. Glycerol-mounted preparations may be made permanent by sealing the edges of the cover slip with nail varnish.

Diaminobenzidine (DAB) may be employed for specific purposes; it is alcohol-resistant and may be subject to staining, dehydration, and mounting in Permount. It also is valuable for the electron microscopist, being electron-dense. For light microscopy some investigators advocate osmication of the DAB reaction product, giving a more intense color. We have not found this necessary for light microscopy; indeed, we feel it may be a disadvantage since background staining also is enhanced, and the end result may be diminished contrast in spite of the more intense staining.

If DAB is used, solutions should be pre-

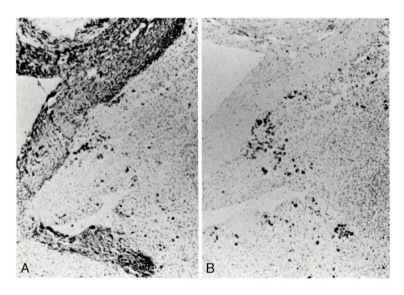

Figure 3–7. Example of the effectiveness of "blocking" nonspecific binding of primary and secondary antibodies. On the left (**A**) is a section of spleen stained for IgG by the PAP method; scattered positive plasma cells (black dots) are seen, but there is heavy staining of collagen bands. On the right (**B**) is the adjacent parallel section treated in an identical fashion except that normal serum from the same species as the linking antibody (in this case normal swine serum to match the swine antirabbit Ig–linking antibody) was added prior to the primary antibody. In this instance the plasma cells are seen even more clearly since the heavy nonspecific staining of collagen is markedly diminished. Paraffin sections, DAB with hematoxylin counterstain (×60).

pared under a hood by a masked, gloved technician. Excess solution should be disposed of with an excess of water. At the working dilution employed, the danger is considered minimal; it is the powdered form that evokes concern. Pre-weighed aliquots in sealed tubes are available from some manufacturers but are expensive.

Alpha-Naphthol pyronin (pink), 4 chloro-1-naphthol (blue), and Hanker-Yates reagent provide other alternatives (see Table 3–9).

BLOCKING OF NONSPECIFIC ANTIBODY BINDING

Antibodies are highly charged molecules and may bind nonspecifically to tissue components bearing reciprocal charges (eg, collagen). Such nonspecific binding will lead to localization of the labelled moiety (conjugate, PAP, etc.) and "false"-positive staining of collagen and other tissue components; this may obscure specific staining (Fig. 3–7a). Nonspecific binding of primary and labelled antibodies may be reduced by prior treatment with an irrelevant antibody or serum that in theory will occupy all charged sites within the tissue section, excluding (or at least reducing) nonspecific attachment of other antibodies added subsequently (Fig. 3–7b). It is customary to use normal serum of the same species as the bridge antibody (in the PAP method) or the secondary antibody (in conjugate and ABC methods) because this serum will neither interfere with nor participate in the immunologic reactions occurring subsequently (see Appendix 1).

4

LYMPHOMA/
HEMATOPATHOLOGY

"Nowhere in pathology has a chaos of names so clouded clear concepts as in the subject of lymphoid tumors."

RUPERT A. WILLIS, 1948

The success of the immunoperoxidase method is limited only by

(a) the quality and specificity of the antibodies available and

(b) the extent to which the antigen under study survives the abuses to which the tissue is subjected during fixation, processing, and sectioning.

As described elsewhere, the advent of monoclonal antibody technology has had a major impact upon the first of these limitations. Regarding the second, many antigens do survive formalin-paraffin processing to a useful degree; those of particular interest to the hematopathologist include cytoplasmic antigens, such as immunoglobulins, lysozyme, hemoglobin, ferritin, and lactoferrin. Other antigens, particularly those present in small amounts on the cell surface, survive routine processing less well and at present are best demonstrated in cryostat sections following brief fixation in acetone. This latter group includes many of the antigens recognized by monoclonal antibodies. Current applications in hematopathology are summarized in Table 4–1.

If only fixed tissues are available, then B5 (or Zenker's) is generally to be preferred over formalin; if only formalin-fixed tissues are available, it may be helpful to predigest sections, prior to immunostaining, with 0.1% trypsin. Full details of these procedures are given elsewhere (see Curran and Gregory, 1978).

The remainder of this chapter presents a pragmatic approach to lymphoma diagnosis. Hodgkin's disease is, however, considered more briefly, since immunohistology is of limited value for the diagnosis of this condition.

70

IDENTIFICATION OF LYMPHOMAS

The classification of lymphomas used in this book is basically that of Lukes and Collins (1975), which was chosen, not because it is correct (for strictly speaking it is not, since it fails to provide a logical place for some of the more recently recognized varieties of lymphoma) but rather because it is accurate in concept. The concept that lymphomas are neoplasms of "immune cells" and that it consequently ought to be possible to recognize various categories of lymphomas corresponding to the various categories of normal leukocytes lends itself well to immunohistologic studies; indeed, as will be seen, it is no longer possible to classify properly many of the lymphomas without resorting to immunologic techniques; flow cytometry; or better, immunohistology on frozen or paraffin sections; or best of all, all three approaches plus morphology.

The Kiel classification based on the work of Lennert and colleagues (1975) is also immune-based and could have been adopted here with equal facility. The "working formulation" of a panel of experts (Rosenberg et al, 1982) is less suitable for this purpose because it ignores some obvious immunologic divisions. It is notable that all three schemes (Lukes-Collins, Kiel, and the experts' formulation), although based to some degree upon immunologic principles, are purely morphologic (or cytologic) in execution and require no immunologic assays for assignment of cases into the various categories. Immunologic studies, including immunohistology, have revealed that morphology alone is not adequate for this purpose and that

Table 4–1. Applications of Immunohistologic* Methods in Hematopathology

Immunoglobulin—
  Paraffin Sections (principally cytoplasmic Ig)
    Distinction of reactive B cell proliferations from B cell neoplasia: myeloma, plasmacytoid lymphocytic lymphoma, follicular center cell lymphoma, immunoblastic sarcoma

    Subclassification of lymphomas; recognition and subclassification of B cell tumors by Ig content

    Recognition of anaplastic tumor as B cell in origin according to content of monoclonal Ig (distinction of immunoblastic sarcoma of B cell type from carcinoma, melanoma, etc)

    Recognition of morphologically unusual tumors as B cell in origin (eg, "signet ring cell" lymphoma)

  Cryostat Sections (principally surface Ig)
    Identification of monoclonal SIg-bearing lymphomas: CLL/small lymphocytic lymphoma, follicular center cell lymphomas

  J Chain—Recognition of B cell nature of normal or neoplastic cells

  Lysozyme—Aid to recognition of reactive & neoplastic granulocytic proliferations; rapid identification of numbers of granulocytes in marrow (marrow granulocyte reserve); recognition of granulocytic sarcoma (paraffin sections); histiocytes less consistently positive

  alpha₁-Antitrypsin—Aid to recognition of reactive & neoplastic histiocytes (paraffin sections)

  Lactoferrin—Aid to assessment of mature granulocytes in marrow (paraffin sections)

  Hemoglobin A & F—Distinction of erythroid precursors from lymphoid cells; specific identification of marrow erythroid reserve; extent of HBF production in marrow in hemolytic diseases (paraffin sections)

  Anti–Common Leukocyte Antigens (CLA)—Recognition of normal and neoplastic leucocytes; include lymphocytes, granulocytes, histiocytes. Distinction of lymphoma from carcinoma, melanoma, etc.

  Anti–T Cell Antibodies—Identification of T cells in sections; recognition of T cell lymphomas; distinction of T cell subsets with specific antibodies against subsets (including use of monoclonal hybridoma antibodies) (frozen sections)

  Antibodies to Ia-(like) Antigen—Identification of B cells in sections; recognition of B cell lymphomas (monocytes and activated T cells also Ia positive) (frozen & paraffin sections)

  Anti-B Cell Antibodies—Monoclonal antibodies to B cells & B cell subsets; most work only on frozen sections; LN series works on paraffin sections

  Antibody to Complement Receptors—B cell and monocytes subsets

  Anti-Terminal Transferase—Recognition of TDT-containing cells (?T cell precursors) in sections (frozen sections)

  Anti-Common ALL Antigen (CALLA)—Recognition of ALL subsets (frozen & paraffin sections); some B cells and B lymphomas

  Research—Powerful investigative tool; widely applicable

  Teaching—Morphologic and functional correlations

*It is now apparent that both immunoperoxidase and immunofluorescence can be used in all of these applications; on paraffin sections, protease digestion is advantageous for demonstration of Ig, especially by immunofluorescence; if good morphology is required, immunoperoxidase—using fixed paraffin sections when possible, otherwise cryostat sections—is preferred. Applications are discussed in detail in the text.

precise categorization of lymphomas, particularly the lymphoblastic and large cell groups, can only be achieved by combining morphologic and immunologic parameters.

IDENTIFICATION OF B CELLS

Surface and Cytoplasmic Immunoglobulin

Immunoglobulin exists on the surface or in the cytoplasm of various B cells or both.

Traditionally, surface immunoglobulin on lymphoid cells has been evaluated on washed live cell suspensions using immunofluorescence, either manual ultraviolet microscopy

or automated cytofluorography with a fluorescent-activated cell sorter (FACS) or a fluorescent cell analyzer (eg, Ortho Spectrum III). Cytoplasmic immunoglobulin is detectable in tissue sections or when lymphoid cells are subjected to some degree of fixation (including air drying) to disrupt the surface membrane prior to addition of the anti-immunoglobulin antibody for labelling.

In staining for immunoglobulin the goals are twofold: first, to demonstrate the B cell nature of the cells in question, and second, to determine whether the putative B cells are monoclonal (monotypic—expressing a single type of light chain and a single class of heavy chain) or polyclonal.

A clear demonstration of monoclonality (monoclonal staining pattern)* may readily be obtained in cell suspension studies of lymphocytes or lymphoid tissues if such tissues are totally involved by B cell lymphoma or leukemia. However, if the neoplastic B cell population constitutes only a small percentage of the total lymph node cell population, as may be the case with many early nodal lymphomas and in extranodal lymphomas, then the residual population of normal lymphoid cells may obscure the presence of a minority monoclonal population. Under these circumstances comparison of kappa with lambda-positive cells (so-called clonal excess) may facilitate the diagnosis of lymphoma of B cell type. Failure to detect the presence of a monoclonal neoplastic lymphocyte population, even when it represents the predominant cell type in the tissue, may also be due to the high death rate of neoplastic cells during the process of suspension, especially observed in certain subtypes of large-cell lymphomas (large cleaved, large non-cleaved); cell death leads to selective enrichment of the normal residual lymphoid population and to falsely low estimates of the number of neoplastic cells.

Selective enrichment of certain types of cells (during separation and suspension) as a result of cell death, different size factors, varying ability to extract different cell types from tissues, or nonrepresentative sampling, may also cause difficulties in interpretation of monoclonality; these types of problems were encountered by Palutke et al (1981), who found monoclonal staining patterns in the lymph node cell suspensions of patients with morphologically "typical" benign follicular hyperplasia. Similar observations have been made in more than a dozen cases from our own institution (Levy et al, 1983). For these reasons it may, at least in some instances, be preferable to study the clonality of human lymphocyte populations by detection of surface immunoglobulin present on lymphocytes in situ (ie, within tissue sections). Under such circumstances focal or localized collections of monoclonal cells may be detected against a polyclonal background.

---

*In immunohistochemistry, the term monoclonal is usually used to denote a cell population all the members of which stain exclusively for one light chain (kappa or lambda) and often also for one heavy chain (gamma, alpha, mu, or delta). This falls short of a more strict definition based on immunoglobulin idiotype or upon genotype.

Demonstration of SIg in Tissue Sections

Surface immunoglobulins and other membrane-related antigens are difficult to demonstrate in paraffin sections, owing in part to the denaturation or masking of immunoglobulin during the fixation-embedding process (see Chapter 3) and in part to the difficulty in obtaining contrast between the small amounts of immunoglobulin on the cell surface and the immunoglobulin present in extracellular fluids. Some investigators have claimed greater success in the identification of surface immunoglobulin in paraffin sections following incubation of the sections with trypsin, which may serve to "unmask" antigen sites (Curran and Gregory, 1978). This method, however, requires careful adjustment of the time of trypsinization; it must not be more than 5 to 10 min, depending on the concentration and purity of the trypsin, in order to avoid loss of antigens from the sections or even loss of the whole section! Also trypsinization facilitates preferential detection of some immunoglobulin classes (mu heavy chain; kappa and lambda light chains), whereas the immunoreactivity of other molecules, such as delta heavy chain, may be largely lost.

Others have claimed success by using special fixation (periodate-lysine-paraformaldehyde, Collings et al, 1984), cold embedding, low melting–point paraffins (eg, cold acetone-paraffin, Tanaka et al, 1984) or by using freeze-dried paraffin sections (Stein et al, 1984) to demonstrate not only surface immunoglobulin but also T cell surface antigens. Such work has yet to be reported widely in the literature, but selected references are given in Tables 4–2 and 4–3. In any event, because these methods require special processing, they are more a substitute for frozen sections than for "routine" paraffin sections. Morphologic detail is particularly good in freeze-dried paraffin sections, and at present this seems to offer the best alternative to orthodox fixation processing methods.

There is now general consensus that surface immunoglobulin may be more reliably detected in frozen sections taken from quick-frozen blocks, cut by cryostat, and briefly fixed in acetone prior to immunostaining. This implies that pathologists should routinely take frozen tissue at the time of biopsy and bank it in liquid nitrogen or in a −70°C freezer for possible use should the need become apparent.

Table 4–2. Selected Bibliography: Non-Hodgkin Lymphomas—Paraffin Sections

Taylor 1976; 1978c, d; 1979a, b, c; 1980c Mason et al 1980b	Reviews of older literature for staining of Ig in paraffin sections
Van Heerde et al 1980	74 cases; light and electron microscopy (EM); Lennert classification
Mori et al 1979	71 cases; 19 showed intracellular Ig
Gourdin et al 1982	EM for surface and cytoplasmic Ig
Taylor & Parker 1981	Several hundred cases; review of methods & results for surface and cytoplasmic Ig and other markers
Hofer et al 1979	Many cases of CLL reclassified as lymphoplasmacytoid lymphoma by immunohistology
Levine et al 1981	Immunoblastic sarcoma of T cell type—clinical features
Maurer et al 1982	Immunoblastic sarcoma of T and B cell types—pathologic features
Merson & Rudens 1981	39 cases; monoclonal immunoglobulin in B cell group
Isaacson et al 1980	185 cases; describe patterns of Ig production in follicular center cells & plasma cells
Syrjänen 1979, 1980	33 cases of B cell lymphoma
Taylor 1979a, b, 1980a	Review and correlation of tissue section immunoperoxidase data with surface marker data and classification
Landaas et al; 1981	83 cases; comparison of surface markers and immunoperoxidase stain; 53% of cases positive for cytoplasmic Ig; PAP method good
Jardon-Jeghers & Reznik 1982	16 CNS lymphomas; 13 probable or definite monoclonal, 9 termed IBS, 4 termed immunocytoma
Azar et al 1980	15 large cell lymphomas; heterogeneous; most of B cell derivation
Laurent et al 1980	Surface and cytoplasmic Ig; comparison of conjugate and PAP methods
Isaacson & Wright 1979	Discussion of "anomalous" staining pattern for Ig
Dell' Orto et al 1982	Post–embedding (EM) immunostaining of Ig on glutaraldehyde-fixed tissues, with trypsinization
Vanden Heule et al 1982	8 lymphomas of rectum; 3 showed monoclonal staining in paraffin sections
Kapadia et al 1982	21 cases thyroid lymphoma
Kojima & Mori 1982	39 patients from Japan, light and EM study; 25 IgM monoclonal
Foucar & Rydell 1980	9 cases of Richter's syndrome; represent "transformation" of the initial CLL
Otto et al 1980	22 intestinal lymphomas; immunostaining of value in diagnosis
Banks 1979	Experience on 400 lymphoma cases; discussion of fixation & specificity
Pangalis et al 1980	Well-differentiated lymphocytic lymphoma vs plasma cell & plasmacytoid lesions
Vernon & Lewin 1980	Fluorescence & peroxidase comparable in study of 23 cases (including 16 lymphomas)
Mason et al 1980b	Surface Ig in smears of non-Hodgkin lymphomas and CLL; most CLL negative when stained as fixed smears (see Laurent et al 1982)
Huber & Gattringer 1983	Review and report of findings in non-Hodgkin lymphomas
Stein et al 1984	Freeze-dried paraffin sections with good preservation of antigens detectable by monoclonals
Collings et al 1984	B and T cell surface antigens in paraffin sections; periodate-lysine-paraformaldehyde fixative
Epenetos et al 1985	An anti-Ia antibody effective in paraffin sections
Epstein A et al 1984	A series of monoclonals effective in paraffin sections; LN2 specific to follicular center cells
Lauder et al 1984	Paraffin sections of 43 lymph node biopsies with anaplastic large cell tumors; staining for keratin and CLA (common leukocyte antigen), valuable
Taylor et al 1978c Allegranza et al 1984	CNS lymphomas; plasmacytoid, lymphocytic, and immunoblastic
Papadimitriou et al 1985 Dragosics et al 1985	Two large series of GI tract lymphomas (61 cases and 150 cases)
Vimadalal et al; 1983	Gastric lymphomas (36 cases)
Ioachim et al 1983	Lymphoid lesions in AIDS and pre-AIDS

Table 4–3. Selected Bibliography: Surface Ig in Frozen Sections and in Cell Suspensions—Methods*

Braylan & Rappaport 1973	Ig in nodular lymphoma vs hyperplasia
Janossy et al 1980c	Immunofluorescence, normal and malignant lymphoid tissue
Janossy et al 1980d	Fluorescence, includes double staining
Levy et al 1977	B cell lymphomas; monoclonal
Tubbs et al 1980c	Peroxidase vs fluorescence
Tubbs et al 1981a	Frozen section; peroxidase method
Curran & Gregory 1978	Trypsinization for SIg
Stein et al 1980	Analysis of normal lymphoid tissue & selected lymphomas
Kazimiera et al 1979	Combined cell suspension and frozen section study
Harris et al 1984	20 cases of orbital lymphoid infiltrates; staining for SIg valuable in demonstrating monoclonality of histologically indeterminate lesions
Hui and Lawton 1984	SIg, B1, and OKT11 in cytocentrifuge preparations
Paradis et al 1984	An immunoperoxidase (ABC) cell preparation method compared favorably with dried flow cytometry
Sandhaus et al 1984	Air-dried smears of leukemia stained for CALLA (BA3, J5)
Moir et al 1983	An immuno–alkaline phosphatase method for routine blood smears; avoids
Erber et al 1984	endogenous peroxidase, no need for separation; good morphology
Falini et al 1984	Immuno–alkaline phosphatase method for frozen sections of undecalcified marrow biopsies. Again avoids problem of endogenous peroxidase; good results with several monoclonals

*For other studies on frozen sections, refer to the section on monoclonal antibodies in lymphomas later in this chapter.

Immunofluorescence and immunoperoxidase techniques give comparable results, with equivalent sensitivity and specificity, when they are applied to frozen sections for the demonstration of surface immunoglobulins (Fig. 4–1). Several reports claiming a higher sensitivity of immunofluorescence techniques for detecting surface immunoglobulins and other membrane-related antigens are, on analysis, more related to differences in fixation and tissue processing than to differences between immunofluorescence and immunoperoxidase methods per se.

That variations in fixation or processing account for the differences described earlier becomes evident when human lymphoid tissues, fixed and processed in a variety of ways, are examined in parallel by immunoperoxidase and immunofluorescence techniques.

Paraffin Sections. Immunoperoxidase staining of paraffin sections of lymph node or tonsil principally detects intracytoplasmic immunoglobulin, surface and extracellular immunoglobulin being less predictably displayed. Typically, mature plasma cells stain positively and are present in the greatest

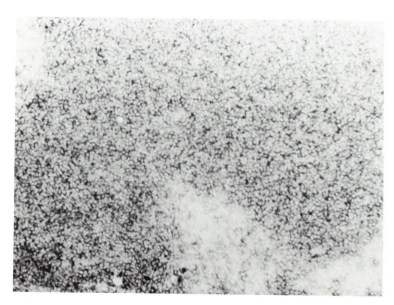

Figure 4–1. Follicular lymphoma with neoplastic cells largely confined to giant coalescent follicles. Anti–lambda chain antibody, frozen section, AEC without counterstain (× 125).

numbers in medullary cord areas of normal lymph nodes. In addition, many transformed B lymphocytes and large cleaved and non-cleaved cells (centroblasts and centrocytes) show cytoplasmic positivity; these cells are distributed within interfollicular areas or in germinal centers of secondary follicles. The number of immunoglobulin-containing cells is variable, depending on the intensity and duration of the antigenic stimulus: chronically reactive nodes may contain numerous positive cells. On the other hand, the small B lymphocytes and small cleaved follicular center cells, constituting the predominant cell population in the cortex and in the primary follicles, stain weakly or not at all, because of the low content or absence of intracytoplasmic immunoglobulins. These cells undoubtedly carry surface immunoglobulins but are not detectable in paraffin sections for reasons given above.

Frozen Sections. A different immunoperoxidase staining pattern is seen in frozen sections of lymphoid tissue in which the overwhelming majority of primary follicular lymphocytes and follicle mantle lymphocytes show a rim of surface IgM (Fig. 4–2) or surface IgD or both, with a few cells bearing surface IgG or surface IgA. IgD cells are concentrated particularly in the mantle zone (Fig. 4–3). In addition, intracytoplasmic immunoglobulins are visualized much as they are in paraffin sections, although localization is less precise owing to diffusion of antigen during freezing or sectioning.

Double-staining techniques show that both surface kappa-positive and lambda-positive cells are present in individual normal follicles at approximately a 2:1 ratio (see Fig. 3–5 and color plate I). Individual B cells bear either kappa light chain or lambda light chain, not both, plus a heavy chain determinant. The presence of both kappa and lambda on or in a cell is generally considered to indicate adsorbed or absorbed polyclonal immunoglobulin; this circumstance is discussed further with reference to Hodgkin's disease. The immunoblasts and the larger germinal center cells may stain more faintly for surface immunoglobulin; plasma cells do not stain for surface immunoglobulin but do stain for cytoplasmic immunoglobulin.

In addition, the cortical (outer) poles of germinal centers usually display a network of positive extracellular staining; with double-staining techniques this network stains both for kappa and lambda light chains and probably represents interstitial polyclonal immunoglobulin, free in the tissue fluids or arranged on the surface membrane of an interlacing network of dendritic reticulum cells. This type of staining pattern is typical of lymph nodes but has been observed in follicular centers of lymphoid tissues throughout the body, including tonsils, intestinal tract, and others.

Methods for Staining Cell Smears or Cytocentrifuge Preparations

The examination of lymphoid cells in direct peripheral blood smears, in either cyto-

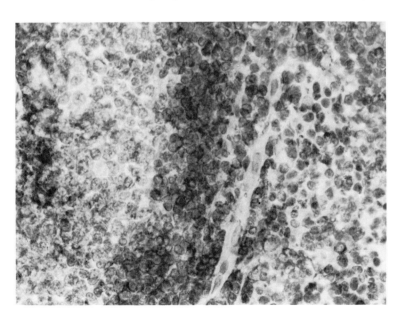

Figure 4–2. Segment of reactive follicle (left) with mantle zone running vertically through the center of the field. SIgM (mu chain) is detectable on a proportion of the follicular center cells (left) and many of the mantle cells. Frozen section, AEC with hematoxylin counterstain (×320).

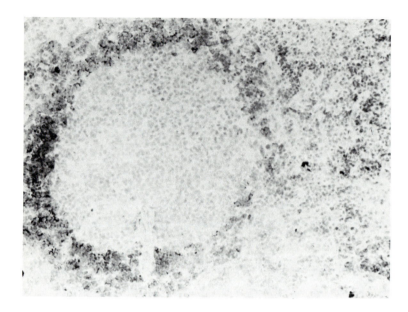

Figure 4–3. Reactive follicle showing distribution of IgD-positive cells in the mantle zone. Frozen section, AEC with hematoxylin counterstain (×125).

centrifuge preparations of buffy coats or gradient-separated lymphocytes, offers an alternative approach to staining for SIg or phenotyping with monoclonal antibodies (see below). Either immunoperoxidase or immuno–alkaline phosphatase may be used, the latter having the advantage of avoiding the problem of endogenous peroxidase activity in leukocytes. Cells are air-dried and may be fixed by various mild procedures to conserve antigens (we use cold acetone for 30 seconds to 5 minutes; Mason [see Moir et al, 1983; Erber et al, 1984] used acetone for 10 minutes, or the buffered formol acetone that we had used for other antigens previously [Ma-

son et al, 1975]). Cytologic detail is good, and a permanent preparation is achieved (Fig. 4–4). Double staining is readily performed.

The method is particularly suitable for study of leukemic cells from peripheral blood or lymphoma cell suspensions from involved lymph nodes, although in the latter instance the method suffers in comparison with frozen sections, since the opportunity to assess the microanatomic distribution of the various cell types is lost. Both conventional antisera [eg, antilysozyme, anti-alpha$_1$-chymotrypsin (granulocytes), anti-immunoglobulins] and many monoclonal antibodies (anti-CALLA and various anti-B and anti-T reagents) may

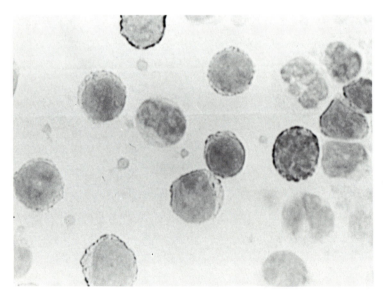

Figure 4–4. Cytocentrifuge preparation of a lymph node suspension prepared on a ficoll-hypaque gradient. A proportion of the lymphocytes show a rim (black) of staining at the cell surface membrane. These are T cells as detected by OKT3. Acetone-fixed preparation, AEC with hematoxylin counterstain (×1200).

be used. Ideally, immunostaining should be performed within 24 hours of slide preparation; however, most antigens are still detectable at 6 days (room temperature) or 6 months (if stored at −80°C).

Selected references are given in Table 4–3. The method developed by David Mason is recommended (see Moir et al, 1983; Erber et al, 1984).

Neoplastic Lymphoid Cells—B Cell Lymphomas

Usually, the behavioral properties of neoplastic lymphocytes resemble to some degree those of their normal counterparts; for reference purposes detailed studies and larger case series studied in paraffin sections are summarized in Table 4–2; Table 4–4 lists small-case series and isolated case reports. Table 4–5 deals with reactive tissue; Table 4–6 with frozen section immunohistology (Tables 4–4 to 4–6 appear later, following discussion of these topics).

The use of frozen sections for immunohistologic investigations has been of special value in those categories of non-Hodgkin lymphomas such as small lymphocytic lymphoma (including CLL) and some follicular center cell lymphomas (mainly small cleaved FCC type) that are characterized by the proliferation of small surface immunoglobulin–bearing (SIg⁺) lymphocytes. It should be noted that the study of these small-cell types of lymphoproliferative disorders on paraffin sections has usually produced negative results

(there are some exceptions as shown in Fig. 4–5). This relative lack of staining is most probably due to the fact that, just as in the normal small lymphocyte and small cleaved cell, so also in their neoplastic derivatives: the small amount of surface immunoglobulin present is denatured or masked by the fixation and embedding procedures that are commonly employed. By contrast, paraffin sections, if optimally fixed, have served well for large cell B lymphomas and plasma cell tumors (large follicular center cell (Fig. 4–6), immunoblastic, plasmacytoid lymphocytic, plasmacytoma, myeloma), for these cell types contain relatively much larger amounts of cytoplasmic immunoglobulin (Fig. 4–7; see also Chapter 5). Burkitt's lymphoma expresses SIg but little cytoplasmic immunoglobulin and is best stained in frozen sections.

In frozen sections of human B cell lymphomas, both immunofluorescence and immunoperoxidase methods may be expected to produce a monoclonal staining reaction that outlines each neoplastic lymphocyte, producing a characteristic honeycomb staining pattern. In follicular or nodular lymphomas, the positively staining cells may be restricted to the neoplastic follicles or may involve both follicles and interfollicular tissue. In diffuse lymphomas the positive neoplastic cells are distributed diffusely, although not necessarily evenly, throughout the section. B cell lymphomas usually show a monotypic, or monoclonal, pattern of staining (exclusively one light chain, one heavy chain, or both); whereas reactive disorders

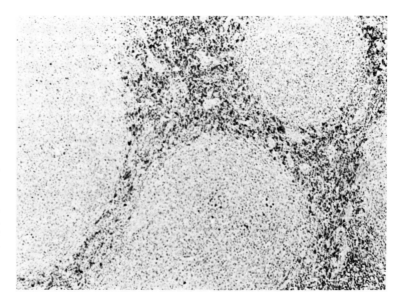

Figure 4–5. Follicular center cell lymphoma with monoclonal plasma cells (black) distributed outside the neoplastic follicles; this is an unusual finding. The cytoplasmic Ig in these plasma cells shows the same light/heavy chain class as the SIg on the neoplastic follicular center cells, suggesting that both populations belong to the same clone. This is a paraffin section: the cytoplasmic Ig in plasma cells is well seen; the surface Ig on the follicular center cells is not (see text). DAB with hematoxylin counterstain (×60).

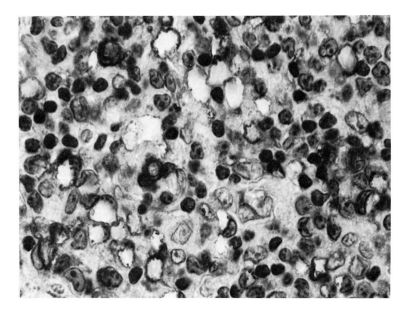

Figure 4–6. "Signet ring" follicular center cell lymphoma; "vacuoles" are outlined in black, representing a positive reaction for lambda light chain (kappa chain was not present). Paraffin section, DAB with hematoxylin counterstain (×650). This is a relatively rare but well-documented variety of follicular center cell lymphoma (see van den Tweel et al, 1978).

such as benign follicular hyperplasia show a polyclonal staining pattern (ie, some of the cells stain for kappa chain and some for lambda chain, with a similar distribution of staining amongst the different anti–heavy chain classes). The most frequently found heavy chain in lymphomas is mu class, followed by gamma. Unlike benign follicular hyperplasia, the follicles in follicular lymphomas do not usually show the presence of a lacy network of polyclonal extracellular immunoglobulin, an observation initially made

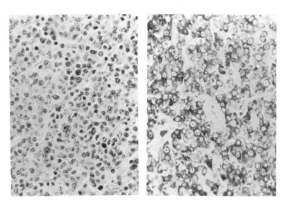

Figure 4–7. Immunoblastic sarcoma of B-cell type showing a "monoclonal" (monotypic) staining pattern, negative for lambda (left) and positive for kappa (right). Positive cells show brown-black staining of the cytoplasm. Paraffin section, DAB with hematoxylin counterstain (×200). See color plate I–3. In this case the "immunoblasts" were small, showing some resemblance to small noncleaved cells; the latter, however, usually express surface Ig but little cytoplasmic Ig. See also Chapter 8 for other examples.

by Braylan and Rappaport a decade ago (1973). It is worth noting that "mantle zone" lymphomas show the interesting condition of monotypic (exclusively kappa and lambda) staining of cells in the mantle region (Fig. 4–8) distributed around reactive centers that are demonstrably polyclonal. Many "mantle zone" lymphomas are IgD positive, resembling the normal mantle (see Fig. 4–3).

Gooi et al (1979) were not able to demonstrate the presence of surface or intracytoplasmic immunoglobulins in paraffin sections of 12 cases of hairy cell leukemia examined with an immunoperoxidase method. Others have, however, succeeded in showing a monoclonal staining pattern in cases of hairy cell leukemia both in frozen sections and at electron microscopy (Martelli et al, 1980). It is our experience that the monoclonality of hairy cell leukemia can readily be demonstrated in frozen sections (eg, Levy et al, 1983), although the intensity of staining is often less than for follicular center cell lymphomas. Studies with monoclonal antibodies (Pallesen et al, 1984b) and the observation of immunoglobulin gene rearrangements in hairy cell leukemia clearly indicate the B cell nature of the process. Our limited studies were reported by Myers et al (1984), but the group with Sklar and Cleary at Stanford has reached similar conclusions in a larger case sample (personal communication 1984).

In lymphoplasmacytoid lymphocytic lymphoma (well-differentiated lymphocytic lymphoma with plasmacytic features, in the Rap-

Figure 4–8. Monoclonal (mono-typic) staining for lambda light chain was confined to the mantle zones, which were expanded. The cells within the reactive centers showed a polyclonal pattern, some reacting for kappa, some for lambda. The heavy chain was IgD; in other cases it may be IgA or IgM. Frozen section, AEC with hematoxylin counterstain (×125). The diagnosis is "mantle zone" lymphoma; this condition may be difficult to distinguish from reactive follicular hyperplasia-absent immunohistologic staining for immunoglobulins. A small group of these tumors has recently been reported from our institution (Samoszuk et al, 1985); the use of immunohistologic techniques is discussed in this paper.

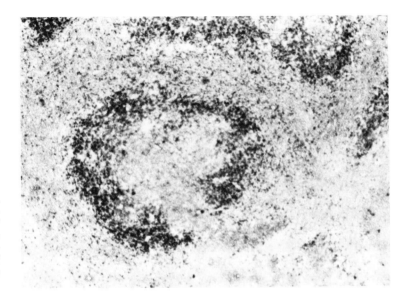

paport classification), immunoperoxidase staining of paraffin sections demonstrates the presence of intracytoplasmic immunoglobulin within the cells showing features of plasmacytic differentiation but typically fails to stain surface immunoglobulin in small lymphocytes (Pangalis et al, 1980). Immunoperoxidase studies on frozen sections clearly show that many mature-appearing small lymphocytes bear surface immunoglobulin of the same light-chain type and heavy-chain class identified in the cytoplasm of the plasma cells. Monoclonality is readily demonstrable: the most frequent heavy chain is mu, followed by gamma and alpha.

Chronic lymphocytic leukemia, involving tissues, presents findings similar to well-differentiated lymphocytic lymphoma. On frozen sections monoclonality is readily established, although the intensity of staining for SIg is generally less than on normal lymphocytes. In paraffin sections these cells will not stain: plasma cells may, however, be present in small numbers to reveal a monoclonal pattern for cytoplasmic immunoglobulin. In our experience, there appears to be a continuous spectrum of appearances from small lymphocytic lymphoma (well-differentiated) to plasmacytoid lymphocytic lymphoma, with an increasing number of plasma cells strikingly revealed by immunostaining. Pangalis and colleagues reported a similar finding (1980). Both small lymphocytic lymphoma and plasmacytoid lymphocytic lymphoma (see later) may form part of a leukemic process; this is much more common in the former

condition in which the leukemia may be predominant (CLL: chronic lymphocytic leukemia, B cell type).

Interestingly, multiple myeloma (generally regarded as a plasma cell neoplasm) may represent the extreme end of the spectrum, with numerous neoplastic plasma cells in the tissue (marrow) but with some circulating small lymphocytes also forming part of the malignant clone (see section on multiple myeloma).

Assessment of Clonality

In general, the proportion of kappa SIg-positive cells compared to lambda SIg-positive cells is assessed by comparison of the staining pattern in adjacent parallel sections stained with anti-kappa and anti-lambda antibodies, respectively (eg, Fig. 4–7; see also Chapter 5). A more rapid and precise assessment may be made by double staining of single sections for both kappa and lambda light chains (or two different heavy chains), utilizing any of the double-staining techniques described earlier in this text (Fig. 3–5 and color plate I–1). It should be noted that although the frequency of occurrence of positive cells with different antibodies is more easily evaluated in double stains than in stains of adjacent sections, the double-staining methods are technically more exacting with an increased risk of misleading cross reactivity and an increased need for adequate controls (Chapter 3).

Double-immunolabelling studies of surface

or cytoplasmic kappa and lambda light chains, enabling one to establish the kappa to lambda ratio directly in one section, may be of particular value in some circumstances. For example, the detection of small foci of cells bearing monoclonal surface immunoglobulin within an overall polyclonal cell response is greatly facilitated by double staining. This is especially critical in recognition of early extranodal lymphomas or of B immunoblastic sarcoma arising in angioimmunoblastic lymphadenopathy; in the latter instance, immunohistologic studies on frozen sections have shown that the "new clone" of malignant transformed lymphocytes expressing monoclonal surface immunoglobulin is detectable by double staining of frozen sections prior to any discernible abnormality of intracytoplasmic immunoglobulin in paraffin sections (Janossy et al, 1980d), prior to diagnostic morphologic changes, and prior to detectable changes in flow cytometry. This also is our experience. We have observed a number of cases of focal monoclonality in apparently reactive nodes (see Fig. 5–5): a proportion of these have progressed to obvious lymphoma in short order; others have not (within a follow-up period of 4 years). Clearly, all such cases should be followed, and the possibility of "benign" lymphomas (ie, true monoclonal neoplasms of the slow-growing type, analogous to benign neoplasms of other cell types) should not be entirely discounted in the face of enthusiasm to embark on some form of therapy.

Nonlymphoid Tissues

Much also has been written concerning detection of immunoglobulin in nonlymphoid tissue (see Table 4–6). As a B lymphocyte marker, SIg has much the same value and significance in other tissues containing lymphocytes or plasma cells as in lymph node or spleen. The demonstration of surface immunoglobulin by immunohistology is for all practical purposes restricted to frozen sections. The detection of cytoplasmic Ig may be accomplished in paraffin sections and is of most value for the recognition of immunoglobulin-producing B cell neoplasms (including myeloma and plasmacytoma as well as some B cell lymphomas) and the distinction of such neoplasms from reactive polyclonal B cell proliferations. This aspect is discussed subsequently in relation to myeloma and the B cell lymphomas.

Identification of B Cells by Use of Monoclonal Antibodies

Limitations of SIg as a B Cell Marker

The detection of SIg has long served as the standard for B cell recognition. However, as other techniques identifying B cells have been described, it has been realized that SIg is not an absolute marker for B cells.

For example, within the B cell series, SIg is not detectable upon plasma cells (which may be considered as fully differentiated functional end–stage B cells); neither is SIg present on cells during the earliest stages of B cell development recognized in the embryo (Fig. 4–9).

Hypothetical Development– Differentiation Pathway for B Cells

Clearly, if lymphoma-leukemia cells mimic their normal counterparts, then only those lymphomas corresponding to virgin or differentiating B cells (Fig. 4–9) would be subject to detection and analysis by staining for SIg. As described subsequently, the advent of a variety of anti–B cell monoclonals now makes it possible to dissect this hypothetical B cell pathway into additional phenotypic divisions.

Surface immunoglobulin does not mark all B cells; likewise, not all cells that bear SIg are members of the B cell family. Just as in studies of SIg in cell suspensions, so also in frozen sections a cell may show detectable surface immunoglobulin by a mechanism other than direct synthesis (B cells express SIg by virtue of in situ synthesis). Cells may passively adsorb SIg upon their surface by a variety of mechanisms. This has been well summarized with regard to cell suspension work (Fig. 4–10), and most of these mechanisms apply equally to frozen sections.

In theory, passive in vivo adsorption of Ig by Fc receptors or by other mechanisms is more of a problem in frozen sections than in cell suspensions, since the latter can be thoroughly washed and incubated in serum-free medium to remove the adsorbed SIg, whereas a frozen section cannot. The problem of adsorption to Fc receptors is encountered more with some antibodies (especially some IgG subclasses) than others. In practical terms, Fc binding appears to be reduced by fixation; thus in fixed paraffin sections it is not a problem, presumably owing to destruction of Fc receptors by fixation or processing.

Table 4–4. Case Reports: Non-Hodgkin Lymphomas, Reactive Hyperplasias

Barr et al 1980	2 cases of cutaneous lymphoid proliferations: 1 reactive, 1 lymphoma
Wright & Isaacson 1981	3 cases of follicular center cell lymphoma in childhood; distinct from Burkitt's
Humphrey et al 1982b	5 patients with rheumatoid lymphadenopathy, including 2 with Sjögren's who showed a monoclonal pattern; both of these developed lymphoma
Pierce et al 1979	Sjögren's, lupus, and immunoblastic sarcoma
Morris & Bird 1979	Immunoblastic lymphadenopathy in a child, becoming immunoblastic sarcoma
Boros et al 1981	Angioimmunoblastic lymphadenopathy to monoclonal immunoblastic sarcoma
Bauer et al 1982	Angioimmunoblastic lymphadenopathy and gastric lymphoma
Merson 1980	5 cases of angioimmunoblastic lymphadenopathy; polyclonal
Bergholz et al 1979	Immunostaining for rubella in angioimmunoblastic lymphadenopathy
Bender & Jaffe 1980	Lymphomatoid granulomatosis, distinguished from a monoclonal lymphoma
Holck 1981	Plasma cell granuloma of thyroid; polyclonal
Matsuta 1982	9 cases of Hashimoto's disease; polyclonal
Von Gumberz & Seifert 1980	Parotitis & lymphoma of the parotid gland
Budka 1982	Hyaline (pseudopsammoma) bodies in meningiomas contain secretor piece & IgA
Hsu et al 1981a	Polyclonal IgA plasma cells in Warthin's tumor
Takahashi et al 1982	Woringer-Kolopp disease (pagetoid reticulosis); immunologically a T cell lymphoma of skin
Ree et al 1980	GI lymphomas and involvement of Walder's ring
Katayama et al 1981	Primary CNS immunoblastic sarcoma
Delsol et al 1982	Warthin-Finkeldey giant cells; believed associated with B cell proliferation
Borowitz et al 1983	A case of lymphoblastic lymphoma with common ALL phenotype
Bogomoletz et al 1983	A case of Lennert's lymphoma; helper phenotype

Table 4–5. Selected Bibliography: Immunoglobulin (Ig)-Containing Cells in Normal and Reactive Tissues*

Nijhuis-Heddes et al 1982	Ig cells in respiratory mucosa in disease
Ali et al 1979	IgE-positive cells in adenoids and tonsils
Rosekrans et al 1981	Ig-positive cells (IgM in jejunal biopsies) increased in active phase gluten enteropathy
Marmar et al 1981	Plasma (Ig positive) cell scores in cervical biopsies in evaluation of infertility
Isaacson 1982a	Plasma cells (IgA, secretor piece) in gut, including dysplastic and carcinomatous gastric epithelium; anaplastic carcinomas lose ability to express secretor piece (and lysozyme)
Matthews & Basu 1982	Ig heavy chains and J chain in tonsils; secretory component absent in tonsillar epithelium
Tsunoda et al 1980	Surface-marker study of expression of germinal centers in tonsil; predominantly B cells
Newell et al 1980	EM localization of Ig in lymphoid cells (restricted saponin digestion of GA–fixed cell suspension); Ig observed in perinuclear space, rough ER, and Golgi area
Curran et al 1982	Study of human reactive lymph nodes, Ig distribution
Straus 1981	Study of phases of production of specific antibody to HRP, following injection of HRP antigen in mice
Matthews 1983	Ig in Russell bodies
Rosekrans et al 1980a Perkkiö 1980	Plasma cells in gut and food allergy
Seo et al 1982	Immunomorphologic study of gut lymphoma
Rosekrans et al 1980b	Plasma cells in ulcerative colitis and Crohn's disease
Togo et al 1981	Immunoglobulins and secretor piece; secretor piece positive in 45% of cancer cases
Morise 1982	Ig cells in gastric cancer and metaplasia

*Additional references appear in Chapter 5.

Table 4–6. Selected Bibliography: Leukocytes and Lymphomas—Frozen Section
Immunohistology

Wood GS et al 1982	25 cutaneous T cell lymphomas; characteristically Leu 3$^+$/Leu 2$^-$ (helper/suppressor), with various admixtures of Ia$^+$ cells and OKT6$^+$ cells
Holden et al 1982	Some loss of T lymphocyte markers in advanced cutaneous T cell lymphomas
Harris & Data 1982	14 "nodular" lymphomas, plus 10 reactive nodes, examined for SIg (light and heavy chains); useful in differential diagnosis of follicular lymphoma vs follicular hyperplasia
Harris et al 1982	46 lymphomas; 15 of 15 "nodular" lymphomas were monotypic (monoclonal), as were 24 of 31 diffuse lymphomas. Emphasized value of this method—it requires no special equipment
Wood GS & Warnke 1982	Details of technique for immunostaining of frozen marrow sections. Results compared favorably with fluorescent-activated cell sorter analysis for phenotyping bone marrow cells (with monoclonal antibodies); excellent practical paper
Tubbs et al 1981b	Comparison of immunohistologic assessment of monoclonality vs cell suspension studies; of 39 lymphomas studied in parallel, 18 (46%) were monotypic (monoclonal) in suspension, against 36 (92%) in sections. Emphasized value of section method; excellent practical paper
Poppema et al 1981	Utilized OKT series antibodies to map distribution of T cell subsets in lymph nodes
Stein et al 1980	Combined frozen and paraffin section study; mapped out distribution of B cell subsets (surface IgM, IgD, C3, etc) in lymph nodes
Gerdes & Stein 1982	Further description of use of anti–C3 receptor antiserum, showing reactivity both with B cells & dendritic reticulum cells of follicles
Schienle et al 1982	Frozen and paraffin sections, monoclonal antibodies reactive with granulocytes (including myelocytes); some positivity with epithelial ducts
Becker GJ et al 1981	PAP method for common leucocyte antigen, plus two anti-monocyte/macrophage-specific antibodies
Wood GW & Travers 1982	Low pH wash to remove polyclonal Ig, improves detection of SIg
Van Ewijk et al 1982a, b	Mouse tissue; interesting study of ontogeny of T cell phenotypes in early gestation (parallels some of Hofman's studies in human embryos)
Kreth et al 1982	T lymphocytes (by phenotype) in frozen sections of brain in multiple sclerosis & subacute sclerosing panencephalitis
Huber et al 1984	Wide range of monoclonals applied to lymphomas and CLL and adult T cell leukemia/lymphoma. Comprehensive but complicated review, includes OKT series, TO15, Leu series, and several unfamiliar reagents
Delsol et al 1984a	Merits of frozen and paraffin sections discussed; includes staining of dendritic reticulum cells in follicular lymphomas
Doggett et al 1984	Stained 95 diffuse large cell lymphomas; most expressed SIg or T markers; 28 showed B1 but no SIg; concluded large cell lymphoma heterogeneous
Borowitz et al 1984	Report of South East Cancer Group study; particularly interesting for use of transport medium to refer specimens
Horning et al 1984	Essentially same data as Doggett et al 1984, but slightly fewer cases (78)
Harrist et al 1983	Histiocytosis X, OKT6- and Ia-positive; also some OKT4 positivity; probably related to Langerhan's cells
Van der Valk et al 1984	T cell, B cell, monocyte, and dendritic cell distribution in normal spleen, including Leu 1,2,3; B1,2; Ia; OKM1; TA1; Na1/34, etc
Von Hanwehr et al 1984	Phenotypic analysis of mononuclear cells infiltrating CNS tumors
McMillan et al 1982	OKT9-positive cells in mycosis fungoides
Fox et al 1982	Phenotypes of reactive lymphoid cells in Sjögren's syndrome (15 patients)—peripheral blood and tissue lymphocytes showed an OKT4/8 ("helper/suppressor") ratio generally in excess of 3 to 1
Naiem et al 1983	Antidendritic reticulum cell antibody; of value in identifying normal and neoplastic follicles
DeWaele et al 1983	OKT3, OKT4, OKT8, and OKM1 in cytocentrifuge preparations compared with cytochemical stains (NSE and phosphatase) with little correlation of subtypes
McMillan et al 1983	OKT6-positive cells in tonsil and lymph nodes; similar distribution to interdigitating reticulum cells
Kilpi et al 1983	OKT series in gastric biopsies of Sjögren's patients
Janossy et al 1982	Review of immunohistologic techniques with monoclonal antibodies, including findings in autoimmune and infective diseases
Parwaresch et al 1983	KiM4 monoclonal antibody recognizes dendritic reticulum cells in follicles, plus rare peripheral blood cells that may be precursor cells
Hofman et al 1983	Variety of B cell monoclonals recognize B cell subsets in reactive lymphoid tissues
Hofman et al 1984a	Early leukocyte phenotypes in fetus

Table 4–6. Selected Bibliography: Leukocytes and Lymphomas—Frozen Section Immunohistology *Continued*

Rao et al 1983	OKT4, 4A, 4B, and 4D recognize different epitopes on the same helper/inducer cell, apparently on a single molecule
Fox et al 1982	IgG, M, complement and fibrinogen in lung disease, including interstitial pneumonia and sarcoidosis
Warnke & Levy 1980	Early monoclonal studies in frozen sections of 6 B and T cell lymphomas
Selby et al 1981a	Conventional antisera vs T cells, plus a mouse monoclonal vs a "human leucocyte antigen"
Huber & Gattringer 1983	Discussion of fluorescence and peroxidase, frozen sections and cell suspensions
Engleman et al 1981	Characterization of an anti–T cell monoclonal (L17F12)
Chechik et al 1981	Detection of adenosine deaminase immunohistologically; cortical thymocytes positive
Hoffman-Fezer et al 1981	Immunoglobulins in tonsils
Checkik et al 1980	Human thymus/leukemia-associated antigen (adenosine deaminase)
Bhan et al 1980	OKT series, Ia, and B2 microglobulin in thymus
Whaley 1980	Complement components in monocytes
Janossy et al 1980b	Immunohistology of thymus
Wright SD et al 1983	C3b receptor on monocytes detected by monoclonal antibody
Weiss LM et al 1985	50 peripheral T cell lymphomas
Miller et al 1984	Distribution of Leu 7 (NK phenotype) and OKT8 (suppressor phenotype) cells in follicular lymphomas; findings not of diagnostic value
Grogan et al 1984	Describe some follicular lymphomas that were negative for SIg, but were B1- and Ia-positive (T negative); possibly different phases of B cell development
Pallesen et al 1984a	Non–B, non–T (E rosette and SIg negative) lymphomas; of 24 cases, 17 showed B cell markers, 6 T cell, 1 apparent double marker (T6, pan-B positive) case; utilized broad panel of monoclonals
Pileri et al 1984	Transferrin receptor (OKT9) positivity correlates with histologic grade
Martin et al 1984	Lymphoma phenotyping by immunocytologic methods; includes fine-needle aspirates
Burns et al 1983	Leu 1 antigen (=T101, =OKT1) in B cell lymphomas (mainly small lymphocytic and intermediate cell types)
Tubbs et al 1983	Large series of lymphomas, plus reactive hyperplasias
Vernon & Lewin 1980	Comparison of fluorescence and peroxidase—frozen sections

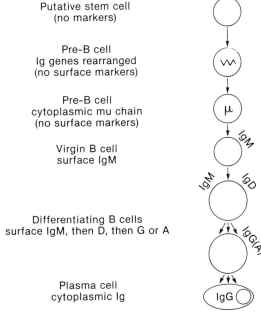

Putative stem cell
(no markers)

Pre-B cell
Ig genes rearranged
(no surface markers)

Pre-B cell
cytoplasmic mu chain
(no surface markers)

Virgin B cell
surface IgM

Differentiating B cells
surface IgM, then D, then G or A

Plasma cell
cytoplasmic Ig

Figure 4–9. B cell markers: postulated sequence of appearance of B cell markers in embryo (up to virgin B cell) and in the immune response (up to plasma cell).

The degree to which Fc receptors present a problem in a particular tissue can be assessed by the "control" preparation, in which a mouse immunoglobulin preparation of corresponding class and concentration is used in lieu of the primary monoclonal antibody. Traces of positivity observed in the control may then be discounted in reading the test section. When the problem persists, we have had some success in reducing adsorption of our monoclonal antibody to putative Fc receptor by preincubation of the section with IgG Fc fragments from an unrelated species.

Elution of in vivo–bound cellular and tissue immunoglobulin with low pH buffer may be of value prior to immunostaining (Wood and Travers, 1982), particularly if such immunoglobulin reflects the presence in the patient's serum of some antibody reactive with surface components of the patient's own cells. These problems relating to the use of SIg as a B cell marker are avoided by the use of monoclonal antibodies against other B cell determinants, since such determinants (anti-

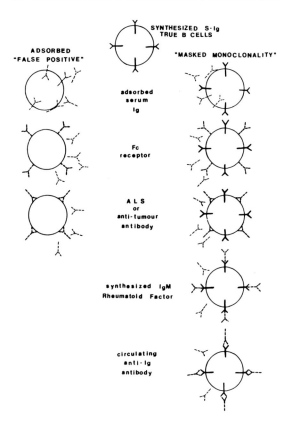

Figure 4–10. Problems of interpreting surface immunoglobulin (SIg) staining of lymphocytes in suspension. These same basic difficulties apply equally to the detection of SIg in frozen sections. The presence of Ig adsorbed to the surface of a cell that normally does not express SIg may lead to false identification as a positive cell (false positive–left side). The adsorption of Ig to a B cell already expressing SIg of a single light chain type and heavy chain class may obscure the characteristics of the original SIg, causing the cell to appear to express both light chains and one or more heavy chains; this circumstance may mask an underlying monoclonal SIg population (masked monoclonality—right side). (Figure is from Linfomi, in Enciclopedia Medica Italiana, Vol VIII, Parker JW, Taylor CR, Levine AM, et al., 1980. Florence, Uses Edizioni Scientifiche with modifications.)

gens) are mostly restricted to cell membranes and are not present in serum or tissue fluids.

Monoclonal Antibodies in the Recognition of B Cells

Just as SIg is not a marker for all B cells, so there is at present no true PAN–B cell antibody, although some come close and will mark a broader spectrum of cells than SIg. As noted above, with most monoclonal antibodies against B cells, the antigen in question is confined to the surface of the B cell; it is not present free in the tissue fluid (as is immunoglobulin). This circumstance eliminates the problem of nonspecific background

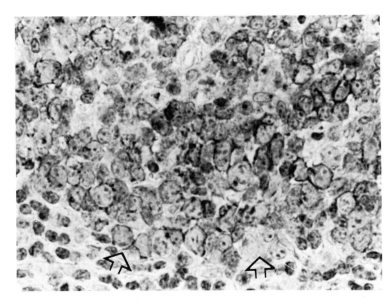

Figure 4–11. Part of reactive (germinal) center within a lymph node showing pattern of reactivity with the monoclonal antibody LN-1 (prepared by Dr. A. Epstein, University of Southern California). The margin of the reactive center is delineated by the large clear arrows. The large follicular center cells show variable cytoplasmic reactivity (gray-black granules and dots in the Golgi area) and surface membrane staining with LN1. The small follicular center cells also stain, but less intensely. Paraffin section, AEC with hematoxylin counterstain (×320).

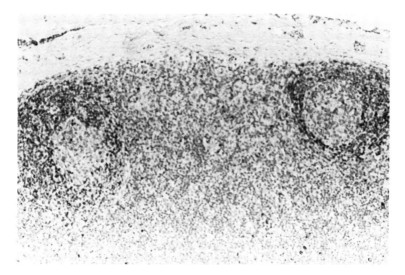

Figure 4–12. LN2 antibody staining B cells in the paracortex and follicles and especially in the mantle zones. Paraffin section, AEC with hematoxylin counterstain (×125). With hematoxylin counterstain the characteristic staining of LN2 is less well seen (in black and white) since it is on the nuclear membrane.

staining observed with anti-immunoglobulin antibodies that detect not only cell surface–bound immunoglobulin, but also immunoglobulin in the tissue fluid. It should be remembered, however, that monoclonal antibodies to cell surface antigens may also be directly bound to Fc receptors (see Fig. 4–10) on B cells or monocytes and histiocytes, giving rise to false interpretation by the unwary.

Note that LN1, LN2, and LN3 are particularly useful since they consistently give good staining in paraffin sections; B5 fixation produces better results than formalin (Figs. 4–11, 4–12, 4–13).

Reactivity of Anti–B Cell Antibodies

The introduction by Ortho Diagnostic Systems of a range of anti–T cell reagents developed by Schlossman and colleagues (see T cell section) offered the promise that a similar range of reagents might be produced against B cells; fulfillment of this promise was soon forthcoming. Many different monoclonal antibodies are now available (Table 4–7) with demonstrable reactivity against several more or less well-defined subsets of B cells (Figs. 4–14 and 4–15). For the present purpose, in assessing the utility of these reagents for cellular identification and diagnosis, it is con-

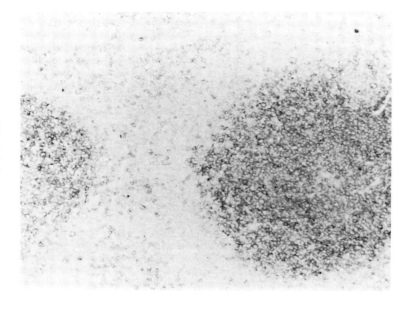

Figure 4–13. LN2 in lymph node reacting with follicular center and mantle zone B lymphocytes. Paraffin section, AEC; counterstain omitted to accentuate pattern of reactivity (×125).

Table 4–7. Anti–B Cell Reagents Available Commercially*†

Anti–Leu 12 Anti–Leu 14	B cells	} Becton Dickinson (Leu 12 ≡ B4)
OKB2 OKB7	B cells/granulocytes B cells	} Ortho (OKB7 ≡ B1)
BA1 BA2	B cells Early B cells	} Hybritech
B1, B2, B4	B cells	Coulter
LN1 LN2 LN3	Follicular center B cells B cells/histiocytes-monocytes B cells/monocytes/some T cells	} Techniclone
Anti–HLA-DR	B cells/monocytes/some T cells	Becton Dickinson

*Note that many other reagents exist; some show identity with one or more of those listed (eg, TO15 = anti–Leu 14). See Appendix 2 for a more complete listing.

†Also, antibodies known for their specificity to non–B cell antigens may show unexpected anti–B cell activity; eg, T101/Leu 1 (a "Pan-T" antibody) reacts with a subset of B cells, with B-CLL and some follicular center cell lymphomas (Al Saate et al, 1984); and CALLA (versus common ALL antigen) reacts with a separate B cell subset plus another subgroup of follicular center cell tumors (Van den Oord et al. 1984).

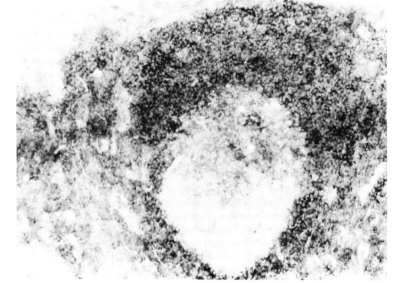

Figure 4–14. BA1 positive cells are distributed partly within the follicle but mainly in the mantle zone and cortex. Frozen section, AEC with hematoxylin counterstain (×320).

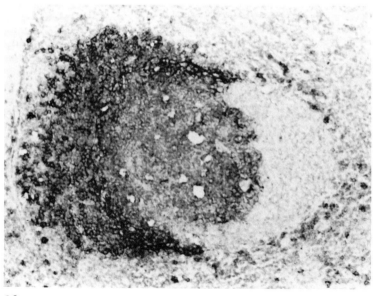

Figure 4–15. Reactive follicle illustrating pattern of reactivity with a monoclonal antibody designated B532 (Dr. S. Baird, University of California, San Diego). Proliferating B cells in the mantle, and within the follicle, appear to stain (black). Frozen section, AEC with hematoxylin counterstain (×200).

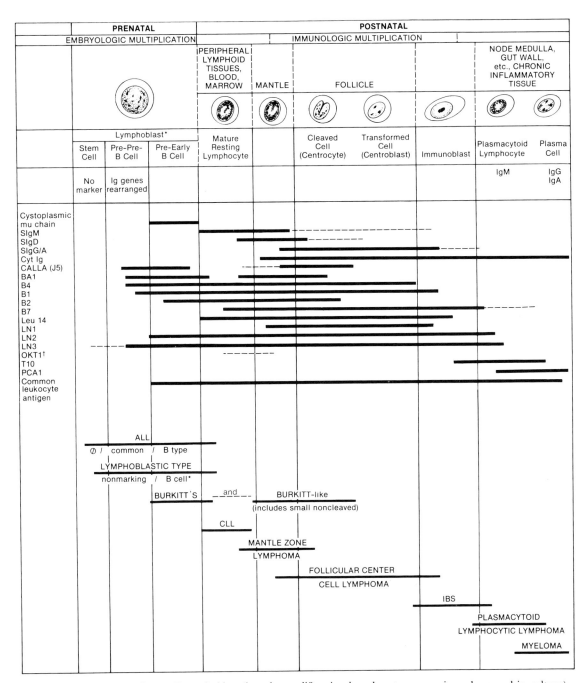

Figure 4–16. B cell antigens. *Lymphoblast (i.e., the proliferating lymphocyte as seen in embryo and in culture). "Lymphoblastic" is used descriptively for lymphomas in which the cells resemble the lymphoblasts of ALL. For the purposes of this discussion this term includes tissue manifestations of ALL, "nonmarking" lymphoblastic lymphomas that are of B cell type by gene rearrangement studies, Burkitt lymphoma, and those follicular center cell lymphomas termed small noncleaved or small centroblastic.

†OKT1 reacts with neoplasms (B-CLL) but not with normal B cells (or possibly with only a small proportion of B cells).

Note: Hairy cells, although they are B cells, are excluded from this "Pathway," because there is no consensus as to their relative position. Hairy cell leukemia has a B cell phenotype (B1[+], To 15[+], Leu 12[+], FMC7[+]) but is negative for BA1; B5; C3bR; Tu 1; OKT3, 4, 6, 8, 10; OKM1; Mo 1; and Mo 2.

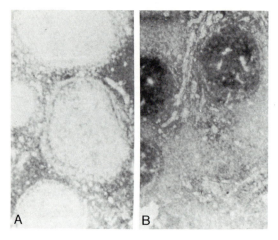

Figure 4–17. Reactive lymph node depicting pattern of reactivity for T cells *(A,* T101 positive) and B cells *(B,* B1 positive). T cells are distributed outside the follicles, B cells within the follicles. Frozen sections, AEC with hematoxylin counterstain (×60).

cell division, lymphocytes actively traverse the cell cycle; undoubtedly there are changes in phenotype during passage through the cell cycle, just as there are also dramatic but ephemeral morphologic changes. The large dividing cell (transformed lymphocyte or immunoblast) reverts back to a typical small lymphocyte during resting phase. The philosophical aspects of these changes and their importance in understanding morphologic and immunologic features of lymphoma have been presented elsewhere (Taylor, 1982a,b). These cell cycle–related changes in phenotype are not well understood and cannot be integrated into the simple scheme presented here.

venient to consider these antibodies in relation to the proposed B cell development-differentiation pathway (Figs. 4–9 and 4–16). It is important to recognize that the pathway is hypothetical and that it is necessarily a straight-line simplification of a complex maturation process that involves multiple cell divisions, both in the embryonic phase and in immunologically activated lymphoid proliferation postnatally. During these phases of

Rudimentary schemes have been developed comparing the microanatomic distribution of B cells (Fig. 4–17 and 4–18) with the pattern of staining of selected anti–B cell monoclonal antibodies (Fig. 4–19). Observed microanatomical distributions are given in Figures 4–20 and 4–21. These findings relate principally to those immunologically competent B cells present in and about the follicles of adult lymphoid tissues. The distribution of lymphocytes showing reactivity in fetal liver, possibly representative of a very early stage of B cell development, were described later (Hofman et al, 1984a; Fig. 4–22). Other investigators have conducted similar studies (Nadler et al, 1984; Anderson et al, 1984)

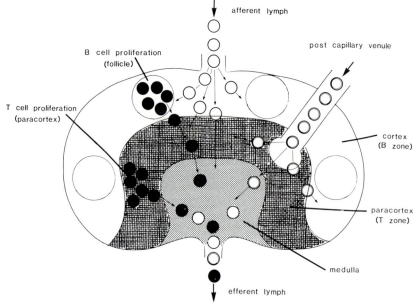

Figure 4–18. Immunotopography of the normal lymph node; postulated on the basis of experimental ablation studies in animals, confirmed by immunohistologic studies with monoclonal antibodies. For further discussion see Taylor, 1982a.

Figure 4–19. Phenotypic expression of B cells during the postulated differentiation and maturation sequence (see Fig. 4–16). Shows observed expression of BA1, CB2 (Dr. R. Billing, University of California, Los Angeles), B1 and B5 (B532, Dr. S. Baird, University of California, San Diego) plus IgD, IgM and IgG mapped here according to their supposed sequence of appearance in the immune tissues of the fetus. (From Hofman FM et al. Analysis of B cell antigens in normal reactive lymphoid tissue using 4 B cell monoclonal antibodies. Blood 4:775–783, 1983, by permission.)

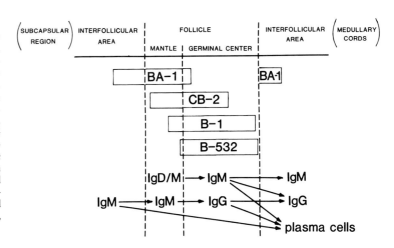

leading to attempts at a more comprehensive scheme (Tubbs and Shebani, 1984).

The diagram given in Figure 4–16 attempts to relate the morphologic recognition of B cell subsets (to the extent that it is possible by judicious application of the Lukes-Collins or the Kiel classification) with immune phenotype as defined by the more commonly available and better characterized anti–B cell antibodies.

It should be emphasized that the listing of

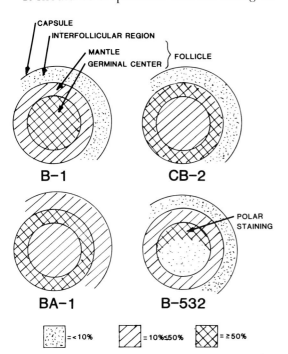

Figure 4–20. The precise microanatomical distribution in the reactive follicle of the different B cell phenotypes is shown by the contrasting shaded areas. (From Hofman FM et al. Analysis of B cell antigens in normal reactive lymphoid tissue using 4 B cell monoclonal antibodies. Blood 4:775–783, 1983, by permission.)

antibodies is not complete and that controversy still exists concerning the precise patterns of reactivity of even these relatively well-characterized reagents.

To some extent, different monoclonal antibodies produced by various manufacturers may have identical specificity, or they may differ to a greater or lesser degree; such differences are not always known. The cross-identity of some of the more commonly employed reagents was summarized, to the extent that it is known, in a recent workshop (see Appendix 3).

There is an additional caveat: namely, two clones producing reagents of identical specificity (eg OKT11 and Leu 5, both versus the E-rosette receptor), developed by two different manufacturers (Ortho and Becton Dickinson), may not behave identically in immunohistologic studies—one or the other may produce more intense staining or may even appear to stain more or fewer cells, and these results may vary from investigator to investigator.

There are several reasons for this variability. First, although two clones developed independently may produce antibody of identical specificity, they do not necessarily produce exactly the same antibody molecule: it may differ in light chain type or heavy chain class or subclass. In an indirect labelling system (such as is used in immunohistologic studies), reagents of different classes or subclasses may be detected with varying facility according to the precise specificity of the secondary or bridging antibody (ie, whether the antibody is directed against IgG1, IgG2a, IgM, etc—remember that even a PAN antiserum directed against whole mouse immunoglobulin will vary in ability to bind the

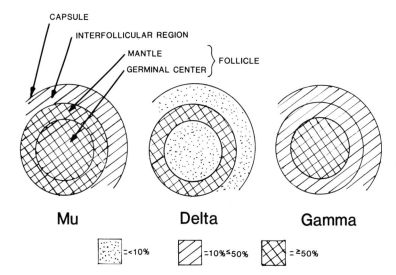

Figure 4–21. This figure similarly depicts the distribution of SIg positive cells in the reactive follicle. (From Hofman FM et al. Analysis of B cell antigens in normal reactive lymphoid tissue using 4 B cell monoclonal antibodies. Blood 4:775–783, 1983, by permisson.)

differing subclasses). Thus OKT11 may produce better results with the PAP method, compared with the ABC or conjugate method, in the hands of one investigator, whereas the reverse may occur in another laboratory utilizing different labelling reagents.

Other factors may also play a role. The dilution (ie, concentration of active antibody) in the reagent available commercially varies from manufacturer to manufacturer, which clearly may have a marked influence, with reagent A producing good results at a dilution of 1:100, whereas reagent B only gives

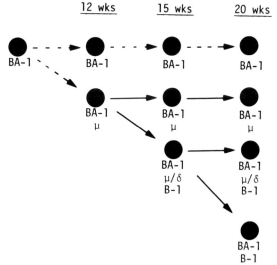

Figure 4–22. The sequential appearance of different B cell antigens is shown as observed in fetal liver at different stages of gestation. (From Hofman FM et al. J Immunol 133:1197, 1984, by permission.)

detectable staining at a dilution of 1:2. This variation reflects the sales philosophy of the commercial corporation as much as anything else. Finally, the degree of background staining also is affected by the type of antibody preparation available, whether ascites (immunoglobulin purified or not) or supernatant, and if supernatant, whether it is prepared in low-serum (low-protein) culture medium or not (a variety of mouse immunoglobulins in mouse ascites and serum immunoglobulins or albumin from other species in supernatants may adversely affect the quality of immunohistologic staining of a given monoclonal antibody).

All of these factors should lead the investigator to select the bare minimum number of reagents required for routine diagnostic studies, preferably from a limited number of suppliers, and having acquired experience in their use, to stick to these reagents and avoid the temptation to flirt with others, since such flirtation tends to lead to complications.

In summary, review of Figures 4–11 to 4–22 clearly shows that monoclonal antibodies reveal phenotypic subdivisions of B cells that are not recognizable morphologically; some investigators have concluded that monoclonal antibodies reveal marked heterogeneity within morphologic groups formerly believed to be homogeneous. The implication is that morphology is thereby devalued.

However, examination of this train of logic reveals that the converse is equally true: within a single phenotypic marker there may be several morphologic (cytologic) expressions—eg, B1 spans a whole range of morphologic expression (normal and neoplastic) from lymphoblastlike cells to small lympho-cytes to variously folded (or cleaved) follicu-lar center cells to immunoblasts and plasma-blasts. This might be interpreted as indicating that morphologic studies yield a much finer discrimination of B cell subtypes than do phenotypic ones.

Clearly the only honest conclusion is that morphology and "phenotypography" are complementary; the judicious use of both is now essential for the precise classification of B cell neoplasms.

Restricted Versus Nonrestricted Antibodies

Those monoclonal antibodies that react only with cells of a single cell line are termed restricted (ie, restricted to reaction with one cell type) by some; antibodies with reactivity to cells of two or more lineages are termed nonrestricted.

By this convention the antibodies B4, B1, B2, PC1, and antibodies versus SIg would be considered restricted (to the B cell line); OKT11, T4, and T8 (or their equivalents) are similarly restricted to T cells. By contrast OKT1 (Leu 1, T101) is nonrestricted (mainly T cells, but also BCLL and some follicular center cell lymphomas [Al Saate et al, 1984]); OKT10 (T cells, but also some maturing B cells) and Ia (B cells, monocytes, and acti-vated T cells) are also nonrestricted.

The designation of restricted versus non-restricted is of limited value, since as addi-tional information becomes available, some restricted antibodies may become nonre-stricted (eg, OKT6, initially restricted to T cells, was later found in Langerhans cells); even restricted OKT4 shows weak reactivity, of unknown significance, with macrophages. For very many antileukocyte antibodies, spec-ificity studies have been limited to blood cells; with exhaustive studies of a wide range of cell types in normal fetal tissues it is likely that other restricted antibodies will forfeit this designation. The term restricted should thus be considered a relative term, limited by the information currently available.

First International References Workshop: Leukocyte Typing (1984)

The most comprehensive, though still in-complete, listings of anti-T, anti-B, and anti–monocyte-granulocyte antibodies are in the recent report of the First International Ref-erences Workshop on leukocyte typing (Ber-nard et al, 1984). The reactivities of more than 100 antileukocyte antibodies were re-viewed, including most of those references in this book. Clearly, many of these antibodies recognize similar or identical epitopes; this is analyzed at some length in the workshop proceedings. Appendix 3 includes a modified listing of the antibodies studied at the work-shop plus the literature sources.

Antibodies to Complement Receptors and Complement Components

Antisera have been prepared against com-plement receptor (Stein et al, 1981a—antiserum; Gerdes and Stein, 1982), and sev-eral monoclonal antibodies are available with specificity for, or cross reactivity against, the C3b complement receptor (eg, IB4, OKM1, OKM9, OKM10—Wright SD et al, 1983). C3 receptor–positive cells include follicular B cells (and some of their corresponding tu-mors), dendritic reticulum cells, and cells of the monocyte-histiocyte series. Whaley (1980) showed the synthesis of the major comple-ment components (C2, C3, C4, C5, and pro-perdin factors B and D) to occur in mono-cytes.

B-Lymphomas—Reactivity with Monoclonal Antibodies

The patterns of reactivity of the principal morphologic types of B cell lymphomas with some of the more commonly used and better characterized monoclonal antibodies are given in Figure 4–16.

In practice, the surgical patholo-gist/cytologist normally first makes a morpho-logic assessment (on lymph node sections, bone marrow aspirates, and so forth), arriv-ing at a differential diagnosis that includes one or more B cell neoplasms plus perhaps some morphologically similar T cell neo-plasms, various other neoplasms (eg, small cell carcinomas, melanomas and the like), and, possibly, reactive lymphoid prolifera-tions.

If the critical decision rests between B cell lymphoma and reactive lymphoproliferative disease, then the most helpful approach will be to stain for surface or cytoplasmic immu-noglobulin or both, seeking evidence of mon-oclonality. For a large cell or plasma cellular proliferation, staining for cytoplasmic Ig in paraffin sections will often suffice; for a small cell proliferation, it will usually be necessary to stain for SIg in frozen sections, as described earlier. In both instances a monoclonal (monotypic) pattern provides staining evidence for a neoplastic process of B cell type; precise categorization (eg, large cleaved versus immunoblastic sarcoma) is by morphologic criteria. If a polyclonal pattern results, it suggests a reactive lymphoid process; remember, however, that lymphocytes and plasma cells infiltrating an underlying neoplasm of any time will appear reactive, and a neoplasm is not thereby totally excluded. Staining with anti–B cell monoclonals is usually of little value in distinguishing benign and neoplastic lymphoproliferative process, since both normal and neoplastic lymphocytes react with these antibodies. Some have argued that the finding of a high population of T cells excludes a B cell neoplasm and is more in keeping with a reactive process. This approach is fraught with danger in that it is not uncommon for follicular center cell lymphomas to contain numerous T cells, 60 percent or more by fluorocytometry. One monoclonal antibody that may be useful in diagnosing a neoplastic process is CALLA; if present in more than 20 percent of a cell population, it suggests malignancy, since CALLA positive cells usually are present only in small numbers.

If the diagnosis of malignancy is obvious by morphologic criteria and the major question relates to definition of the type of malignancy, then the B cell antibodies may be very useful. A simple approach is to screen first with antibody to common leukocyte antigen (CLA) (Figs. 4–23 and 4–24) or with pan–B and pan–T cell antibodies (ie, the broadest spectrum reagents available; Fig. 4–17) then, if B cell positive, to focus down on subset antibodies that may further help define the process (Fig. 4–25). With the exception of ALL, in which cytoplasmic mu, SIg, CALLA and BA1 may help categorize the process more precisely, it must be admitted that the most useful subdivisions (clinically) are still to be made morphologically (Fig. 4–16). Table 4–6 lists some of the more helpful T and B cell frozen section studies; additional T cell studies are considered later.

Burkitt's lymphomas and lymphoblastic lymphomas that apparently are of B cell type are discussed later in relation to T cell lymphoblastic lymphoma. Typical phenotypic findings in the other B cell lymphomas are shown in Figure 4–16. For example, it may be seen that B-CLL typically bears SIg, IgM, IgD, or all of these and reacts with a variety of anti–B cell monoclonals (including B1, B2, B4, B7, Leu 12, and sometimes BA1); more surprisingly B-CLL also reacts with OKT1 (T101 or Leu 1), better known as Pan–T cell marker (eg, Al Saate et al, 1984; Huber et al, 1984) and sometimes shows positivity for CALLA (Van den Oord et al, 1984).

Hairy cell leukemia clearly falls within the B cell family on the basis of phenotype, reacting with several B cell antibodies (B1, To15, Leu 12, FMC 7), and also showing Ia positivity (Pallesen et al, 1984b; Meijer et al 1984).

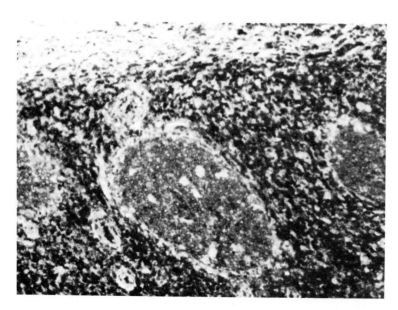

Figure 4–23. Staining for common leukocyte antigen (CLA) in normal lymph node. B cells, T cells, histiocytes, and granulocytes are positive. Vessels and connective tissue elements are not. Paraffin section, AEC with hematoxylin counterstain (× 125).

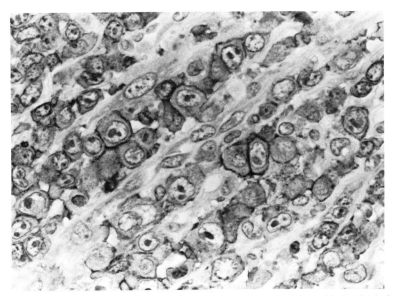

Figure 4–24. Anaplastic tumor showing intense surface membrane staining (black rims) for CLA (common leukocyte antigen). The final diagnosis was immunoblastic sarcoma of B cell type. The patient was one of a series of AIDS patients with B cell lymphoma. Paraffin section, AEC with hematoxylin counterstain (×500).

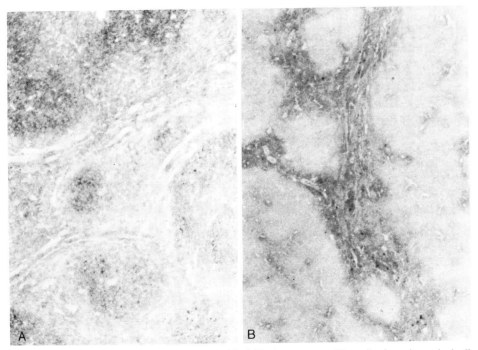

Figure 4–25. *A*, Follicular center cell lymphoma with follicular pattern. B1 antibody stains principally the cells within the follicles; *B*, BA1 antibody stains principally cells outside the follicles. Staining for SIg revealed the same monoclonal pattern both inside the follicles and out, showing that this neoplastic clone expresses two phenotypes (B1+, BA1− in follicles and B1−, BA1+ outside follicles). This appears to mimic the pattern of reactivity of these antibodies in normal follicles. Frozen sections, AEC with hematoxylin counterstain (×60). See Figures 4–14 and 4–17 for comparison with normal follicles.

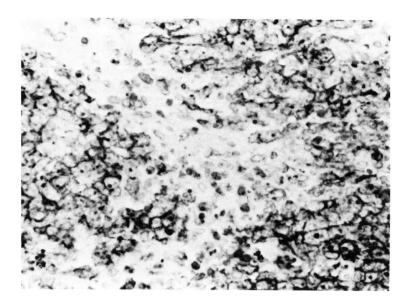

Figure 4–26. Large cleaved follicular center cell lymphoma with residual follicular pattern showing intense reactivity of the large follicular center cells with LN1. Paraffin section, AEC with hematoxylin counterstain (×200).

Anti–CLA (common leukocyte antigen) antibody and LN1 and LN2, versus follicular center cells (and the corresponding lymphomas) are particularly valuable since they are effective in paraffin sections (Figs. 4–23, 4–24, 4–26 and 4–27; for further discussion see Chapter 14).

IDENTIFICATION OF T LYMPHOCYTES IN TISSUE SECTIONS

E Rosette in Suspension

Traditionally, the identification of human T lymphocytes (from tissues) has been accomplished by assay of E rosette formation (Fig. 4–28) using cell suspensions obtained by disaggregation of tissues using mechanical or enzymatic means (review, Taylor and Parker, 1981). This method has several disadvantages:

(a) Although a cell suspension is easily produced from peripheral blood, preparation from lymphoid organs is less straightforward and less predictable; any degree of fibrosis within the tissue may lead to difficulty in extracting some of the cells. Digestion of the tissue with trypsin may increase the yield, but, unfortunately, it may remove or alter

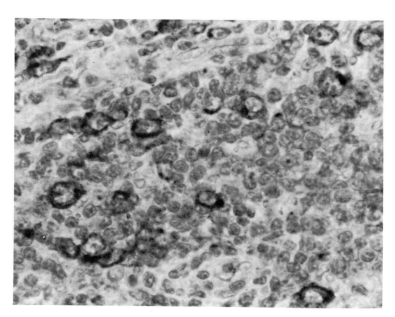

Figure 4–27. Follicular center cell lymphoma, small cleaved (centrocytic), in which the presence of scattered large follicular center cells is highlighted by staining (black) with LN1 antibody. Paraffin section, B5 fixed, AEC with hematoxylin counterstain (×500).

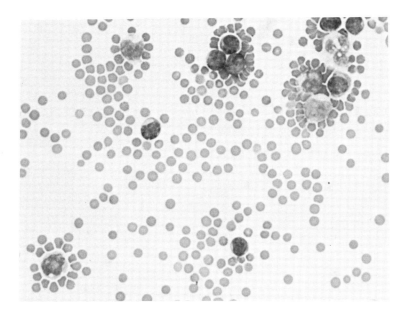

Figure 4–28. E rosette cytocentrifuge preparation of a T cell leukemia. Positive cells are surrounded by a "rosette" of closely apposed sheep red blood cells. Wright's stain (×500).

surface antigens; for this reason, the use of enzyme collagenase has been advocated, although there is no surety that similar problems will not be encountered.

(b) Nonlymphoid organs, in general, present a problem, especially if the lymphocyte infiltration is sparse or focal. The yield of cells may be particularly low in certain tissues (eg, skin), because of the small size of the sample, the presence of collagen fibers, and the relatively small number of lymphoid cells present.

(c) Finally, the topographical distribution of T lymphocytes and their microanatomical interrelationships with other cellular components of the lymphoid tissue cannot be studied in cell suspensions.

There are thus several theoretical advantages to the direct demonstration of T cells in tissue sections.

E Rosette–Tissue Section Method

Some investigators have been able to identify T lymphocytes by direct use of an E rosette technique in tissues; the method involves incubating frozen sections with aminoethylisothiuronium bromide hydrobromide (AET)–treated sheep erythrocytes and washing to remove non-attached cells ("open technique") or incubating the sections in small closed chambers, using gravity to remove unattached indicator cells.

Unfortunately, E rosette methods applied to tissue sections possess several intrinsic disadvantages:

(a) Although it is generally possible to distinguish areas containing many T cells from areas containing few T cells, discrimination between individual cells is not possible, and the underlying tissue and cellular architecture is obscured.

(b) Because of the labile nature of the receptor for sheep erythrocytes, the success of these rosetting techniques is initially dependent upon carefully controlled experimental conditions; different investigators have found it difficult to obtain reproducible results.

(c) The technique fails to demonstrate "immature" T cells that do not express the ability to form E rosettes, and does not discriminate between other subpopulations of T lymphocytes.

Histochemical Identification of T Cells

Some investigators have claimed that the histochemical demonstration of punctate paranuclear staining for acid alpha-naphthyl acetate esterase (alpha ANAE) activity is more reliable and more easily performed than the E rosette assay. Although this claim may have some merit, the specificity of the method falls far short of techniques using monoclonal antibodies. Preservation of ANAE enzyme activity is optimal in cryostat sections prepared from formol-sucrose–fixed tissue blocks, which have been maintained in Holt's syrup. There is some agreement that the demonstration of ANAE activity may be a reliable enzymatic marker of circulating, fully mature normal T lymphocytes and perhaps their neoplastic counterparts; however, ANAE activity is inconsistently present or absent in immature human thymocytes and their neoplastic counterparts (the lymphoblastic lymphomas and some of the acute leukemias), limiting the utility of the method. Punctate paranuclear staining for acid phosphatase has, in our experience, similar limitations.

Use of T Cell Antibodies

In theory, immunologic methods using antibodies against T lymphocytes represent the most specific and reliable means of identifying T cells in tissue sections, in cell suspensions, or in cell smears or imprints.

A variety of conventional heteroantisera have been prepared utilizing different sources of T cell antigens, such as fetal and infant thymus, monkey thymocytes (sharing cell surface antigens with human thymocytes), T cell enriched blood lymphocytes, peripheral blood lymphocytes from Bruton-type agammaglobulinemic patients, cultured T lymphoblasts, T cell leukemia cells, and human brain (containing an antigen in common with some T cells). In order to produce T cell specificity, these reagents must be extensively absorbed with a panel of other cell types, specifically excluding T cells; these may include human kidney, liver, erythrocytes, malignant B cells, or lymphoblastoid B cell lines. The human membrane-related T

differentiation antigens recognized by these heterologous antisera are poorly characterized; collectively they are referred to as human thymic lymphocyte antigens (HTLA). Some of these antisera appeared to recognize different phenotypic subsets of normal and malignant T lymphocytes, suggesting that marked functional heterogeneity existed in the T cell compartment, although final definition proved difficult with conventional antibodies.

The concept of T cell phenotypic, and perhaps functional, heterogeneity has, however, been substantiated by the introduction of monoclonal antibodies directed against antigens that appear to define specific subsets of human T lymphoid cells (Tables 4–6, 4–8, 4–9). Unlike conventional antisera, these monoclonal antibodies identify a single class of determinant on a cell. The use of these reagents has fostered the belief that the various stages of human normal T cell differentiation may be defined according to sequential expression of different T cell antigens (Figs. 4–29, 4–30). Some understanding of the normal pathway of T cell differentiation is critical for the immunologic characterization of T cell malignancies, for the neoplastic T cells appear to retain many of the behavioral properties of their normal counterparts. On this basis, the use of monoclonal antibodies versus T cell-related antigens already has spilled into "diagnostic" studies; it must be admitted, however, that interpretation of the clinical or therapeutic significance of the phenotypic definition of lymphoma cells is still uncertain.

Initial enthusiasm in support of the belief that individual monoclonal antibodies, react-

Table 4–8. Anti–T Cell Reagents Available Commercially

Antibody	Specificity	Similar Clones
Leu 9	"Pan-T"	3A1
OKT1	"Pan-T"	Leu 1, T101, 10.2
OKT3	"Pan-T"	Leu 4
OKT4	Helper-inducer	Leu 3a, Leu 3b, OKT4a, T4
OKT6	Thymocyte	Leu 6, NA 1/34
OKT8	Suppressor–cytotoxic	Leu 2a, Leu 2b, OKT5, T8
OKT9	Transferrin receptor, proliferating cell	Transferrin receptor reagents
OKT11	"Pan-T," E rosette receptor	Leu 5, T11, 9.6
OKT10	Early T cells, stem cells, activated cells, some B cells	
OKIa1	Most B cells, monocytes, activated T cells	Anti-Ia reagents
OKM1	Monocytes, granulocytes, natural killer cells, some T cells	Leu 15, Mac1
Leu 7	Natural killer cells	Natural killer cell reagents, Leu 11 (overlaps)

NB. Not all of these reagents show reactivity restricted to the T cell types shown; eg, OKT1 (Leu 1, T101) reacts with a subset of B cells, all B-CLL, and some follicular center cell lymphomas (Al Saate et al., 1984), and Leu 7 reacts not only with T cells but also with neuroendocrine cells (See Chapter 7). For additional information see Appendix 2.

Table 4–9. Selected Bibliography: T Cell Markers, T Cell Lymphomas

Huber et al 1984	Excellent comprehensive study includes phenotypes of principal T cell lymphomas; some reagents used are unfamiliar
Brubaker & Whiteside 1977	E rosette in tissues
Greaves & Janossy 1976	Need for absorption of conventional anti–T cell antibodies
Gutman & Weissman 1972	Mouse T cells
Hoffman-Fezer et al 1976	Mouse T cells
Bhan et al 1980	Monoclonal anti–T cell antibodies on thymus
Janossy et al 1980a, b, 1981	Monoclonal anti–T cell antibodies, normal tissues
Kung et al 1979	
Reinherz et al 1979, 1980a, b	Monoclonals versus T cell subsets
Reinherz & Schlossman 1981	
Stein et al 1980	Immunohistology of lymphoid tissue
Levine et al 1981	IBS T-cell type
Edelson 1980b	Lymph node and cutaneous–based T cell lymphoma
Collins et al 1979	T cell lymphoma
Maurer et al 1982	Distinction of T-IBS from B-IBS by morphology
Warnke et al 1980	Monoclonal antibodies and T lymphoma
Yamanaka et al 1981	Heterologous antibodies and T lymphoma
Warnke et al 1980	Large cell lymphoma phenotype (no T cell cases)
Watanabe et al 1980	Five adult T cell lymphomas
Edelson 1980a	Cutaneous T cell lymphomas
Lutzner et al 1975	Cutaneous T cell lymphoma—concept
Claudy et al 1976	T cells in cutaneous lymphoma
Miller RA et al 1980	T cell migration patterns
Rappaport & Thomas 1974	Cutaneous involvement in mycosis fungoides—morphology only
Broder et al 1976	Sezary syndrome helper T cells
Boumsell et al 1981	Sezary cell phenotype
Haynes et al 1981	Cutaneous T cell lymphoma—phenotype
Kung et al 1981	Cutaneous T cell lymphoma—phenotype
Weiss LM et al 1985	50 peripheral T cell lymphomas (excluding MF): 64% helper phenotype, 12% suppressor, 8% mixed, 16% negative for helper and suppressor phenotype; 75% were Ia positive; most had lost one or more of the "Pan-T cell" antigens
Hoffmann-Fezer et al 1981	Immunotopography of tonsil (B and T cells)
Engleman et al 1981	Anti-T cell monoclonal (L17F12) antibodies
Rao et al 1983	Helper/inducer cell epitopes; at least 5 distinct epitopes recognized
Poppema et al 1983	NK (phenotype—Leu 7) cells within reactive centers
Swerdlow & Murray 1984	NK (phenotype—Leu 7) in reactive centers and in follicular center cell lymphomas
Meissner et al 1983	Sezary syndrome OKT8 positive; also increased numbers of OKT6-positive Langerhans's cells

ing with separate antigenic determinants, identify distinct and separate subsets of T cells, has given way to tacit recognition of the fact that functional subsets of T cells are not strictly defined by surface phenotype, although broad correlations are possible. These limitations should be kept in mind when venturing into manuscripts that describe T cell distribution in normal and pathologic tissues. When the term helper or suppressor cell is used, it applies to the usually ascribed phenotype and does not necessarily imply that such cells display the corresponding function.

It should also be recognized that these initial concepts of the organization of the human T lymphocyte compartments were derived from cytofluorographic analysis or cytotoxicity tests performed on suspensions of living lymphocytes obtained from different lymphoid organs. More recently, panels of monoclonal antibodies have been employed for in situ identification of T lymphocyte subpopulations in frozen sections of normal human lymphoid organs, providing more precise information as to the relationship of the various T cell subtypes to one another and to their microenvironments, including other cell types (histiocyte, reticulum cells, B cells, and so forth).

As with anti–B cell monoclonal antibodies, so with anti–T cell antibodies: it is important to recognize that diverse sources exist for these antibodies. It is not always clear to what extent reagents from one source are equivalent to those from another source. In the following description, the Ortho reagents are utilized: corresponding antibodies from other sources may be found by reference to Table 4–8 and the Appendix.

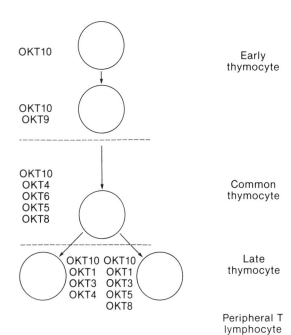

Figure 4–29. Thymic maturation as reflected by the OKT series. Modified from Reinherz and others. Proposed sequential appearance of T cell phenotypes as detected by the OK (Ortho) series of monoclonal antibodies. The OKT4 positive cells are commonly termed helper cells and the OKT8 positive cells, suppressor cells.

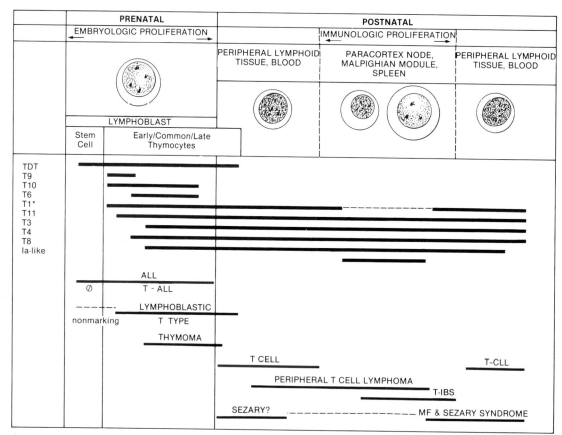

Figure 4–30. T cell antigens. *T1 (Leu 1) reacts with some B cell neoplasms (B-CLL) but is said not to react with normal B cells.

Note: The diffuse small and large cleaved lymphomas that Tubbs and Sheibani (1982) place in the T cell group should, in my view, be held in reserve until this morphologic phenotype is much more clearly defined, since some diffuse cleaved cell lymphomas clearly are formed by monoclonal B cells. T4 (Leu 3) identifies the so-called helper cell, and T8 (Leu 2) the suppressor cells.

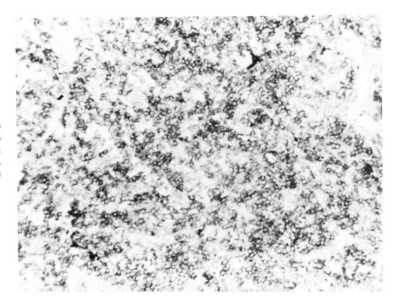

Figure 4–31. Leu 3 positive cells in thymic cortex. Most lymphocytes are positive with some variation in intensity of staining. Frozen section, AEC with hematoxylin counterstain (×200).

Distribution of T Cell Phenotypes in Normal Human Lymphoid Tissue

Human Thymus. The thymus consists of two main lobes encapsulated by connective tissue. Its parenchyma is partially subdivided by septa into lobules composed of darkly staining cortex and lightly staining medulla. The thymic cortex is composed predominantly of small T lymphocytes (Fig. 4–31); the thymic medulla contains obvious thymic epithelial cells and small lymphocytes that are arranged less compactly than in the cortex. This histologic pattern is observed in the thymus during infancy and childhood; with age, marked involution occurs (decrease in overall size, decrease in number of lymphoid cells).

Immunohistologic studies of human thymus with monoclonal antibodies have shown that the T cells corresponding to the stage II ($T1^-$, $T3^-$, $T4^+$, $T5^+$, $T8^+$, $T6^+$, $T10^+$) phenotype in the Reinhertz differentiation scheme (Fig. 4–29) are mainly located in the thymic cortex, whereas the cells present in the thymic medulla belong to stage III (ie, more mature thymocytes showing the phenotype $T1^+$, $T3^+$, $T4^+$, $T5^+$, $T6^-$, $T8^+$, $T10^+$). It would appear that in human as well as in mouse thymus, the change of phenotype closely parallels the migration of T lymphocytes from the cortex to medulla. Moreover, the presence in the thymic medulla of a large percentage of $T4^+$ cells and a small percentage of $T8^+$ cells suggests that the segregation of T lymphocyte helper or suppressor sub-

populations occurs during the last phase of thymocyte development, although these cells only acquire the ability to display their specific functions after migration to the peripheral lymphoid organs.

Thymomas typically contain thymocytes with phenotypes closely resembling those found in normal thymus (eg, Chilosi et al, 1984); the epithelial cells however may be abnormally distributed. Note that thymic and thymoma epithelial cells are keratin-positive and may also be stained with antibodies against thymic epithelium (distinct from keratin) and thymosin (van den Tweel, 1979).

Human Peripheral Lymphoid Organs

Direct in situ evidence that human T and B cells are predominantly located within separate compartments, the T cells largely restricted to the paracortical areas and the B cells limited to the follicles and cortex of lymph nodes, was obtained using heterologous anti–T cell antisera for immunohistologic studies; later the use of monoclonal antibodies permitted refinement of these findings (Fig. 4–17 and 4–32). The potential value of immunohistologic techniques in permitting localization of individual positively stained cells within the microarchitecture of the lymphoid tissues was revealed by the observation that some T cells also may be found within the follicles. Furthermore, T cells appear to possess a differential pattern of localization within follicles, being numerous in the centrocyte-rich pale-staining zone

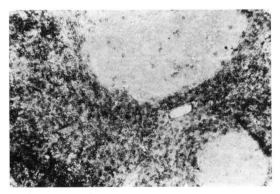

Figure 4–32. Normal lymph node stained with a "pan-T cell" antibody (T101—Hybritech) showing positively stained T cells (small brown-black rings) in an extrafollicular distribution. Frozen section, DAB, no counterstain (×125). See color plate I–4.

(cortical or outer pole) of reactive germinal centers and relatively few in the centroblast-rich dark zone (medullary pole).* Similar findings have also been reported in mouse lymphoid tissues by several authors.

These studies have been taken a stage further by the use of those monoclonal antibodies that purport to identify various T cell subsets (Fig. 4–33; Tables 4–6 and 4–9). For example, it has been shown that the majority of T cells (T1$^+$, T3$^+$, or both) in the paracortical areas of lymph nodes and tonsils appear to express the "helper phenotype" (T4$^+$, T8$^-$); whereas cells displaying the suppressor phenotype (T4$^-$, T8$^+$) are fewer in number and are situated particularly around the periphery of the follicles (see Fig. 4–39). The predominant T cell subpopulation in the human bone marrow and intestinal lamina propria reacts with OKT8 monoclonal antibodies, the so-called suppressor-cytotoxic phenotype (OKT8$^+$, OKT4$^-$).

In addition, immunohistologic studies have shown that most of the T cells identified within the germinal centers of the secondary follicles express the helper phenotype.

Our own experience suggests that all of these findings will be subject to some reappraisal in the light of further data; early follicles (in the initial stages of reactive hyperplasia) contain predominantly helper phenotype cells; whereas "late" regressing

follicles may show a conspicuous "suppressor cell" content. It is tempting to speculate that these types of studies may eventually enhance our understanding of the tissue immune response.

The distribution of natural killer (NK cells) at least as recognized by Leu 7 has been well described by Swerdlow and Murray (1984). Natural killer cells particularly are present in the pale zone of reactive centers and are rare in the interfollicular zone (Fig. 4–34). Follicular center cell lymphomas often contain many NK cells within the neoplastic follicles. Note that Leu 7 also stains selected nonlymphoid cells (neuroendocrine cells—Chapter 7).

The proposal that only mature T lymphocytes are found in lymph nodes receives some support from demonstration that monoclonal OKT6 antibody, which reacts with a major immature thymocyte population, usually stains few or no lymphocytes in lymph nodes. However, exceptional cases of OKT6-positive lymphocytes in adult lymph nodes do occur (Fig. 4–35); the significance is at present unknown. In addition, the cytoplasm of large stellate cells scattered through the paracortical areas shows diffuse staining with OKT6, leading to the postulate that these positive cells might represent Langerhans cells (or a closely related cell type). This point of view is given some credence by the fact that the Langerhans cells in the skin react with monoclonal OKT6 antibodies (see Chapter 13). It has been proposed that these Langerhans cells migrate from skin to node; there is, however, no reason why migration, if it occurred at all, should not have been in the reverse direction. Nor can the possibility be excluded that OKT6 antibody, which already is known to react with two totally distinct cell types (thymocytes and Langerhans cells), reacts independently with a third cell type.

This type of interpretive problem is being encountered with increasing frequency as diverse new monoclonal antibodies are applied to a wide variety of tissue (cell) types. Just because a monoclonal antibody has, by definition, a single specificity does not mean that it will bind only to one particular type of molecule or cell. It may react with two or more identical determinants situated on unrelated molecules, or it may show reaction with unrelated cell types that express the same molecule in common, or two different determinants may show enough similarity for the antibody to cross-react.

Centrocyte is the term used in the Kiel classification for follicular center cells with folded nuclei—the equivalent of cleaved cells in the Lukes-Collins scheme. *Centroblast* is the term for the transformed type of cell (noncleaved cell) within the center (for detailed descriptions and illustrations see Robb-Smith and Taylor, 1981).

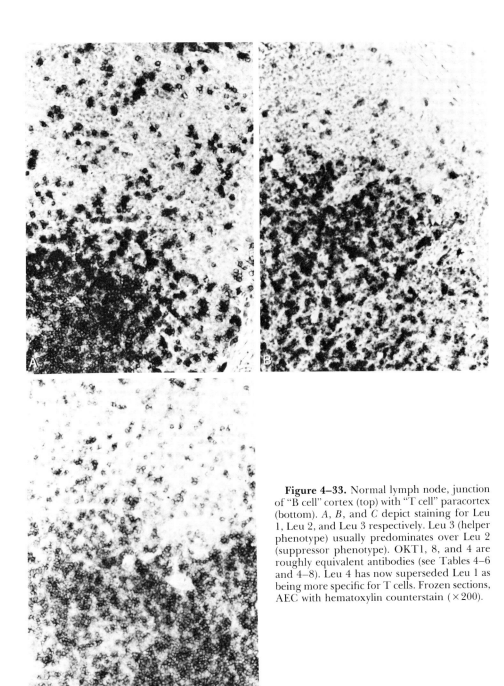

Figure 4–33. Normal lymph node, junction of "B cell" cortex (top) with "T cell" paracortex (bottom). *A*, *B*, and *C* depict staining for Leu 1, Leu 2, and Leu 3 respectively. Leu 3 (helper phenotype) usually predominates over Leu 2 (suppressor phenotype). OKT1, 8, and 4 are roughly equivalent antibodies (see Tables 4–6 and 4–8). Leu 4 has now superseded Leu 1 as being more specific for T cells. Frozen sections, AEC with hematoxylin counterstain (×200).

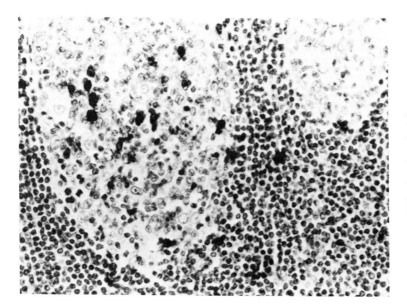

Figure 4–34. Reactive lymph node showing part of two reactive centers. Cells with dense black cytoplasm, mostly present within the centers, are positive for Leu 7 (HNK1), "human natural killer cell" antibody. Paraffin section, DAB with hematoxylin counterstain (×200). Note that Leu 7 also stains melanoma cells and certain neuroendocrine cells (see Chapters 13 and 7).

The wealth of data generated by numerous investigators using monoclonal antibodies versus T cell determinants is both exciting and frustrating: exciting because there is the promise of new understanding, frustrating because this new understanding presently remains beyond our grasp.

AIDS—Acquired Immunodeficiency Syndrome

It is convenient at this point to describe the immunohistologic findings in AIDS and progressive generalized lymphadenopathy (so-called pre-AIDS syndrome). In the stage of atypical follicular hyperplasia in lymph nodes, the irregular follicles are clearly demarcated by anti-B cell antibodies; LN1 stains them well in paraffin sections, and B1 in frozen sections. The mantle zone typically is moth-eaten and depleted; this condition is visible on hemotoxylin and eosin (H and E) section but is enhanced by staining with LN2 in paraffin sections and BA1 or IgD in frozen sections. As the disease progresses, disruption and disorganization of the follicles is clearly seen using anti–B cell monoclonal antibodies (Fig. 4–36 and 4–37). The most characteristic feature is related, however, to changes in distribution and frequency of T cells (Fig. 4–38 and 4–39).

In AIDS and pre-AIDS there is a progressive decrease in the numbers of helper

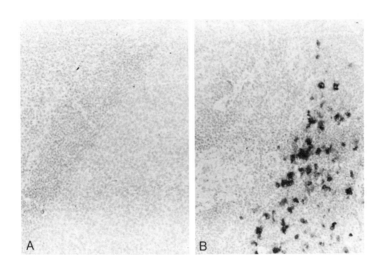

Figure 4–35. *A,* Normal lymph node contains few or no OKT6 positive cells. *B,* OKT6 positive cells in lymph node of a patient with AIDS (on right); OKT6 positive cells often are increased in numbers in this condition. Frozen sections, AEC with hematoxylin counterstain (×125).

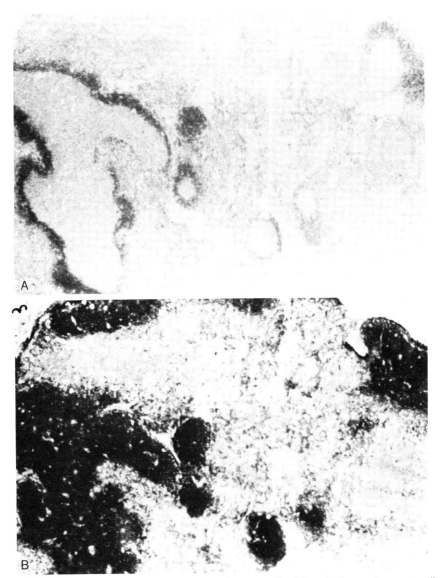

Figure 4–36. Lymph node from a patient with progressive generalized lymphadenopathy, eventually developing classical AIDS (acquired immunodeficiency syndrome). *A,* Staining for IgD (delta chain specific) outlines some residual small reactive follicles and a large bizarre follicle. *B,* The adjacent parallel section stained with B1 shows staining especially within follicles. Frozen sections, AEC with hematoxylin counterstain (×60).

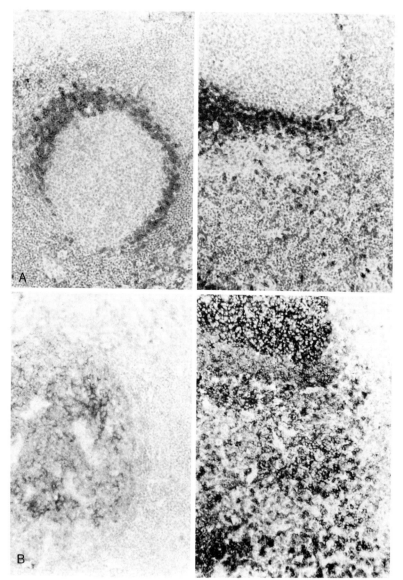

Figure 4–37. *A*, Staining for IgD revealed disruption and loss of mantle zone in a case of AIDS, with dispersion of delta positive cells into the paracortex. *B*, Staining with B1 (pan-B cell) antibody (parallel field to *A*) reveals the full extent of disruption of the follicle with spread of B cells into the paracortex. In each instance the pattern of staining in a normal follicle (left) is given for comparison. Frozen sections, AEC with hematoxylin counterstains (×200). This patient developed a B cell lymphoma, although the lymphocytes were not monoclonal at the time of this biopsy. This process appears to represent a progressive hyperplasia, with a high risk of evolution to lymphoma.

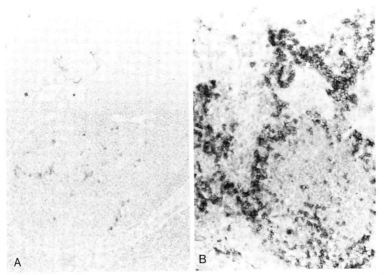

Figure 4–38. *A*, Normally lymph nodes contain few OKT10 positive T cells. *B*, OKT10 positive T cells (small black donuts) clustered around a reactive center in a lymph node from a patient with progressive generalized lymphadenopathy (sometimes termed pre-AIDS). Frozen sections, AEC with hematoxylin counterstain (×125).

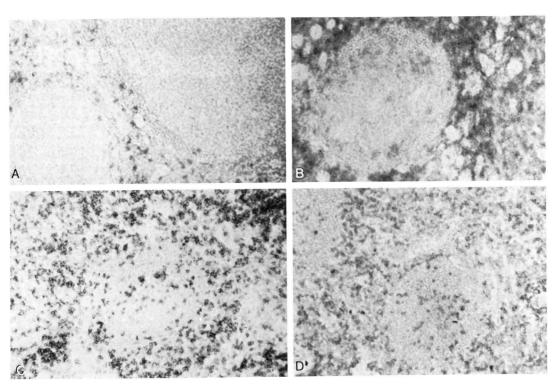

Figure 4–39. Staining for suppressor and helper T cell phenotypes. *A* and *B*, suppressor and helper cells respectively (red-black) in normal reactive lymph node. Helper cells predominate, with occasional cells within the reactive center but most cells outside the follicles. *C* and *D* show suppressor and helper cells respectively (red-black), in lymph node from a patient with AIDS. Note that in comparison with the normal lymph node there is a decrease in helper cells and an increase in suppressor cells such that the latter predominate; suppressor cells also are present within the B cell follicle (*C*). Frozen sections, OKT4 (helper), OKT8 (suppressor), AEC with hematoxylin counterstain (×50). See color plate I–5.

phenotype T cells (OKT4) and an increase in suppressor phenotype T cells (OKT8), so the latter come to predominate. This change parallels the reversal of the helper to suppressor cell ratio seen in peripheral blood but may be seen in lymphoid tissues prior to detectable changes in the blood. An additional feature is the presence of suppressor cells actually within reactive centers as well as clustered about the periphery of centers. These findings although characteristic of AIDS are not diagnostic, for they may occur in various degrees in nodes reactive to viral infections. Such findings, however, justify a strong suspicion of AIDS or pre-AIDS; the lack of these changes almost excludes the diagnosis. For a more detailed description of the immunomorphology of pre-AIDS see Meyer et al (1985).

Human T Cell Malignancies

Two concepts are particularly important in understanding the biology of human T lymphocyte malignancies.

First, although malignant T cells frequently express one or more of the phenotypic markers that characterize their normal counterparts, they also retain some degree of phenotypic heterogeneity that is possibly reflective of different phases of maturation or the presence of cells in different stages of the cell cycle. Thus it is possible to analyze T cell malignancies immunologically by using antibodies directed against normal T cell differentiation antigens, but not all of the neoplastic cells will necessarily display the same phenotype (ie, the antibodies cannot be used as markers for the presence of an expanded or neoplastic clone in the way that anti-immunoglobulin markers may identify clonal B cells).

Second, the propensity of lymphocytes to "home" to the B cell or T cell regions of normal peripheral lymphoid tissues is also observed in many malignant lymphomas of B and T cell origin. In other words, malignant T cells tend to migrate preferentially to the T cell zones of lymphoid tissues and ultimately produce effacement of normal lymphoid architecture.

To these considerations must be added the caveat that any neoplastic T cell population observed within the tissues will be intermingled with residual normal T cells (and B cells), and apart from morphology, which is unreliable, we have no method of setting these two populations apart.

T Cell Acute Lymphoblastic Leukemia and Lymphoblastic Lymphoma

These two conditions are discussed together, because clinically, morphologically, and immunologically they appear to represent different parts of a single spectrum of disease; such separations as do exist are somewhat arbitrary, based upon the classic clinico-pathologic picture at either end of the spectrum.

The problem of cellular recognition is well revealed in the study of tissue involvement by a lymphoblastic lymphoma or by the related process of acute lymphoblastic leukemia. In such a case, morphologists have generally assumed (rightly or wrongly) that all of the cells with the cytologic features of lymphoblasts are malignant and, correspondingly, that all cells in the malignant clone look like lymphoblasts; as a corollary, of course, all cells that do not look like lymphoblasts are considered neoplastic. This assumption is unlikely to be valid. Experience of B cell lymphomas, in which individual clones may be morphologically diverse (see Taylor, 1982b), leads us to expect that similar diversity will also be found in T cell lymphomas. In the study of T cell lymphomas, we are handicapped by the fact that in spite of the plethora of T cell markers we lack a clonal T cell marker corresponding to monoclonal surface immunoglobulin (or, even better, a specific immunoglobulin idiotype) for B cell lymphomas.

T cell lymphoblastic lymphoma-leukemia typically expresses the early thymic markers as revealed by the OKT series of monoclonal antibodies (Fig. 4–30). Although some variations in phenotype have been reported, these do not appear to lead to clinically useful distinctions. However, it is important to distinguish this process from NULL cell, or common ALL (acute lymphoblastic leukemia) and morphologically similar lymphoblastic processes that express B cell markers. Clinically, there are important behavioral and therapeutic reasons for separating the definite T cell cases from the definite B cell cases and the so-called common ALL category (although the great majority of these turn out to be members of the B cell series, as is described later in the chapter). There are also, of course, implications concerning understanding the differentiation pathways of these cell types.

Of cases of lymphoblastic lymphoma (defined morphologically as consisting of "lymphoblasts"), many will show some T cell markers (one or more of T1, T4, T8, T3, and T11), but there will be quite variable expression of the "intrathymic" T cell markers (T9, T6, and T10); some lymphoblastic lymphomas may show almost 100 percent of cells positive for T6, others, morphologically identical, may show 10 percent or less of positive cells. In addition, some morphologic lymphoblastic lymphomas do not bear detectable T cell markers and appear to correspond to the non-B, non-T unclassifiable group; some of these cells are of B cell lineage, expressing early B cell markers, or showing evidence of immunoglobulin gene rearrangement. Most T cell cases will show positive nuclear staining for TDT, as will some NULL and pre–B cell cases.

It has become clear that within the general category of lymphoblastic lymphomas and acute lymphoblastic leukemias, the time-honored morphologic distinctions are not reliable. Cases of B cell ALL and the related condition of Burkitt's lymphoma (which some would classify as a subset of small noncleaved follicle center cell lymphoma) must also be considered closely related to lymphoblastic lymphomas on the basis of immunologic phenotyping, and the morphologic distinctions that have been made to separate these tumors appear to be somewhat artificial.

Thus, although a classic Burkitt's lymphoma (classic in terms of its minute morphology) generally will mark as a monoclonal B cell proliferation, occasional cases have been observed that apparently are of T cell type. Similarly, within the lymphoblastic lymphomas (whether convoluted or not), some cases will mark as T cells, but other cases will display B cell markers with monoclonal surface immunoglobulin. Still other cases will show neither T nor B cell markers but will show evidence of immunoglobulin gene rearrangement, assigning them to the early stages of the B cell pathway. The principal distinctions the pathologist must make are those the clinicians presently demand, that is, the recognition of T cell ALL and T cell lymphoblastic lymphoma as one therapeutic category, the recognition of B cell ALL and Burkitt's lymphoma as another, and the distinction of both from the common ALL group and the related non-B, non-T lymphoblastic lymphoma. These distinctions can be made far more reliably by immunologic phenotype than by morphology. Beyond these broad categories, although it is theoretically possible to further subdivide B and T cell diseases by the expression of phenotypic markers within each series, there is at this point no generally accepted clinical purpose for so doing. Staining for CALLA (common acute lymphoblastic leukemia antigen) may however be extremely useful in identifying neoplastic lymphoblasts in tissues (Fig. 4–40).

Cossman (1985), in a recent review of diffuse aggressive lymphomas, basically concurs with this viewpoint.

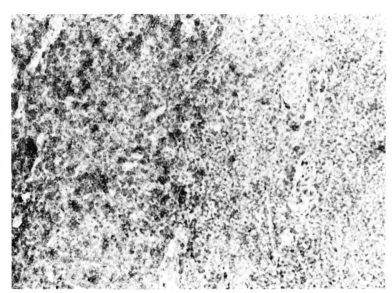

Figure 4–40. Lymph node showing encroachment by CALLA (common ALL antigen) positive lymphoblasts in a case of ALL. Positive cells appear as small black donuts (left side). Frozen section, AEC with hematoxylin counterstain (×200). CALLA positivity is seen in some cases of ALL, some lymphoblastic lymphomas and, rather surprisingly, some follicular center cell tumors (see Fig. 4–16).

Immunoblastic Sarcoma of T Cell Type (T-IBS) (Node-Based T Cell Lymphoma—Peripheral T Cell Lymphoma) (See Tables 4–6 and 4–9.)

These lymphomas are at this time incompletely described and are not clearly delineated one from another. All appear to arise from T cells in the lymph nodes and peripheral lymphoid tissue. For the purpose of the present discussion, T immunoblastic sarcoma (T-IBS), in which large immunoblasts predominate, is regarded as a subset of "peripheral T cell lymphoma," which displays a rather broader range of morphologic appearances. The concept that the lymph nodes represent the primary site of this disease is based upon clinical data showing that the majority of patients with T-IBS present initially with lymph node enlargement; by comparison, approximately half of the patients with B-IBS present with extranodal disease, usually in the gastrointestinal tract or lungs.

Although the histopathologic picture in a few cases seems to be characteristic (ie, presence of a diffuse proliferation of immunoblasts with typical "water-clear" cytoplasm admixed with small and medium-sized lymphocytes having dense contorted nuclei, with absence of plasmacytoid features), in other cases the picture is less distinctive and differentiation of T-IBS (or peripheral T cell lymphoma) from immunoblastic sarcoma of B cell type, from large noncleaved FCC lymphoma, and from lymphocyte-depleted varieties of Hodgkin's disease may be impossible on histologic grounds alone (Schneider et al, 1985). Under these circumstances, it is necessary to use additional methods (immunologic, cytochemical, and ultrastructural) for the confirmation of the diagnosis.

E-rosette formation by lymphocytes of various sizes, including immunoblasts, appears to be characteristic of this lymphoproliferative disorder. At this time there have been few reports utilizing anti-T cell antibodies on frozen sections or cell suspensions of T-IBS. A single case of node-based T cell lymphoma was reported to react with monoclonal antibodies both against mature and immature T lymphocytes (Warnke et al, 1980). Yamanaka et al (1981) used heterologous anti–human T cell antisera in conjunction with immunofluorescence to identify malignant T cells on frozen sections of 44 non-Hodgkin lymphoma cases. The two antisera employed in their study were prepared by immunizing

rabbits with human thymocytes (ATS-T) or human lymph node cells (ALS-T) obtained by the nylon wool column method. All the cases of lymphoblastic lymphoma in the series reacted with ATS-T antiserum, recognizing an immature T lymphocyte population; whereas 6 of 19 (about 30 percent) of large cell lymphomas were positive for ALS-T antiserum, identifying a more mature T lymphocyte population. The high incidence of T cell lymphomas reported in this study contrasts with another study (Warnke et al, 1980) in which no cases of T cell lymphoma were detected in a series of 33 cases of large cell lymphomas studied immunohistologically with monoclonal antibodies against T cell subsets. This discrepancy may reflect the higher incidence of T cell malignancies observed in Japan as compared with the United States, particularly the Stanford case population.

Watanabe et al (1980) performed cytotoxicity tests on lymph node cell suspensions of five cases of adult T cell lymphomas with hypergammaglobulinemia and found that the neoplastic cells were invariably killed in each case by anti-MOLT (an acute lymphocytic leukemia-derived T cell line) serum, indicating the presence of T differentiation antigens on the surface of the neoplastic population. One of these cases also showed the presence of other antigens as defined by heteroantisera anti-Raji (Burkitt's lymphoma–derived cell line), anti-AML (acute myeloid leukemia), and anti-AMoL (acute monocytic leukemia). The reported expression of Ia-like antigens on the surface of normal T cells appears to be a marker of T cell activation, since these antigens are not present on the surface of resting T cells; Ia reactivity has also been seen in some T immunoblastic sarcomas. These immunologic data give some support to the morphologist's concept that T immunoblastic sarcoma is a neoplasm of activated (transformed) T-lymphocytes presumably having limited capability for differentiation to smaller effector cells, a characteristic somewhat analogous to the presence of plasmacytoid cells (effector B cells) in immunoblastic sarcoma of B cell type.

T lymphocyte effector activity has not been extensively studied in this type of lymphoma. Some clinical and immunologic data however suggest that, at least in some circumstances, these tumors may display helper function. Clinically, 41 percent of patients with T-IBS demonstrate diffuse hyperglobulinemia (Levine et al, 1981), and five cases with similar findings have been recently described in Japan (Watanabe et al, 1980). Lawrence et al (1978) have reported a patient with Sezary syndrome whose malignant T lymphocytes were shown to have helper activity. Five months after the initial diagnosis, the patient presented with lymphadenopathy; biopsy revealed an evolution to immunoblastic sarcoma of the T cell type. The malignant T immunoblasts in this case were demonstrated to have retained their helper cell activity.

Our own experience at the University of Southern California also reflects a selected case population but includes approximately 20 cases of immunoblastic sarcoma of T cell type from among a total of more than 500 lymphomas studied by immunohistologic methods on frozen sections. These cases showed intense reactivity with anti–Pan T antibodies (eg, Leu 1, Leu 4, OKT3), and variable reactivity with OKT6, OKT10 (thymocyte related) and antibodies against the helper-inducer and suppressor-cytotoxic phenotypes (Leu 3, OKT 4 and Leu 2, OKT8); in some cases individual cells appeared to react with several different antibodies (eg, OKT10, OKT8 [Leu 2], and OKT4 [Leu 3] positive), a feature ascribed to the intermediate phases of T lymphocyte maturation in the thymus. Rather than conclude that this therefore is a "thymic"-type neoplasm, a more realistic concept might be to regard appearance of these thymic markers as expressions of oncofetal antigens, somewhat analogous to CEA and alpha-fetoprotein in other tumors.

A greater number of cases must be examined and followed over a prolonged period before attempting to draw definite conclusions with regard to diagnostic or prognostic significance. Nonetheless, even with our present rudimentary knowledge, it is possible to assign cases to the T cell lymphoma category with some confidence, on the basis of a combination of morphology and the pattern of reactivity with these antibodies.

Cutaneous T Cell Lymphomas

Mycosis fungoides and Sezary syndrome are neoplasms of thymus-derived lymphocytes that express thymic markers and are part of the broad spectrum of cutaneous T cell lymphomas (CTCL).

Definitive evidence that these tumors are T cell–derived came from the demonstration that neoplastic populations in blood, skin, and lymph nodes form E rosettes and react with anti-T heteroantisera. Although the majority of these investigations have been performed in cell suspensions, putative malignant T cells may also be identified in situ by using heterologous or monoclonal anti-T sera in conjunction with immunoperoxidase or immunoflourescence techniques (Table 4–9). When applied to unfixed frozen sections of cutaneous lesions, these techniques show a positive labelling on the surface both of the cells infiltrating the dermis and of those constituting the Pautrier's microabscesses in mycosis fungoides.

These immunohistologic studies engender some doubt concerning the effectiveness of certain therapeutic modalities such as photochemotherapy, for scattered neoplastic cells appear to be present in the dermis at a level deeper than the known penetration of longwave ultraviolet light; such cells appear to possess the morphologic, immunohistologic, and ultrastructural characteristics of the typical Sezary's cells.

The T cell nature of these neoplasms fits well with the tissue-infiltration pattern observed in patients with cutaneous T cell lymphomas (ie, preferential involvement of the skin, the paracortical areas of the lymph nodes, and the periarteriolar sheaths of the spleen with minimal or absent bone marrow infiltration).

In analogy with their normal T cell counterparts, these neoplastic cells also show a propensity to recirculate through tissues; the lymph nodes do not appear to be an obstacle to spread of the disease once the cells leave the skin. The understanding of this migration pattern has an important clinical implication, because histologic demonstration of microscopic involvement of lymph nodes indicates a need for a systematic therapy; immunohistologic techniques with frozen sections have proven valuable in uncovering lymph node involvement. Again, recognition of the Sezary's cells in lymph nodes involves use of a combination of morphologic and immunologic criteria, since there is no "Sezary"-specific antibody.

Several studies indicate that the neoplastic cells of cutaneous T cell lymphomas may stimulate immunoglobulin production in vitro (ie, helper cell function) in both normal B cells and B cells from some patients with immunologic deficiencies. In addition, studies with monoclonal antibodies directed

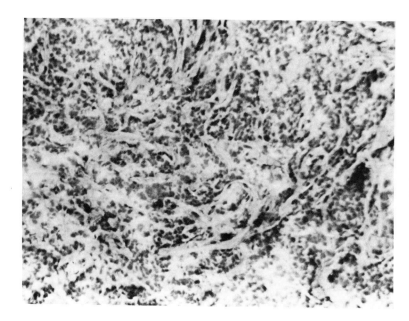

Figure 4–41. Diffuse cutaneous T cell lymphoma showing positive reactivity with Leu 3 antibody (helper phenotype). Frozen section, AEC with hematoxylin counterstain (×125).

against normal "T cell differentiation antigens" have shown that the neoplastic population of both leukemic and aleukemic cutaneous T cell lymphomas express T1 or T3 and T4 (helper) antigens or a combination of all three; these are regarded as "mature" T cells (Fig. 4–41). These cells do not usually react (occasional cases do) with monoclonal antibodies recognizing mature suppressor T cell subpopulations or immature T cell subpopulations. In concert these findings suggest that most cutaneous T cell lymphomas are composed of T lymphocytes displaying helper function (ie, inducing the differentiation of B lymphocytes into immunoglobulin-secreting plasma cells); this circumstance may explain both the observations of elevated serum immuoglobulins, particularly of the T cell dependent classes of IgE and IgA in many patients, and the relative infrequency of serious infections induced by encapsulated organisms in this condition.

The immunologic characterization of cutaneous lymphomas using monoclonal antibodies has also provided other important information on the biology of these neoplasms.

First, neoplastic cells showing helper phenotype (ie, $T1^+$ and/or $T3^+$, $T4^+$, $T8^-$) do not necessarily exhibit helper function in tests in vitro. Second, the helper phenotype may be lost during the final phases of the disease, possibly due to the emergence of de-differentiated malignant T cell subclones (possibly concurrent with so-called blastic transforma-

tion of mycosis fungoides). This phenomenon may be similar to the loss of capability for producing lysozyme or immunoglobulin observed with anaplastic forms of malignant histiocytosis and myeloma or B immunoblastic sarcoma, respectively.

T-Zone Lymphoma

This nodal lymphoma, first described by Lennert (1978), is characterized by neoplastic proliferation of the small T lymphocytes, with relative sparing of the follicular center apparatus. Transformation to a blastic process (usually designated T cell immunoblastic sarcoma) has been noted. The few cases studied have shown that 20 to 85 percent of the suspended cells form E rosettes. The neoplastic nature of the rosetting cells has been confirmed, at least by cytologic features, in cytocentrifuge preparations.

Immunohistologic studies of this type of lymphoma have confirmed the initial impression that T zone lymphomas are composed of neoplastic T cells admixed with some residual normal B cells which, at least in the early phases of lymph node involvement, are sharply compartmentalized. The follicular structures, like those of normal or hyperplastic lymph nodes, bind AEC rosettes (complement receptor positive) and show a polyclonal staining pattern for surface and cytoplasmic immunoglobulins. In contrast, the neoplastic cells located in the T-dependent areas of the lymph node strongly react with anti-T het-

Table 4–10. Selected Bibliography: Lichen Planus and Reactive T Cells in the Skin

Alario et al 1978	Anti-HTLA antiserum
Edelson et al 1973	Mononuclear cell differentiation, early study
Harrist et al 1981	Lymphomatoid papulosis and granulomatosis
Walker 1976	Lichen planus
McMillan et al 1981	Lichen planus T cells

eroantisera (HTLA) and with monoclonal PAN T cell antibodies. These T cells show widely variable expression of helper-suppressor phenotypes in different cases studied to date. A certain percentage of these cells also bear surface Ia-like antigens, suggesting that they may be activated (transformed) neoplastic T lymphocytes. The Ia-positive malignant T cells, like their normal activated T cell counterparts, show little propensity to recirculate.

Benign Skin Conditions

Immunohistologic studies (Table 4–10) with heterologous anti-T serum on frozen sections have shown that most of the cells of the infiltrates of Lichen planus and other "chronic inflammations" of the skin are T lymphocytes. Recent studies using monoclonal antibodies to identify T cell subpopulations directly on frozen sections have demonstrated that the infiltrate of Lichen planus consists predominantly of helper T cells. In this condition, as in mycosis fungoides, an increased number of Ia-positive Langerhans cells is also detectable.

Immunohistologic studies per se will not distinguish Sezary's syndrome or mycosis fungoides from conditions characterized by dense infiltration of lymphocytes into the dermis as part of the chronic inflammatory process.

IMMUNOHISTOLOGIC TECHNIQUES IN THE DIAGNOSIS OF HODGKIN'S DISEASE

Two quite extensive reviews representing somewhat contrasting viewpoints of the nature of Hodgkin's disease have recently been published (Kadin, 1983; Taylor, 1983b). Although there is much of academic interest, immunologic studies of Hodgkin's disease have not contributed greatly to diagnosis, which still depends, as for the past 100 years, upon the recognition of Reed-Sternberg cells or acceptable "variants."

Staining for Immunoglobulin

That Reed-Sternberg cells and mononuclear Hodgkin's cells frequently contain immunoglobulin is no longer in dispute (Figs. 4–42 and 4–43). Characteristically, individual Reed-Sternberg cells contain both kappa and lambda light chain and usually gamma heavy

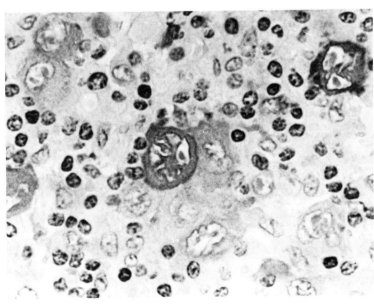

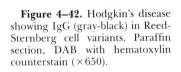

Figure 4–42. Hodgkin's disease showing IgG (gray-black) in Reed-Sternberg cell variants. Paraffin section, DAB with hematoxylin counterstain (×650).

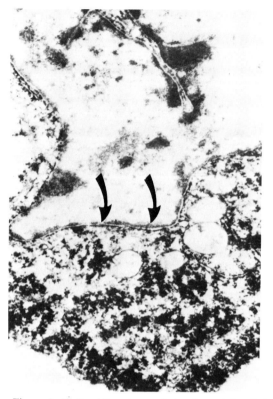

Figure 4–43. Reed-Sternberg cell showing staining for immunoglobulin (IgG—intense black granules) by electron microscopy with a pre-embedding immunoperoxidase method. At the top is the nucleus; the cytoplasm (lower field) contains numerous positive granules, including some arranged as a rough endoplasmic reticulum. The nuclear membrane (arrows) also stains for IgG. This pattern is suggestive of ribosomal IgG synthesis in at least some Reed-Sternberg cells (slide by Dr. T. Dura).

chain (IgG), demonstrable in paraffin sections (Fig. 4–44). Rarely, a monotypic-monoclonal pattern is seen in Reed-Sternberg–Hodgkin's cells in a case of morphologically acceptable monoclonal Hodgkin's disease; however, in general, the finding of a monoclonal monotypic light chain pattern should steer one to a diagnosis of immunoblastic sarcoma, poorly differentiated myeloma (plasmacytoma), or large cell follicular center cell tumor rather than Hodgkin's disease; all of these conditions may display occasional large multilobulate or multinucleate cells that resemble Reed-Sternberg calls. In Hodgkin's disease staining for immunoglobulin (in paraffin sections) also reveals variable numbers of polyclonal reactive plasma cells.

In frozen sections stained for immunoglobulin, there may be extensive background due to extracellular tissue-fluid immunoglobulin. Extensive collagen formation may produce some nonspecific background staining. Variable numbers of SIg-positive B cells are, however, apparent. In most instances the B cells, like the plasma cells for cytoplasmic Ig, are polyclonal. Often these B cells cluster together, in a manner reminiscent of primary follicles. Monoclonal staining of Reed-Sternberg cells has however been described in lymphocyte-predominant Hodgkin's disease (HD-LP) (Poppema et al, 1979b), an indication that this form of Hodgkin's disease may be separate from the other types (nodular sclerosis, mixed cellularity, and lymphocyte depleted; see also the following section).

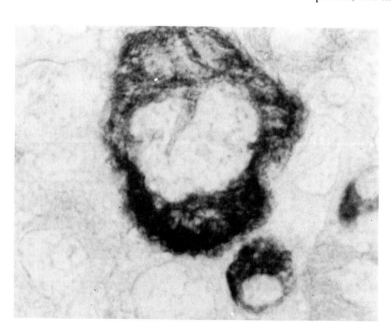

Figure 4–44. Reed-Sternberg cell containing both kappa and lambda light chains in a double stain. Two plasma cells also are present. Kappa was stained brown by immunoperoxidase with DAB, and lambda was stained blue by immunoglucose oxidase. Paraffin section, no counterstain (×1200). In this black and white photomicrograph, kappa appears pitch black and lambda gray.

Staining with T and B Cell Monoclonal Antibodies

Staining of frozen sections of Hodgkin's disease for T and B cells typically shows a preponderance of T cells (Pan–T or E rosette OKT11-positive; Table 4–11).

In some instances this may be much more marked than in "normal" reactive lymph nodes (ie, >80 percent T cells). In lymphocyte-predominant Hodgkin's disease, T cell scores of 90 percent are not infrequent. The distribution of helper phenotype to suppressor phenotype (OKT4:T8 ratio) is usually within normal range for lymph nodes (1 to 3.5). Occasionally, however, helper cells may predominate to such a degree (90 percent), that this on may give rise to suspicion of a T cell lymphoma, in which an excess of helper cells is more typical. In such cases the final decision will rest with a careful morphologic judgment. Anti–B cell antibodies reveal clusters of B cells, sometimes apparently forming primary follicles; this grouping resembles the pattern of staining seen for SIg but is generally cleaner owing to absence of these B cell antigens in the tissue fluids. Isolated reports have described the reactivity of Reed-Sternberg cells with some anti–B cell antibodies (eg, B1; Table 4–11). This reactivity has not been widely confirmed. Pinkus and Said (1985) reported the presence of B cell–specific antigens and common leukocyte antigen on L and H cells (ie, the Reed-Sternberg variants found in lymphocyte-predominant Hodgkin's disease). In other types of Hodgkin's disease the Reed-Sternberg cells showed no evidence of B cell antigens but did react with Leu M1 (vide infra). Dorreen et al (1984) also noted that Reed-Sternberg cells in some cases reacted with B1, although their positive cases were nodular sclerosis or lymphocyte-depleted types. They also noted positive reactivity of Reed-Sternberg cells for OKT9 and Ia, a finding echoed by Watanabe and colleagues (1984). On the basis of their study, Dorreen concluded that the Reed-Sternberg cell may have a follicular center

Table 4–11. Selected Bibliography: Hodgkin's Disease

Taylor 1983b } Kadin 1983 }	Lengthy reviews of immunohistologic findings in Hodgkin's disease up to 1983
Poppema 1980	Staining with anti-Ig and anti–alpha₁-antitrypsin; concluded Reed-Sternberg cells related to histiocytes
Poppema et al 1979a	Earlier study of SIg & E rosettes in frozen sections
Poppema et al 1979b	Felt that some Reed-Sternberg cells were lymphocyte-derived in lymphocyte-predominant Hodgkin's disease
Balázs 1981 } Balázs & Kelenyi 1980 }	IgG-staining in Hodgkin's disease; Reed-Sternberg cells positive
Borowitz et al 1982	Study of 15 cases of Hodgkin's disease with monoclonal antibodies; most lymphocytes marked as T cells; frozen sections
Herva et al 1979	Case study including DNA synthesis led to conclusion that "immunoblasts, Hodgkin cells and Reed-Sternberg cells formed part of a continuous DNA synthesizing series"
Stuart et al 1983	Monoclonal antibodies with anti–B cell specificity (FMC1 and B1) react with Reed-Sternberg cells
Möller et al 1983	Fibronectin-positive fibroblasts are more numerous in Hodgkin's disease; Reed-Sternberg cells do not contain fibronectin
Stein et al 1982	Anti–Reed-Sternberg cell antibody (Ki 1)
Ree et al 1981a, b	Paraffin sections—lysozyme in histiocytes in Hodgkin's disease
Payne et al 1982	Alpha₁-antitrypsin, paraffin sections; concluded that Reed-Sternberg cells resemble histiocytes
Möller 1982	Peanut lectin and Hodgkin cells
Poppema et al 1982	T cells predominate in Hodgkin's disease
Poppema et al 1985	Hodgkin (Reed-Sternberg) cell line—B cell on basis of immunologic and genetic analysis
Forni et al 1985	B and T lymphocytes in frozen sections of Hodgkin's disease
Okon et al 1985	Staining of Reed-Sternberg cells with LN2, and occasionally LN1
Hsu & Jaffe 1984 } Hsu et al 1985 }	Leu M1 staining in Hodgkin and Reed-Sternberg cells
Warhol et al 1985	Leu M1 in Reed-Sternberg cells and granulocytes
Kornstein et al 1985	Leu M1 and S100 in lymphomas and Hodgkin's disease
Watanabe et al 1984	OKT9 and Ia activity in Reed-Sternberg cells
Dorreen et al 1984	30 cases; helper T cells and NK cells (Leu 7) clustered around Reed-Sternberg cells; in 2 cases Reed-Sternberg cells reacted with B1
Pinkus & Said 1985	Lymphocyte-predominant Hodgkin's disease showed B cell markers

origin. Of more practical value for diagnosis are the reported findings in paraffin sections with three monoclonal antibodies, Leu M1, LN1 and LN2.

Leu M1 stains some Reed-Sternberg cells in some paraffin sections in the hands of some investigators (Table 4–11). The ability to obtain satisfactory staining is very much technique-related and probably very much dependent upon optimal fixation of the tissues; both formalin and B5 have been reported as giving satisfactory results. Overall, 60 to 70 percent of cases show moderate Leu M1 staining of more than 25 percent of the Hodgkin and Reed-Sternberg cells. Another 10 to 20 percent show weak reactivity or only rare positive cells, or both. In about 10 percent there is no detectable staining. In all cases, negative Reed-Sternberg cells can be seen alongside positive ones. Staining is weakest and least frequent in the lymphocyte-predominant type. Leu M1 marks cells of the monocyte-histiocyte series; the staining of Reed-Sternberg cells has been used as an argument for the histiocytic nature of these cells. In tissue sections, granulocytes stain with Leu M1, and reactive histiocytes show variable staining. The staining of Reed-Sternberg cells is usually cytoplasmic or paranu-

clear. In our experience, non-Hodgkin's lymphomas have given negative reactions. Little data is available on the pattern of reactivity of true histiocytic tumors. A positive stain for Leu M1 in multilobulate or multinucleate cells certainly raises the suspicion of Hodgkin's disease. It is, however, not of itself diagnostic; equally, a negative result does not exclude Hodgkin's disease.

LN2 is a monoclonal antibody developed by Dr. A. Epstein (Department of Pathology, University of Southern California). In normal tissues it reacts with the majority of B lymphocytes and with some histiocytes. LN2 does not stain T cells or granulocytes. It stains almost all Reed-Sternberg cells (Fig. 4–45) in nearly all cases, intensely (Table 4–11). LN2 staining is, in our experience, of real value in searching for the presence of some Reed-Sternberg cells in tissues (eg, spleen and marrow in early stage III and stage IV disease or in lymphocyte-predominant Hodgkin's disease), since the staining of these cells contrasts so markedly with the surrounding cells that they are readily located in a low-power scan. Because LN2 reacts both with B lymphocytes and histiocytes, it sheds little light upon the question of the origin of Reed-Sternberg cells.

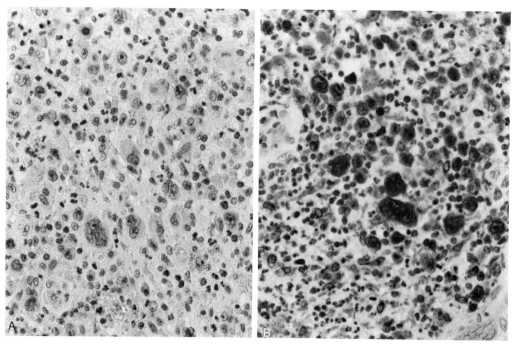

Figure 4–45. H&E section (**A**) reveals typical Hodgkin's disease with many Reed-Sternberg cell variants. These are even more clearly seen when stained for LN2 (**B**), which produces cytoplasmic and nuclear membrane staining. Paraffin section, B5 fixed, AEC with hematoxylin counterstain (×200).

LN1, by contrast, in normal lymphoid tissue stains only follicular center B lymphocytes; T cells, histiocytes, granulocytes, and other cells are nonreactive. Small and large cleaved and noncleaved cells stain in paraffin sections; staining is localized to the cell surface and the area of the Golgi apparatus. Optimal results are obtained in B5-fixed tissues, with formalin fixation giving more variable results. Many B cell lymphomas, including large cell follicular center cell lymphomas and immunoblastic sarcomas, show strong reactivity with LN1; T cell lymphomas and histiocytic tumors are nonreactive. In Hodgkin's disease the Reed-Sternberg (and Hodgkin cells) are negative in most cases of nodular sclerosis, mixed cellularity, and lymphocyte-depleted disease but are consistently positive in the lymphocyte-predominant type. In our experience positivity has been observed in all B5–fixed lymphocyte-predominant cases; in formalin-fixed material (fixed in various ways, often unknown, since many were outside referrals), results are less clear-cut, with positive reaction in more than half of the lymphocyte-predominant cases (Okon et al, 1985).

LN1 is thus a helpful diagnostic stain, facilitating recognition of the infrequent Reed-Sternberg cell variants in this form of disease and abetting the distinction of HD-LP from the other subtypes. Positivity with LN1, which otherwise stains only follicular center cells, also provides evidence suggesting that HD-LP may be a B cell–derived process, possibly closely related to the follicular center cell lymphomas. This would incidentally provide a logical explanation for the fact that HD-LP may occur in a nodular (should we say "follicular"?) form and fits in with the recent concept that "progressive transformation of reactive centers" may precede lymphocyte-predominant Hodgkin's disease (Poppema et al, 1979c).

Finally, in support of this concept, some investigators have observed that Reed-Sternberg cells show reactivity with other B cell antibodies in frozen sections (eg, B1—Linch et al, 1985; Dorreen, et al 1984; Stuart et al, 1983). This observation has also been our experience with certain anti–B cell monoclonal antibodies (eg, LYM1, prepared by Dr. A. Epstein), although most available anti–B cell reagents have in our hands shown no reactivity with Reed-Sternberg cells. It is of interest that the study of Linch et al (1985) also reported Ig gene rearrangement (a good B cell marker) in cells believed to be Reed-Sternberg cells.

5

MULTIPLE MYELOMA AND RELATED DISEASES

"Pathology has been released from the anomalous and isolated position which it has occupied for thousands of years. . . . It is no longer merely applied physiology, it has become physiology itself."

RUDOLF VIRCHOW, 1821–1902

MULTIPLE MYELOMA

Diagnosis of multiple myeloma is generally based on concurrent clinical, radiographic, and laboratory findings (serum or urinary monoclonal immunoglobulin or both and bone marrow plasmacytosis). These criteria establish the correct diagnosis in many cases, especially in more advanced disease. There are, however, cases in which a modest degree of bone marrow plasmacytosis and absence of a definite monoclonal immunoglobulin make it difficult to establish whether a plasma cell population in the bone marrow is reactive or neoplastic. The use of immunofluorescence or immunoperoxidase to demonstrate the monoclonality or polyclonality (within the limits of the definition given in the preceding chapter) of cytoplasmic immunoglobulin in the plasma cell population may be extremely useful in these situations (Table 5–1).

Immunostaining of suspected "myeloma populations" may be performed either on cell smear preparations of marrow aspirates, smeared and fixed briefly in buffered formol acetone or Baker's fixative, or upon paraffin sections of pelleted aspirates or sections of marrow biopsies. In the latter instance, attention should be paid to fixation (which should be minimal, in either formalin or, better, B5) and to decalcification (prolonged exposure to acid decalcification or EDTA may denature immunoglobulin, giving a lack of positive staining).

A monoclonal staining pattern for immunoglobulin (ie, monotypic staining—exclusively kappa or lambda light chain, with a single heavy chain) correlates well with the diagnosis of multiple myeloma, a malignant process; whereas a polyclonal staining pattern is indicative of reactive plasmacytosis. Anomalous staining patterns (ie, reactions of individual cells both with anti-kappa and anti-lambda sera) have been observed in association with poorly differentiated myelomas and in poorly fixed tissues. It has been suggested that this may reflect the synthesis of incomplete (or fragmented) light chain, which cross-reacts with the usual anti-kappa and anti-lambda antibodies, or that this phenomenon reflects an artifact of autolysis and delayed fixation. Such cases are fortunately rather rare and, in our experience, occur only in neoplastic plasma cell proliferations, not in reactive plasmacytosis.

In multiple myeloma the majority of the plasma cells within a marrow specimen show positivity for one light chain, with very few plasma cells staining for the other light chain; ie, there is a marked disturbance of the ratio of kappa-containing cells to lambda-containing cells. This ratio normally is approximately 3:2; a ration of 10:1 or 1:4 would clearly suggest neoplasia, but it is not possible to construct a rigid range of values defining neoplastic and normal populations in tissue sections. Indeed, in early disease the neoplastic change may be focal, with a localized area containing plasma cells showing a markedly abnormal kappa:lambda ratio, whereas the majority of the biopsy shows a scattering of cells with a normal "reactive" distribution of light chain types.

Although we usually screen suspected mye-

Table 5–1. Selected Bibliography: Immunohistologic Studies in Myeloma

Bartl et al 1982	Marrow biopsies in 200 myelomas, 50 benign monoclonal gammopathies, 40 reactive plasmacytoses and 20 solitary plasmacytomas—emphasizes value of immunohistologic studies
Martelli et al 1982	Marrow biopsies in myeloma
Zarrabi et al 1981	IgG myeloma; 2 cases described plus literature review
Clausen et al 1979	Marrow biopsies from 34 myelomas
Johansen & Jensen 1980	Marrow smears in 25 patients with myeloma; found some differences in pattern in benign monoclonal gammopathy but distinction not sharp
Sun et al 1979	Light chain myeloma evolving to "histiocytic lymphoma" (better classified as immunoblastic sarcoma of B cell type)
Spiers et al 1980	Meningeal myeloma
Gorin et al 1979	Nonsecretory myeloma
Tschen et al 1980	Cutaneous involvement in myeloma (see also PLASMACYTOMA)
Metz & Leder 1980	Myeloma with immunohistochemically distinct populations (some cells exclusively kappa, some exclusively gamma)
Beckstead et al 1981	Good "techniques" paper; various fixation procedures and thin sections
Biberfeld et al 1979	Circulating idiotype-positive cells (lymphocytes and lymphoplasmacytoid cells) in myeloma provide method of monitoring progress of disease
Morell et al 1978 Taylor et al 1978b Clausen et al 1979 Johansen & Jensen 1980 Pinkus & Said 1977 Taylor & Mason 1974 Taylor 1978c	Clonality—reactive versus myeloma and related conditions
Canale & Collins 1974	Morphologic features of myeloma

lomas only with anti-kappa and anti-lambda antibodies (plus controls), it is useful to remember that a borderline abnormal distribution may be further investigated by staining for heavy chain class. With monotypic (monoclonal) light chain staining, it is usually also possible to demonstrate a monoclonal pattern of staining for one of the heavy chain classes: the exception of course is in light chain disease in which heavy chains typically are absent. It should be emphasized that monoclonal plasma cells, particularly in early myeloma, are not always cytologically abnormal (ie, they may be indistinguishable from the usual Marschalko-type plasma cells and may lack the "immature" nuclei that the traditional hematopathologists believe denote and define myeloma cells); indeed, the proportion of "immature" dividing cells in early myeloma may be very small, rising only in the latter stages of the disease as the proportion of the clone in active cycle increases (Taylor, 1982a).

The preceding is simply another way of stating that a diagnosis of myeloma may be made by immunohistologic means at an earlier stage than is possible by traditional histologic methods, even when using such fine morphologic criteria as those established by Canale and Collins (1974).

Thus, in multiple myeloma the immunostaining pattern is monoclonal, contrasting with the polyclonal pattern of reactive marrow plasmacytosis (Fig. 5–1).

In benign monoclonal gammopathy, there is a plasmacytosis, usually of "mature"-appearing plasma cells, but occasionally including a sprinkling of cells with more "primitive" nuclei and nucleoli. By definition, a stable monoclonal spike (usually IgG) of less than 1.0 gm/100 ml is detectable in serum. In such cases the marrow plasma cell population shows a polyclonal distribution (ie, ratio of kappa to lambda light chain and the different heavy chains in near normal proportions) in spite of the presence of a detectable monoclonal immunoglobulin in serum. Presumably in these cases, those plasma cells responsible for the production of the monoclonal spike are distributed diffusely among the population of reactive polyclonal plasma cells in numbers that are insufficient to noticeably change the overall kappa to lambda ratio.

In myeloma it is the suppression of a background of reactive polyclonal plasma cells that is a characteristic feature; this suppression of course permits a more ready visualization of the monoclonal neoplastic population. To put it another way, in multiple myeloma the kappa or lambda monoclonal

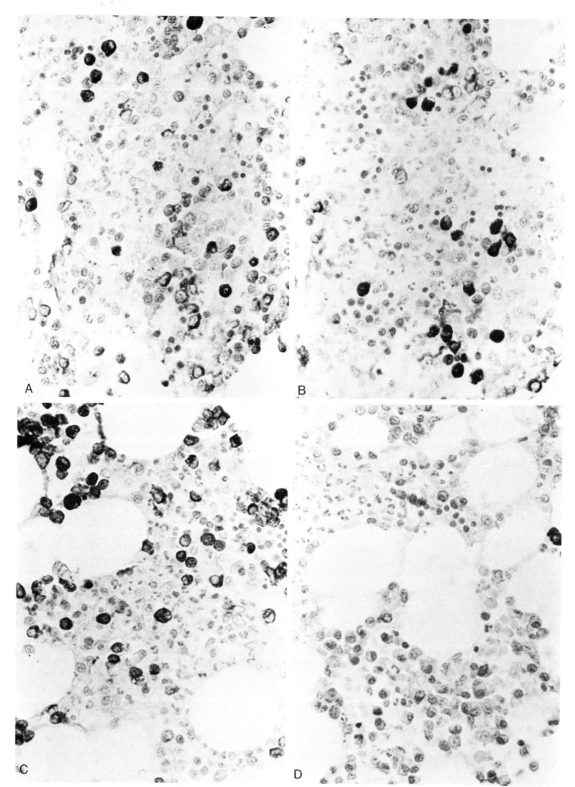

Figure 5–1. Two cases of bone marrow plasmacytosis, neither fulfilling the Canale-Collins criteria for myeloma. *A* and *B* show first case stained for kappa and lambda respectively. Positive (black) cells are revealed in approximately equal numbers with both antisera. In spite of the fact that some of the plasma cells have large nucleoli and appear "blastic," this probably is a reactive population (i.e., admixture of kappa and lambda cells). Contrast this observation with *C* and *D*, again stained for kappa (*C*) and lambda (*D*) light chains. There is marked predominance of kappa positive cells (*C*) and a dearth of lambda positive cells (*D*, only one positive cell). This predominance of one light chain, particularly with the relative lack of the alternate light chain, strongly suggests myeloma. Paraffin sections, DAB with hematoxylin counterstain (×200).

118

cells usually involve 90 to 100 percent of the cytoplasmic immunoglobulin-containing cells, regardless of the degree of bone marrow plasmacytosis and the level of the serum monoclonal pattern.

In the great majority of cases of multiple myeloma, the light chain type and heavy chain class, as determined in myelomatous tissues by immunoperoxidase procedures, correspond to the serum, to the urine monoclonal protein type, or to both. In light chain disease, however, it is sometimes possible to demonstrate both light and heavy chains within the myeloma cells in spite of the fact that only light chain is detectable in the serum. This immunohistologic finding has been interpreted as a partial loss of functional organization of the neoplastic plasmacytes (ie, failure to secrete heavy-chain component into the serum). Nonsecretory myeloma may represent the extreme manifestation of this phenomenon; in this condition other features typical of myeloma are present, but it is not possible to identify a monoclonal paraprotein, despite careful study of both the serum and urine. In these nonsecretory myelomas, the diagnosis is established by a combination of marrow examination, radiographic findings, and clinical features. If the clinical presentation is atypical or if the neoplastic cells are undifferentiated by light microscopy, the differential diagnosis between a nonsecretory plasma cell dyscrasia and carcinomatous or leukemic infiltration of the bone marrow, with associated skeletal destruction, may be extremely difficult. Immunohistologic demonstration of a monoclonal intracytoplasmic immunoglobulin within the "undifferentiated" cells is then of great value in recognizing the plasmacytic character of the neoplastic population. Immunocytologic investigations have permitted the recognition of two types of nonsecretory myelomas: those that do not synthesize immunoglobulin components ("nonproducers," ie, cells containing no detectable immunoglobulin) and those that apparently do synthesize some immunoglobulin but do not secrete it in detectable amounts (ie, cells containing detectable immunoglobulin by immunocytochemical methods [Fig. 5–2]). In these cases of "true" nonsecretory myeloma, the diagnosis may be established by immunohistologic staining; the monoclonal cytoplasmic immunoglobulin is mostly of IgG-kappa type, and the neoplastic plasma cells typically stain more intensely (brightly) for gamma heavy chain than for kappa light chain. Intracytoplasmic IgM has been detected by the immunofluorescence method in at least one case of nonsecretory myeloma.

In more usual cases of multiple myeloma, the neoplastic plasma cells contain IgG with either kappa or lambda light chain; IgA myeloma is encountered less often, followed in frequency by cases with the immunohistologic pattern of light-chain disease. Intracytoplasmic IgM has also been detected by immunocytochemical techniques in patients with typical multiple myeloma (typical classi-

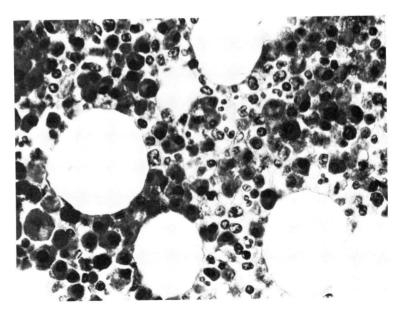

Figure 5–2. "Nonsecretory" myeloma showing intense cytoplasmic (black) staining of large plasmacytic cells in bone marrow for alpha chain (IgG-kappa). Paraffin section, DAB with hematoxylin counterstain (×320).

cal features, multiple lytic bone lesions, and morphologic myeloma–type plasma cells in the marrow). These patients have been reported in the past literature as cases of Waldenström's macroglobulinemia with associated osteolytic lesions and hypercalcemia. They are, however, distinct from the usual cases of Waldenström's disease, which are associated with a different morphologic type of cell proliferation, namely a malignant lymphoma (plasmacytoid lymphocytic lymphoma) involving primarily extramedullary tissues, rather than with a marrow-centered plasma cell proliferation. It should be realized that typical multiple myeloma may occasionally secrete IgM, just as morphologically typical plasmacytoid lymphocytic lymphoma may produce IgG or IgA in lieu of the usual IgM. The distinction between these related lesions should be made on the basis of the cytology of the cells, the distri-

bution of the lesions, and the clinical picture, rather than on the class of immunoglobulin produced. The class of immunoglobulin produced will of course determine the risk of hyperviscosity syndrome (macroglobulinemia), regardless of morphologic cell type.

Immunoglobulin-Containing Cells in Reactive Tissue

The same techniques that have been employed for the recognition of neoplastic immunoglobulin-containing cells in myeloma and some of the B cell lymphomas have been successfully employed for the study of reactive immunoglobulin-containing cells (primarily plasma cells) in a variety of tissues. Selected studies are summarized in Tables 5–2 and 5–3. It should be noted that most of the studies are informational-investigative and that they contribute little to diagnosis

Table 5–2. Selected Bibliography: Immunoglobulin (Ig)-Containing Cells in Normal and Reactive Tissues, Including "Auto-Immune" Diseases

Nijhuis-Heddes et al 1982	Ig cells in respiratory mucosa in disease
Ali et al 1979	IgE-positive cells in adenoids and tonsils
Marmar et al 1981	Plasma (Ig positive) cell scores in cervical biopsies in evaluation of infertility
Matthews & Basu 1982	Ig heavy chains and J chain in tonsils; secretory component absent in tonsillar epithelium
Tsunoda et al 1980	Surface marker study of expression of germinal centers from tonsil; predominantly B cells
Newell et al 1980	EM localization of Ig in lymphoid cells (restricted saponin digestion of GA-fixed cell suspension); Ig observed in perinuclear space, rough endoplasmic reticulum (ER), and Golgi area
Curran et al 1982	Study of human reactive lymph nodes, Ig distribution
Straus 1981	Study of phases of production of specific antibody to HRP, following injection of HRP antigen in mice
Callihan & Jaffe 1980	Identification of crystal deposits as Ig
Matthews 1983	Ig in Russell bodies
Martin et al 1980	IgM deposits in arteries of giant cell arteritis
Schmidt et al 1980	PAP more sensitive than fluorescence for detection of antiplatelet IgG antibodies
Fritz et al 1980	Distinguished osteoarthritis from rheumatoid arthritis by immunoglobulin deposition in joint capsule in the latter
Inouet et al 1979	Lupus pneumonitis—immunoglobulin deposition in the interstitium of the alveolar walls and in alveolar capillaries by fluorescence and immunoperoxidase at light and EM; C3 and DNA also present in these immune complexes
Hasselbacher 1979 ⎫ Hasselbacher et al 1980 ⎭	Antigen-induced arthritis (in rabbits) as a model for rheumatoid arthritis, using egg albumin/antibody complexes
Boyer et al 1980	Ig deposits in choroid plexus in patients with lupus or rheumatoid arthritis
Fulthorpe & Hudgson 1982	IgG- and IgM-positive cells in polymyositis
Esiri 1980	Immunoglobulin-containing cells in poliomyelitis
Newell et al 1982	Ultrastructural study demonstrating sites of Ig production in perinuclear membrane, rough ER, and Golgi membranes
Fleischer et al 1980	Immunocytochemical analysis of the cellular response to parotid gland carcinomas
Wijesinha & Steer 1982	Studied "defunctioning" colostomies and concluded that the presence of large numbers of plasma cells is dependent upon continued antigenic stimulation

Table 5–3. Selected Bibliography: Immunoglobulins in Gut

Brown WR 1980	IgA across colonic epithelium
Hsu & Hsu 1980	IgA and secretor piece in hepatocytes
Crifò & Russo 1980	IgA across nasal mucosa
Jos et al 1979	IgA and secretor piece in jejunum
Isaacson 1982b	IgA, secretor piece, and J chain in gut and in carcinoma
Rosekrans et al 1980a ⎱	Plasma cells in gut and food allergy
Perkkiö 1980 ⎰	
Perkkiö and Savilahti 1980	Development of plasma cells in neonatal gut
Seo et al 1982	Immunomorphologic study of gut lymphoma
Rosekrans et al 1980b	Plasma cells in ulcerative colitis and Crohn's disease
Togo et al 1981	Immunoglobulins and secretor piece; secretor piece positive in 45% of cancer cases
Isaacson 1982a	Comprehensive study of Ig-positive cells in normal dysplastic and neoplastic colon; secretory component appeared increased in epithelium of ulcerative colitis but reduced in areas of precancerous dysplasia and in cancer; the number of IgA-positive plasma cells showed a correlation with staining for secretory component, suggesting that one may induce the other
Morise 1982	Ig cells in gastric cancer and metaplasia
Rosekrans et al 1980c	Allergic proctitis distinguished by many IgE-positive cells
Kingston et al 1981	Plasma (Ig positive) cell counts in jejunal biopsies
Rosekrans et al 1981	Ig-positive cells (IgM in jejunal biopsies) increased in active phase gluten enteropathy

other than to separate the "monoclonal" conditions.

One interpretative problem should be considered: namely, that macrophages (histiocytes) may contain significant amounts of immunoglobulin, especially if immune complexes are present (Fig. 5–3). Individual histiocytes contain both kappa and lambda light chains, whereas individual reactive plasma cells, like neoplastic cells, contain either kappa or lambda, not both. Finally, degenerating cells, normal or neoplastic, suffer a relative and progressive loss of surface membrane integrity and may permit the passive passage of serum protein into the cytoplasm: such cells may stain for immunoglobulin (both kappa and lambda in single cells). The presence of albumin or other serum protein in the cells provides a clue to this being a passive leakage phenomenon. A number of investigators therefore "routinely" stain one parallel section with antialbumin antibody as a control, seeking to reveal the extent of leakage within a particular section under

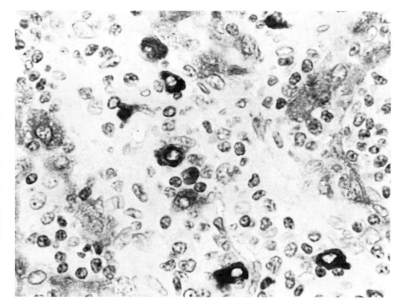

Figure 5–3. Medullary sinuses and cords of lymph node depicting intense staining (black) for IgG in plasma cells and weak granular staining (gray) in sinus histiocytes. The former staining is believed to represent synthesis, the latter, phagocytosis (of immune complexes). These appearances are quite distinctive under the microscope and with experience will rarely cause confusion in normal cells, although in neoplastic cells the problem is more difficult. Paraffin section, AEC with hematoxylin counterstain (×750).

study (see discussion of anomalous staining in the preceding chapter).

PLASMACYTOMAS (AND EXTRAMEDULLARY MYELOMA)

Extramedullary "plasmacytomas" often represent secondary deposits of multiple myeloma, but primary extramedullary plasmacytomas do occur.

Isolated plasmacytomas (not associated with myelomas) are most often located in the upper respiratory tract, although various body sites may be involved. Usually neither detectable serum, nor urinary monoclonal immunoglobulin is present, probably owing to the small size of the tumor cell mass (insufficient secreting cells to produce a level of monoclonal immunoglobulin detectable above normal serum content). Occasionally, however, a monoclonal spike may be present; it usually disappears after surgical removal or radiation therapy of the tumor mass.

When a well-differentiated (ie, consisting of mature "normal"-appearing plasma cells) plasmacytoma primarily involves lymph node, it must be distinguished from benign conditions in which a high number of plasma cells are found, including lymphadenopathy associated with rheumatoid disease, the plasma cell variant of giant lymph node hyperplasia (Castleman's disease), various chronic immune reactions (eg, syphilis), and abnormal immune responses.

If the plasmacellular lesion is poorly differentiated (ie, composed of cells that morphologically show little resemblance to plasma cells or indeed any other normal cell—anaplastic), it may be misdiagnosed as granulocytic sarcoma or undifferentiated carcinoma. Assuming some discernible morphologic resemblance to plasma cells or immature plasma cells, some pathologists would classify such a lesion as poorly differentiated plasmacytoma. Others would dub it immunoblastic sarcoma of B cell type. In my view, these are two names for the same thing: I prefer the latter (vide infra; see also Fig. 4–7).

In all of these situations, the identification of a monoclonal pattern of staining for immunoglobulin by immunoperoxidase techniques establishes both the plasmacellular nature of the lesion and its neoplastic character (Fig. 5–4). Similar criteria may be utilized to differentiate plasmacytoma of the respiratory

or gastrointestinal tract from so-called plasma cell granulomas, the latter consisting of an admixture of reactive plasma cells of kappa or lambda light chain type and various heavy chain classes (Table 5–4).

It should be noted, however, that plasma cell variants of Castleman's disease may rarely be associated with a monoclonal plasma cell reaction (Fig. 5–5); such a finding raises the index of suspicion for an eventual neoplastic outcome, but cases have not been followed for a sufficient length of time to predict the long-term course. In one reported case of primary plasmacytoma of the lymph node, both neoplastic plasma cells and infiltrating macrophages contained crystalline inclusions consisting of the same monotypic immunoglobulin as the serum paraprotein (IgG-kappa; Addis et al, 1980); presumably, the macrophages had phagocytosed immunoglobulin released by dying myeloma cells; we too have observed this phenomenon in several cases. Occasionally, the "crystals" are to be seen within the large neoplastic plasma cells (Fig. 5–6).

Assessment of clonality may also be extremely useful in patients with solitary myeloma of the bone in which one solitary lytic lesion may be detected and shown histologically to be a plasma cell tumor, with no evidence of other lytic lesions or bone marrow plasmacytosis and no serologic or urinary abnormalities. In such cases, biopsies of "uninvolved" marrow may be examined by immunohistologic techniques in order to rule out the presence of a sparse infiltrate of monoclonal cells throughout the marrow (ie, the case is truly multiple myeloma, with more extensive growth in one focal area).

Solitary plasmacytoma, as distinct from an extramedullary deposit of multiple myeloma, undoubtedly exists and indeed has in the past been underdiagnosed owing to difficulties in distinction on morphologic grounds from plasma cell granuloma (Table 5–4). By immunohistologic techniques solitary "well-differentiated" plasmacytoma is readily identifiable and is apparently a relatively benign lesion. In a few cases, we have observed progression to a more aggressive lesion, immunoblastic sarcoma of the B cell type. This simply represents a shift in the kinetics of the monoclonal B cell (plasma cell population) toward a greater proportion of cells in the dividing phase of the cell cycle (ie, immunoblasts); this shift inevitably alters the morphology (because of the increased pro-

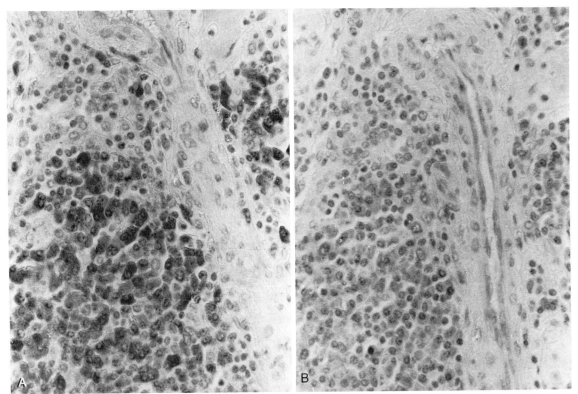

Figure 5–4. *A*, Plasmacytoma showing monoclonal staining pattern, positive for IgA-kappa and *B*, negative for IgG, IgM, and lambda chain. Paraffin section, DAB with hematoxylin counterstain (×200).

Table 5–4. Selected Bibliography: Immunohistologic Studies of Plasmacytoma

Soffer & Siegal 1982	Dural plasmacytoma
Hara et al 1979	Gastrointestinal plasmacytoma in a transplant patient: multiple lesions
Humphrey et al 1982a	Pharyngeal plasmacytoma; value of monoclonal pattern
Gleason & Hammar 1982	Colonic plasmacytoma (lambda only), in a 10-year-old
Rygaard-Olsen et al 1982	Small intestinal plasmacytoma, local reaction, no recurrence at 5 years
Seddon et al 1982	Conjunctival plasmacytoma
Aufdemonte & Humphrey 1982	Mandibular plasmacytoma (in a patient with myeloma)
Okada et al 1982	Bronchial plasmacytoma; no paraprotein
Addis et al 1980	Lymph nodal plasmacytoma; with crystalline inclusion in macrophages
Urbanski et al 1980	Intrasellar plasmacytoma; solitary lesion, death in 3 years
Toccanier et al 1982	9 cases of plasma cell "granuloma" of lung
Edwards and Zawadzki 1967	Extraosseous lesions in myeloma
Pasmantier & Azar 1969	Extraosseous lesion in myeloma
Wiltshaw 1976	Primary plasmacytoma—review
Sun et al 1979	Poorly differentiated plasmacytoma
York et al 1981	"Monoclonality" in Castleman lesion
Falini et al 1982b	Myeloma evolving to immunoblastic sarcoma
Holt & Robb-Smith 1973	Evolution of myeloma to sarcoma (would term this immunoblastic sarcoma)
Taylor 1978c	Changing concepts in lymphoma classification—review
Taylor 1982a	Pathobiology of lymphocyte transformation—review
Kirshenbaum & Rhone 1985	Plasmacytoma of breast

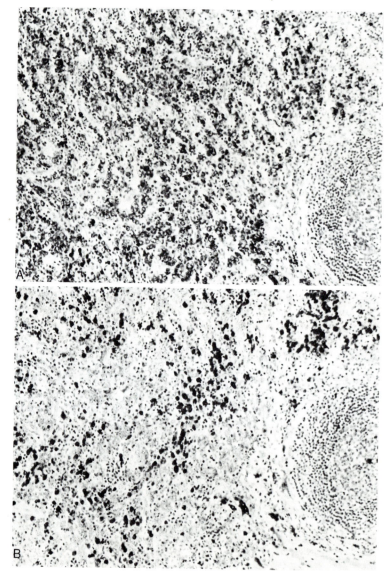

Figure 5–5. Diagnosis of giant lymph node hyperplasia, plasmacellular type (Castleman-Iverson lesion—for further description see Robb-Smith and Taylor, 1981). Typical hyperplastic reactive follicles are present (lower right). Most of the plasma cells reacted with anti-lambda antibody (*A*); only about 15% reacted with anti-kappa antibody (*B*). This marked predominance of lambda over kappa (6:1—the normal is 2:3) suggests the development of a monoclonal proliferation, presumably neoplastic (remember it could be a "benign" plasmacytoma or lymphoma). Some of these cases may evolve to frank lymphoma (usually immunoblastic sarcoma); the outcome in others is not known. Paraffin sections, DAB with hematoxylin counterstain (×125). The follicles show a reactive (polyclonal) pattern, somewhat analogous to the situation in mantle zone lymphoma (Chapter 3).

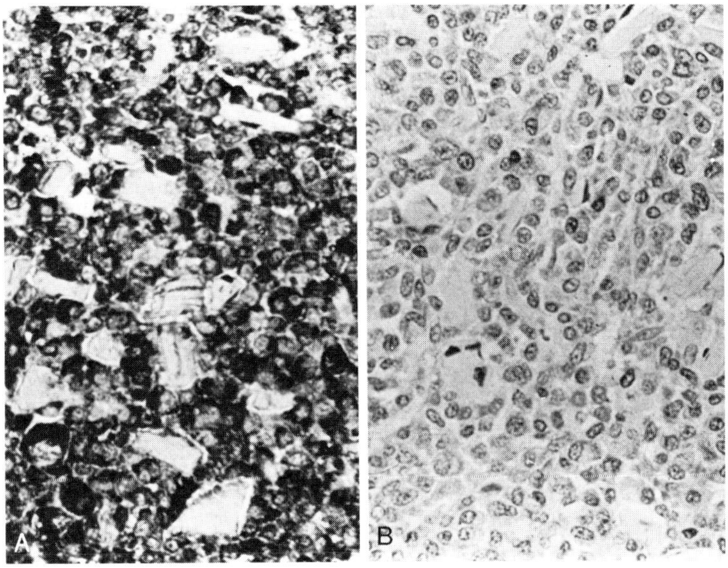

Figure 5–6. Immunoblastic sarcoma of B cell type. The large plasmacytoid immunoblasts react intensely with anti-kappa antibody (**A**), but not at all with anti-lambda antibody (**B**). Peculiar crystals, well seen in **A**, do not stain for kappa, except slightly at edges. Paraffin sections, DAB with hematoxylin counterstain (×200).

portion of cells with the "immature" nuclei, typifying late steps of the cell cycle) much as may occur in myeloma (vide infra). Other cases of apparently solitary plasmacytomas are later found to be associated with myeloma, either at diagnosis or during the course of the disease; the presence of coexistent myeloma should always be sought by immunohistologic staining of marrow biopsies from patients with "solitary" plasmacytoma. Still other cases remain localized and relatively benign, without associated multiple myeloma. Finally, we have observed rare cases consisting of "well-differentiated" plasma cells embedded in pink "amyloid" (congo red–positive) material—examples of amyloid tumors; on examination of such cases, diffuse marrow involvement by monoclonal plasma cells may sometimes be demonstrated (Fig. 5–7, A to F). Immunohistologic studies are critical in defining these lesions as has been emphasized in many recent reports (Table 5–4).

UNDIFFERENTIATED MYELOMA, ANAPLASTIC MYELOMA, RETICULUM CELL SARCOMA, IMMUNOBLASTIC SARCOMA OF B CELL TYPE, AND RELATED DISEASES

The appearance, during the course of multiple myeloma or plasmacytoma, of large masses with sarcomatous characteristics, with or without infiltration of the bone marrow or adjacent connective tissues by highly anaplastic cells resembling "reticulum cells," is a phenomenon well known to pathologists (Table 5–4). Histologically, these lesions may or may not show recognizable plasmacytoid features, but immunohistologically, they have been shown to contain the same monoclonal cytoplasmic immunoglobulin that is present within the original myeloma cell population and in the serum or urine or both (Figs 4–7, 5–6, and 5–8).

Morphologic and immunohistologic investigations support the concept that these tumors, described in the past literature as reticulum cell sarcoma, plasmacytic reticulum cell sarcoma, plasma cell sarcoma, histiocytic lymphoma, and dysplastic myeloma are all examples of a single phenomenon best termed immunoblastic sarcoma of B cell type (Fig. 5–9; Falini et al, 1982b), arising de novo or supervening upon a preexisting B lymphocyte neoplasm—namely, multiple myeloma or, less often, plasmacytoma. As such, these tumors represent a metamorphosis of the original myeloma process rather than the emergence of a second genealogically unrelated neoplasm suggested by some authors. This point of view is in agreement with the modern concepts concerning the histogenesis of multiple myeloma (Taylor, 1978c, 1982b) and its close relationship to other B cell neoplasms (Fig. 5–10). It is now believed that in multiple myeloma the actively dividing cell responsible for the perpetuation and expansion of the neoplastic clone is the transformed B lymphocyte or immunoblast (some

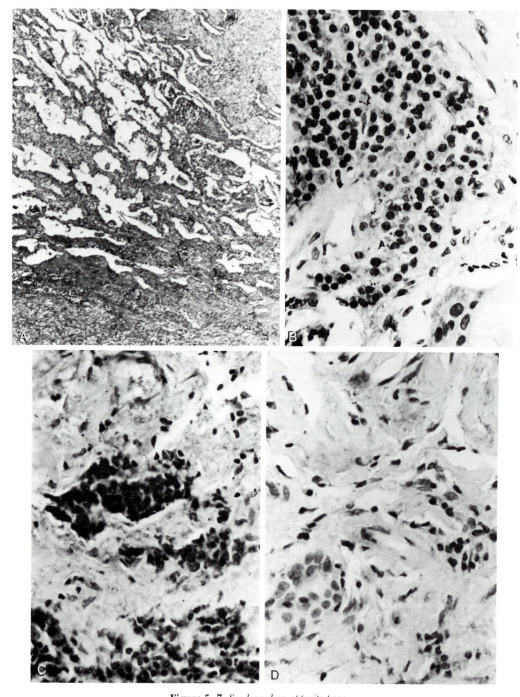

Figure 5–7. *See legend on opposite page*

Illustration continued on opposite page

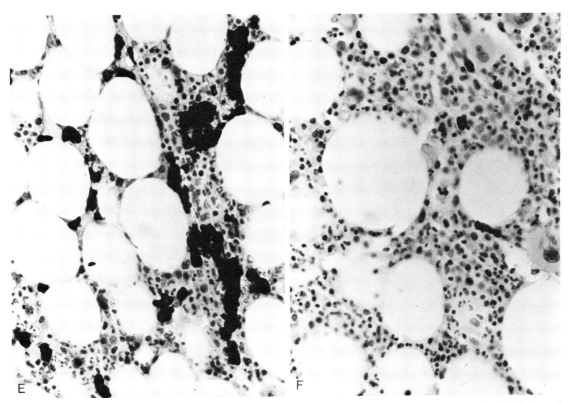

Figure 5–7. Case 116-81: Amyloid tumor of lung. H&E sections showing part of a small solitary dumbbell-shaped lung nodule (**A**) that gave the histochemical staining reactions for amyloid and contained clusters of mature-appearing plasma cells (**B**) with occasional foreign body giant cells (**A**, ×60; **B**, ×320). **C**, Immunoperoxidase stain of "tumor" shows clusters of lambda-positive (black) cells with **D** a singular lack of kappa-staining cells (monoclonal or monotypic pattern suggesting a neoplastic plasma cell population). **C**, The amyloid itself shows patchy granular staining for lambda. Paraffin sections, AEC with hematoxylin counterstain (×320). **E**, Section of B5 fixed bone marrow aspirate shows a number of intensely stained lambda positive cells scattered within the marrow. **F** is the adjacent parallel section stained for kappa chain showing only a single positive plasma cell. Although the morphologic features alone do not permit a diagnosis of myeloma, the monoclonal (monotypic) pattern strongly suggests the diagnosis. It is the lack of the alternate light chain (in this case kappa) that is particularly persuasive. Paraffin sections, AEC with hematoxylin counterstain (×200). This stain demonstrates marrow involvement in what initially was thought to be a solitary lung lesion (amyloid tumor).

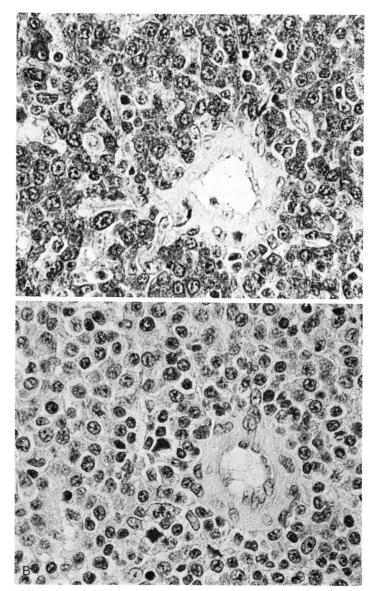

Figure 5–8. Immunoblastic sarcoma (B cell type) with pronounced plasmacytic features; in the presence of known myeloma, this might equally well be termed "poorly differentiated myeloma." *A*, Anti-kappa antibody produces intense reactivity, whereas anti-lambda antibody *B*, is nonreactive—a so-called "monoclonal" pattern. Paraffiin section, DAB with hematoxylin counterstain (×320). Tumor was present in lymph node; there was a prior history of myeloma "in remission." The myeloma protein type was identical to that detected in the immunoblastic sarcoma, as usually is the case.

Figure 5–9. Anaplastic large cell tumor classified as immunoblastic sarcoma of B cell type on the basis of content of "monoclonal" immunoglobulin (IgG-kappa). Paraffin section, DAB with hematoxylin counterstain (×320). This case was in the Oxford files as "reticulum cell sarcoma"; it could equally well have been termed histiocytic lymphoma by others, or poorly differentiated extramedullary myeloma if developing in a patient with pre-existing myeloma. Such lesions have commonly been misdiagnosed as carcinoma (see Chapter 14).

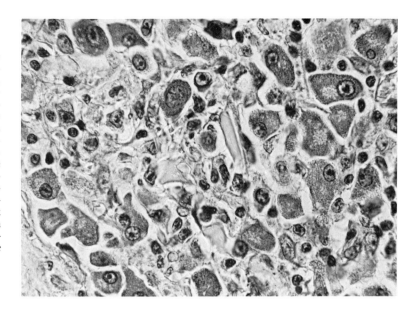

might term it a plasmablast). In the bone marrow of patients with typical multiple myeloma, these immunoblasts constitute only a small portion of the neoplastic population and are intermingled with the predominant population of myeloma (plasma) cells (for which the tumor is named) and a small number of lymphocytes, some of which also belong to the neoplastic clone (Fig. 5–10). These morphologically innocuous small lymphocytes circulate in the peripheral blood of myeloma patients, where they are indistinguishable from normal small lymphocytes unless special techniques are used (Biberfeld

Figure 5–10. Diagrammatic representation of cell types in four morphologically diverse B cell lymphomas (CLL, chronic lymphocytic leukemia; FCC, follicular center cell lymphoma; IBS, immunoblastic sarcoma of B cell type, and myeloma). A simplified schematic representing the different forms that the B cell takes during transformation and maturation to the plasma cell is given at the top; small lymphocyte → follicular center cell → immunoblast → plasma cell. The radically different morphologic appearances of these lymphomas can be explained by postulating that each proliferation consists of B cells but that the predominant phase of the maturation process differs as depicted in the graphs. (Reprinted from Taylor CR, Parker JW, Pattengale PK, et al. Malignant lymphomas: an exercise in immunopathology. *In* Advances in Medical Oncology, Research, and Education. Proceedings of the 12th International Cancer Congress, Buenos Aires, 1978. Vol VII, Leukemia and Non-Hodgkin Lymphoma, DG Crowther, ed. Elmstead, N.Y., Pergamon Press, 1978. See also Taylor 1980a)

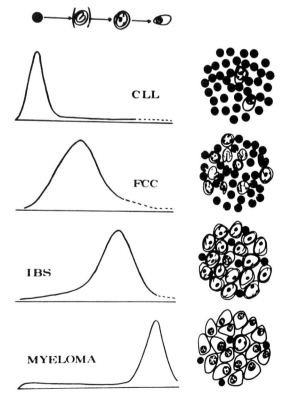

CLL

FCC

IBS

MYELOMA

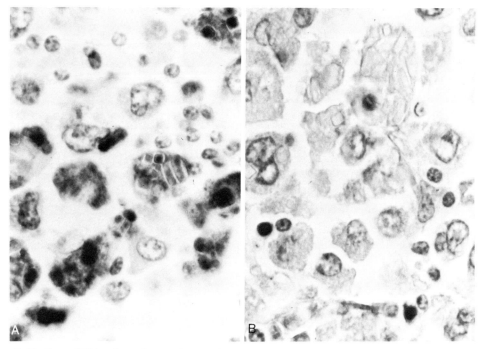

Figure 5–11. Case of Richter's syndrome, CLL evolving to an aggressive large cell tumor (immunoblastic sarcoma). The large bizarre cells contain rod and brick-shaped crystalline inclusions that stain for lambda chain, **A**, but not kappa chain, **B**. The CLL population expressed SIg of lambda type, suggesting that both CLL cells and immunoblasts belong to the same neoplastic clone. For discussion see Taylor 1982a. Paraffin sections, DAB with hematoxylin counterstain (×650).

et al, 1979). It is thus proposed that the morphologic change to B immunoblastic sarcoma (formerly reticulum cell sarcoma) is the result of the increase in the number of these immunoblasts, which in turn produces a change in the overall histologic picture (Falini et al, 1982b; see reviews, Taylor, 1978c, 1982a).

The progression of multiple myeloma to B immunoblastic sarcoma represents a transition from a low-turnover neoplasm (with few dividing cells) to a kinetically more aggressive tumor of transformed lymphocytes or B immunoblasts (dividing cells), with a correspondingly poor prognosis. Progression of CLL to Richter's syndrome is analogous (Fig. 5–11).

As noted above, in many cases of myeloma, it has been possible to demonstrate that some of the circulating normal-appearing small lymphocytes belong to the myeloma clone (Biberfeld et al, 1979). This relationship was shown by preparing an antibody to the myeloma protein, specific for the variable end of the molecule (anti-idiotype), and demonstrating that this anti-idiotype antibody reacted with the SIg of some small lymphocytes in the peripheral blood. Furthermore, following

stripping, these small lymphocytes were able to resynthesize this same SIg. Myeloma is thus revealed as a B cell clonal proliferation containing diverse morphologic forms (small lymphocytes, immunoblasts, and plasma cells) in which plasma cells predominate.

PLASMACYTOID LYMPHOCYTIC LYMPHOMA

Plasmacytoid lymphocytic lymphoma represents a B cell proliferation in which the neoplastic cells show some differentiation toward immunoglobulin-secreting plasma cells; however, the degree and extent of plasma cell differentiation falls short of that observed in multiple myeloma or in plasmacytoma. According to the schema of B cell maturation and differentiation presented earlier, one would postulate an arrest at the IgM stage prior to the "heavy chain" switching necessary to produce IgG and IgA. Typically, the critical cells have nuclei more closely resembling those of lymphocytes than those of plasma cells, but the cytoplasm is more extensive and more basophilic than that of small

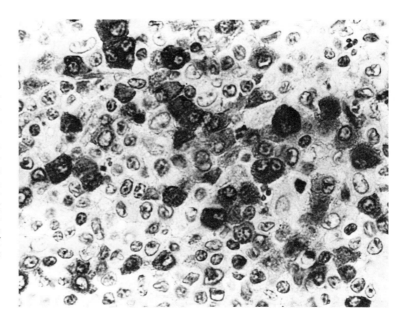

Figure 5–12. Monoclonal plasma cells, stained for lambda chain (gray-black), in an "unclassifiable" B cell lymphoma showing mixed features of follicular center cell tumor, plasmacytoid lymphocytic lymphoma, plasmacytoma, and immunoblastic sarcoma. Paraffin section, DAB with hematoxylin counterstain (×500). This is an example of a B cell lymphoma lacking predominance of any particular form of B cell, thus making classification difficult; minor degrees of morphologic admixture are common in lymphomas if searched for by immunologic methods.

lymphocytes, giving a "lymphoplasmacytoid" appearance; a variable admixture of small lymphocytes, plasma cells, and immunoblasts is also typically present. Thus, this also is a "multimorphic" process, like myeloma, in which the clone contains B cells at several different stages of maturation (Fig. 5–12).

A monoclonal staining pattern is observed in a high percentage of cases. In the great majority, the heavy chain class is IgM; in a lesser number of cases, IgA or IgG has been demonstrated, in each case corresponding to the serum monoclonal protein class. In these cases the majority of the immunoglobulin-containing cells are of plasmacytoid type (Fig. 5–13), but the proportion of these cells varies greatly in different tumors. Positive cytoplasmic staining of small lymphocytes is usually not observed in paraffin sections, although immunoblasts, plasma cells, and cells with intermediate morphology (ie, the lymphoplasmacytoid cells) do show staining. In frozen sections, however, the small lymphocytes present in the mixture appear to bear detectable surface immunoglobulin with a monoclonal staining pattern matching that

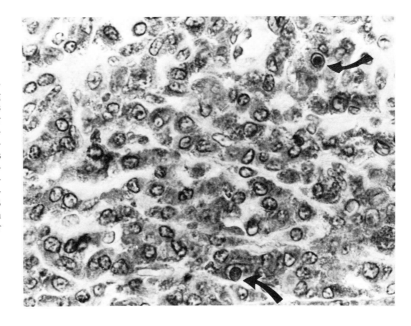

Figure 5–13. Plasmacytic tumor stained for IgM depicting cytoplasmic reactivity (gray) plus Dutcher bodies (intranuclear black globules—arrows). This tumor produced IgM and hyperviscosity but morphologically was not the classic plasmacytoid lymphocytic lymphoma that is usually associated with this condition. Paraffin section, DAB with hematoxylin counterstain (×320). Two obvious Dutcher bodies are present (arrows).

seen in the cytoplasm of the more plasmacytoid cellular component.

The neoplastic clone thus is of B cell origin but consists of a variable mixture of lymphocytes, lymphoplasmacytoid cells, plasma cells, and immunoblasts. In frozen sections stained with anti–T cell antibodies, positive cells (T cells) may be seen in surprisingly large numbers within tissue that morphologically had been judged to be totally involved by the B cell neoplasm.

In lymphoplasmacytoid lymphocytic lymphoma, it is not unusual to find a certain percentage of cells with intranuclear inclusions (Dutcher bodies, Fig. 5–13). Immunofluorescence and immunoperoxidase staining have shown that Dutcher bodies are composed of immunoglobulin and represent invaginations of immunoglobulin-rich cytoplasm into the nucleus. These inclusions, like the intracytoplasmic immunoglobulin, mark monoclonally for light chain and usually also for IgM (Fig. 5–13), although staining for other heavy chains has been described. The percentage of positively stained Dutcher bodies is variable. A certain percentage of cells may contain a central unstained nuclear vac-

uole; this vacuole probably reflects loss of reactivity of immunoglobulin contained in the vacuole, or alternatively, it may reflect loss of immunoglobulin from the vacuole during processing or sectioning.

Once again it is important to recognize that the histologic picture of plasmacytoid lymphocytic lymphoma, once considered typical of Waldenström's macroglobulinemia, has been seen in patients with IgG (Fig. 5–14), IgA, and IgD monoclonal gammopathy in addition to the more typical and much more common IgM-producing cases. It is the physical nature of the secreted IgM that leads to the manifestations of Waldenström's disease (macroglobulinemia). Apparent nonsecretory cases and cases of light chain disease with similar morphologic features have also been recognized by immunohistologic studies (Table 5–5).

Plasmacytoid lymphocytic lymphoma is related to chronic lymphocytic leukemia of B cell type. As discussed in Chapter 4, the distinction between these two diseases is usually based on the degree to which the neoplastic clone circulates and the number of plasma cells and plasmacytoid lymphocytes

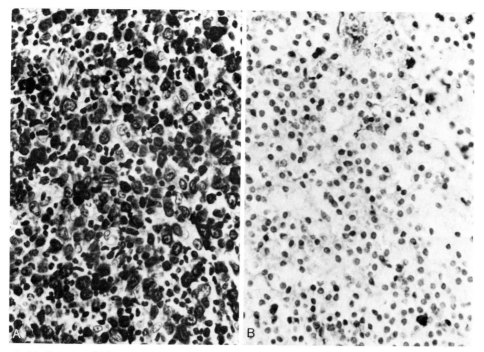

Figure 5–14. Plasmacytoid lymphocytic lymphoma producing IgG. Numerous plasmacytoid and plasmacytic cells show positive reactivity for gamma chain (**A**); staining for mu chain in a parallel section shows only one or two positive cells (**B**—residual normal plasma cells). Paraffin sections, DAB with hematoxylin counterstain (×200). Note the admixture of different forms of the B cell; this form of lymphoma most often produces IgM and may result in hyperviscosity (Waldenström's) syndrome.

Table 5–5. Selected Bibliography: Plasmacytoid Lymphocytic Lymphoma

Pangalis et al 1980	Well-differentiated lymphocytic lymphoma (CLL) and plasma cells
Tabilio et al 1981	Light chain plasmacytoid lymphocytic lymphoma
Boyd 1980	Immunostaining of Dutcher bodies
Brisbane et al 1981	Orbital lymphoma
Astarita et al 1980	Orbital lymphoma
Levine et al 1980	IgG, IgA, and IgM in lymphoplasmacytoid lymphomas
Alberti & Neiman 1984	Partially follicular variant

observed in the lesions; it has become obvious that morphologic assessment alone leads to gross underestimation of the number of plasma cells or plasmacytoid cells present, leading to a falsely high number of cases diagnosed as CLL. If immunohistologic techniques are employed (Pangalis et al, 1980), then a diagnosis of plasmacytoid lymphocytic lymphoma, as opposed to CLL or small lymphocytic lymphoma, may be made more often. It will also be recognized that many cases of plasmacytoid lymphocytic lymphoma are associated with a lymphoplasmacytoid cell leukemia or a chronic lymphocytic leukemia if plasmacytoid features are slight. Clearly, the distinction between these two conditions is somewhat arbitrary, since they do represent a continuous spectrum (Taylor, 1982a); however, the opposite poles do show different clinical and prognostic features, and in this respect immunohistologic staining provides a valuable means of making the distinction.

The distinction of IgM-producing plasmacytoid lymphocytic lymphoma from the rarer case of multiple myeloma–producing IgM has been discussed with respect to myeloma; the distinction is made, not on the type or class of immunoglobulin produced, but on the basis of cytologic appearances (Fig. 5–15) and clinicopathologic features, including the principal sites of the lesions.

Plasmacytoid lymphocytic lymphoma is a frequently observed histologic picture in orbital or adnexal lymphomas. On histologic criteria alone, the "error rate" in the differential diagnosis of this kind of extranodal lymphoma from benign "pseudolymphomatous" lesions is estimated to lie between 20 and 50 percent. Assessment of the monoclon-

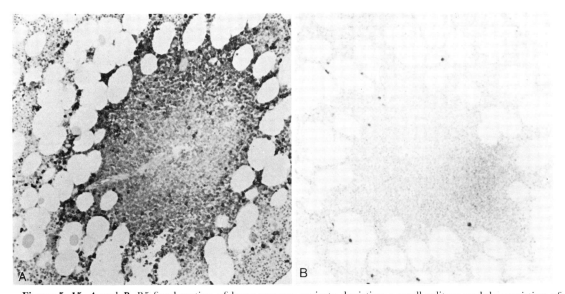

Figure 5–15. *A* and *B*, B5-fixed section of bone marrow aspirate depicting a small solitary nodule consisting of lymphocytes and occasional plasmacytoid lymphocytes, with scattered plasma cells around it. Many of the lymphoid and plasmacytoid cells reacted strongly with anti-lambda antibody (*A*). Anti-kappa reacted only with scattered plasma cells outside the nodule (*B*, small black dots). This patient eventually was shown to have a solitary plasmacytoid lymphocytic lymphoma in the small intestine (also lambda type). Paraffin sections, DAB with hematoxylin counterstain (×125). There was no serum paraprotein detectable at this time; presumably the number of tumor cells was insufficient for production of a detectable paraprotein; however, a "monoclonal" IgM appeared later in the course.

ality or otherwise of the lymphoid population may provide conclusive evidence of the neoplastic or reactive nature of the lesion. The superiority of immunohistologic investigation (in paraffin and frozen sections) compared with the functional studies in cell suspensions is also particularly evident in these lymphomas. Frequently, foci of monoclonal malignant lymphoma cells are surrounded by an extensive polyclonal cell response that may serve to mask the minor monoclonal population in cell suspension studies; in many cases the small size of the biopsy specimen precludes cell suspension studies.

HEAVY CHAIN DISEASES

The term *heavy chain disease* was coined as a parallel to *light chain disease* for a group of conditions characterized by production of free heavy chain, as opposed to free light chain. Heavy chain diseases are further subdivided according to the class of heavy chain produced, since the different classes are associated with marked clinical differences—unlike light chain disease, in which it matters little whether the type is kappa or lambda.

Alpha Chain Disease (Table 5–6)

The designation *alpha chain disease* has been applied to any phase of a spectrum of events ranging from a plasma cell hyperplasia, usually involving the lamina propria of the intestine, through some form of progressive hyperplasia to frank neoplasia, all in association with a detectable monoclonal serum–urine immunoglobulin component that contains alpha chain (fragments) but no light chain.

The term *immunoproliferative small intestinal disease (IPSID)* has also been proposed for this condition (or spectrum of conditions).

In most instances the monoclonal alpha-chain component is detectable in serum by protein electrophoresis and immunoelectrophoresis, reacting with anti–alpha-specific antibodies but not with antibodies to kappa or lambda light chains; in some cases detection is difficult consequent upon diffuse migration of the alpha-chain component, owing to polymerization, structural abnormality, or fragmentation. In addition, "nonsecretory" cases lacking detectable serum monoclonal proteins, at least by the usual techniques, have been described.

Immunohistologic techniques provide a powerful alternative method of diagnosis, avoiding the difficulties inherent in serologic diagnosis and permitting simultaneous assessment of the morphologic characteristics of the cellular infiltrate (ranging from a bland, "normal-appearing" plasma cell population to a more mixed population with varying proportions of immunoblasts) and immunologic features (ie, a cell population staining for alpha chain in the absence of corresponding staining for kappa and lambda light chains (Fig. 5–16). Experience indicates that these immunohistologic techniques are superior to serologic methods in achieving a diagnosis.

Immunoperoxidase studies have also proved particularly valuable in investigating the relationship between alpha-chain disease and the so-called Mediterranean lymphoma, or immunoproliferative small intestinal disease (IPSID). Three histologic stages of the disease have been described. The initial nontumor phase is characterized by a diffuse plasma cell infiltrate (rarely with an admixture of lymphocytes) limited to the lamina propria; morphologically this infiltrate appears benign, but immunohistologic staining reveals an alpha–chain restricted pattern. This stage is succeeded by morphologic prelymphoma with some cytologic atypia and infiltration beyond the lamina propria, but

Table 5–6. Selected Bibliography: Alpha-Chain Disease

Isaacson 1979b	Middle East lymphoma and alpha-chain disease
Brouet et al 1977	Alpha-chain disease and immunoblastic sarcoma—common clonal origin
Pangalis & Rappaport 1977	Common clonal origin
Haghighi et al 1978	Immunohistologic patterns
Rambaud et al 1980	Nonsecretory alpha-chain disease
Skinner et al 1976	Alpha-chain disease and plasmacytoma
Cho et al 1982	Alpha-chain disease and colonic lymphoma
Nemes et al 1981	Alpha-chain disease and follicular center cell lymphoma
Rambaud et al 1978	Alpha-chain disease—review of 120 cases
Seligmann 1979	Heavy chain disease—review

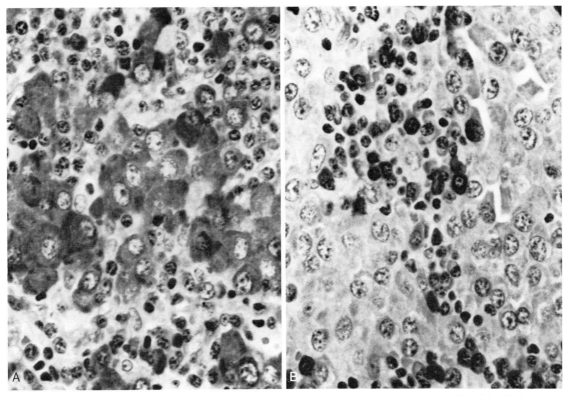

Figure 5–16. "Tumor" in gut wall composed of large plasmacytic cells that react positively for alpha chain (gray-black) (**A**) but are nonreactive for gamma chain (**B**). A few residual normal IgG-containing plasma cells are present. Paraffin sections, AEC with hematoxylin counterstain (×500). There was no detectable light chain in the large alpha-positive cells.

still the features of "destructive" lymphoma are lacking. In the final stage, that of frank lymphoma, the morphologic features of cellular atypia and destructive invasion are present; such cases, with a high content of alpha–chain-containing immunoblasts, have been termed (morphologically) immunoblastic sarcoma of B cell type (formerly, they would have been placed under the category of reticulum cell sarcoma or histiocytic lymphoma).

Immunohistologically, the benign-appearing lesions of the early stage show the presence of a high number of "mature" plasma cells containing alpha and J chains, but no other heavy or light chains. Isaacson P et al (1979) have pointed out that it may be necessary to utilize a higher titer of the primary antibody (ie, antialpha heavy chain) to label the plasma cells in alpha-chain disease compared with the plasma cells of a classic IgA multiple myeloma. This finding may reflect a lower content of alpha heavy chains, a molecular abnormality of this alpha-chain determinant, or some form of intracellular

cross linkage that interferes with antigen-antibody recognition. A similar monoclonal staining pattern for alpha chain has been observed within the neoplastic cells of the prelymphomatous and lymphomatous lesions of later stages. These immunohistologic findings support the concept of the common clonal origin of the lymphoplasmacellular infiltrate of alpha-chain disease and the supervening large cell lymphoma that eventually evolves (immunoblastic sarcomas of B cell type) (Pangalis and Rappaport, 1977; Brouet et al, 1977).

It should be noted that this point of view has recently been questioned by Isaacson P (1979b), who in some cases was not able to demonstrate alpha and J chains in the cytoplasm of the lymphomatous lesions of late stages. Failure to detect intracytoplasmic immunoglobulin in these cases may have been the result of fixation denaturation or low intracellular concentration of immunoglobulins in these tissues. Our experience and that of other investigators has served to reinforce the concept of a common clonal origin.

Gamma and Mu Chain Diseases

Gamma and mu chain diseases are rare, even in comparison with alpha chain disease. The principal features and immunologic characteristics have been well summarized elsewhere (Seligmann, 1979). Mu chain disease occurs most often as a CLL-like process. Gamma chain disease tends more often to manifest as a solid lymphoproliferative lesion, with admixtures of lymphoid cells and plasma cells; some of the early cases were misdiagnosed as Hodgkin's disease. In our experience, immunohistologic studies showing staining only for gamma chain have rendered this diagnosis in the absence of any detectable serum abnormality, although the serum monoclonal protein (gamma chain) became detectable a year or more later.

Possible J chain disease has also been recognized by immunohistologic methods (vide infra).

J Chain Disease

J (joining) chain is an elongated polypeptide of about 15,000 molecular weight, linked to IgA and IgM immunoglobulins by disulfide bonds. It was identified by study of the fast-moving bands observed following reduction and alkylation of polymeric IgA and IgM immunoglobulins. The unique "acid" property of J chain is responsible for its high electrophoretic mobility. With the advent of antisera with specificity for J chain, investigations of the cellular localization of this polypeptide became feasible.

J chain appears to be folded within the polymeric structure of intact immunoglobulin molecules, which means that only a few antigenic determinants remain exposed. In consequence, it is not easy to elicit anti–J chain antibodies by immunizing animals with native IgA and IgM, and purified J chain must be used. Purified J chain may be obtained by first completely reducing and alkylating the IgA and IgM immunoglobulins and then separating the J chain from the light and heavy chains by stepwise elution on DEAE cellulose columns at pH 8 to 9 or by elution on alkaline–urea polyacrylamide gels. The relative efficiency of these two methods depends on the magnitude of the· charge difference between J chain and the other components in the reduced and alkylated mixture. Unfortunately, J chain and light chains may show a similar charge distribution in some species, so that clean separation may be impossible; light chain contaminants may be removed using the appropriate anti–light chain antibodies. Antisera against human J chain cross-react with J chain of a variety of mammalian species, especially primates.

It is now clear that the J chain expression is not limited to cells that produce IgM and IgA polymeric immunoglobulins. For example, J chain has been detected not only in cells that contain IgA and IgM, but also in IgG- and IgD-containing cells. J chain appears to be present in a large proportion of the immunoglobulin-positive cells in germinal centers of tonsils and lymph nodes (Fig. 5–17). It is, however, not detectable in

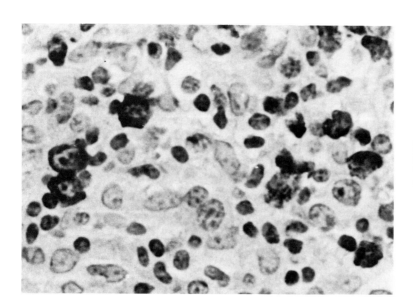

Figure 5–17. Plasma cells and immunoblasts showing reactivity for J chain. Paraffin section, DAB with hematoxylin counterstain (×500).

Table 5–7. Selected Bibliography: J Chain Disease

Brandtzaeg 1976a	J chain—review of structure and function
Meinke & Spiegelberg 1974	J chain as an antigen
Brandtzaeg 1976b	J distribution in B cells
Brandtzaeg et al 1981	J distribution in B cells
Kutteh et al 1980	J synthesis
Mestecky et al 1980	J synthesis
Isaacson 1979b	Diagnostic studies in fixed tissue
Mason DY & Stein 1981	Lymphomas—J chain disease
Stein et al 1981b	Lymphomas and J chain
Poppema 1980	J chain in some Reed-Sternberg cells
Laurent et al 1981	J chain detectable in a minority of B cell lymphomas

most of the "mature" IgG–containing plasma cells found in tonsils or in chronically inflamed tissues. Presumably, B cell clones express J chain at an early stage of differentiation, with expression persisting in those cells destined to produce IgA or IgM but ceasing in IgG- and IgD-producing plasma cells. The findings that both J chain and immunoglobulin are detectable at about the same time— during the first six days—in pokeweed-stimulated B lymphocytes and that J chain–staining subsequently diminishes whereas staining for IgG persists at the tenth day seem to support the above hypothesis (Brandtzaeg, 1976a, b).

Brandtzaeg and colleagues (Table 5–7) were the first to demonstrate that the IgG myeloma cells frequently contain J chain. Later, Mestecky et al (1980) studied a large series of patients with various lymphoproliferative disorders and found that J chain is present in normal and malignant lymphoid cells that produce monomeric (IgG, IgD, IgA) as well as polymeric (IgA, IgM) immunoglobulins. They also found J chain in light and heavy chain disease and in cases of nonsecretory myeloma.

P. Isaacson (1979a) pioneered direct demonstration of J chain in formalin-fixed, paraffin-embedded tissues by the immunoperoxidase technique after trypsinization of the sections. Käyhkö (1980) has since shown that trypsinization is unnecessary if the tissues are fixed in Bouin's fluid at room temperature for 1 to 5 hours. The introduction of immunoperoxidase techniques for J chain identification has made it possible to reveal this antigen in paraffin sections of various lymphomatous conditions. J chain was detected in all cases of B cell lymphoma and plasmacytomas that displayed a monoclonal light chain staining pattern in Isaacson's series, whereas the neoplastic cells of patients with malignant histiocytosis and the Reed-Stern-

berg cells of patients with Hodgkin's disease were J chain-negative. Some investigators believe that staining for J chain is a more reliable marker for B cells than staining directly for immunoglobulin, since IgG may be present within cells by absorption or phagocytosis.

Several authors have been able to detect J chain, but not intracytoplasmic immunoglobulins, in certain malignant and reactive immunoblastic proliferations. The term *J chain disease* was proposed for at least some of these conditions; 3 of 90 "high-grade" lymphomas tested by Mason and Stein (1981) fell into this possible category. The presence of intracellular J chain should therefore be considered a B cell marker, regardless of whether intracellular immunoglobulins are present or not. A possible explanation of these findings is that neoplastic or normal proliferating B immunoblasts may contain, at an early stage of B cell differentiation, an intracellular concentration of J chain that greatly exceeds the concentration of immunoglobulins; thus J chain may be detected, whereas immunoglobulin levels fall beneath the threshold for demonstration by the immunoperoxidase method. Mather and Koshland (1977) have reported that intracellular J chain synthesis is far greater than that of IgM in the early stages of mitogen-induced B cell differentiation.

Poppema (1980) has recently demonstrated monoclonal staining for light chain along with the presence of J chain in Reed-Sternberg cell variants of lymphocytic-predominant Hodgkin's disease (nodular pattern); he concluded that these cells were probably B immunoblasts and that they differed from the Reed-Sternberg cells found in other subtypes of Hodgkin's disease in which Reed-Sternberg cells typically manifest IgG, kappa and lambda light chains, and $alpha_1$-chymotrypsin positivity, but not J chain.

The study of J chain by ultrastructural immunoperoxidase techniques has resulted in additional important findings:

1. Both intracellular J chain and IgM are present in small lymphocytes prior to any morphologic evidence of blast transformation; the failure to detect J chain and immunoglobulins in the cytoplasm of "mature" small lymphocytes by the common immunocytochemical methods probably reflects the limits of sensitivity or visual resolution of these techniques in comparison with immunoelectron microscopy; and

2. J chain is located primarily in the rough endoplasmic reticulum, suggesting that this is the site in which J chain and immunoglobulins combine (Yasuda et al, 1980).

AMYLOID

Amyloid, named for its tinctorial resemblance to starch, is no longer regarded as a single substance; rather, the different amyloids are composed of various fibrillary deposits of different proteins, principal among which are the immunoglobulin fragments.

The traditional histochemical stains for amyloid, such as congo red or methyl violet, are useful in a general screening sense but do not facilitate the distinction of amyloid subtypes. Neither is the usual clinical definition of primary and secondary amyloid useful in this respect. In view of the possibility of therapeutic intervention, the distinction of amyloid subtypes based upon the dominant component of the amyloid in a particular case is of growing importance.

This may be achieved, at least partially, by immunohistochemical techniques, with useful results even in paraffin sections (Table 5–8).

The current nomenclature for amyloid proteins is a curious hybrid of immunologic information and clinical features: eg, AL (amyloid light chain fragments), AA (amyloid-associated protein), AF (amyloid familial), AS (amyloid senile), AE (amyloid endocrine). It seems likely that this system will soon be replaced by a more complete immunologic-immunohistologic scheme.

Already AL and AA are readily distinguishable by use of the appropriate antibodies, and with the availability of monoclonal

Table 5–8. Selected Bibliography: Amyloidosis

Fujihara 1982	Good review of approach to classification of amyloid in paraffin sections
Fujihara and Glenner 1981	Eleven cases of primary localized amyloidosis in GI tract; 9 contained A lambda fibril components
Fujihara et al 1980	Principles of identification and classification of amyloid in paraffin sections, human and murine
Livni et al 1980	Principles of classification of amyloid in paraffin sections; antibody versus murine AA protein cross-reacts with human AA
Linke and Nathrath 1980, 1982	Definition of 3 amyloid types (AA, A lambda, and A kappa) with antisera in cryostat and paraffin section
Linke 1984	Monoclonal antibody to amyloid AA protein; useful for routine diagnosis in paraffin sections
Westmark et al 1981, 1982	Amyloid "AP" positive, distribution by anti-AP antibody
Hardy et al 1979	Plasma cells associated with amyloidosis showed monoclonal pattern
Mornaghi et al 1982	Amyloid A (AA) and L (AL) in kidney
Wheeler and Eiferman 1983	Immunohistochemical demonstration of A protein in "lattice dystrophy"
Hind et al 1983	Demonstration of amyloid A protein and P component in systemic amyloidosis
Feurle et al 1984	Amyloid neuropathy; IgA lambda amyloid in some cases, prealbumin in related AF-amyloid in others; distinguishable by immunohistochemistry
Rowe et al 1984	Demonstration of AP amyloid in cerebrovascular amyloid
Breathnach et al 1982	AP amyloid in skin diseases
Eto et al 1984	Staining with antikeratin antibodies suggested that skin-limited amyloids may be keratin-derived
Dalakas et al 1984	Lambda amyloid in polyneuropathy with an amyloid positive hypernephroma
Dyck et al 1980	Amyloid P component in the endothelial aspect of the glomerular basement membrane
Ishii & Haga 1984	Immunoglobulins in amyloid of "senile" plaques of Alzheimer's disease

antibodies that are effective in paraffin sections (eg, Linke, 1984, monoclonal to AA proteins), it appears likely that this method will become the standard approach. In addition, some cases of AF (familial) amyloid react with antibodies to prealbumin, some skin-restricted amyloids react with selected anti-keratin antibodies, and some AE (endocrine) amyloids react with antibody to the corresponding hormone (eg, amyloid in medullary carcinoma of the thyroid frequently reacts with anti-calcitonin antibodies). Some cases of AS (senile) amyloid show reactivity for prealbumin, others stain for immunoglobulin.

In general, AL amyloid is associated with plasma cell dysplasia or lymphoma and with the concept of *primary* amyloid. AA amyloid is associated mainly with so-called secondary amyloid and some familial cases.

It is particularly important to identify cases of immunoglobulin-containing amyloid (AL) for two reasons. First, some have shown dramatic improvement, even remission, with cytotoxic therapy (melphalan). Second, plasma cell dyscrasias are identifiable in many cases. Tissue sections from such cases, when they contain plasma cells, should be stained for kappa or lambda light chains (and heavy chains if necessary) to determine whether or not the plasma cells are monotypic (monoclonal). If monoclonal, they should be viewed as neoplastic and potentially malignant, and a thorough search should be made for B cell lymphoma or multiple myeloma. This search should include immunohistologic staining of sections of bone marrow aspirates, which may reveal "monoclonal" plasma cells even when present in small numbers.

The case of "amyloid tumor" shown in Figure 5–7 illustrates how immunohistologic staining may contribute to the diagnosis and radically change the prognosis and therapy. "Amyloid tumors" are relatively uncommon, consisting of local, more or less circumscribed, soft tissue masses that are composed of amorphous hyaline material with the tinctorial properties of "amyloid." Typically, such lesions contain a focal collection of normal-appearing lymphocytes, plasma cells, and plasmacytoid lymphocytes admixed with the amyloid material. Foreign body giant cells are present in some cases. The case depicted in Figure 5–7 manifested as a solitary nodule in the lung; the plasma cells and plasmacytoid cells within the amyloid, although innocuous in appearance, were clearly monoclonal (IgA lambda). Bone marrow examination was requested; this tissue contained a small number of plasma cells that upon immunostaining were also monoclonal (IgA lambda). There was no detectable serum protein.

IMMUNOHISTOLOGIC LOCALIZATION OF TWO ANTIGENS IN THE SAME SECTION: ITS ROLE IN HEMATOPATHOLOGY

Double immunoenzymatic techniques for the simultaneous detection of two different antigens in the same section allow rapid assessment of the relative frequency and the topographical relationship of two cell populations with separate antigens; this technique is of particular value in exploring the clonality of lymphocyte–plasma cell populations (see color plates I–1 and I–2).

For example, patients with benign monoclonal gammopathy characteristically yield bone marrow biopsies that contain a mixed population of kappa-positive and lambda-positive plasma cells; whereas in patients with multiple myeloma, the majority of the plasma cells present in a marrow biopsy appear to stain either for one light chain or the other (monoclonal, or monotypic, staining) (Taylor et al, 1978a). These differences are more readily appreciated in double-stained preparations than by examination of serial sections.

Double-staining techniques for the simultaneous identification of kappa and lambda light chains may also be applied to the sequential bone marrow biopsies of myeloma patients in order to monitor the response to therapy (ie, the reappearance of a small number of "monoclonal" plasma cells, which indicates an impending relapse). Finally, double staining for one of the light chains and for lysozyme or hemoglobin A or F is of value in recognizing cases of myelomonocytic leukemia or erythroleukemia arising during the course of multiple myeloma.

The demonstration of the kappa:lambda surface or cytoplasmic immunoglobulin ratio directly in tissue sections, either by immunofluorescence or immunoperoxidase methods, has certain advantages over the more traditional assessment of membrane immunoglobulin by staining of viable cells in suspension (reviews—Taylor and Parker, 1981; Taylor et al, 1982; Lukes et al, 1978). In the first place, the risk of falsely low scores in cell suspensions, due to a very high neoplastic cell death rate, especially in large cell lymphomas, is avoided. Second, the problem of a selective bias in extracting cells from tissues for preparation of cell suspensions is also circumvented. The difficulties of interpreting the finding of apparent monoclonality in cell suspensions derived from tissues that carry an unequivocally benign morphologic diagnosis (eg, Palutke et al, 1981—monoclonality in giant lymph node hyperplasia) may be resolved by direct study of the ratio of kappa to lambda cells (surface, cytoplasm, or both) in situ in tissue sections; double-labelling methods afford the means for achieving this.

The association of Hodgkin's disease with a non-Hodgkin's lymphoma, or the occurrence of two morphologically distinct non-Hodgkin's lymphomas in the same mass or organ, has long been recognized. Custer (1954) proposed the term "composite lymphoma" for this phenomenon. Immunoperoxidase studies seem to indicate that at least some of the so-called composite lymphomas are, in fact, composed of closely related neoplasms with a common lymphocytic progenitor (van den Tweel et al, 1979). Certainly, this situation appears to be the explanation in the majority of those cases in which two non-Hodgkin's lymphomas occur together (eg, "reticulum cell sarcoma" and CLL—Richter's syndrome; each component is a different morphologic expression of a B cell neoplasm derived from a single clonal precursor). However, this is not always the case, and immunohistologic studies, preferably those using double-staining techniques, should be performed in order to confirm or deny that the two neoplastic populations that seem to be more or less closely related on morphologic grounds are, in fact, also functionally related.

In addition, simultaneous double-staining may reveal small foci of neoplastic cells containing monoclonal intracytoplasmic immunoglobulin among a larger population of reactive plasma cells. The frequency and the biologic significance (benign versus malignant) of these focal monoclonal proliferations have not been extensively studied; yet the evidence in certain high risk groups (eg, angioimmunoblastic lymphadenopathy and pre-AIDS and AIDS lymphadenopathy) is that focal monoclonality presages the development of overt B cell lymphomas in these conditions (see Janossy et al, 1980b). Such

studies are important, because the finding of monoclonality is usually considered to be synonymous with malignancy, although some monoclonal proliferations are regarded as "benign," exemplified by transitory paraproteinemias (Van Camp et al, 1980) or so-called benign monoclonal gammopathy.

Double or sequential immunoenzymatic techniques can be employed not only for identifying two or more antigens in different cell populations, but also for demonstrating the presence of two different antigens in the same cell, as judged by the formation of a mixed colored reaction (Mason and Sammons, 1978). For example, Joseph and Sternberger (1979) used the double–PAP immunostaining technique to demonstrate that both adrenocorticotropic hormone (ACTH) and beta lipotropin (beta-LPH) are located in the same pars intermedia cell and that they are probably derived from a common 31,000-dalton precursor.

We have used both sequential techniques and double-labelled antigen techniques with some success. The double-labelled antigen method (Chapter 2) is elegant and specific but is not widely applicable owing to the necessity for preparing labelled antigen reagents. Sequential techniques, although less demanding in terms of availability of the necessary reagents, always leave open the possibility of occurrence of some unsuspected cross reactivity of antibody or chromogen. In practice, the choice of method for double labelling is usually dictated by the reagents available, and only if the need for assurance of absolute specificity is pressing is one forced to resort to the more sophisticated and esoteric labelled antigen method, which requires the preparation of unique reagents.

Sequential double-staining methods and double-labelled antigen methods have confirmed the presence of both kappa and lambda light chain reactive moieties in individual Reed-Sternberg cells (see section on Hodgkin's disease). Some Reed-Sternberg cells (and incidentally, some other neoplastic giant cells in non-Hodgkin's lymphomas and in carcinomas) also contain serum proteins (eg, albumin), encouraging the belief that the presence of kappa and lambda may be accounted for by passive absorption of serum proteins into "sick" cells. Some Reed-Sternberg cells do not contain other serum proteins yet are positive for kappa and lambda, negating the above proposal and perhaps favoring the idea of adsorption by an Fc receptor and subsequent absorption, or even supporting the proposal of antibody attack in which the Reed-Sternberg cells are presumed to be attacked by a specific anti–Reed-Sternberg cell antibody. A further possibility that the immunoglobulin in Reed-Sternberg cells cross-reacts with both anti-kappa and anti-lambda antibodies, whether as a result of imperfect synthesis, partial degradation, or denaturation by fixative, cannot be proved or denied by immunohistologic methods alone. These matters are discussed more fully with reference to Hodgkin's disease (Chapter 4).

Double immunoenzymatic labelling for IgG or IgM and J chain has increased our knowledge of the biology of human lymphocytes: It has shown that (1) double-stained IgM/IgG cells (ie, those cells caught in the act of switching the class of immunoglobulin they secrete) are rare both in benign and in neoplastic lymphoid tissue; (2) J chain is present in the cytoplasm of cells that contain immunoglobulin regardless of the class (similar results have also been obtained with double immunofluorescence techniques); (3) a normal J^+/Ig^- immunoblast population as well as its neoplastic counterpart can be detected by double immunoenzymatic procedures (Stein et al, 1981b)—a not unexpected finding, since under certain circumstances J chain synthesis can precede Ig synthesis (Kutteh et al, 1980). This means that J chain can be considered a B cell marker of lymphoma whether intracytoplasmic immunoglobulins are present or not and that the existence of a J chain lymphoma becomes predictable and eventually is found (see J Chain—Chapter 5).

Finally, the introduction of immunoperoxidase techniques for revealing the enzyme terminal deoxynucleotide transferase (TDT) in peripheral blood smears (Hecht et al, 1981), frozen sections (Janossy et al, 1980a; Rouget and Penit, 1980), and paraffin sec-tions (Janossy et al, 1980b, c) means that the relationship between the cellular content of TDT and the stage of T cell differentiation can be studied by the simultaneous application of different antibodies. For example, double-staining techniques for TDT, Ia, common ALL antigen, and HUT1a antigens can help to differentiate directly in frozen sections thymic acute lymphoblastic leukemia ($TDT^+/HuT1A^+$/common ALL antigen$^-$) from common type acute lymphoblastic leukemia ($TDT^+/HuT1A^-$/common ALL antigen$^+$) (Janossy et al, 1980a). Furthermore, double immunoenzymatic studies in paraffin sections for TDT, IgM, lysozyme, and hemoglobin A and F should provide some information on the morphologic type of blast crisis in chronic myeloid leukemia (CML) and its relationship with the ability to express the enzyme.

Double-labelling studies for surface antigens are better performed in frozen than in paraffin sections. Double immunofluorescence techniques have been widely used for this purpose; more recently, double immunoenzymatic techniques using peroxidase and alkaline phosphatase as enzyme markers have been successfully applied to frozen sections for the detection of membrane-associated antigens (see color plate I–2).

Double-immunostaining techniques for kappa and lambda light chains in frozen sections are particularly useful for assessing clonality of B cell populations in situ in tissue sections. The importance of performing immunohistologic studies in frozen rather than paraffin sections has been particularly stressed by Janossy et al (1980d), who demonstrated, in a case of immunoblastic sarcoma arising in preexisting angioimmunoblastic lymphadenopathy, that the new clone of malignant transformed lymphocytes expresses a monoclonal surface immunoglobulin before the monoclonal intracytoplasmic Ig is detectable.

6

OTHER "HEMATOPOIETIC CELL" MARKERS

"Curiouser and curiouser!"
Alice, in her Adventures in Wonderland

LEWIS CARROLL, 1832–1898

Ia-LIKE ANTIGENS

Ia antigens are reviewed briefly because initially it was thought that they might serve as B cell–specific markers; this view is no longer tenable.

Two groups of polymorphic cell surface glycoproteins, the major transplantation antigens (coded by the HLA-A, HLA-B, and HLA-C loci) and the HLA-D or Ia (immune-associated antigens), which appear to be the equivalent of the murine Ia antigens, are under the direct control of the major human histocompatibility complex (HLA in humans). The availability of specific antibodies against the human Ia-like antigens has provided a means of examining the cell and tissue distributions of these molecules; several approaches have been employed.

Originally, alloantisera (from subjects alloimmunized during pregnancy, organ transplant, or blood transfusion) were used for immunologic studies. Unfortunately, antisera from these sources are usually of low titer and are in short supply; in addition, as human antibodies, they are not easily employed for immunohistologic studies of human tissues for reasons described earlier. Subsequently, the high immunogenicity of the Ia-like molecules has facilitated the production of heterologous anti-Ia antibodies in both rabbits and chickens. In addition, many monoclonal anti-Ia antibodies have been developed; the latter do not require lengthy absorption procedures and have the advantage that they can be directed against common or variable parts of Ia molecules.

Antibodies specific for these antigens are known by a variety of names: anti-B cell because of the initial findings that B lymphocytes carry Ia-like antigens; anti-"Ia-like" because of the similarity to the antigens of the murine Ia region; anti-DR (or HLA-D–related), for the relationship of the antigens to the HLA-D locus; or anti-p28,33 antigens because of the molecular weight of glycoprotein components in the mouse system. The patterns of immunohistologic reactivity of these different reagents are at this time not clearly defined, and these antibodies with their various designations should not be assumed to be identical. Certain generalizations are, however, possible.

Normal Human Tissue

Early reports suggested that the expression of Ia-like antigens was restricted to cells associated with the immune response (principally B lymphocytes and some monocytes-histiocytes). Immunohistologic studies using immunofluorescence or immunoperoxidase techniques have shown, however, that Ia antigens in animals as well as in humans have a wide distribution in normal adult tissues, being present in both lymphoid and nonlymphoid organs (Table 6–1). On the other hand, available evidence suggests that Ia-like antigens may be restricted to a limited number of cell types in early stages of fetal life (at least in animals). For example, in 15-day-old mouse embryo, no Ia-positive cells were observed in the skin (Natali et al, 1981b), possibly owing to the fact that the Ia-positive Langerhans cells, thought to originate in the bone marrow (Frelinger et al, 1979), have not yet migrated to this body site. It must be

Table 6–1. Selected Bibliography: Ia-Like (Immune-Associated) Antigens

Winchester & Kunkel 1979	Review
Seymour et al 1980 (p. 28–33)	(Ia-like) antigens
Janossy et al 1980c	Analysis, lymphoid tissue by phenotype
Brodsky et al 1979	Monoclonal antibodies and HLA
Bhan et al 1980	T cell and HLA antigens in thymus
Naiem et al 1981	Analysis of lymphomas
Scott et al 1980	Intestinal cells
Danilovs et al 1982	HLA-DR (Ia in fetal pancreas)
Ammirati et al 1980	Ia in reactive T cells
Poppema et al 1981	T cell subsets in lymph nodes
Janossy et al 1980a	Distribution helper/suppressor cells and Ia cells
Selby et al 1981b	T cells and histocompatibility antigens in gut wall
Hofman et al 1982	Surface and cytoplasmic Ia
Rowden 1980	Ia in Langerhans's cells
Streilen & Bergstrasser 1980	Ia in Langerhans's cells
Lampert et al 1980	OKT6 and Langerhans's cells
Knowles 1980	Non-Hodgkin's lymphomas
Warnke et al 1980	Immunologic phenotype of large cell lymphomas
Stein et al 1980	Normal and neoplastic lymphoid tissue
Kadin 1980	Ia in differential diagnosis of lymphoma
Pizzolo et al 1980	Ia in differential diagnosis of lymphoma
Wilson et al 1984	Ia on melanoma and lung cancer
Thomas JA et al 1982	Ia in nasopharyngeal carcinoma
Bernard et al 1984	Ia in breast cancer
Bröcker et al 1984	High grade and metastatic melanoma shows more Ia positivity
Natali et al 1981c	Human non-lymphoid tissues; Ia positive melanoma

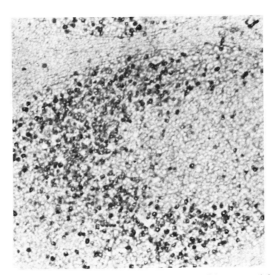

Figure 6–1. Frozen section of spleen with tangential cut of Malpighian nodule showing distribution of Ia-positive cells around a reactive center; positive cells are a mixture of B lymphocytes and histiocytes. Frozen section, DAB, no counterstain (× 125).

admitted that knowledge of Ia distribution in the fetus is even more limited than for adult tissues; inevitably, these views will change as new data are added. Even in our own laboratories, the observation of Ia-DR–positive "dendritic" cells in human fetal pancreas (Danilovs and collaborators, 1982) heralds changes in our concept as to the significance of Ia for cell and tissue recognition.

Peripheral Lymphoid Tissue

In peripheral blood and lymph node suspensions, Ia antigens are present on B cells and monocytes. Only a small percentage of mature peripheral T lymphocytes (about 1 to 4 percent) are Ia-positive. Ia-like antigens appear, however, on activated T lymphocytes (Table 6–1).

Immunohistological studies show that Ia-positive B cells are mainly located in reactive follicles (Fig. 6–1): the small lymphocytes of the mantle zone stain more intensely than do the large germinal center cells. In contrast, the T lymphocytes in the paracortex of

lymph nodes and tonsils are negative. However, double-labelling studies on frozen sections have shown the presence of few Ia-positive T lymphocytes in both the paracortex and the follicles of tonsils. Whether these cells are the tissue counterparts of the small percentage of Ia-positive "activated" T lymphocytes detectable in peripheral blood suspensions is unclear.

Several large scattered cells in the paracortex of tonsils and lymph nodes show intense cytoplasmic staining for Ia antigens, apparently in the cytoplasm (Fig. 6–2). These cells probably correspond to the interdigitating reticulum cells described in the T-dependent areas of rabbit and human and lymphoid organs. Janossy et al (1980e) have demonstrated varying numbers of Ia positive cells within the human lympho-hemopoietic tissues. Ia-positive "dendritic"* cells are numerous in those lymphoid areas that contain large numbers of phenotypic helper T cells—for example, the thymic medulla, the paracortex of the lymph nodes and tonsils, and the intestinal lamina propria. However, these dendritic cells are few in normal human

---

*Histologists distinguish dendritic reticulum cells, confined to the B cell follicles, and interdigitating reticulum cells, occurring in the T cell paracortex (Muller-Mennelink and Kaiserling, 1980; van den Tweel, 1980); immunologists use the term *dendritic cell* for a conceptual antigen-handling cell that may include both of the aforementioned types. Both are Ia-positive.

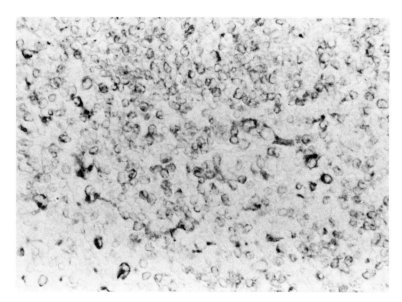

Figure 6–2. Staining for Ia showing margin of reactive center top with Ia-positive B cells, plus scattered, more intensely stained Ia-positive "interdigitating" reticulum cells in the underlying paracortex. Frozen section, AEC, no counterstain (×200).

bone marrow and gut epithelium, where suppressor-cytotoxic T cells (determined by phenotype) appear to predominate. The close association of Ia-positive "dendritic"* reticulum cells with T lymphocytes is considered by some to suport the view that these cells are intimately involved in binding and presenting antigens to T cells; this concept is a leap in logic that not all are prepared to make.

Antibodies claimed to react specifically with follicular dendritic reticulum cells (Parwaresch et al, 1983) are probably of more value for study of this cell type than Ia, which, as will be seen, is ubiquitous.

The principal diagnostic application of immunostaining for Ia thus is in the recognition of B lymphocytes (usually Ia-positive, although plasma cells, which in effect are highly specialized differentiated B cells, are usually Ia-negative) as distinct from T lymphocytes (usually Ia-negative, although "activated" T cells show positively).

It should be pointed out that these distinctions, tenuous as they are, hold only for normal B and T lymphocytes; in our experience neoplastic lymphocytes do not always obey these rules.

In addition, staining for Ia cannot be used to distinguish lymphocytes from cells of the monocyte-histiocyte series, since both may be positive.

Recent studies (Hofman et al, 1982) have revealed yet another complication. The great

majority of studies reporting the cellular specificity of anti-Ia antibodies have been based upon studies of cells in suspension, detecting cell surface Ia. Hofman, by study of tissue sections and fixed cytocentrifuge preparations, has reported the presence of Ia antigens within the cytoplasm also (Fig. 6–3), and it appears that the distribution in cytoplasm does not parallel cell surface distribution.

Thus, immunoperoxidase or immunofluorescence techniques applied to tissue sections may reveal different populations of positive cells compared with studies using identical antibodies in cell suspensions. As is described later, these factors combine to limit the practical value of Ia staining for diagnostic purposes. The reports that advocate the demonstration of Ia positivity as a valuable criterion distinguishing lymphomas (may be positive or negative) from carcinomas (negative) and other sarcomas (negative) appear liable to gradual erosion as the distribution of Ia antigens is explored in more detail (vide infra).

Skin

Human dermal cell suspensions contain a low percentage of cells (2 to 4 percent) that form EA (IgG) and EAC rosettes (ie, bear Fc and C3 receptors) and react with alloantisera from multiparous women (ie, appear to bear Ia antigens). Recently, several investigators have shown by immunofluorescence or immunoperoxidase methods that histiocytes

---

*See footnote on page 143.

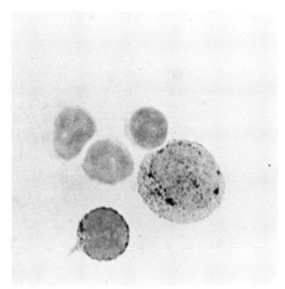

Figure 6–3. Cytocentrifuge preparation from lymph node shows positive granular (black) staining for Ia on and in cells. AEC with hematoxylin counterstain (×900).

and Langerhans's cells in situ in human skin express Ia-like antigens (Fig. 6–4; Table 6–1). In frozen sections of skin, the Ia-positive cells accounted for approximately 2 to 4 percent of the total number of epidermal cells, thus confirming previous cell suspension studies. Immunoelectron microscope studies have furnished conclusive evidence that these positive cells are Langerhans's cells (easily recognizable by the Birbeck granules). In contrast, keratinocytes and normal melanocytes are consistently Ia-negative. A similar im-

munohistologic pattern has also been observed in mouse. Quantitative binding studies using radioiodinated anti-Ia monoclonal antibodies support the view that Langerhans's cells in mouse skin express Ia antigens in quantities larger than expressed by small B lymphocytes.

Interestingly, Langerhans's cells appear to react also with anti-T6 monoclonal antibody, which recognizes an immature thymocyte population and some cells in the paracortical zone of normal lymph nodes. The significance of this circumstance is at present obscure; it may be merely coincidental (see Chapter 13). It has been suggested that Langerhans's cells are the "dendritic cells" of the skin and, like the dendritic cells in lymph node or spleen, play some role in antigen presentation to T lymphocytes.

Other Human Tissues

High levels of Ia antigens have been found in cell homogenates of various tissues, including human kidney and liver. Immunohistologically, the Ia-positive cells in these organs appear to be glomerular and peritubular renal endothelial cells and Kupffer's cells.

The presence of Ia-like antigens on Langerhans's cells as well as in certain cellular components of kidney and pancreas may have some clinical importance (eg, induction of anti-Ia antibodies and consequent graft rejection). A number of tumors also show Ia positivity (vide infra).

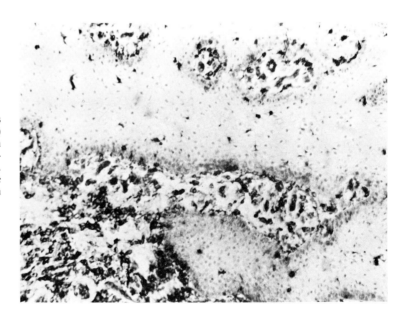

Figure 6–4. Ia-positive cells (Langerhans cells and histiocytes) appear in increased numbers in the epidermis and dermis in granulomatous diseases; this is leprosy. Paraffin section, LN3 anti–Ia-like antibody, DAB with hematoxylin counterstain (×125).

Pathologic Tissues

Malignant Lymphomas

Early reports of restrictions of the Ia-like antigens to B lymphocytes and perhaps "null" cells resulted in attempts to utilize Ia antibodies to discriminate between neoplasms of these cell types and all other neoplasms.

Studies of Ia-like antigens in cell suspensions of non-Hodgkin's lymphomas have shown that the majority of these neoplasms are indeed Ia-positive. In B cell lymphomas the majority of the neoplastic cells, like their normal B lymphocyte counterparts, express Ia-like antigens as well as surface immunoglobulins (especially of IgM type). A low percentage of neoplastic cells that appear to bear Ia antigens but not surface immunoglobulins has also been observed. It may be that these two phenotypically different populations represent cells that belong to the same neoplastic clone but are at different stages of maturation.

Some authors believe that, in contrast with acute lymphoblastic leukemia, the expression of Ia-like antigens alone in absence of T cell markers and surface immunoglobulins is rare in non-Hodgkin's lymphomas. On the other hand, other investigators frequently found Ia-like antigens in cases of human lymphomas with no other lymphocyte markers ("null" cell lymphomas; Table 6–1). These apparent "null" cell lymphomas have been claimed to represent 25 to 50 percent of all non-Hodgkin's lymphomas and are pre-sumed by some to belong to the B cell series. Warnke et al (1980) studied 30 cases of large cell lymphomas by an immunofluorescence technique on frozen sections and found that only half of the cases expressed monoclonal surface immunoglobulins. Of the remaining cases, 13 showed the presence of Ia-like antigens, but neither surface immunoglobulin nor T cell differentiation antigens were detectable.

T cell lymphomas have been reported to be Ia negative; however, exceptions clearly exist (Fig. 6–5). Halper et al (1980), in their series of 33 non-Hodgkin's lymphomas, mentioned a single patient whose neoplastic cells lacked surface immunoglobulins but formed E rosettes and stained positively for Ia-like antigens. Stein et al (1980) showed that neoplastic cells in frozen sections of T-zone lymphomas may express T cell differentiation antigens as well as Ia-like antigens. SM Fu et al (1978) had previously observed that leukemic T cells in a number of different leukemias might be Ia-positive.

Since only 1 to 4 percent of mature resting T lymphocytes are Ia-positive, whereas up to 75 percent of T cells express the antigen following pokeweed mitogen stimulation, it appears possible that "activated" T lymphocytes may represent the "normal counterparts" of at least some of the Ia-positive T cell lymphomas. This point of view is supported by two circumstantial observations: high numbers of Ia-positive T cells are frequently observed in the peripheral blood in association with infectious mononucleosis

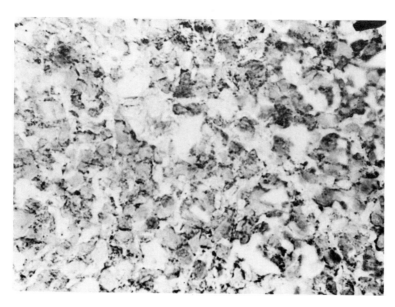

Figure 6–5. Anaplastic large cell tumor showing positive surface membrane reactivity with an anti-Ia antibody. The eventual diagnosis was immunoblastic sarcoma of T cell type. Frozen section, AEC with hematoxylin counterstain (×320). Staining for Ia is not all that helpful, positivity also being observed in histiocytic tumors, B cell lymphomas, melanomas, and some carcinomas.

(Tatsumi et al 1980) or following a simple booster shot of tetanus toxoid (Winchester and Kunkel 1979), ie, under circumstances that cause T cell activation in vivo.

Benign and malignant T cell proliferations derived from mature T lymphocytes (mainly displaying helper function), such as dermatopathic lymphadenopathy and mycosis fungoides, are frequently associated with the presence in involved tissues of numerous Ia-positive (and OKT6-positive) dendritic reticulum cells or Langerhans's cells. This immunohistologic pattern may reflect the close association between Ia-bearing dendritic cells and helper T lymphocytes that is seen in certain compartments of normal human lymphoid tissue. Some have cited this as evidence supporting the occurrence of some perturbation of the immunoregulatory mechanisms in these conditions.

Finally, detection of Ia-like antigens has been advanced as of particular value in distinguishing large cell lymphomas (usually positive) from undifferentiated epithelial and connective tissue tumors, on which they are seldom detectable (Kadin, 1980; Pizzolo et al, 1980). It should be noted, however, that melanomas are an exception, because they are often Ia-positive (Table 6–1). For example, Natali et al (1981a) found Ia-like antigens in all the cases of frozen melanoma tissue sections (primary, recurrent, and metastatic lesions) that they examined by an immunofluorescence technique. Interestingly, the lowest percentage of Ia-positive melanoma cells was found in the primary lesions, whereas Ia expression was increased in those lesions with the highest degree of invasion and in metastatic lesions. Likewise, Bröcker and colleagues (1984) found that 18:24 melanomas that metastasized were Ia-positive. Whether these immunohistologic findings have some prognostic value (in melanomas) is, at this moment, unclear (see Chapter 13). Other tumors showing definite Ia positivity include squamous carcinomas, breast cancer, and lung cancer (Table 6–1).

In our experience immunostaining for Ia is subject to so many qualifications as to be of little value in cell recognition or tumor recognition and classification.

HEMOGLOBINS A AND F

Hemoglobin is not strongly antigenic; nonetheless, it is possible to produce antisera

Table 6–2. Selected Bibliography: Hemoglobin Immunohistochemistry

Taylor & Skinner 1976	HbF in fetal thymocytes; distinction of erythroblast from lymphoblast
Neiman 1980	Extramedullary erythropoiesis
Pinkus & Said 1981	Erythroleukemic and marrow dysplasias
Forni et al 1983	Neoplastic erythropoiesis shows an increase in HbF-positive cells (oncofetal expression)
Underwood & Dangerfield 1981	Extramedullary and bone marrow erythropoiesis
Kaplan et al 1982	HbF shows presence of fetal rbc in intervillous thrombi
Isobe et al 1981	Transferrin in immature erythroid cells (in mitochondria)
Albrechtsen et al 1980	HbA and HbF in yolk sac tumors, in erythroid and epithelial type cells
Keifer et al 1984	Erythroleukemic infiltrates in lymph node

with differential specificity for adult (HbA) and fetal (HbF) hemoglobins (Table 6–2).

The detection of hemoglobins A and F in paraffin-embedded tissues by the immunoperoxidase technique was introduced by Taylor and Skinner (1976), who succeeded in revealing a variable percentage of hemoglobin-containing cells in the human fetal thymus, thereby furnishing evidence that this organ may contain significant numbers of erythropoietic elements (as had already been demonstrated in animals) (Fig. 6–6). Individual nucleated red cell precursors (hemoglobin-positive) were not distinguishable morphologically from thymic lymphocytes or lymphoblasts; the reality of this conclusion is underlined by the consistent failure of successive generations of pathologists to make this very distinction in fetal thymus.

A fundamental weakness in the application of traditional morphologic methods is thereby revealed, for all too often cells are identified and distinguished as much by their tissue location or by the "company they keep" as by their fine cytologic features; small round cells with dense but "immature" nuclei and scant basophilic cytoplasm are erythroblasts in the marrow, but lymphoblasts in the thymus. Immunohistologic techniques staining for hemoglobin provided a more accurate and more reliable distinction.

Underwood and Dangerfield (1981) have confirmed these observations and have shown that in human fetal tissues most of the hemoglobin-producing cells are located within the red pulp of the spleen and the hepatic vascular sinusoids, small erythropoietic islands being also present in the lung and kidney.

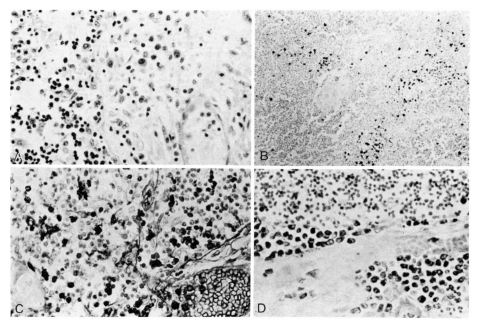

Figure 6–6. Composite figure relating to a study of hemopoiesis in the fetal thymus (Taylor and Skinner, 1976). Perivascular pyroninophilic cells (*A*—H&E, ×125) had been identified as plasma cells but were shown to contain muramidase (black dots, ***B***—×35). This finding resulted in a tentative classification of these cells as fetal myeloblasts and myelocytes, and was confirmed by a chloroacetate esterase stain (***D***—intense black cells are positive). Fetal erythropoiesis was then demonstrated by staining with an anti-HbF antibody (***C***—black cells are positive in an intravascular and perivascular location). It should be noted that, using morphologic criteria alone, scattered erythroblasts within the thymic cortex COULD NOT BE DISTINGUISHED from lymphoblasts. Paraffin sections, DAB with hematoxylin counterstain.

Hemoglobin A is also readily identifiable by immunoperoxidase techniques in paraffin sections prepared from bone marrow aspirates or biopsies. Detailed studies have shown that hemoglobin is detectable not only in the cytoplasm of normal erythroid cells at all stages of maturation, but also in the cytoplasm of erythroid cells with megaloblastic features. Pinkus and Said (1981) have discussed the rationale and basis of this approach in some detail:

Studies of hemoglobin production during erythropoiesis readily explain the reason intracellular hemoglobin represents an excellent marker for erythroid cells. Hemoglobin synthesis begins at the stage of the proerythroblast, the earliest cell of erythrocytic maturation, which has a hemoglobin content of 0–14.4 μg per cell. This cell undergoes a series of divisions and maturation stages which include basophilic normoblasts, polychromatophilic normoblasts, "orthochromatic" normoblasts, reticulocytes, and finally the erythrocytes. During the maturation sequence, erythroid precursors continue to synthesize hemoglobin. The most rapid rate of hemoglobin synthesis occurs at stages of proerythroblast and basophilic erythroblast (0.5 μg/cell/hour) and progressively decreases at subsequent stages of maturation to a

rate of 0.1–0.2 μg/cell/hour in the reticulocyte. At the stage of a mature erythrocyte, the hemoglobin content reaches 30–34 μg/cell. In megaloblastic erythropoiesis, although nuclear-cytoplasmic maturation is dyssynchronous, hemoglobin synthesis still occurs. [See Lajtha, 1965.]

The value of being able to detect hemoglobins in paraffin-embedded tissues has become obvious in at least some instances. Important clinicopathologic applications include the identification of small cell infiltrates of unknown origin and the distinction of erythroid cell precursors from immature cells of the lymphoid and myeloid series. For example, cases of blastic transformation in chronic myeloid leukemia that until recently would have been tentatively diagnosed as of "erythroid nature" on the basis of morphologic criteria can now be easily identified by immunoperoxidase staining for intracellular hemoglobin as a specific marker (Neiman, 1980). In addition, immunohistologic investigations also may help differentiate sideroblastic anemia from both myeloblastic leukemia and "immunoblastic sarcoma" occurring during the course of multiple myeloma.

"Erythroid bone marrow reserves" can be

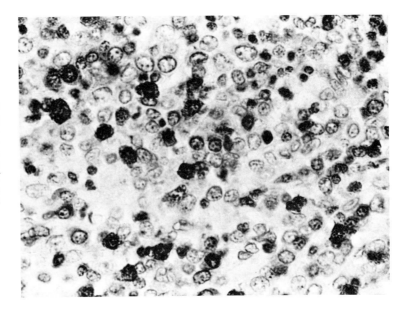

Figure 6–7. Erythropoiesis in spleen; positive (black) staining with antihemoglobin F antibody. Paraffin section, AEC with hematoxylin counterstain ($\times 500$). HbA-positive cells were present in lesser numbers. A predominance of HbF-positive cells commonly is seen in neoplastic states; this was erythroleukemia (Di Guglielmo).

better evaluated in the bone marrow of postchemotherapy patients, in which the hemoglobin-containing cells are easily distinguished from the residual lymphoblasts or myeloblasts.

In erythroleukemia, immunohistologic detection of hemoglobin in paraffin sections of bone marrow biopsies has shown that a high percentage (average 42 percent) of the dysplastic or megaloblastic erythroid neoplastic cells or both contain hemoglobin; a variable number of lysozyme-positive myeloid precursors and unstained blast cells are also present; the latter presumably are representative of these cells at an early stage of differentiation prior to the synthesis of detectable amounts either of hemoglobin or lysozyme (Pinkus and Said, 1981).

Meyer, Forni, and other members of our group at the University of Southern California have taken this approach one step further (Forni et al, 1983). They have shown that neoplastic erythroid proliferations contain a predominance of HbF-positive cells (Fig. 6–7) in marked contrast to the "reactive" or physiologic erythroid hyperplasias such as may occur in recovering marrow, which typically contains HbA-positive cells. Some of

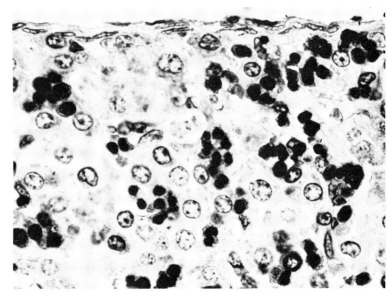

Figure 6–8. Extramedullary erythropoiesis in spleen, in a case of myelofibrosis. Red cells and red cell precursors are stained with antibody to HbA (hemoglobin A). Paraffin section, DAB with hematoxylin counterstain ($\times 500$).

the dyserythropoietic disorders, such as pernicious anemia, contain an admixture of HbA- and HbF-positive cells. The presence of HbF in the neoplastic cells may be considered analogous with the expression of oncofetal antigens by other neoplasms (eg, CEA by colonic neoplasms; alpha-fetoprotein by hepatomas).

Finally, immunohistologic methods clearly reveal foci of extramedullary erythropoiesis (Fig. 6–8). For example, Underwood and Dangerfield (1981) found an unsuspected high incidence of fetal-type extramedullary erythropoiesis in patients with non-Hodgkin's lymphomas, leukemias, and myeloproliferative disorders with splenic involvement, but not in those suffering from Hodgkin's disease.

One other practical application stems from the work of Albrechtsen et al (1980), who were able to demonstrate, by immunoperoxidase technique, that both the epithelial cells and the erythroidlike cells in the human yolk sac contain hemoglobins A and F. This observation may have some diagnostic importance in relation to germ cell tumors; those with yolk sac differentiation, but not those of other types, may also contain hemoglobin in the neoplastic cells.

TERMINAL DEOXYNUCLEOTIDYL TRANSFERASE (TDT)

Terminal deoxynucleotidyl transferase (TDT) is a DNA polymerase that catalyzes the polymerization of deoxynucleotides at the 3'-hydroxyl ends of oligo- or polydeoxynucleotide initiators in the absence of template. This enzyme is present at high levels in cortical thymocytes but is found at low levels in some bone marrow lymphocytes (about 2 percent of bone marrow cells). It is not detectable in circulating or mitogen-stimulated lymphocytes. During normal thymic maturation, TDT activity disappears before the T cells become immunologically competent; the enzyme would appear primarily to be located in an early T cell precursor, perhaps a prothymocyte.

Populations of TDT-positive cells are therefore usually found in the neoplastic disorders that arise from or mimic the early thymocyte (prothymocyte) compartment, eg, acute lymphoblastic leukemia and lymphoblastic lymphoma (Table 6–3). In addition, high levels of TDT have been identified in

Table 6–3. Selected Bibliography: Terminal Deoxynucleotidyl Transferase (TDT)

Goldschneider et al 1977 Stass et al 1979 Okamura 1980 Stass et al 1982	Detection of TDT by immunohisto-logic method
Stass et al 1982	Advantages of immunoperoxidase versus immunofluorescence for TDT detection
Halverson et al 1981	Enhanced sensitivity of detection of TDT in paraffin sections
Braziel et al 1983	TDT detectable in 25/25 lymphoblastic lymphomas; rarely in other lymphomas
Jäger 1981	PAP method for TDT detection
Steinmann et al 1981	TDT in MOLT4 (a T lymphoblastic line) shown cytoplasmic by EM!
Ho et al 1982	TDT in leukemias; comparison of biochemical fluorescence and peroxidase methods, preferred PAP
Thomas JA et al 1984	TDT in 95% of ALL: immunostaining possible in formalin paraffin sections (but not Bouin's or Carnoy's) with DNase pretreatment; frozen sections did not require DNase
Kawakami et al 1981	TDT distribution with age in rat thymus
Muehleck et al 1983	TDT staining (ABC and PAP) in 169 cases using marrow smears. Scattered TDT-positive cells in normals may be hematogones; presence of these cells means TDT-positive cells do not denote relapse of ALL
Racklin et al 1983	ABC method for TDT; frozen sections and cell smears: normal marrow up to 5% positive cells; ALL 30%–90%.
Jäger and Lau 1982	CALLA and TDT in normal mononuclear blood cells
Hecht et al 1981	TDT staining (letter to N Engl J Med)
Sasaki et al 1984	TDT-positive intranuclear granules in ALL; methanol-treated cell smears, one fourth cases of CML in blast crisis also positive
Tavares de Castro et al 1984	TDT in nucleus of PAP method, with simultaneous staining of membrane antigens by immunogold

about one third of patients with chronic myeloid leukemia in blast crisis; this last observation raises the question as to whether TDT activity is also present in a primitive multipotent hematopoietic cell or a very early B cell lymphoid precursor.

TDT activity is usually assayed biochemically in crude cell extracts following chromatography. Unfortunately, the relatively large numbers of cells (up to 10^8) required for this biochemical assay preclude satisfactory TDT testing when involvement occurs in extramedullary sites, such as skin. In other situations the ratio of TDT-containing cells (abnormal cells) to the total cell population may be so low that the normal cells "dilute out" the enzyme activity of the blast cells. Furthermore, the tissue distribution of TDT-containing cells cannot be studied by the biochemical method, and enzymatically inactive forms of the enzyme (if they exist) will not be detected.

Only when anti-TDT antibody became available (Bollum, 1975) was it possible to directly identify the enzyme in situ by immunocytochemical techniques. Much of the current information concerning the nature and distribution of TDT-positive cells has come through the use of antibody raised in rabbits or mice against calf thymus TDT. Such antibody shows a broad species reactivity, permitting its use in immunocytologic studies on birds and many mammals, including humans.

Strong supporting evidence for the conservation of TDT structure in different species has recently been furnished by Bollum et al (1981). Crude extracts of TDT derived from thymus and from malignant cell lines (human and mouse) were separated by SDS gel electrophoresis, then transferred to a nitrocellulose membrane and subsequently labelled by immunoperoxidase technique, using rabbit anti-TDT antiserum. Using this procedure, which permits solid-phase immunoassay of peptide structures with simultaneous estimation of molecular weights, it was possible to show that the most common form of TDT (in various animal species) is a 60K peptide having immunologic determinants in common with the 32K form originally isolated from calf thymus gland.

A number of the early studies utilized indirect immunofluorescence with affinity purified rabbit anticalf TDT. With this technique, simple methanol-fixed smears and frozen sections can be analyzed for TDT, making possible large studies of clinical material (Goldschneider et al, 1977; Stass et al, 1979; Okamura et al, 1980). A single TDT-positive cell can be detected by indirect immunofluorescence or immunoperoxidase techniques among a population of ten thousand or more TDT-negative cells, making this technique far more sensitive than biochemical assays of extracts prepared from heterogeneous cell populations. Immunoperoxidase techniques have recently been used for the identification of TDT in cell smears, frozen sections and paraffin sections (Table 6–3). Remarkably, paraffin sections appear in some respects to be more suitable than frozen sections for immunohistologic studies, because in the lat-

ter situation the enzyme tends to diffuse out of the nucleus, leading to false-negative results or obscure diffuse positivity.

In order to increase the sensitivity for detection of traces of TDT in individual cells using immunoperoxidase staining, several authors have advocated treatment of paraffin sections with deoxyribonuclease for 4 to 6 hours at room temperature, coupled with overnight incubation with primary anti-TDT antibody and repeated additions of the bridge antibody and PAP reagent (Halverson et al, 1981).

Both immunofluorescence and immunoperoxidase staining of normal thymus glands from different species have produced similar staining patterns, ie, marked positivity of the cortical thymocytes (Fig. 6–9) and little or no evidence of reaction in the thymic medulla. As expected, using rabbit anticalf TDT antibody, the intensity of staining in human cortical thymocytes is less than that observed with calf and rat thymus. Disagreement still exists as to the exact intracellular location of the enzyme. The majority of the authors have observed a nuclear staining pattern in cortical thymocytes as well as in TDT-positive neoplastic cells. In contrast, other investigators favor a cytoplasmic or a cytoplasmic and an intranuclear location of the enzyme. Two

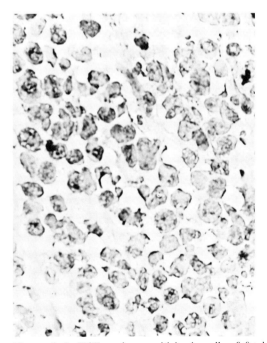

Figure 6–9. TdT nuclear positivity in cells of fetal thymic cortex. Frozen section, no counterstain (×500).

lymphoblastoid cell lines (including MOLT 4) have been shown to exhibit cytoplasmic fluorescence or cytoplasmic ultrastructural immunoperoxidase staining for TDT (Tanaka et al, 1980). Furthermore, Cibull et al (1981) have reported both fluorescent cytoplasmic and intranuclear TDT staining in the peripheral blast cells of two patients with chronic myeloid leukemia undergoing blast crisis. In the rat embryo, TDT is strictly nuclear in bone marrow cells and immature subcapsular thymocytes but may be nuclear, cytoplasmic, or both within the thymic cortex. These different staining patterns do not seem simply to represent technical artifacts, but may correspond to differences in maturational stage; indeed, in chicken embryo thymus, the variability in intensity of staining has been correlated with thymocyte maturation (Sugimoto and Bollum, 1979). That T cell leukemias stain more intensely in the nucleus than "null" cell leukemias may also reflect the supported differences in maturity of these two forms of acute lymphoblastic leukemia (Steinman et al, 1979).

Immunohistologic investigations have also shown that cortical thymocytes and TDT-positive lymphoblasts show a variable degree of intensity of nuclear staining, probably reflecting a different content of enzyme from cell to cell. This point of view is supported by the observation that there is no correlation between the number of TDT-positive cells and quantitative enzymatic activity; eg, high levels of terminal transferase by biochemical assay are not always associated with a high percentage of cells reacting with anticalf TDT, therefore the intensity of cellular staining must also be considered.

At the present time intracellular detection of TDT is of some diagnostic value in selected situations, as described below.

Diagnostic Uses of TDT Staining

The histopathologic and cytologic criteria for the differential diagnosis of lymphoblastic lymphoma, Burkitt's lymphoma, noncleaved follicular center cell lymphomas, and the various forms of acute lymphoblastic leukemia are now quite well recognized and permit the correct diagnosis in many cases (review text—Robb-Smith and Taylor, 1981).

However, in other cases characterized by the absence of nuclear convolutions (non-convoluted T lymphoblasts), presentation in anomalous body sites (eg, T lymphoblasts

without mediastinal involvement), or occurrence in older patients, it may be extremely difficult to make the correct diagnosis on morphologic grounds alone. In these instances either the ability of the neoplastic cells to form E rosettes or the demonstration of positivity for acid phosphatase may facilitate recognition of the T cell nature of the disorder. Similarly, demonstration of SIg would permit recognition of B cell cases, and positive reaction with antibody (monoclonal or conventional) versus common ALL antigen (CALLA) might help define the null cell group.

For example, double immunofluorescence techniques on frozen sections have been used by Janossy et al (1980 c, d, e) to differentiate directly in situ, thymic ALL blast cells (TDT$^+$, HuTLA$^+$, CALLA$^-$) from common or "null" ALL blasts (TDT$^+$, HuTLA$^-$, CALLA$^+$). If these surface markers are not expressed because of the immaturity of the neoplastic lymphoblasts, then the demonstration of high levels of TDT may be important in establishing the thymic origin of the lymphomatous cells. In these circumstances immunocytochemical demonstration of intracellular TDT (in sections or imprints) is more practical than the biochemical assay of the enzyme in lymph node cell suspensions, especially when the diagnosis is unexpected or if the biopsy specimen is small (Table 6–3).

TDT, besides showing positivity in ALL (acute lymphoblastic leukemia), shows distinctive positivity in the closely related condition, lymphoblastic lymphoma. This should not be surprising because lymphoblastic lymphoma and ALL are simply the two ends of a continuous spectrum of disease; in many cases separation is arbitrary. Lymphoblastic lymphomas consist of cells that resemble the lymphoblasts of ALL. Most cases are of T cell type as noted in Chapter 4; these typically show "immature" T cell markers (see Fig. 4–30). Approximately one third are "non-B non-T" type (ie, they lack the usual surface markers). These include cases of B cell type (strictly pre-B: SIg negative, but cytoplasmic mu chain–positive) and "null" type (common ALL antigen positive). Most authorities now believe that the presence or absence of convolutions is of little value in separating these different types. The distinction of lymphoblastic lymphoma from Burkitt's lymphoma and non-Burkitt's lymphoma (diffuse small cleaved follicular center cell lymphomas) may often be made morphologically; immunohistologic studies with anti–B cell monoclonals are more reliable, whereas TDT is negative in all but the lymphoblastic group, with rare exceptions (see Braziel et al, 1983).

Other applications include the immunocytochemical detection of TDT to search for subclinical bone marrow involvement in patients with common type acute lymphoblastic leukemia—remember, of course, that the small number of TDT-positive lymphocytes normally present in the marrow cannot be distinguished by this technique from ALL-positive blast cells. Also, immunohistologic techniques may be extremely useful in displaying increased numbers of positive (leukemic) cells and may detect any focal infiltrates of leukemic cells in extramedullary sites, including cerebrospinal fluid and testicles, in which TDT-positive cells are not normally found (Table 6–3).

Immunostaining on paraffin sections may also be utilized to demonstrate TDT in bone marrow and extramedullary tissues of chronic myeloid leukemia patients undergoing blast crisis. Double immunoenzymatic techniques using anti-TDT antibody in combination with antilysozyme, anti-mu chain cytoplasmic, and anti-HbA antibodies (markers respectively of myeloblastic, pre-B and erythroblastic types of blast transformation) may provide important information regarding the natural history and interrelations of these diseases. Immunocytochemical recognition of TDT–positive blast crisis appears to have some prognostic value, for these patients have been reported to respond well to treatment with vincristine and prednisone (Marks et al, 1978).

ADENOSINE DEAMINASE (ADA)

Adenosine deaminase (ADA) catalyzes the conversion of adenosine or deoxyadenosine to produce ammonia and inosine. Two forms of ADA with apparent molecular weights of 35,000 to 45,000 and 200,000 to 300,000 have been distinguished. The low molecular weight form of the enzyme, purified from erythrocytes and thymus, has been utilized to raise antibody anti-ADA in animals. Chechik et al (1980, 1981), using an immunoperoxidase technique, have been able to detect the enzyme ADA in paraffin sections. ADA appears to be located mainly within the cortical thymocytes. Peripheral blood and tonsil cells are heterogeneous with respect to the expres-

sion of the enzyme. The utility of this enzyme as a T cell marker is limited by the fact that only quantitative differences exist from cell to cell, and by our collective lack of experience of the distribution of this marker in normal and neoplastic cells.

HISTIOCYTES AND MONOCYTES— LYSOZYME, ANTITRYPSIN, ANTICHYMOTRYPSIN

Lysozyme, described by Alexander Fleming in the 1920's as "tear antiseptic," otherwise known as muramidase, is an enzyme with a low molecular weight (about 15,000 daltons); it catalyzes the hydrolysis of the beta-(1,4)-glycosidic linkage between N-acetylmuramic acid and N-acetyl-D-glucosamine in bacterial cell walls and hence has bacteriocidal properties. Lysozyme also facilitates the digestion of chitin.

This enzyme is present in certain human secretions such as milk, tears, and saliva, and also in myeloid, histiomonocytic, and certain epithelial cells (Mason and Taylor, 1975; Reitamo et al, 1978) (Table 6–4; Fig. 6–10). Because the lysozyme isolated from different tissues of the same species has an identical structure, it can be separated from the milk, saliva, or urine of patients with myelomonocytic leukemia for the purpose of raising heterologous antisera; these antisera can then be utilized in immunocytochemical studies of the tissue distribution of lysozyme.

Immunocytochemical methods represented a considerable improvement over the previously available methods for assessing tissue distribution of lysozyme, first overlaying fresh frozen sections with a growth lawn of *Micrococcus lysodeicticus* (a lysozyme-susceptible organism) or with "chitin soup," then searching for focal areas of lysis that betray the presence of an underlying lysozyme-containing cell.

Glynn and Parkman (1964) used immunofluorescence techniques for the demonstration of lysozyme directly in tissue sections. Since then, many investigators have used immunofluorescence techniques for demonstrating lysozyme in situ, but it was not until the advent of the immunoperoxidase techniques (Table 6–5) that some of the problems inherent in immunofluorescence were overcome. The high resistance of the lysozyme molecule to a number of fixatives and processing techniques (Reitamo, 1978) is partly

Table 6–4. Distribution of Lysozyme in Human Tissues

Normal Tissue	Lysozyme (Muramidase) Activity	Normal Tissue	Lysozyme (Muramidase) Activity
Digestive System		**Lymphatic and Hematologic Tissue**	
Stomach	Negative		
Small bowel	Paneth's cells positive	Lymph nodes	Histiocytes positive
Colon	Negative	Spleen	Histiocytes positive
Liver	Kupffer's cells positive	Peripheral blood	Polymorphs and monocytes positive
Pancreas	Negative		
		Bone marrow	Myeloid cells positive
Endocrine System			
Adrenal	Negative	**Respiratory System**	
Thyroid	Negative	Lung	Alveolar lining cells and iron/carbon-containing macrophages negative
Genitourinary System			
Testis	Negative	Bronchial epithelium	Mucus-secreting cells negative
Ovary	Negative		
Prostate	Negative	**Integument**	
Kidney	Proximal tubular cells positive	Skin	Sweat and sebaceous glands positive
Uterine cervix	Negative, including endocervical glands		
Endometrium	Negative		

Pathological Tissue	Lysozyme (Muramidase) Activity
Exocrine Glands	
Reactive	
Lacrimal	Positive
Granulation tissue	Histiocytes positive
Salivary	Serous elements positive
Fat necrosis	Giant cells positive
Bronchial	Serous elements positive
Tuberculosis, sarcoidosis, and Crohn's disease	Epithelioid histiocytes and giant cells positive
Sebaceous	Negative
Sweat	Negative
Lipid-containing phagocytes	
Mammary Tissue	
Nonlactating	Negative
Xanthoma	Giant cells positive
Lactating	Positive
Gaucher's disease	Histiocytes positive
Musculoskeletal System	
Miscellaneous	
Striated muscle	Negative
Histiocytoma	Negative
Smooth muscle	Negative
Giant cell tumor of tendon sheath	Negative
Myocardium	Negative
Cartilage	Positive
Eosinophilic granuloma	Eosinophils and histiocytes positive

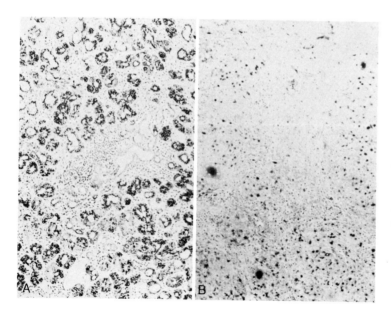

Figure 6–10. Lysozyme (or muramidase—tear antiseptic) was identified in tears by Alexander Fleming 60 years ago. **A,** The secretory elements of the lacrimal gland stain strongly for lysozyme (black acini). **B,** Many histiocytes also contain lysozyme in detectable amounts, as typified by the epithelioid histiocytes and giant cells of sarcoidosis. Paraffin sections, hematoxylin counterstain (×60).

Table 6–5. Selected Bibliography: Lysozyme, Alpha₁-Antitrypsin, Alpha₁-Antichymotrypsin

Isaacson et al 1982	Malignant histiocytosis of intestine
Carbone et al 1981	Malignant histiocytosis; histochemistry/immunohistochemistry
Bellomi & Gamoletti 1981	Case report—malignant histiocytic tumor
Jothy et al 1981	Malignant histiocytosis involving kidney—2 cases
Mendelsohn et al 1980c	Lysozyme and histiocyte differentiation in malignant histiocytosis
Risdall et al 1980	Lysozyme and histiocyte differentiation, light and EM study in malignant histiocytosis
Koh et al 1980	Lysozyme and alpha₁-antichymotrypsin staining revealed one "true" histiocytic lymphoma among 41 childhood cases
Nash 1982	Lysozyme in macrophages in a variety of human tumors
Nathrath & Meister 1982 / Meister & Nathrath 1980	Lysozyme and alpha₁-antichymotrypsin as histiocyte markers
Carr et al 1980	Lysozyme in granulomas; release into serum and lymph
Burgdorf et al 1981b	Histiocytosis X, juvenile xanthogranuloma, positive for lysozyme; fibrous histiocytoma, dermatofibroma negative
Seo et al 1982	4 lysozyme-positive tumors among 22 "lymphomas" of stomach
Ducatman et al 1984	Malignant histiocytosis; lysozyme and alpha₁-antitrypsin
Howard & Batsakis 1982	Peanut agglutinin marks more histiocytes than does lysozyme
Tubbs et al 1980b	Giant cell myocarditis—giant cell negative
Klockars et al 1979	Lysozyme-positive cells in renal graft indicate poor prognosis
Kami et al 1981	Staining of leukocytes
Ogawa et al 1979	Nasal mucosa
Heitz & Wegmann 1980 / Reitamo et al 1981	Paneth's cells in intestinal carcinomas
Ree et al 1981a / Ree et al 1981b	Lysozyme in Hodgkin's disease; many positive cells indicate better prognosis
Payne et al 1982	Alpha₁-antitrypsin and macrophage origin of Reed-Sternberg cells
Motoi et al 1980	Lysozyme, antichymotrypsin, antitrypsin in lymph node cells
Papadimitriou et al 1980	Antichymotrypsin and antitrypsin in lymph node cells
Aozasa & Inoue 1982	Lethal midline granuloma—16 cases—evidence that critical cells are truly histiocytic (lysozyme-positive)
Kerdel et al 1982	Lysozyme, antitrypsin, antichymotrypsin in histiocytic infiltrates of dermis
Pinkus & Said 1977	Lysozyme in normal and neoplastic tissues
Mason & Tatlor 1975	Tissue distribution of lysozyme
Tahara et al 1982	Lysozyme in about 40% of cases of gastric carcinoma

responsible for the successful application of the immunoperoxidase method in cell smears fixed in buffered formol-acetone, as well as in tissue specimens fixed in formalin or Zenker's fluid. The PAP and protein A immunoperoxidase techniques both are more sensitive than the conventional indirect antibody technique, which, in early studies, gave poor results in the detection of lysozyme; the labelled antigen method (peroxidase-labelled lysozyme) has also been used with success.

Distribution of Lysozyme in Human Tissues

Table 6–4 shows the wide distribution of lysozyme in normal human tissues as revealed by immunoperoxidase staining. Because the importance of lysozyme detection in surgical pathology is mainly related to its utilization as a marker for cells of the myeloid and histiocyte-monocyte series, the staining pattern of normal lymphoid and hematopoietic tissues is discussed more extensively.

Lysozyme is present in the myeloid cells of normal human bone marrow at various stages of maturation from the promyelocyte to the segmented forms; cell fractionation studies have shown that the primary granules are responsible for about 50 percent of the lysozyme activity in human myeloid cells, and secondary granules are responsible for the rest.

Lysozyme is also a marker of cells of the histiocyte-monocyte series and is a major secretory product of blood monocytes; epithelioid histiocytes contain large amounts of lysozyme (Figs. 6–10 and 6–11). Histiocytes, including "starry-sky" macrophages, epithelioid cells, and certain sinus lining cells, have all proven to be lysozyme-positive in normal human lymphoid tissues (Fig. 6–11); whereas lymphocytes, dendritic reticulum cells, interdigitating reticulum cells and the "reticulum cells" of the bone marrow (Fig. 6–12) are consistently lysozyme negative. The mononuclear phagocytes of the central nervous system (glia) and the lung alveolar macrophages also appear to be lysozyme negative. Granulocytes, neutrophils, and eosinophils are lysozyme positive, as are mast cells (Table 6–4).

Lysozyme is stored in the granules of granulocytes and liberated after cell death or degranulation; whereas in the mononuclear phagocytes it is synthesized and released continuously, and this is probably the reason for weaker staining for lysozyme in monocytes than in myeloid cells. It may also explain (a) why the staining is stronger near the cell surface, and (b) why there is a brown halo around these latter cells after immunoperox-

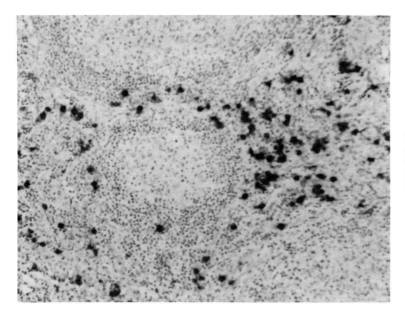

Figure 6–11. Lymph node in leprosy. Positively stained (black) cells are epithelioid histiocytes reacting with antilysozyme antibody. Paraffin section, AEC with hematoxylin counterstain (×125).

idase staining, especially noticeable in frozen sections and in cell smears.

Applications

Granulocyte Proliferations—Granulocytic Leukemias, Granulocytic Sarcoma

Immunocytochemical detection of lysozyme may be of particular value in separating granulocytic sarcoma (Fig. 6–13) from other undifferentiated large cell malignancies, because a significant number of the neoplastic cells are positive for lysozyme at immunope-

roxidase staining; this tumor has often been misdiagnosed as reticulum cell sarcoma (Wiernik and Serpick, 1970) or nonsecretory myeloma (Carmichael and Lee, 1977). Since neoplastic histiocytes may also be lysozyme-positive, it is essential that immunohistochemical investigations be backed by confirmatory studies or staining for lactoferrin to distinguish granulocytic sarcoma from the very rare "true" histiocytic lymphoma (ie, large cell tumors of histiocytic origin as opposed to large cell tumors of transformed lymphocytes, now called immunoblastic sarcoma, but formerly termed histiocytic lymphoma or reticulum cell sarcoma). Confirm-

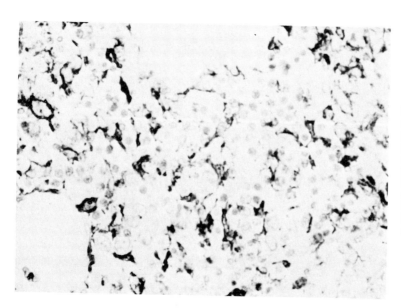

Figure 6–12. Lysozyme-negative histiocytes often can be detected by demonstration of an absorbed or phagocytosed product, for example, ferritin. Section of bone marrow aspirate fixed in B5 showing a positive immunostain for ferritin in marrow histiocytes (reticulum cells); patient had cirrhosis and iron overload. Paraffin section, DAB with hematoxylin counterstain (×200).

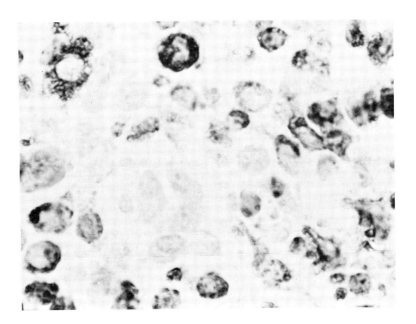

Figure 6–13. Granulocytic sarcoma demonstrating lysozyme reactivity within primitive myeloid cells. Paraffin section, DAB with hematoxylin counterstain (×900).

atory stains for granulocytes include immunohistochemical stains for lactoferrin (Mason and Taylor, 1978; Briggs et al, 1983) or histochemical stains for chloroacetate esterase (Leder's stain—effective in paraffin sections).

Studies on the distribution of lysozyme in acute myeloid leukemias have brought conflicting results. Some authors (eg, Mason, 1977) have been able to detect lysozyme in mature-stage myeloid cells in cases of acute myeloblastic leukemia but have failed to detect the enzyme in leukemic myeloblasts. This failure may be due to the fact that the primary granules, which contain about 50 percent of the lysozyme, first appear during the promyelocytic stage; whether or not the so-called blasts are lysozyme positive would depend on the degree of maturation (eg, most of the "blast cells" in acute promyelocytic leukemias are lysozyme-positive).

Other investigators (Pinkus and Said, 1977; Kageoka et al, 1977) claim to have detected lysozyme in the cytoplasm of a percentage of myeloblasts. The degree of staining was variable and probably reflected a fluctuation in the enzyme content from cell to cell. These observations agree with the finding of Karle et al (1974), who reported the extraction of lysozyme from leukemic myeloblasts, and with the immunofluorescence studies of Greenberger et al (1977), in which intracytoplasmic lysozyme was demonstrated in 80 to 95 percent of blast cells in eight of ten acute myeloblastic leukemia patients. Green-

berger and colleagues previously had demonstrated that lysozyme is synthesized by primitive myeloblasts in experimental myelocytic leukemia in rats. The raised levels of serum lysozyme encountered in acute leukemias may be the result of an increased production and destruction of myeloid, monocytic cells, or both. These discrepancies most probably are of no real consequence, reflecting differences in criteria for designating cells as blasts or promyelocytes or perhaps reflecting asynchrony of nuclear and cytoplasmic maturation in the leukemic cell population.

The immunohistologic detection of lysozyme in bone marrow biopsies is of particular clinical value in diagnosing myeloblastic and myelomonocytic leukemias (Fig. 6–14) arising during the course of multiple myeloma or Waldenström's macroglobulinemia or other lymphomas in the marrow. Under these circumstances immunohistologic studies in combination with cytochemical and ultrastructural investigations help to distinguish myeloid cells from "undifferentiated" plasma cells (ie, the neoplastic transformed B lymphocytes that represent the proliferating cell population in patients with myeloma; see Chapter 5).

Histiocytic Disorders

Epithelioid histiocytes and multinucleated giant cells in granulomatous disorders such as sarcoidosis, tuberculosis, and Crohn's dis-

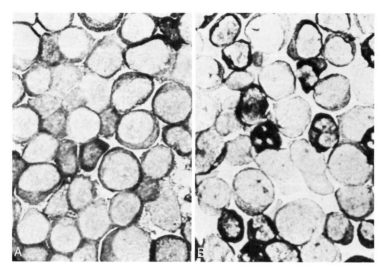

Figure 6–14. Marrow smears in a case of acute myelo-monocytic leukemia (M4) identifying the granulocytic lineage of the cells by staining for lysozyme (muramidase) in immature cells, *A*, and lactoferrin in mature cells, *B*, (both, black cytoplasmic staining). Lysozyme is present in granulocytes and histiocytes, lactoferrin in granulocytes only. DAB with hematoxylin counterstain (×900).

ease contain large amounts of lysozyme that is demonstrable by immunoperoxidase methods in paraffin sections (Table 6–5).

Certain other giant cells, such as Warthin-Finkeldey cells, first identified in 1931 by Warthin and Finkeldey and thought to be specific of measles but now identified in many benign and malignant lymphoid disorders (Kjeldsberg and Kim, 1981), do not contain lysozyme; it is believed that they may be of lymphocytic origin rather than derived from histiocytes.

The granulomas of lepromatous leprosy have been found to be strongly lysozyme-positive, whereas those of tuberculoid leprosy contain lesser amounts. Foreign body granulomas have been reported to be negative or faintly positive (Table 6–5). Immunoelectron microscope studies of experimental rat granulomas and human sarcoid granulomas (Lobo et al, 1978) have shown that lysozyme is located within electron-dense bodies of various sizes in the cytoplasm of macrophage and giant cells. A possible explanation of the variability with which epithelioid cells in granulomas stain for lysozyme is that these cells contain different amounts of enzyme, depending on their stage of differentiation, the rate of synthesis, and the rate of release of lysozyme.

Florid epithelial cell reactions are sometimes observed in association with non-Hodgkin's lymphoma (Fig. 6–15), Hodgkin's disease, multiple myeloma, and solid tumors.

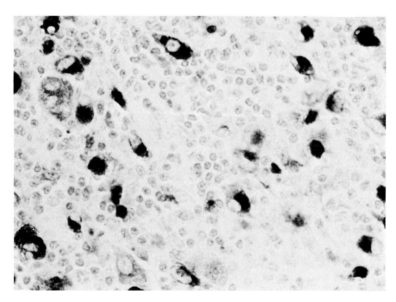

Figure 6–15. Non-Hodgkin lymphomas: a case of lymphoepithelioid cell lymphoma (a T cell lymphoma sometimes termed Lennert's lymphoma) stained for lysozyme (muramidase). The cells with positive cytoplasmic staining are the "reactive" epithelioid histiocytes. The neoplastic T cells are not positive. Paraffin section, DAB with hematoxylin counterstain (×200).

Immunohistologic studies of tissue distribution of lysozyme in different subtypes of Hodgkin's disease have been recently reported by Ree et al (1981b); these authors found positivity for lysozyme in benign histiocytes, epithelial cells, granulocytes, and eosinophils but not in the Reed-Sternberg cells or mononuclear variants. The most intense staining reaction for lysozyme was observed in patients with the most favorable clinical course (eg, absence of general symptoms and stages I and II disease). This immunohistologic staining pattern has therefore been interpreted as expression of host resistance to the tumor, although conflicting evidence does exist.

Reactive histiocytes, multinucleated giant cells, and eosinophils present in eosinophilic granuloma are usually lysozyme-positive.

Langerhans's cells, present in variable numbers in the epidermis, are usually negative, although some contrary claims have been made. Immunohistologically, Langerhans's cells appear to differ from histiocytes, lacking detectable lysozyme (Elema and Atmosoerodjo-Briggs, 1984) but showing a positive reaction with a monoclonal antibody, designated anti-T6, that recognizes an immature population of thymocytes (see Chapter 4).

Burgdorf et al (1981b) used immunoperoxidase techniques to investigate the distribution of lysozyme in different types of cutaneous lesions of uncertain cellular origin (eg, histiocytosis X, multicentric reticulohistiocytosis, juvenile xanthogranuloma, "fibrous" dermatofibroma, dermatofibrosarcoma protuberans, and malignant fibrous histiocytoma). The majority of the cells of juvenile xanthogranuloma and the reactive histiocytes and multinucleated giant cells present in histiocytosis X appeared to contain lysozyme. Histiocytosis X is, however, readily distinguishable from other "histiocytic" disorders in showing strong reactivity with OKT6 (monoclonal antibody in frozen sections) as well as with anti–HLA-DR (Ia) reagents; OKT6 reactivity has been the justification for claims that histiocytosis X is derived from the Langerhans's cell or a close relative thereof (Bos et al, 1984). The cells of the other conditions were lysozyme-negative, suggesting an origin from cells other than histiocytes or, alternatively, the loss of capability to produce lysozyme as a result of cell dedifferentiation.

A number of researchers (Table 6–5) consider lysozyme to be a marker of histiocyte-derived tumors (Tubbs et al, 1977b), eg, malignant histiocytosis, including the condition termed histiocytic medullary reticulosis by Scott and Robb-Smith (see Robb-Smith and Taylor, 1981). Elevated levels of serum lysozyme have been observed in a percentage of histiocytic medullary reticulosis patients, and in some cases the more mature-appearing histiocytes are strongly lysozyme-positive by immunohistologic staining. More immature-appearing cells most often appear to be lysozyme negative but often show positive reactions with antibodies to alpha$_1$-antitrypsin (Fig. 6–16) or chymotrypsin, advanced by some as valid histiocyte markers (Table 6–5).

Meister et al (1980; Meister and Nathrath,

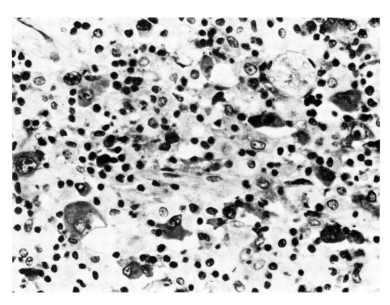

Figure 6–16. Alpha$_1$-antitrypsin reactivity of varying intensity (pale to dark gray) within malignant histiocytes of a case of histiocytic medullary reticulosis (malignant histiocytosis). The better-differentiated cells tend to stain most intensely; this is a better-differentiated area. Paraffin section, DAB with hematoxylin counterstain (×200).

1980), using an immunoperoxidase procedure, succeeded in demonstrating intracytoplasmic lysozyme in 16 cases of malignant histiocytosis. Cytoplasmic lysozyme was detected in the neoplastic histiocytes, regardless of the stage of differentiation, in all four cases of malignant histiocytosis studied by Tubbs et al (1977a) using a similar technique, whereas Mendelsohn and colleagues (1980c) found intense positive staining for lysozyme in the group I (minimal cytologic atypia and rare erythrophagocytosis) cases but little or no staining in group II (minimal cytologic atypia with extensive erythrophagocytosis) and group III (marked cytologic atypia and rare erythrophagocytosis). Serial biopsies of one of these patients appeared to show a loss of ability to synthesize lysozyme concomitant with a progressive dedifferentiation of the malignant cells. Risdall et al (1980) reported three cases that were morphologically similar to Mendelsohn's group III patients and were lysozyme-negative; diffuse cytoplasmic staining for nonspecific esterase and acid phosphatase was observed in the tumor imprints of all three. These findings suggest that lysozyme is mainly present in the relatively more differentiated cases of malignant histiocytosis and that it is absent from the relatively more dedifferentiated form. The greater the differentiation of histiocytic lesions, the greater the lysozyme expression, and this circumstance is considered by some authors to indicate a favorable prognosis.

This finding places some restrictions on lysozyme as a histiocyte marker, because it is the more anaplastic forms of malignant histiocytosis that are difficult to distinguish from large cell lymphomas and from undifferentiated carcinomas, neither of which usually contains lysozyme. The situation is further complicated. The degree of differentiation of neoplastic histiocytes would also seem to affect the degree to which enzymatic markers such as nonspecific esterases and acid phosphatase are expressed, the well-differentiated cells being strongly positive and the undifferentiated cells only slightly positive (Vilpo et al, 1980).

It is now known that the majority of non-Hodgkin's lymphomas that were previously classified as reticulum cell sarcomas (histiocytic lymphomas in Rappaport's classification) are in fact a heterogeneous group of tumors that usually originate from lymphocytes of the B, T, or null cell type. "True" histiocytic lymphomas as defined by cytologic and immunologic criteria are quite rare (Groopman and Golde, 1981). In the series of 425 cases of non-Hodgkin's lymphoma studied at our institution (Lukes et al, 1978), only a single case of "true" histiocytic lymphoma appeared. Another single case has been reported by Koh et al (1980) in his series of 41 cases of childhood malignant "histiocytic lymphoma." In other immunohistologic studies of large cell lymphomas, not one case of "true" histiocytic lymphoma was detected (Stein et al, 1981b).

However, it should be noted that not all researchers agree on the rarity of histiocytic malignancies. For example, 33 of the 66 cases of gastrointestinal lymphomas studied with immunoperoxidase techniques by Isaacson and colleagues were interpreted as lysozyme-positive and thus were presumed to be of histiocytic origin. Twenty-two of these positive cases were designated intestinal malignant histiocytosis; the other 11 were diagnosed as "true" histiocytic lymphomas (Isaacson et al, 1979, 1982). Also, 10 cases of non-Hodgkin's lymphoma described by van der Valk (1981) fulfilled the morphologic, ultrastructural, cytochemical, and immunohistochemical criteria of "true" histiocytic lymphoma. Histologically, these tumors were composed of large, often multinucleated cells with abundant basophilic cytoplasm. The nuclei varied from oval to kidney-shaped, and there was a variable degree of erythrophagocytosis in all cases. Half of the patients presented a clinical picture different from the one classically observed in malignant histiocytosis; instead of the characteristic organ dissemination, there was involvement of a single lymph node station. Although lysozyme could be detected in all cases, the staining was more intense when there was a high degree of differentiation—that is, when the number of lysosomes present in the cytoplasm was high at electron microscopy. The authors proposed the term "histiocytic sarcoma" for these tumors.

Reactivity for lysozyme does not necessarily imply a histiocytic derivation. As already described, granulocytic sarcomas are lysozyme-positive. Also, there are theoretical grounds for expecting that certain carcinomas derived from epithelial cells that normally may secrete lysozyme might be lysozyme-positive. Such tissues include lacrimal gland, salivary gland, breast, stomach, and intestine (Paneth cells). Positivity for lysozyme has indeed been reported in the corresponding tumor cells

Table 6–6. Occurrence of Lysozyme, Alpha₁-Antitrypsin (AAT), Alpha₁-Antichymotrypsin (AACT), Albumin, and Transferrin in Various Lymph Node Cells*

Type of Cell	Lysozyme	AAT	AACT
Neutrophils	+ + +	+	–
Eosinophils	+ + +	na	–
Mast cells	+ +	+/+ +	+
Histiocytes of the pulp	+/+ +	–	–/+ +
Starry-sky cells	+/+ +	–	+/+ +
Sinus histiocytes	–	–	+/+ +
Sinus-lining cells	–	–	+
Epithelioid cells	+/+ +	–/+	+
Giant cells of Langerhans's type	+/+ +	–/+	+
Dendritic reticulum cells	–	–	–
Interdigitating reticulum cells	–	–	–
Lymphocytes	–	–	–
Immunoblasts	–	–	–
Germinal center cells	–	–	–
Plasma cells	–	–	–

*Modified from Motoi et al. Virchows Arch (B) 35;73, 1980.

(Table 6–5). This positivity also is distinct from the reported presence of reactive histiocytes infiltrating tumors (Nash, 1982), a finding particularly prevalent in intestinal cancers.

Alpha₁-Antitrypsin and Alpha¹-Antichymotrypsin

Recognizing the shortcomings of lysozyme as a histiocytic marker, some investigators have explored the utility of alpha₁-antitrypsin (AAT) (Fig. 6–16) or alpha¹-antichymotrypsin (AACT) for this purpose (Table 6–5). Overall, this approach has not proved much more successful. However, when used in con-

junction with staining for lysozyme, these antibodies are of value, often giving reactivity in histiocytes when lysozyme does not, and vice versa (Table 6–6). It should be remembered that both AAT and AACT also are found in cells other than histiocytes (liver cells, hepatomas, germ-cell tumors). We have used a combination of staining for lysozyme, AAT, and AACT as a valuable indicator of myeloid differentiation in the acute leukemias (Krugliak, 1985).

Other Histiocytic Markers

A number of monoclonal antibodies with reactivity against cells of the histiocyte-mon-

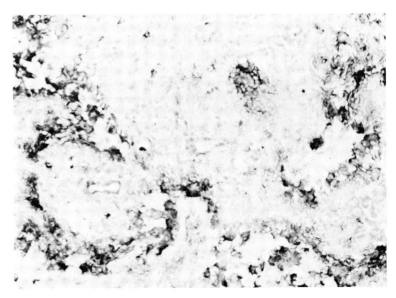

Figure 6–17. Lymph node medulla showing reactivity of sinus histiocytes (black) with an antimonocyte monoclonal antibody (Leu M2). Frozen section, glucose oxidase, no counterstain (×200).

Table 6–7. Monoclonals with Activity Against Cells of the
Macrophage-Monocyte-Histiocyte Series

Anti-	Cell Types Showing Reactivity	Source
Ia (various antibodies)	Some monocytes (histiocytes) B lymphocytes Activated T cells Null cells, other cell types (Chapter 6)	Various manufacturers
OKM1,Mol	Monocytes (histiocytes) Granulocytes, "suppressor" T cells "Null" cells (NK cells)	Ortho, Coulter (possibly equivalent to Leu 15)
OKM5	Monocytes (histiocytes), platelets	Ortho
LeuM1	Monocytes (histiocytes) Granulocytes	Becton Dickinson
LeuM2	Monocytes (histiocytes), platelets	Becton Dickinson
LeuM3, Mo2	"Mature" monocytes (histiocytes)	Becton Dickinson, Coulter
OKT9 (antitransferrin receptor)	Activated lymphocytes Some monocytes, other cells	Various manufacturers

ocyte series have become available. Most are effective only in frozen sections, although LeuM1 does give reactivity in paraffin sections.

The specificity of these reagents is still under investigation. Much of the published work relates to normal peripheral blood monocytes, with relatively little data on tissue phagocytes (histiocytes), Kupffer's cells, littoral cells, glial cells, and so forth (Figure

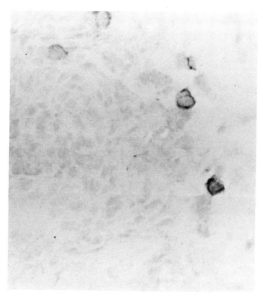

Figure 6–18. Part of a large sarcoid granuloma, bordered by a few cells showing reactivity with an interleukin 2 (IL2) antibody. Frozen section, AEC with light hematoxylin counterstain (×320) (see Modlin et al, 1984a). Presence of IL2 and Tac-positive cells is thought to indicate an ongoing active immune response.

6–17) and even less data on neoplastic histiocytes. These reagents should thus be used with caution in support of orthodox cytologic methods for cell recognition. Table 6–7 lists some of the widely available reagents (Ortho, Becton Dickinson, Coulter, and others). Other "custom-made" reagents have also been described (Becker GJ et al, 1981– PHM1, 2, and 3, recognizing certain blood monocytes). The manufacturers are usually pleased to provide the latest literature on the application of their own products. Still other reagents may detect histiocyte or lymphocyte products (eg, anti-interleukin 2) and are the subject of intense investigation (Figure 6–18).

The potential utility of antimacrophage monoclonals is well shown by the report of Harrist and colleagues (1983) showing phenotyping similarities between histiocytosis X and Langerhans's cells (OKT6$^+$, Ia$^+$). Anti-Ia antibodies mark most histiocytes but also mark B cells and other cell types as described earlier.

Mast Cells

Human platelet factor 4 (HPF4) binds to heparin in mast cell granules. Utilized in conjunction with anti-HPF4 antibodies, HPF4 provides an effective immunohistologic method for the specific staining of mast cells in paraffin and Epon-embedded tissues (Shaw et al, 1982; McLaren et al 1980; Giddings et al, 1982b). Factor VIII antigen has also been described in mast cells (Kindblom, 1982; Giddings et al, 1982b).

7

THE DIFFUSE NEUROENDOCRINE SYSTEM OF THE GASTROINTESTINAL TRACT

"The adventurous physician goes on, and substitutes presumption for knowledge. From the scanty field of what is known, he launches into the boundless region of what is unknown."

THOMAS JEFFERSON, 1743–1826

The presence of a population of endocrine cells within the gastrointestinal tract has long been recognized; morphologically, they appear as scattered clear "paracrine" cells. There has been, however, considerable uncertainty concerning their embryologic origin, their anatomic distribution, and their function; it also is unclear if they represent a homogeneous population of cells or a series of subpopulations subserving different functions.

On hematoxylin and eosin preparations, these cells are relatively inconspicuous and morphologically homogeneous (clear cells). However, following fixation in formalin, considerable heterogeneity is demonstrable with respect to silver staining (argentaffin and argyrophil cells), autofluorescence, and metachromasia. Subsequently, the realization has grown that many of these cells contain biologically active polypeptides or biogenic amines, and attempts have been made to correlate the different histochemical reactions with these cell products.

Initially, success was rather limited until Pearse, in 1968, introduced some organization into what had become a rather confused field with his concept of the APUD (amine precursor uptake and decarboxylation) sys-

tem. Pearse noted that all of the APUD cells had the capacity to produce one or more biogenic amines or polypeptide hormones; furthermore, the corresponding neoplasms frequently displayed similar capabilities.

The embryologic origin of these cells remained controversial, some investigators favoring origin from the neural crest, others supporting the idea of direct origin by differentiation from endodermal stem cells. It was generally accepted that these "neuroendocrine" cells, dispersed throughout the stomach, small intestine, and colon, were closely related to cells forming the islets of Langerhans and shared common histochemical characteristics. The paper by Bryant and colleagues (1982) charting the time of appearance and distribution of positive cells in the human fetus is of particular value in documenting the microanatomic relationship of the various hormone-producing cells, and the report of Lewin and colleagues (Ulich et al, 1983) postulating a spectrum of tumors from typical adenocarcinoma to typical carcinoid (see later) is of interest in suggesting derivation of endocrine cells from the gut endoderm. Likewise, the occurrence of APUD cells in ovarian and testicular teratomas is best explained by the proposition that

163

they differentiate in situ from endodermal elements within the teratoma (Bosman and Louwerens, 1981). Vuitch and Mendelsohn (1981) advance a similar argument to explain the presence of neuroendocrine elements (ACTH-producing) in a case of prostatic carcinoma. These elements also have been reported in bile duct carcinoma (Yamamoto et al, 1984), cervical and endometrial carcinomas, and ovarian tumors (see Table 7–4). The corresponding cell in the skin is believed to be the Merkel cell, from which neuroendocrine carcinomas (Merkel cell carcinomas) may or may not arise (Silva et al, 1984b).

The demonstration of cytokeratin in carcinoids suggests that these tumors and their progenitor neuroendocrine cells are derived from epithelium (Höfler and Denk, 1984).

RECOGNITION OF NEUROENDOCRINE (APUD) CELLS

The introduction of immunocytochemistry with the capability of identifying specific biogenic amines and polypeptide hormones in situ revolutionized the approach of pathologists towards recognition of these "neuroendocrine" cells and their corresponding neoplasms. The suspicion that the basic histochemical reactions (argentaffin, argyrophil, masked metachromasia, enterochromaffin) are relatively nonspecific, in terms of categorizing cells according to the type of hormone they produce, was confirmed. Gradually it has become clear that the only reliable approach towards classification of these cells and their corresponding neoplasms is by hormone immunocytochemistry.

Most of the hormones produced by these cells are relatively small polypeptides that often show remarkable similarities in sequence from one to another; this resemblance is both fortunate and unfortunate with regard to immunocytochemistry. The fortunate aspect relates to the relative reistance of polypeptide hormones to the adverse effects of fixation and processing; thus the majority of these cell products are demonstrable in routinely processed paraffin sections. The less fortunate aspect is that, because many of these polypeptides share amino acid sequences, the antibodies prepared against them may also show considerable cross reactivity. For example, antibodies to glucagon often show cross reactivity with somatostatin

and almost always show some reactivity with enteroglucagon (glicentin). Likewise, many antibodies against gastrin show considerable cross reactivity with cholecystokinin.

With some limitations, therefore, immunocytochemistry provides the ability to identify the individual neuroendocrine cells by their hormonal content and to relate corresponding neoplasms to the normal cell types.

One further point must be made; individual cells may produce more than one hormone, both in the normal state and in neoplasms. This ability, of course, has also been observed in the cells of the pituitary, in which ACTH, beta-lipoprotein, and MSH may be found in single cells, and the thyroid, where calcitonin may be present along with somatostatin, ACTH, or both.

Fifteen or more different neuroendocrine cells, based on the type of granule observed by electron microscopy, the silver stain reaction, and more recently upon immunohistochemical demonstration of the cell products, have now been distinguished within gut and pancreas. The functional interrelations of these cells are still not fully resolved, but there is a general consensus in favor of a neuroendocrine control matrix whereby the products of each of these cells have regulatory effects on neighboring cells, either via long cellular processes or via release of the active product into the local tissue milieu. The finding of some hormones in common in brain, peripheral nerves, and gut reinforces this neuroendocrine concept.

The principal cell types, distinguishable by immunocytochemistry, are listed in the accompanying tables (Tables 7–1 and 7–2).

It is also worth considering the intestinal neuroendocrine cells in relation to similar cells elsewhere in the body (the other cells of the APUD system). There has been considerable controversy, of course, as to exactly which cells belong to the system. Today, as described previously, the category of gastrointestinal endocrine cells recognized by Pearse (1968), by Tischler et al (1977), and others has been enormously expanded and diversified, whereas other cell types included initially within the APUD series may not properly belong there. Indeed, the overall usefulness of the concept of APUD cells has considerably diminished in the face of new knowledge, derived from immunocytochemistry, of the precise products of this diverse but interrelated family of cells.

The majority of neoplasms of the gastroin-

Table 7–1. Intestinal Neuroendocrine Cells

		Location					
Designation	Product	Body of Stomach	Antrum	Duo-denum	Jejnum Ileum	Colon	Rectum
G	Gastrin	−	+ + +	+	±	−	−
D	Somatostatin	+ +	+ + +	+	+	±	±
D_1	VIP-(like)	+	+	±	±	+	±
E*	5HT	+ +	+ +	+ +	+ +	+ +	+ +
I	Cholecystokinin	−	−	+ +	±	−	−
P	"Bombesin"	±	+	+	±	−	−
PP	Pancreatic polypeptide	−	±	±	±	±	+
K	GIP	−	−	+	±	−	−
L	GL1	−	−	±	+ +	+	+ +
N	Neurotensin	−	−	−	+ +	−	−

*Subsets of E have been distinguished: EC_1 contains 5HT plus substance P and occurs in small and large intestine; EC_2 contains 5HT and motilin and is restricted to the upper small intestine. *NB*: E cells are argentaffin; all cells are argyrophil (depending on method).

Table 7–2. The Neuroendocrine System—Immunohistochemical Definition*

Type	Product	Location	Possible Embryologic Origin
I. Diffuse Gastrointestinal Tract			
A	Glucagon	Stomach	
D	Somatostatin	Stomach, intestine	
E	Substance P/motilin/5HT	Stomach, intestine	
G	Gastrin	Stomach, duodenum	Endodermal
D_1	VIP	Intestine	
I	Cholecystokinin	Intestine	
L	Enteroglucagon (glicentin)	Intestine	
K	GIP	Intestine	
II. Pancreatic			
A	Glucagon, 5HT		
B	Insulin, 5HT		
D	Somatostatin	Islets	Endodermal
D_1	VIP		
P	"Bombesin"		
PP	Pancreatic polypeptide		
III. Thyroid/Parathyroid			
C	Calcitonin	Thyroid	Endodermal, or possibly
Chief	PTH	Parathyroid	neural crest
IV. Peripheral Neural/Ganglia and the Like			
Chromaffin	Adrenalin, nor-adrenalin	Adrenal medulla	
Melanocytes?	Melanin	Skin	? Neural crest
Glomus	Nor-adrenalin	Carotid body	
E	5HT	UG tract	
V. Neural			
Nuclear	Various releasing factors, soma-tostatin, oxytocin, vasopressin	Hypothalamus	
Pituitary	Growth hormone, prolactin, LH, FSH, ACTH, TSH, MSH, dopamine	Pituitary	Neuroectoderm
?Pineal	Luteinizing hormone, releasing factor, 5HT	Pineal	
VI. Other			
Trophoblast	hCG, ACTH	Placenta	Extraembryonic ectoderm

*Composite table (includes the so-called APUD cells).
From Larsson LI. Scand J Gastroenterol 14(Suppl 53):1, 1979.

Table 7–3. APUD Cells, APUDomas, and Ectopic Polypeptide Hormones Produced by APUDomas*

Cell	Putative Tumor[1]	Ectopic Hormone/Product
Hypothalamic neurosecretory	None identified	
Pinealocyte	Pinealoma	Unknown
Adenohypophyseal	Pituitary adenoma	Unknown
Autonomic neuron	Neurocytoma	ACTH; vasoactive intestinal peptide (VIP)
Chromaffin	Pheochromocytoma	ACTH; follicle-stimulating hormone; calcitonin; insulin
Carotid-body and other paraganglion cells	Paraganglioma; chemodectoma	ACTH; calcitonin
Thyroid C	Medullary carcinoma of thyroid	ACTH; insulin
Bronchial Kulchitsky	Bronchial carcinoid; oat cell carcinoma	ACTH; ADH; calcitonin; insulin; growth hormone; prolactin, glucagon
Gastrointestinal endocrine[2]	Intestinal carcinoid	ACTH; ADH; 5HT; serotonin; VIP, somatostatin, "bombesin", etc.
Pancreatic islet	Islet cell tumor	ACTH; ADH; VIP
Melanocyte	Melanoma	ACTH; gastrin
Germ cells[3]	Ovarian and testicular teratomas and teratocarcinomas	Various polypeptides

*Modified from Tischler AS et al in The New England Journal of Medicine (Vol 296, 1977, p. 219), by permission.
[1]Multiple endocrine adenoma (MEA) syndromes may include two or more of these tumors occurring concurrently.
[2]Adenomas and carcinomas of these cells may, of course, produce any of the polypeptide hormones normally produced by the cell type.
[3]Germ cell tumors have been described as containing APUD cells, presumably differentiating from endodermal elements in these tumors (Bosman and Louwerens, 1981).

testinal neuroendocrine cells and of the embryologically closely related cells in the bronchi, are termed carcinoid tumors (the aggressive form in the lung is called oat cell carcinoma). They appear to have a close relationship to other of the neuroendocrine tumors sometimes occurring alone or as part of the multiple adenoma syndromes (Table 7–3).

Immunostaining and the Need for Controls

O'Briain and Dayal (1981) have written, "immunohistochemical staining techniques using antibodies specifically directed against biogenic amines or polypeptide gut hormones currently represent the most reliable, sensitive, and specific means for the identification and localization of a particular endocrine cell type in tissue sections."

Some reservations are, however, in order. As emphasized elsewhere, the demonstration of molecules by immune-labelling methods is contingent upon the preservation of antigenicity, which in turn means preservation of molecular stucture. Autolysis, fixation, and other stages of tissue-processing may all have adverse effects on the immunoreactivity of tissue antigens. As noted earlier, it is fortun-ate that the majority of products of the neuroendocrine cells are polypeptide hormones and that these are remarkably resistant to the adverse effects of fixation and the various processing and embedding methods. Nonetheless, fixation and paraffin-embedment does result in the loss of some antigen, and maximum presevation of antigen appears to be achieved in tissues that are snap-frozen, freeze-dried, or subject to special processing (Kendall et al, 1971). Less elaborate and requiring less in terms of special equipment or expertise is simple cryostat sectioning of rapidly frozen tissues; good results are obtainable with a number of fixatives.

Much of the work that has been published has utilized tissues fixed in buffered formalin and embedded in paraffin or, alternatively, fixed in Bouin's fixative or picric acid-paraformaldehyde. These last methods, though less efficient than the frozen section approach, do appear to permit detection of polypeptide hormones with a high degree of sensitivity and reproducibility. According to O'Briain and Dayal (1981), mercury and chromate-based fixatives result in loss of some antigenicity and are to be avoided.

Immunoperoxidase techniques, with the intrinsic advantage of excellent morphology, have been preferred over immunofluorescent methods and, in general, the PAP method has been the most widely reported immunoperoxidase procedure for demonstration of gastrointestinal neuroendocrine cells.

Multiple staining methods have also proved popular in the assessment of two or three different hormones in single tissue sections, usually achieved by sequential double or triple immunostaining utilizing different substrates (commonly diaminobenzidine first, followed by alpha naphthol pyronine, 4-chloro-1-naphthol, or amino-ethyl carbazole). The possible drawbacks of using sequential double or triple staining methods in terms of possible cross reactivity and the need for careful control of such stains have been discussed in detail in Chapter 3.

Availability of Reagents

Primary antisera with specificity against gastrin, somatostatin, and VIP are quite widely available from reputable commercial sources, and antibodies against secretin, cholecystokinin, 5-hydroxytryptamine, neurotensin, and bombesin may also be obtained, although the choice of suppliers is less extensive.

One major problem after the antiserum is purchased is assessment of its specificity. Information concerning the specificity tests utilized by the manufacturer is of considerable value, but ultimate assessment of suitability for immunohistochemical studies should be based upon immunohistochemical controls—that is, upon the staining of tissues of known type, fixed and processed in exactly the same manner as tissues that later are to be subject to assay.

With some knowledge of the distribution of the different neuroendocrine cell types in different parts of the gastrointestinal tract (Table 7–1), it is possible to gain a good idea of the specificity of an antibody by staining sections taken at different levels throughout the gastrointestinal tract and assessing the numbers of positive cells. For example, an antigastrin antibody should give easily detected positive cells in sections taken from normal pyloric antrum and lesser numbers of cells in sections from duodenum and small intestine; there should, however, be no positive cells in gastric fundus and none in colon or rectum. If positive cells are observed in these latter situations, then the possibility of cross reactivity with one of the other poly-

peptide hormones such as somatostatin should be considered.

Corresponding control of specificity of an antisomatostatin antibody may be somewhat more difficult, since somatostatin-containing cells may be distributed throughout the gastrointestinal tract, and cross reactivity of such an antibody against gastrin, for example, would be less obvious. However, staining of parallel sections both with antibodies against gastrin and with somatostatin should show differences in numbers and distribution if these two antibodies are indeed picking up separate cell populations.

A more certain way of visualizing that two antibodies in fact do stain distinct cell populations, even though there may be some overlap, is of course by performing double staining; and this procedure should be carried out if suspicion of cross reactivity still lingers. The performance of such biologic controls may of course be time consuming and tedious, but is nonetheless essential to reliable interpretation of immunohistochemical staining reactions on unknown tissues, particularly when staining neoplasms in an attempt to determine the hormonal product, if any, of the neoplastic cells.

If one is using immunostaining kits such as those widely available from Ortho (formerly Immulok), Dako, and Miles (see Appendix 2), one may be a little more confident in terms of specificity, since the reagents used will have been selected particularly with immunohistologic studies in mind and dilutions will have been chosen to give an optimal combination of specificity and sensitivity. Nonetheless, the ultimate responsibility for control of specificity is incumbent upon the user; stained biologic controls that from past experience have been shown to contain known numbers and distributions of the various neuroendocrine cell types should always be utilized in parallel with any new tissues that are being examined.

Neuron-Specific Enolase (NSE)

Although the separate individual types of neuroendocrine cells are identifiable by staining for their separate products, it clearly is not possible to screen putative neuroendocrine tumors with a panel of 10 to 15 different antipolypeptide antibodies. Thus a "pan"-neuroendocrine stain would be helpful. Neuron-specific enolase (NSE) has been advo-

Table 7–4. Selected Bibliography: Neuroendocrine System of the Gastrointestinal Tract

Dubois 1980 Buchan & Polak 1980 Facer et al 1980	Good review of immunohistology of polypeptide hormones Immunocytochemical approach to diagnosis and classification—good review
Nielsen et al 1980b Fujimoto et al 1980	Gastrin: G cell numbers as predictor of response to cimetidine and relationship to cimetidine–oxo test meals; the more G cells, the less likelihood of response to cimetidine therapy
Nielsen et al 1980a	Morphometric methods for quantitation of gastrin cells in antrum
Nielsen et al 1979	Gastrin and enteroglucagon cells in intestinal metaplasia in antrum; enteroglucagon present in areas of intestinal metaplasia (but never in normal antrum); gastrin not present in metaplasia (but present in normal antrum)
O'Briain et al 1982	Hormonal profile of rectal (hindgut) carcinoids; the majority contain PP (pancreatic polypeptide), whereas slightly under half contain enteroglucagon
Askew et al 1980	Found no correlation between number of G cells and measurements of gastrin release
Lehy et al 1979	Gastrin cells few at birth (in rat); somatostatin cells, few at birth, appear rapidly in neonatal period
Long et al 1980	Zollinger-Ellison syndrome and a gastrin-positive ovarian cystadenoma
Taxy et al 1980	Serotonin in rectal carcinoids
Krajs et al 1979	Somatostatinoma syndrome
Grube & Aebert 1981	Good review of specificity controls for polypeptide hormones; includes use of serial dilutions of reagents and a high salt PBS dilution buffer; nonspecific ionic binding may be a problem for the unwary
Lehy et al 1981	Compared classification of colonic neuroendocrine cells by EM and granule size, versus immunocytochemistry; noted pancreatic polypeptide and enteroglucagon in same cells
Wahlström & Seppälä 1981	Luteinizing hormone releasing factor and alpha subunit of the glycoprotein hormones present in all carcinoid tumors
Leduque et al 1981	Motilin and secretin in fetal gastrointestinal tissue
Larsson et al 1979	Somatostatin cells as local controls for release of other neurohormones
Vaalasti et al 1980	VIP in nerves of prostate
Larsson 1980	ACTH—corticotrophs and melanotrophs of pituitary and in cerebral nerves plus ACTH fragment in gastrin-positive cells of gut
Reinecke et al 1981	VIP reactivity by PAP method; true VIP in nerves, VIP-like substance in neuroendocrine cells of gut
Wilander et al 1979	Substance P and enteroglucagonlike immunoreactivity in argentaffin and argyrophil midgut carcinoid tumors
DeLellis & Wolfe 1981	Neuroendocrine cells producing polypeptide hormones; corresponding neoplasms
Ueda et al 1984a, b	Neuroendocrine cells in cervical adenocarcinoma
Silva et al 1984a	"Endocrine" carcinoma of cervix; 5HT, VIP; somatostatin
Aguirre et al 1984	Endometrial carcinoma with neuroendocrine cells; ACTH; somatotatin
Bannatyne et al 1983	Endometrial carcinoma with neuroendocrine cells; ACTH, calcitonin; no correlation with grade or stage
Sweeney et al 1983	Sertoli–Leydig cell tumor with gastrin cells
Warren et al 1984 Berger et al 1984a	Bronchial carcinoids most frequently contain 5HT, followed by VIP, gastrin, somatostatin, and calcitonin; keratin is present; almost all stain for Neuron-specific enolase (NSE)
Sheppard et al 1982 Springall et al 1984	NSE-positive in bronchial carcinoids and small cell tumors of lung; other types of lung cancer negative; also valuable in staining cells in effusions
Nakajima et al 1984	NSE in pituitary adenoma, retinoblastoma, and brain tumors
Huntrakoon et al 1984	Thymic carcinoid—NSE- and ACTH-positive
Kasurinen & Syrjänen 1984	Immunostaining of APUDomas by kits (gut, lung, thymus)
Ulich et al 1983	Spectrum of cases from adenocarcinoma to carcinoid; multiple cell products present
Wells et al 1985	Presence of 5HT; good stain for carcinoid tumor
Dayal et al 1980	Review of polypeptide hormone profiles in carcinoids
Dayal et al 1983 Griffiths et al 1984	Psammomatous somatostatinomas
Viale et al 1985	VIP in pheochromocytoma
Bostwick et al 1984	"Bombesin" equivalent to gastrin-releasing polypeptide of mammals
Saito et al 1982	Paraganglionoma producing catecholamines and somatostatin

Table 7–4. Selected Bibliography: Neuroendocrine System of the
Gastrointestinal Tract *Continued*

Hassoun et al 1984	Variety of polypeptides in pheochromocytomas
Shioda et al 1984 ⎫	
Lipinski et al 1983 ⎬	Leu 7 (HNK1) positivity in neuroendocrine cells
Caillaud et al 1984 ⎭	
Inokuchi et al 1983	Immunohistochemistry superior to silver methods for identification of neuroendocrine cells
Yamamoto et al 1984	Neuroendocrine cells in bile duct carcinoma
Höfler & Denk 1984	Cytokeratin in carcinoids

cated by some as such a stain (Table 7–4).
Neuron-specific enolase staining is present in
neuronally derived neoplasms, including
neuroblastoma (Ishiguro et al, 1982, 1983a;
Tsokos et al, 1984), as well as in neuroendocrine tumors (Simpson S et al, 1984). Most
of the gastroenteropancreatic neuroendocrine tumors (carcinoids, islet cell tumors)
are positive for NSE (Figs. 7–1 and 7–2), as
are pituitary adenomas, pheochromocytomas, lung carcinoids and oat cell carcinomas,
and Merkel cell tumors of skin (Table 7–4).
Staining is usually achievable in paraffin sections but is diminished by prolonged fixation
in formalin. Staining for NSE thus serves as
a valuable screen for this general group of
tumors, to be followed by staining for specific
polypeptides.

It should be noted that serum levels of
NSE do not correlate well with tissue staining;
generally, quite extensive disease is necessary
before serum levels are elevated.

Note that rarely has NSE positivity been
described in non-neuroendocrine tumors (eg,
Asa et al, 1984—one breast carcinoma, one
ovarian carcinoma, and one lymphoma). In
our experience this occurrence is unusual
and does not interfere with interpretation in
most cases.

A separate application of NSE staining has
been to facilitate the search for ganglion cells
in investigation of Hirschsprung's disease.
Hall and Lampert (1981) used both S100 and
NSE: NSE gave positive staining of ganglion
cells, and S100 stained the Schwann cells,
thus highlighting the nonreacting ganglion
cells. Paraffin sections were employed; the
study included material from 27 patients.
Tsuto et al (1982) also demonstrated absence
of VIP-positive nerve endings in the agan-
glionic segment, contrasting with the readily
demonstrated VIP reactivity in adjacent normal bowel.

Histaminase

Histaminase has also been investigated as
a possible pan-neuroendocrine marker. Although it is present and stainable in paraffin
sections of most carcinoids, it is also found
in a wide variety of carcinomas (lung, stom-

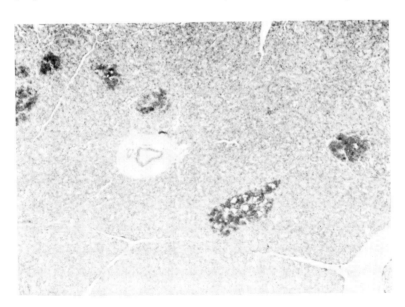

Figure 7–1. Section of pancreas treated with antibody to
neuron-specific enolase (NSE);
the islets of Langerhans stain intensely (black). Normal pancreas
makes an excellent "biologic control" for NSE staining; this is
from a fresh autopsy. Paraffin
section, AEC with hematoxylin
counterstain (×60).

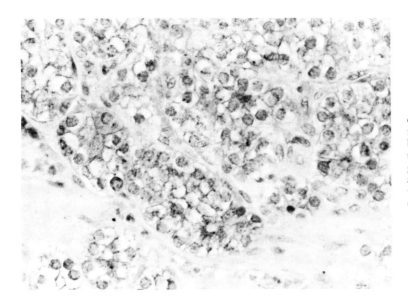

Figure 7–2. Neuroendocrine adenoma in duodenal wall; diffuse reactivity was observed with antibody to NSE. There were also scattered cells positive with antiglucagon antibody and an anti-VIP antibody. Paraffin section, AEC with hematoxylin counterstain (×320).

ach, thyroid, ovary—about 30 percent positive) but, interestingly, not in sarcomas.

HNK1 (Leu 7)

Finally, serendipity has put at our disposal one other possible pan-neuroendocrine marker, namely, HNK1 antigen—the antigen defined by antibody HNK1, which is best known as a marker of human natural killer (hence HNK) cells and is also known as Leu 7 in the current terminology. Lipinski and colleagues (1983; Caillaud et al, 1984) have shown that HNK1 antibody (Leu 7) consistently and reliably stains a "common neuroendodermal" antigen in paraffin sections. In normal tissues (both adult and fetal), positive cells were observed in the central nervous system, the adrenal medulla, and the islets of Langerhans, while the cells of the APUD system in lung and gut also reacted strongly. Of more than 150 tumors studied, positivity was the norm in astrocytomas and ependymomas; in neuroblastomas, retinoblastomas, and neuroepitheliomas; and in carcinoids, paragangliomas, pheochromocytomas, and medullary carcinomas of thyroid. Occasional cases of Ewing's sarcoma, granular cell myoblastoma, and melanoma also were positive. Other sarcomas, including lymphomas, were negative, and no reactivity was seen in squamous cell carcinomas or adenocarcinomas or in embryonal carcinomas. Subsequent publications by Shioda et al (1984) and Bunn et al (1985), using anti–Leu 7,

confirmed the essence of this work. In Shioda's work, insulin-containing cells were said to be Leu 7–negative; most other neuroendocrine cells were positive. The paper by Bunn, particularly, showed the value of staining in small cell carcinoma of lung. Again, the stain is effective in formalin-fixed, paraffin-embedded tissues.

Gastrin

Gastrin is a 17–amino acid polypeptide hormone with a molecular weight of 2100, produced primarily by the G cells of the pyloric antrum. Lesser numbers of gastrin-containing cells are demonstrable in the duodenum, still fewer in the jejunum and ileum; these cells are classed as G cells by some authorities and as D cells (somatostatin-producing) by others. Human gastrin (17–amino acid polypeptide) differs from gastrin of other mammals by only one or two amino acid groups. Other molecular forms of gastrin containing 13, 34, or 45 amino acid groups also exist; these forms are referred to as mini-gastrin, big gastrin, and big-big gastrin, respectively, with the usual 17–amino acid type enjoying the term *little gastrin*. It is generally accepted that antibodies raised against the 17–amino acid gastrin show a high degree of cross reactivity with the other molecular forms. Likewise, antibodies against gastrin from many animals show signifiant cross reactivity with human gastrin. In addition, for immunohistochemical studies, it must be remembered that gastrin has significant amino acid sequences in common with cholecystokinin and that conventional antisera to gastrin usually shows significant cross reactivity with cholecystokinin; theoretically, such cross reactivity could be avoided by the selection of suitable monoclonal antibodies.

G Cells of the Pyloric Antrum

Gastrin induces HCl secretion by gastric parietal cells through a mechanism that appears to involve mediation by histamine. Other effects of gastrin include stimulation of insulin secretion, production of pepsinogen and pancreatic bicarbonate, and probably increase in bile flow. Release of gastrin itself is dependent upon vagal activity or the direct presence of food substances within the stomach.

Within the pyloric antrum, the G cells occur either singly or in small clusters towards the bottom of the glands. They appear as small pyramidal cells situated close to the basement membrane (Fig. 7–3), though it is thought that all G cells do, in fact, have cytoplasmic extensions that reach the lumen of the gland.

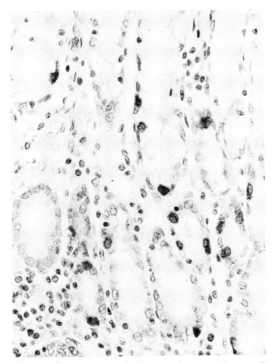

Figure 7–3. Scattered G (gastrin-containing) cells (black cytoplasm) within pyloric antrum. G cell scores have been used to predict clinical response in patients with peptic ulcer. Paraffin section, AEC with hematoxylin counterstain (×200).

Within the duodenum they are present in small numbers scattered along the villi, the crypts, and within Brunner's glands (Table 7–1). Reports of the presence of G cells in islets of Langerhans (of adults) have not been confirmed by other workers, a discrepancy probably relating to differences in specificity of the antisera employed.

G cells have been reported prior to the twentieth week of gestation. Postnatally, the number is thought to remain relatively constant, decreasing after the fourth decade. Studies of the numbers of G cells by immunohistologic methods have not always correlated well with serum gastrin levels, although in certain disease states in which there is marked G cell hyperplasia, the correlation is good.

G Cell Hyperplasia

In some conditions G cell hyperplasia appears to represent a secondary response to decreased production of hydrochloric acid by the gastric mucosa; this for example is seen in pernicious anemia and atrophic gastritis.

In other circumstances, as in the case of Zollinger-Ellison syndrome, the G cell hyperplasia appears to represent the primary abnormality. In this latter instance, the G cell hyperplasia is considered etiologically important in the development of multiple ulcers that may occur in this syndrome. The pathogenic role of G cell hyperplasia in duodenal ulcers in general is more debatable. Nonetheless, some investigators advocate the importance of G cell counts in patients with peptic ulcer as a means of predicting whether or not such patients are likely to respond to medical therapy (cimetidine; Nielsen et al, 1980b). If G cell counts are high, a response to cimetidine is improbable; but if G cell counts are low, then a cimetidine response is commonly seen, and it is usually not necessary to resort to surgery.

Overall G cell hyperplasia has been observed not only in pernicious anemia, atrophic gastritis, and Zollinger-Ellison syndrome, but also in duodenal ulcers, several of the multiple endocrine adenomatosis syndromes, pyloric stenosis, gastric carcinoma, acromegaly, hyperparathyroidism, and hypercalcemia.

G Cell Neoplasia (Gastrinomas)

Gastrinomas, unlike some of the other neoplasms of the neuroendocrine cells, are often

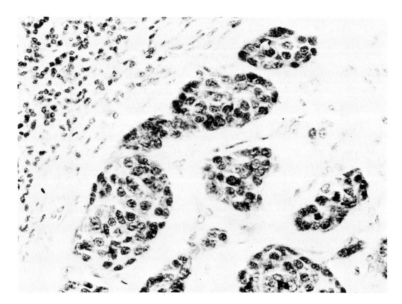

Figure 7–4. Gastrinoma in duodenal wall showing variable cytoplasmic staining for gastrin (gray-black) within clumps of tumor cells. Many of the gastrointestinal neuroendocrine tumors are morphologically similar and are best distinguished by immunohistochemical techniques. Paraffin section, AEC with hematoxylin counterstain (×320).

malignant and commonly metastasize. Frequently, they are associated with Zollinger-Ellison syndrome, a result of the production of large amounts of gastrin. Primary gastrinomas may be single or multiple and may occur in the pancreas, pyloric antrum, or duodenum. Varying proportions of the tumor cells show positive immunohistologic reactivity with antibodies against gastrin in paraffin sections (Fig. 7–4). The proportion of cells stained may vary markedly in different areas of the tumor and in different tumors from the same patient. Such tumors are, of course, commonly argyrophilic, but there is not a good correlation between the degree of argyrophilia and the extent of immunoreactivity for gastrin.

Immunohistochemistry has also revealed that many gastrinomas produce polypeptides in addition to gastrin; these include pancreatic polypeptide (in up to 50 percent of cases), ACTH, insulin, glucagon, and growth hormone (or cross-reacting polypeptides).

Gastrin, like most other polypeptide hormones, appears relatively stable upon fixation, although in our experience prolonged fixation in formalin does produce a reduction in immunoreactivity.

Somatostatin

Somatostatin, so called because of its inhibitory effect upon release of growth hormone, is a 14–amino acid polypeptide that is distributed widely throughout the gastrointestinal tract and the central and peripheral nervous systems. It is believed to act as a local neuroendocrine inhibitor with a wide variety of regulatory effects, including inhibition of release of insulin, glucagon, secretin, cholecystokinin, and gastrin.

Immunohistologic studies have done much to define the distribution of somatostatin-producing cells throughout the body. Users of immunohistochemical methods should, however, remember that antibodies against somatostatin may show cross reactivity against other polypeptide hormones, particularly gastrin, and that such cross reactivity is often difficult to detect. Antibodies raised in different species generally show good cross reactivity with somatostatin from other species.

Somatostatin was first isolated from hypothalamus and can be demonstrated within the hypothalamus by immunoperoxidase techniques. Within the gastrointestinal tract somatostatin is present within the D cells; these are most numerous in the stomach, including both the fundus and the pyloric antrum, with decreasing frequency in the duodenum, the remainder of the small intestine, and the colon (although small numbers of positive cells may be detected as far down as the rectum) (Table 7–1). Within the stomach somatostatin-positive cells appear as flattened pyramids between the basement membrane and the overlying gastric epithelial cells, and it is thought that many of the D cells have no direct contact with the lumen. In the pyloric antrum, the D cells are often somewhat bigger and may show luminal extensions. One characteristic of D cells is that they possess cytoplasmic processes that subtend upon neighboring cells of the neuroendocrine system and upon epithelial cells and may mediate their inhibitory effects by local release of somatostatin. Silver staining of these cells is somewhat variable according to method; they do, however, have distinctive granules identifiable by electron microscopy. Currently, the simplest and most reliable way of demonstrating somatostatin–producing D cells is by immunocytochemistry.

In addition to their presence throughout the gut proper, somatostatin–positive D cells are to be found in the endodermally derived pancreas (D cells of the islets of Langerhans) and in the thyroid (derived from the endodermal thyroglossal duct). In the thyroid somatostatin may even be present in the same cells as calcitonin (demonstrated in some species).

Pathology of D Cells

D cell hyperplasia has been observed in the islets of Langerhans in juvenile diabetes by Rahier et al (1980). Apart from this observation, reports of variations in the numbers of D cells are somewhat anecdotal, and significant pathological hyperplasias and hypoplasias have yet to be described.

Somatostatin-producing neoplasms have however been recognized, albeit in small numbers. The majority of these neoplasms appear to have originated in the islet of Langerhans, but primary intestinal somatostatinomas have been described more recently. Actively secreting somatostatinomas are associated with a distinctive syndrome of achlorhydria, steatorrhea, gall bladder disease, and diabetes mellitus (Krajs et al, 1979), possibly due to inhibition of insulin, gastrin, and pancreatic secretions. Histologically, somatostatinomas resemble other islet cell tumors, having a trabecular pattern or having cells occurring in small nests or, occasionally, in organized acinar-type structures. The histochemical Grimelius's stain is usually negative, whereas the alcoholic silver nitrate method (Hellstrom and Hellman) may be positive. Immunohistologic staining reveals somatostatin-positive cells in varying proportions, and there may be minor populations of cells that immunocytologically show positivity for ACTH, gastrin, or calcitonin; occasionally these subpopulations may produce

hormone in sufficient amounts for the appropriate clinical signs to develop (Cushing's syndrome, peptic ulceration, or hypocalcemia).

The converse occurs much more frequently, with somatostatin cells being found quite frquently as minor components of other APUDomas, including medullary C cell carcinoma of the thyroid and carcinoid tumors in the gut. Indeed, DeLellis and colleagues have suggested that immunocytochemical staining for somatostatin (and for pancreatic polypeptide, glucagon, calcitonin, and gastrin) may be essential to the recognition and precise classification of gastrointestinal carcinoid tumors (Dayal et al, 1980). In their study, the majority of foregut carcinoids were somatostatin-positive, whereas midgut carcinoids were positive less than 15 percent of the time, and hindgut carcinoids about 50 percent of the time. Almost all hindgut carcinoids were positive for pancreatic polypeptide. Enteroglucagon occurs in midgut and hindgut carcinoids in varying proportions according to different reports.

Recently, another variant of somatostatin-containing tumor has been recognized—the so-called psammomatous glandular carcinoid of the duodenum. These tumors are morphologically unique with conspicuous psammoma bodies in the lumina of those areas of the tumor showing glandular differentiation (Griffiths et al, 1984—four cases; Dayal et al, 1983—three cases). Somatostatin is readily demonstrable within tumor cells, but other polypeptide hormones are reported absent (in contrast with most other carcinoids that typically contain two or more products).

Glucagon and Enteroglucagon

Glucagon has a molecular weight of 3500 and is a 29–amino acid polypeptide. It is secreted by the alpha (A) cells of the islets of Langerhans in the pancreas; the principal stimulus for release is hypoglycemia. Glucagon acts to elevate glucose levels by facilitating glycogenolysis and accelerating protein and lipid catabolism. Release is inhibited by somatostatin.

Enteroglucagon, a substance having glucagonlike reactivity, is produced within a distinctive cell (the so-called L cell; glucagon-producing A cells of the islets of Langerhans and L cells are distinguishable by EM). L cells are present throughout the small gut but are most numerous in ileum and rectum. The structure of enteroglucagon has not been clearly defined, but it appears to consist of several polypeptide units, one of which has been termed glicentin; antisera against glicentin cross-react with pancreatic glucagon. It is, however, possible to prepare antisera against pancreatic glucagon that do not react with enteroglucagon (these antisera are thought to be directed against the C-terminal end of the pancreatic glucagon molecule).

Glucagon-positive A cells, demonstrable by immunohistochemistry, are confined in humans to the pancreas, in which they are distributed in the islets of Langerhans, particularly toward the peripheral part of the islet (see Chapter 8). In the normal pancreas, they are less numerous than insulin-positive cells (at least as demonstrated by immunohistochemical methods). Interestingly occasional hormone-positive (insulin-, glucagon-, or somatostatin-positive) cells may be observed outside the islets, apparently within exocrine pancreas, a phenomenon that has been described more often in neonatal pancreas. This occurrence may simply reflect the pattern of embryologic development of the pancreas in the fetus, in which, initially, both ventral and dorsal pancreatic buds consist of branching trees of fine ducts. Some of these ducts then pinch off to become islets, whereas those remaining in contiguity become the exocrine pancreas. The occurrence postnatally of cells positive for insulin, glucagon, or somatostatin within the exocrine system may simply reflect this common embryologic origin.

Islet cell adenomas, producing glucagon, are described in the section relating to pancreas (Chapter 8). Tumors producing enteroglucagon, associated with clinical syndromes of malabsorption and extreme hypomotility of large and small intestine, have only been recognized much more recently. As noted previously, a varying proportion of carcinoid tumors of the midgut and hindgut contain cells that react positively with antibodies against enteroglucagon. Pathologic states associated with hyperplasia or hypoplasia of this cell type have yet to be recognized.

Secretin

Secretin was the first of the gastrointestinal polypeptides to be clearly recognized. It is a 27–amino acid polypeptide secreted by the S cells within the mucosa of the duodenum and upper jejunum. The amino acid sequence shows partial homology with that of vasoactive intestinal polypeptide (VIP) and glucagon, and antisera to those polypeptides may be cross reactive. Secretin, however, differs from many of the other intestinal polypeptides in that it is less readily demonstrable in fixed paraffin sections (whether fixed in formalin, Bouin's or Zenker's fluid, or glutaraldehyde). Thus, studies defining the numbers and distribution of secretin-positive cells have been performed on frozen sections, often with fixation in carbodiimide.

The inability to demonstrate secretin in routinely processed tissues has severely limited studies of numbers of secretin-positive cells in disease states. Thus there are no published reports of secretin-producing APUDomas and only one or two descriptions of numbers and distribution of secretin-positive cells in pathologic states. Hypersecretinemia has, of course, been observed in Zollinger-Ellison syndrome and in patients with chronic duodenal ulceration, in whom the increase in secretin production is thought to be secondary to gastric hyperacidity. It has, however, not proved possible up to this time to study tissue distribution in a detailed fashion. The few studies that have appeared have reported secretin distribution only in small random biopsies and are subject to such sampling errors that at this time there is no clear understanding as to whether hyperplasia of secretin cells exists.

Secretin functions as an inhibitor of gastric acid secretion, a stimulus for bile and intestinal secretion, and a potent releasing factor for alkaline pancreatic juice. The release of secretin is stimulated by intestinal acid and is inhibited by somatostatin.

Cholecystokinin

Cholecystokinin exists in several molecular forms, of which a small octapeptide is most active and most common; the other two forms described contain 33 to 39 amino acids respectively.

There is marked structural homology between cholecystokinin and gastrin, and this is reflected both in the common cross reactivity observed of antibodies for one against the other and in some of their common physiologic actions. It should be noted that cholecystokinin and pancreazymin are now considered a single hormone and that the name cholecystokinin is preferred. Cholecystokinin stimulates contraction of the gall bladder and secretion of pancreatic enzymes and, like some of the other intestinal polypeptides, appears to serve also as a local neurotransmitter, since it is found not only throughout the gastrointestinal tract but also in central nervous tissues.

Within the gastrointestinal tract, the cholecystokinin-containing cell is known as the I cell; it is present in the duodenum and jejunum but not in stomach, colon, or pancreas (Tables 7–1 and 7–2). Cholecystokinin-positive cells are to be found toward the bases of the villi and within the crypts. Silver reactions vary according to the technique. These cells can be reliably demonstrated by immunohistologic methods in frozen tissues; following fixation demonstration is considered less reliable. The preferred fixative, for prospective studies is picric acid paraformaldehyde (Zamboni's fixative).

Regarding pathologic states, knowledge of cholecystokinin-producing cell numbers and distribution is limited by the difficulty in demonstrating this hormone in routinely processed tissues. Thus, cholecystokinin-producing APUDomas have not been described by immunohistochemical methods, and there is a corresponding dearth of information concerning hyperplastic states. It is, however, known that certain conditions are associated with increased circulating levels of cholecystokinin; these include Zollinger-Ellison syndrome, chronic pancreatitis, and chronic renal failure. The gastrin-producing adeno-

mas responsible for Zollinger-Ellison syndrome may also co-produce cholecystokinin, though this has yet to be proven; the source of cholecystokinin production in the other conditions remains unknown.

Vasoactive Intestinal Polypeptide (VIP)

Vasoactive intestinal polypeptide exists in at least four molecular forms, the exact structure of which is yet to be defined; the most common variety appears to be a polypeptide with 28 amino acids. Like cholecystokinin it is quite widely distributed and is present both in gastrointestinal tract and in neural tissue. There currently is some debate as to whether the different forms of VIP are distributed differently within neural tissues and the gastrointestinal tract. Antibodies raised against VIP may react predominantly with one component, and this circumstance may to some extent explain discrepant results reported in the literature, and also the ability of antisera to demonstrate VIP in some tissues and not in others.

Vasoactive intestinal polypeptide-positive cells are present throughout the gastrointestinal tract (the so-called D_1-type cells), but have also been described in the exocrine pancreas and pancreatic islets (Tables 7–1 and 7–2; Fig. 7–5). The precise function of VIP is not clearly understood, but like many of the other polypeptides, it may have both neurotransmitter and local endocrine effects,

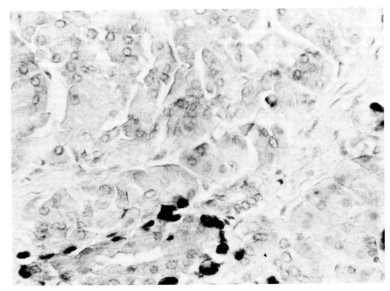

Figure 7–5. VIP (vasointestinal polypeptide) positive cells (black) arranged around a small duct in the head of the pancreas. VIP positivity may also be seen along small nerve tracts. Paraffin section, AEC with hematoxylin counterstain (×400).

regulating neighboring neuroendocrine cells. Vasoactive intestinal polypeptide is demonstrable within routinely processed tissues, although not equally well by all antisera.

A number of patients with VIP-producing tumors have been descibed, the tumors occurring either in the islets or in an extrapancreatic site. In certain cases immunohistologic studies reveal presence of VIP-reactive cells in varying proportions within the tumor; many cases also show elevations of VIP levels in serum. Classically, a functioning VIP-producing tumor is associated with a clinical syndrome of watery diarrhea and hypochlorhydria (Verner-Morrison), in which the hypochlorhydria is associated with hypocalcemia, hypotension, and often hyperglycemia and hypercalcemia. The role of VIP in induction of this syndrome has not fully been clarified since not all patients show elevated levels of VIP, and in some instances VIP-producing tumors have not been detectable, or other substances have been identified (eg, serotinin—Nishiyama et al, 1984—two cases).

Pathologic consequences or associations of VIP cell hyperplasia or hypoplasia have not yet been clearly described. Vasoactive intestinal polypeptide with the associated clinical syndrome may also be produced by tumors other than "carcinoids," particularly adrenal tumors (adrenal ganglioneuroblastoma—Yagihashi et al, 1982; and pheochromocytoma—Viale et al, 1985).

Substance P, Motilin, Gastric Inhibitory Peptide (GIP), Pancreatic Polypeptide (PP)

These are four additional polypeptides ranging in size from 11 amino acids (substance P), 22 amino acids (motilin), 36 amino acids (pancreatic polypeptide), up to 43 amino acids (gastric inhibitory peptide). The cellular distribution and designation of the corresponding neuroendocrine cell is given in Table 7–1. The biologic function of these polypeptides has not been clearly characterized, and there is little data currently available concerning normal distribution of the respective neuroendocrine cells or any changes that may occur in pathologic states. Regarding the development of the corresponding neoplasms, only pancreatic polypeptide has been described at all frequently; it was reported in six of seven rectal carcinoids but appears not to be present in carci-

noids of foregut or midgut (O'Briain et al, 1982). Pancreatic polypeptide also occurs quite commonly as clusters of positive cells in islet cell tumors that predominantly produce (contain) gastrin, insulin, or glucagon.

Bombesin

Antibodies developed against bombesin, a small polypeptide found in amphibian skin, show significant immunostaining of scattered neuroendocrine cells in the gut, the highest concentration of positive cells being seen in the pyloric antrum and in the duodenum. Bombesin-positive cells have been observed in some neuroblastomas and in a small number of gastric or pancreatic neuroendocrine tumors. There have also been rumors of bombesin positivity within oat cell carcinoma of the lung (see Chapter 11), with claims that this positivity may be of value in identifying these cells histologically (eg, distinguishing oat cells from lymphoma cells).

More recent work indicates that gastrin-releasing polypeptide (GRP), a 27–amino acid polypeptide, may be the mammalian analogue of bombesin. Of 20 cases of carcinoids studied by Bostwick et al (1984) using antisera to GRP, most showed strong positivity (small intestine and appendix 13/15, but colon only 1/5). Formalin paraffin sections were employed with good results.

5-Hydroxytryptamine

5-Hydroxytryptamine, a biogenic amine rather than a polypeptide, nonetheless qualifies for consideration as a gastrointestinal hormone; it has a range of ill-defined effects upon secretion of intestinal epithelial cells and also reduces gastric motility. The demonstration of 5-hydroxytryptamine using specific antisera is readily achieved under ideal circumstances (freeze-dried, vacuum-embedded tissue, according to O'Briain and Dayal, 1981). It may also be demonstrated in frozen sections and, less reliably, in routinely processed, formalin-fixed, paraffin-embedded material (Table 7–4).

The difficulty in achieving consistent immunocytochemical demonstration of 5-hydroxytryptamine in formalin paraffin sections has severely restricted studies of the distribution of 5-hydroxytryptamine–positive cells in normal intestine, in pathologic states, and in intestinal neoplasms. Thus, many of the current perceptions of the distribution of 5-hydroxytryptamine–containing cells are based upon the fact that these cells give a positive argentaffin reaction, whereas the other neuroendocrine cells are considered argentaffin-negative, though they show variable argyrophilic reactions according to method. On this basis it is accepted that many carcinoid tumors contain 5-hydroxytryptamine (they show positive argentaffin reactions), particularly those carcinoids derived from the midgut.

It is now recognized, however, that any of the neuroendocrine cells within the intestine are potentially capable of producing neoplasms that would be classified morphologically as carcinoids and that precise designation as to the cellular origin of an individual tumor depends upon immunohistochemical studies in addition to conventional histochemical silver stains.

The classic midgut carcinoid, composed of 5-hydroxytryptamine–producing cells, may of course be associated with clinical carcinoid syndrome.

APPROACH TO RECOGNITION OF CARCINOIDS

In subclassifying carcinoid tumors and in distinguishing these tumors from less well-differentiated adenocarcinomas, immunostaining has evolved into an important ancillary tool. Many investigators advocate combining several approaches in a sequential fashion to achieve the correct diagnosis. This combination approach involves H&E staining plus silver staining techniques, and it may extend to the categorization of tumors according to the type of secretory granule visible by electron microscopy. Immunostaining appears increasingly useful, even when only routinely processed tissues are available, for many of these antigens survive to a sufficient degree to permit their demonstration following fixation and processing. Immunocytochemical staining, when successful, is of course more rapid and more cost-effective than electron microscopy as well as more practical for smaller hospitals.

In summary, staining for NSE (or Leu 7 or both) serves as a screen, effective in paraffin sections. This may be followed by staining for the specific poypeptide in paraffin sections when appropriate or, better, in frozen tissues. In practice, a case may only be pursued to this degree if clinical symptoms are present that require elucidation.

OTHER NEUROENDOCRINE NEOPLASMS: ADRENAL

Immunohistochemical techniques have found extensive application with regard to the investigation of hyperplasias and neoplasias of a variety of other endocrine tissues. Pearse (1983) gives a good discussion of the role of histochemical and immunohistochemical techniques in the so-called neuroendocrine tissues, including not only the major endocrine organs discussed separately above, but also other APUDomas that he lists in two categories.

Among APUDomas of neural origin, Pearse includes pheochromocytoma, neuroblastoma (and ganglioneuroblastoma), medullary carcinoma of thyroid, pituitary and pineal tumors, Merkel cell tumors, and melanomas.

In the second category of APUDomas, presumably of endodermal origin, Pearse includes carcinoids of the gastrointestinal tract, pancreas, and bronchial tree, as well as a variety of small cell carcinomas, particularly those of the lung (the oat cell carcinoma and its relatively benign cousin the bronchial carcinoid, generally accepted to be derived from the Kulchitsky's cells of the bronchial mucosa).

All of these tissues, both normal and neoplastic, have in various studies been claimed to show some degree of positivity with neuron-specific enolase, although detailed data in large numbers of cases is not always available. However, with the rapid accumulation of immunohistologic studies utilizing antibodies against neuron-specific enolase, this method has now superseded electron microscopic demonstration of neuroendocrine type granules as the simplest and most reliable means for recognition of this category of cells.

The cells of the adrenal medulla and their derivative neoplasms have been reported to show consistent positivity with antibodies against "neurofilaments," which otherwise appear largely restricted to functioning neurons (Chapter 16).

Classically, the cells of the adrenal medulla (and nonadrenal paraganglion cells) produce catecholamines; these have not been convincingly demonstrated by immunohistologic methods, though the precursor enzymes may be more readily demonstrated. Adrenal medullary cells and their derivative neoplasms (pheochromocytomas) have also been reported as showing immunoreactivity for enkephalins, somatostatin, VIP, ACTH, and calcitonin (Table 7–4; additional polypeptide hormones have been detected in other species). Neuron-specific enolase is positive, as is Leu 7, and immunohistologic staining with monoclonal antibodies versus "endocrine granules" has also been described in preliminary reports (Lloyd and Wilson, 1983). These latter stains obviously will not distin-

guish pheochromocytomas from tumors of the "enterochromaffin" cells, but they may be of value in separating these tumors from metastatic anaplastic carcinoma. In children, neuroblastomas (and ganglioneuromas) show moderate to strong positivity for cathepsin D; lymphomas, Wilms's tumor, and rhabdomyosarcomas are usually nonreactive. Cathepsin D can be demonstrated in paraffin sections, B5 being preferred to formalin (Parham et al, 1985).

Aldosterone has been demonstrated in tumors of the adrenal cortex, and is present in the so-called spironolactone bodies in paraffin sections (Hsu et al, 1980).

ENDOCRINE SYSTEM: PANCREAS, THYROID, PITUITARY

8

*"Physicians of the utmost fame
were called at once, but when they came
they answered, as they took their fees,
'There is no cure for this disease.'"*

HILAIRE BELLOC, 1870–1953

ENDOCRINE PANCREAS

The hormone-producing cells of the pancreas, concentrated within the islets of Langerhans, are developmentally and physiologically related to the diffuse neuroendocrine cells of the gut. The principal cell types distinguishable within the human islet of Langerhans by immunocytochemical methods are, in decreasing order of frequency, insulin producers (B cells), glucagon producers (A cells), somatostatin producers (D cells), and small numbers of cells producing pancreatic polypeptide and vasointestinal polypeptide (Tables 7–1, 7–2, and 8–1). Gastrin-producing cells are present only in small numbers or not at all in the adult but are normally present in the fetal and neonatal pancreas.

Whereas the majority of hormone-containing cells within the adult pancreas are confined to the islets of Langerhans, immunohistochemical techniques have led to the recognition that hormone-producing cells may also occur in small numbers within the acini and ducts of the exocrine pancreas. This is particularly true of somatostatin, pancreatic polypeptide, and vasointestinal polypeptide-containing cells, but occasional glucagon or insulin-positive cells, or both, may also be observed outside the confines of a recognizable islet. This cellular distribution is perhaps more reasonably understood by reference to the pattern of islet cell devel-opment in the early fetus, in which immunohistologic techniques have revealed that the islets of Langerhans develop from the branching duct system present in the eight-week human embryo. A number of these branches are apparently pinched off, losing their contiguity with the lumen, and these separated branches develop into hormone-producing islets of Langerhans. Clearly early pancreatic cells appear to have dual potency, either for exocrine or endocrine function, and this ambivalence may occasionally be manifest in later life. The relative proportions of A, B, and D cells at different phases of fetal development are given by Clark and Grant (1983) and Bryant et al (1982).

In the normal adult islet of Langerhans, insulin-producing cells are most numerous and are situated more centrally; glucagon-producing cells are next most frequent and are distributed more around the periphery, at least in the human islet. The pancreatic hormones are quite hardy and usually can be demonstrated in paraffin sections (Fig. 8–1).

Having a close developmental relationship to the neuroendocrine cells of the intestine, the cells of the islet of Langerhans also display a number of the histochemical features that characterize the APUD cells, and they contain endocrine granules that can be differentiated by electron microscopy. Islet cells, like other neuroendocrine cells, are neuron–specific esterase (NSE)- and Leu 7–positive in paraffin sections. These stains therefore

Table 8–1. Selected Bibliography: Pancreatic Hormones

Mukai K 1983	Excellent review of immunohistology of islets
Mukai K et al 1982	Excellent study of 77 pancreatic endocrine tumors (including Zollinger-Ellison syndrome, hypoglycemia, watery diarrhea, and asymptomatic patients): glucagon, insulin, gastrin, VIP; poor correlation with histologic subtypes; one third of tumors produced more than one hormone, with different patterns in separate tumors in same patient
Cohen & Budgeon 1982	Use of commercial kits in 13 islet cell tumors: glucagon, somatostatin, insulin, gastrin; excellent results
Klempa et al 1980	Study of 24 pancreatic endocrine tumors plus 14 carcinoids: insulin, glucagon, VIP, cholecystokinin, motilin, neurotensin, PP (pancreatic polypeptide), somatostatin, and ACTH; half the tumors contained more than one hormone, though symptoms related only to one
Wright J et al 1980	Case report: somatostatin-positive tumor with scattered insulin-positive cells
Lloyd RV et al 1981	Case report and review of diffuse adenomatosis with admixture of insulin, glucagon, and somatostatin-positive cells
Ruttman et al 1980	5 patients with glucagon-positive adenomas (2 were symptomatic, 3 silent)
Asa et al 1980	Islet cell carcinoma positive for gastrin, somatostatin, calcitonin, ACTH, and alpha endorphin—with all 5 hormones apparently present in same cells
Bussolati et al 1984	Antibody to prealbumin stains islet cell tumors and intestinal carcinoids, possibly because of amino acids in common with polypeptide prohormones
Clark ES & Carney 1984	7 cases of Cushing's syndrome with ACTH-producing islet cell tumors
Tomita et al 1980	"Pancreatic polypeptide cell" hyperplasia; relationship of Verner-Morrison syndrome
Kasajima et al 1980	Watery diarrhea syndrome with pancreatic carcinoma positive for VIP
Cooney et al 1980	Bronchial carcinoid (ACTH-positive) associated with islet cell tumor (insulin-positive) and "C" cell hyperplasia of thyroid (calcitonin-positive)
Jennette et al 1982	A case of islet cell hyperplasia (insulin-positive) apparently secondary to presence of an anti-insulin receptor antibody in scleroderma (systemic sclerosis)
Matsuba et al 1982	"Clonal" growth of islet cells in culture revealed that the cells of each "clone" made only one hormone
Falkmer 1979	Phylogeny of islet; insulin present in invertebrates, later in evolution somatostatin-glucagon-pancreatic polypeptide appear
Fujii 1979	Ontogeny of islets (in rat); glucagon first, followed by insulin, pancreatic polypeptide, somatostatin, and gastrin; predominantly foregut derivation in small clusters from "exocrine" tubules
Bryant et al 1982	Ontogeny of islets (in man); with emphasis on polypeptides: gastrin, secretin, motilin, inhibitory peptide, VIP, glucagon, somatostatin all present at 8 weeks; adult pattern by 20 weeks; VIP confined to nerve tracts
Wirdnam & Milner 1981	A and B cell development in human islets from 12-week fetus to puberty
Teitelman et al 1981	Study in mouse utilized immunoperoxidase methods to demonstrate origin of islet cells from dopaminergic precursors; suggested common embryonic origin for peptide-producing cells of skin, brain, and gut (including APUD cells)
Gould VE et al 1983	Nesidioblastosis of infancy
Kenney et al 1981	Demonstration of B cell destruction at autopsy following poisoning with a phenylurea compound
Baskin et al 1982	Demonstration of insulin at EM
Saito et al 1982	Somatostatin in a paraganglionoma
Ravazzola et al 1979 } Garaud et al 1980 }	Antiglucagon and antiglicentin antisera show positive cells concentrated at the periphery of the islets (within the same cells—type A); both also positive in so-called "L" cells of small intestine
Amouric et al 1982	Kallikrein present in zymogen granules of pancreatic acinar cells

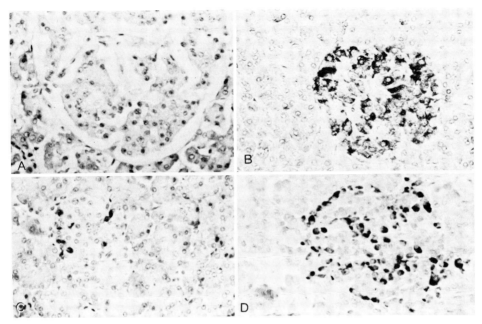

Figure 8–1. Normal islets of Langerhans in autopsy pancreas following formalin fixation. Four parallel sections were treated with nonimmune serum. *A*, negative control; *B*, anti-insulin antibody; *C*, antiglucagon antibody; and *D*, antisomatostatin antibody. Insulin-positive cells are most numerous, somatostatin-positive cells the fewest. Note that occasional "hormone-positive" cells may be found outside of the islets, more often in the neonate than in the adult. Paraffin sections, AEC with hematoxylin counterstain (×60).

serve as useful screens for suspected islet cell tumors; if positive, staining for the specific hormones described below follows. It is also worth noting that sections of pancreas (from a reasonably fresh autopsy) serve as excellent controls for NSE and Leu 7 staining, since the normal islets react well with both (see Chapter 7).

There have been several independent reports describing the production of antibodies against antigens that may be specific to the exocrine pancreas or to carcinoma derived from the exocrine cells. These are discussed in Chapter 11.

Gastrin

The association of islet cell adenomas with excessive production of gastrin and with the Zollinger-Ellison syndrome provides strong circumstantial evidence for the production of gastrin by islet cell adenomas and hence for the presence of gastrin-producing cells or their progenitors within the normal islet. A number of investigators have searched for gastrin-containing cells using immunocyto-chemical methods, and the general consensus seems to be that G cells, if present in the

normal islets, are present at very low frequency. In our own experience, we have observed occasional cells reacting with anti-gastrin antibodies within islets and also, rarely, within pancreatic ducts. Conceivably, these cells could represent the origin of pancreatic gastrinomas; alternatively, some residual pluripotent cell within the islet of Langerhans might serve as the progenitor for such a neoplasm. Suffice it to say that gastrin-producing neoplasms whether they arise in the pancreas or in the gastrointestinal tract are readily identifiable by immunostaining techniques (see Table 8–1 and also Chapter 7).

Glucagon

Glucagon is a polypeptide consisting of 29 amino acids produced and secreted by the A cells of the islets of Langerhans. Traditional histochemical methods for distinguishing A cells have been superseded by immunohisto-chemical methods utilizing antibodies against glucagon. It should however be noted that electron microscopic studies combined with immunocytochemistry have shown other polypeptides within the A cells, including

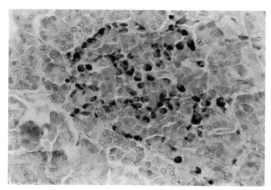

Figure 8–2. Autopsy pancreas showing glucagon-positive cells (redbrown-black) within an islet of Langerhans; note that occasional glucagon-positive cells may be found isolated in the exocrine pancreas (bottom right). Paraffin section, AEC with hematoxylin counterstain (×200). See color plate I–6.

gastric inhibitory peptide, cholecystokinin, ACTH, and glicentin or a variety of cross-reacting molecules. Glicentin is considered a precursor in the synthetic pathway for glucagon. Substances present in a subpopulation of diffuse neuroendocrine cells in the small intestine show cross reactivity with various antiglucagon antibodies and have been termed enteroglucagon; these substances are discussed in conjunction with the diffuse neuroendocrine system of the gut (Chapter 7).

Glucagon-containing cells normally constitute approximately 10 percent of the islet cells (Fig. 8–2). Their numbers may be observed to be increased in some forms of pancreatitis, in acromegaly, and in some forms of the multiple endocrine adenopathy syndrome (specifically, MEA type I with islet cell hyperplasia). There have been some reports of decreased numbers of A cells following administration of certain organic compounds to experimental animals, but this occurrence has not been well documented by immunohistochemical techniques.

Glucagonomas

Neoplasms of the islets of Langerhans may produce sufficient amounts of glucagon to produce clinical effects, and in such cases glucagon is usually demonstrable within tumor cells by immunohistochemical methods. Such tumors are frequently termed glucagonomas. As with the other islet cell tumors, the morphology may resemble to a degree the normal islet, or it may show resemblance to carcinoid tumors occurring in the small intestine (Fig. 8–3). Cytologic atypia or even cellular pleomorphism may be present to a marked degree but is not considered predictive of malignant behavior. As with other islet cell tumors, the ultimate criterion for malignancy is extensive invasion or metastasis.

It should also be noted that glucagonomas, although they classically show immunostaining for glucagon, may also show variable

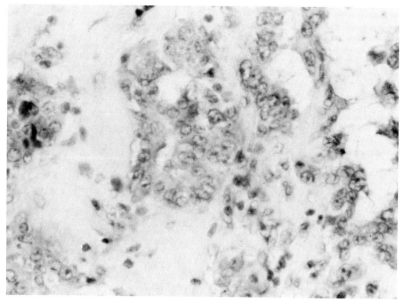

Figure 8–3. Aggressive islet cell tumor with a "pseudoglandular" pattern showing moderate staining for glucagon (gray cytoplasm) in most tumor cells. Paraffin section, AEC with hematoxylin counterstain (×320).

proportions of cells with immunostaining for other islet cell hormones (insulin, somatostatin, gastrin, and others) and pancreatic polypeptide (Table 8–1). With sufficiently sensitive techniques, some investigators believe the latter to be present in all cases, albeit in a small subpopulation of the tumor cells. As described previously, islet cell tumors also show positivity for neuron-specific enolase, with relatively uniform staining of a high proportion of cells.

Insulin

In the normal islet, insulin-producing cells predominate but typically are markedly reduced in numbers in juvenile diabetes. There is less consistent reduction in proportion of stainable insulin-containing cells in pancreatitis. It should be noted that the number of cells staining positively for insulin may be markedly increased in the newborn, and in these circumstances insulin-positive cells are frequently observed within the ducts and acini of the exocrine pancreas. This condition has been termed nesidioblastosis (Grampag et al, 1974). It was felt by some investigators that this condition might be responsible for hypoglycemia in childhood that is associated with elevated insulin levels; however, the frequency with which this phenomenon is observed in neonatal pancreas casts some doubt upon the hypothesis.

Insulinomas

Insulinomas are defined by immunocytochemical staining for insulin, or by the demonstration of increased insulin levels within the serum. They represent the most common form of islet cell tumor, and the great majority are benign. However, as in glucagonomas, cytologic features are unreliable for distinguishing benign from malignant lesions, and the ultimate definition of malignancy is the demonstration of metastasis. Histologically, insulinomas may resemble in structure rather bizarre islets, or they may show an organoid pattern or one reminiscent of carcinoid tumors. Immunohistologic staining with antibody against insulin reveals variable degrees of cytoplasmic staining within tumor cells (Fig. 8–4), but these cells usually constitute only a minority of the total cell population (Table 8–1). Immunohistochemical staining for insulin appears to be a more reliable method for identification of these tumors than electron microscopic examination of granules or various histochemical silver-staining methods. It should however be noted that insulinomas, even those with clinical evidence of hyperinsulinism, may also show the production of other polypeptide hormones

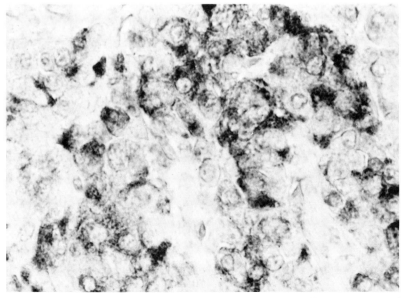

Figure 8–4. Islet cell adenoma displaying positive reactivity (black) for insulin in a portion of the tumor cells. Paraffin section, AEC with hematoxylin counterstain ($\times 500$).

within minority subpopulations of the tumor cells.

Somatostatin

Somatostatin-containing neoplasms are relatively rare in the pancreas, and morphologically and behaviorally they resemble other islet cell neoplasms. A number of cases described have been associated with a clinical syndrome of achlorhydria, anemia, steatorrhea, and diabetes, these clinical features being explained by the inhibitory effects of somatostatin upon gastrin, cholecystokinin, and insulin. It should be noted that although somatostatinomas morphologically resemble other islet cell tumors, their behavior in most cases observed to date has been malignant, with extensive metastasis at the time of diagnosis of the pancreatic tumor. On immunostaining the percentage of positive cells may vary from 20 to almost 100 percent, and as with other islet cell tumors, subpopulations of the cells may also show immunostaining for other islet hormones and occasionally for calcitonin or ACTH-like molecules. Somatostatinomas have been described in the duodenum, in which they appear to exhibit distinctive features (Chapter 7).

VIP

The normal function of vasoactive intestinal polypeptide (VIP) has not been clearly defined, but the clinical syndrome associated with VIP-producing tumors is well recognized, and more than 100 cases have been described. Variously termed watery diarrhea, syndrome, pancreatic cholera syndrome, or Verner-Morrison syndrome, it shows a characteristic constellation of clinical features, including voluminous watery diarrhea, hypochlorhydria, and hypochloremic acidosis. Hypercalcemia and hyperglycemia are variably present. The associated neoplasm is usually to be found within the pancreas and morphologically resembles other islet cell neoplasms. Immunohistochemically, it is possible to demonstrate VIP in a variable proportion of tumor cells, although it should be noted that other polypeptide hormones, particularly pancreatic polypeptide, frequently are also present in significant numbers of

cells (Table 8-1). Behaviorally, it is important to note that at least half of the VIP-producing tumors have shown malignant behavior. These tumors also occur in the gut (Chapter 7).

Distribution of VIP in the normal pancreas is of interest, being found in a small percentage of islet cells, in cells scattered throughout the exocrine ducts and acinar tissues in small numbers, and in association with recognizable nerve fibers running through the pancreas. Changes in the number and distribution of VIP-producing cells in pathologic states have not been clearly documented.

Pancreatic Polypeptide

In the human pancreas, pancreatic polypeptide has been shown to be present, by immunocytochemical methods, within a small percentage of islet cells and in rare cells within the exocrine pancreas. The number and distribution of pancreatic polypeptide–containing cells in the normal pancreas and in pathologic states has not been extensively documented, though there are preliminary reports of increased numbers in some forms of pancreatitis, in juvenile diabetes, and in association with some islet cell tumors (Table 8–1). In some instances, the pancreatic polypeptide–producing cells also appear to be part of the tumor cell population. As noted previously, some investigators believe that pancreatic polypeptide may be detachable in a minority of the cells of all islet cell tumors if sufficiently sensitive techniques are employed.

Islet cell neoplasms staining exclusively for pancreatic polypeptide are relatively rare and are not associated with any clinical recognizable state; elevated levels of pancreatic polypeptide have been observed in some instances of the watery diarrhea syndrome, as noted earlier, and some authorities believe that some instances of this syndrome may be attributable to the effects of pancreatic polypeptide rather than to VIP production. Tumors producing pancreatic polypeptide have usually been solitary, except in multiple endocrine adenomatosis type I, and are usually benign. There are also some suggestions that increased numbers of pancreatic polypeptide cells are particularly associated with familial varieties of islet cell tumors.

Other Polypeptides and Biogenic Amines

A small number of islet cell tumors have been described in association with production of clinically detectable amounts of 5-hydroxytryptamine and 5-hydroxytryptophan. Immunocytochemical studies of these tumors currently are anecdotal, and it is presumed that they are derived from small numbers of 5-hydroxytryptamine–producing (APUD) cells distributed within the exocrine pancreas rather than from the islet cells proper.

In addition, other polypeptide hormones not produced by normal islets of Langerhans have been described in association with islet cell tumors. In cases in which immunohistochemical studies have been performed, it appears that these "ectopic" polypeptides are products of subpopulations of the tumor cells (eg, production of calcitonin, ACTH, gastrin, and the like, in tumors that are classifiable on the basis of the majority of cells as insulinomas or glucagonomas, and so forth (Table 8–1).

THYROID

The thyroid gland contains two hormonally active components. The thyroid follicular cells proper are responsible for the production of thyroglobulin, a glycoprotein that contains the active thyroid hormones T3 (triiodothyronine) and T4 (thyroxine). The follicular C cells are present in smaller numbers, in an apparent extrafollicular situation and are responsible for the production of calcitonin. Embryologically, the thyroid is of endodermal derivation and is formed from a downgrowth of the epithelial cells at the base of the tongue during the first few weeks of development of the embryo. The precise embryologic interrelations of the follicular thyroglobulin–producing cells and the parafollicular C cells have been the subject of contention.

Thyroglobulin

Human thyroglobulin is a relatively good antigen and, following isolation and injection into rabbits or other animals, produces good antibody titers. It is claimed that most antibodies prepared in this way show specific reactivity with thyroglobulin, with little cross reactivity with triiodothyronine or thyroxine.

As an antigen, thyroglobulin appears to be well preserved within tissue sections following a variety of fixation and processing procedures (Table 8–2). Thyroglobulin can be detected immunohistologically in tissues fixed routinely in 4% formalin (even following fixation for several days), in B5 solution, or in Bouin's fixative. The procedures for immunostaining do not differ from those described earlier. The PAP method has been most widely employed in reported studies, but good results have been obtained with indirect conjugate methods.

The thyroid gland does not normally contain endogenous peroxidase activity except

Table 8–2. Selected Bibliography: Carcinoma of Thyroid

Böcker et al 1981	Excellent general survey of thyroglobulin staining, techniques, and interpretation
Permanetter et al 1982	Papillary carcinoma strong for keratin, weak for thyroglobulin; follicular carcinoma, reverse; medullary carcinoma and undifferentiated carcinoma, negative for both
Burt & Goudie 1979	Thyroglobulin positive in 30/30 well differentiated papillary and follicular carcinomas but in only 1 of 20 anaplastic tumors; valuable in recognition of thyroid carcinoma
Kawaoi et al 1982	Staining for thyroglobulin, thyroxine (T4), and triiodothyronine (T3) in 97 nontoxic thyroid tumors; T4 positive in 60%, T3 in 80%. T4 correlated well with thyroglobulin localization; T3 sometimes differed
Inoue M et al 1980	Follicular adenoma developing in a benign cystic teratoma
Gould SF et al 1983	Thyroglobulin in papillary carcinoma within ovarian teratoma (strum ovarii)
Mambo & Irwin 1984	Utilized thyroglobulin, calcitonin and immunoglobulin antibodies to study 10 anaplastic "small cell tumors;" concluded 6 were lymphomas; 2, follicular carcinomas; and 2, undesignated
Stefaneanu et al 1984	Thyroglobulin in thyroiditis, Graves's disease, and carcinoma
Franssila et al 1984	Mucoepidermoid cancer of thyroid; thyroglobulin negative
Nishiyama T et al 1983	Histaminase in primary and metastatic cancers of lung, colon, thyroid, pancreas, carcinoids etc; overall 28/84 epithelial malignancies were positive compared with 1/22 sarcomas and 0/19 benign lesions. Degree of positivity did not correspond to degree of cellular differentiation

for red cell pseudoperoxidase; staining of red cells with the substrate system does not usually present a problem in interpretation, and procedures for the blocking of endogenous peroxidase activity are thus generally unnecessary in attempting to interpret immunostaining within the thyroid.

Commercial kits are available for the demonstration of thyroglobulin, and, in our experience, give excellent results. If commercial antisera are obtained from other sources, or if the pathologist makes his own antisera, then it is necessary to perform a checkerboard titration to determine the optimal dilution for use of the antibody in immunohistologic studies. The commercial kits contain pretitered reagents.

Background staining due to nonspecific binding of antisera is generally not a serious problem in immunohistologic studies of the thyroid, but in the event that sclerosis is present, it is advisable to pretreat sections with normal serum as described in Chapter 2.

Patterns of Thyroglobulin Staining

In normal thyroid the colloid within the follicles generally shows no staining or light diffuse staining; the larger follicles lined by flattened epithelial cells show minimal or absent staining of colloid and minimal staining of the lining epithelium. Smaller follicles within the same thyroid often show more staining of the colloid, on occasion intense, whereas the cuboidal cells lining these follicles may show very intense staining (Fig. 8–5). In a normally active thyroid, the immediate- to small-sized follicles predominate and consistently show a positive reaction to thyroglobulin. The discrepancy in staining pattern between the colloid present in the smaller follicles (staining intensely) and in the larger follicles (staining lightly or not at all) is in present terms inexplicable, but in simplistic terms it seems that active follicles with active laying down and removal of thyroglobulin are stained, whereas inactive follicles are inert. Consequently, in simple thyroid goiters in which there typically is extensive "colloid storage," one normally sees absence of staining of colloid in these large follicles and an absence of staining in the flattened lining epithelium, but scattered among the large follicles are variable numbers of very small follicles with cuboidal epithelium and dense cytoplasmic staining.

By contrast, in Graves's disease, the thyroid shows evidence of diffuse hyperactivity with intense staining of the majority of the epithelial elements, some of which are arranged in small tight follicles, whereas others form larger follicles with infoldings of the epithelium. The colloid often stains intensely.

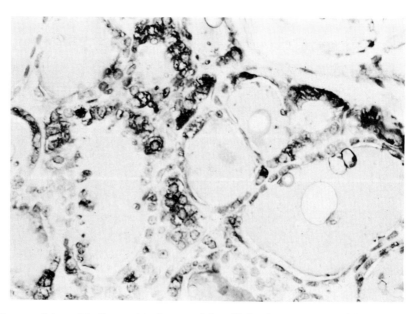

Figure 8–5. Pattern of thyroglobulin reactivity in normal thyroid showing some areas of thickened active epithelium staining strongly (black cytoplasm) for thyroglobulin. Colloid itself shows little staining. Paraffin section, AEC with hematoxylin counterstain (×320).

The immunohistologic staining patterns are more variable in hypothyroid states, but are readily distinguishable from hyperactive thyroid and from normally active thyroid, though clearly a spectrum of intermediate forms exist between the normally active and the functionally hypoactive thyroid. In autoimmune (Hashimoto's) thyroiditis, the thyroid typically contains a dense lymphocytic and plasma cell infiltrate with variable numbers of distinct thyroid follicles, some composed of atrophic follicular cells, others of larger granular eosinophilic cells resembling so-called Hürthle cells.

Böcker and colleagues (1981), on the basis of immunohistologic staining for thyroglobulin, have distinguished two varieties of cells within this Hürthle cell group. The majority are deeply eosinophilic granular cells lining small imperfectly formed follicles; these cells show variable degrees of thyroglobulin staining. A minority of cells, less than 10 percent, are less densely eosinophilic and show no evidence of thyroglobulin synthesis. It should also be noted that in one study these or closely associated cells were shown to contain somatostatin and neuron-specific enolase, possibly bespeaking a different origin (see Dhillon et al, 1982a) (and Table 8–3).

In the more advanced stage of the disease, the number of thyroglobulin-containing cells appeared to decrease progressively. In any event, the number of thyroglobulin-containing cells appears to correlate with the clinical thyroid status.

When stained for immunoglobulin, plasma cells in Hashimoto's thyroiditis show a typical polyclonal pattern, though it must be emphasized that rarely have monoclonal immunoblastic proliferations been detected as part of a transformation of this lymphocytic proliferation to an aggressive immunoblastic sarcoma (Maurer et al, 1979).

Other forms of thyroiditis, such as Riedel's thyroiditis and granulomatous thyroiditis, in which there may be variable destruction of the follicles, show a decreased total number of follicles, and those that are present often show intense staining, suggesting that there is increased cellular activity of the residual thyroid epithelium.

Thyroid Adenoma

In the strict sense, the term *adenoma* should be utilized for benign neoplastic growths of the thyroid follicular epithelium. In practice it is difficult, on the one hand, to distinguish adenomas from hyperplastic nodules within nodular goiters and, on the other hand, to distinguish certain adenomas from carcinomatous growths.

Thyroid adenomas are classified on a morphologic basis into three broad categories: follicular; papillary; and others, the so-called atypical adenomas.

True papillary adenomas, that behave in a benign fashion, are particularly difficult to differentiate from papillary carcinomas that have metastasized.

Follicular adenomas are further subdivided according to microscopic pattern or cytologic features of the cells that make up the follicles; subcategories include embryonal adenomas, fetal adenomas, microfollicular and macrofollicular adenomas, and so-called Hürthle cell adenomas in which the cells of the epithelium have the typical abundant granular pink cytoplasm ascribed to Hürthle cells.

The functional potential of these various adenomas in terms of production of thyroid hormone is variable and unpredictable. Adenomas may cause hyperthyroidism, or a hyperfunctioning nodule commonly turns out to be an area of focal nodular hyperplasia within a multinodular goiter. Recently, immunohistologic studies have shed some light upon the functional capacity of the thyroid neoplasms and have led to some suggestions for modifications of the classification system described above. This classification is based on the immunomorphologic features of thyroid adenomas stained with antisera to thyroglobulin (see Böcker et al, 1981).

Immunohistologic Classification of Thyroid Adenomas

1. Adenomas of main cell type
   a. Trabecular/normofollicular
   b. Macrofollicular
   c. Microfollicular (Autonomous)
2. Adenomas with specific cytologic differentiation
   a. Oxyphilic
   b. Clear cell
   c. Gastroplasm-rich cell
   d. Mitochondrion-rich cell

Overall, the great majority of the adenomas show positivity for thyroglobulin, thyroxine (T4), or triiodothyronine (T3), commonly for all three. T3 is positive in about 80 percent of adenomas, T4 in 60 percent, the distribution and localization of T4 correlating

Table 8–3. Selected Bibliography: Medullary Carcinoma of Thyroid

DeLellis & Wolfe 1981	Polypeptide hormone neuroendocrine cells and their neoplasms; excellent detailed review
Becker KL et al 1981	Calcitonin in Kulchitsky's cells (K cells) of bronchial wall; increased in emphysema and pneumonitis; present in carcinoids and small cell carcinomas (both perhaps K cell–derived)
Burtin et al 1979	CEA and NCA positive in medullary C cell carcinoma
Cox et al 1979	CEA and calcitonin combined markers of malignancy in medullary C cell carcinoma
Talerman et al 1979	Medullary C cell carcinoma positive both for CEA and calcitonin, although distribution different in individual tumors
Deftos et al 1980	59 thyroid C cell neoplasms (human and rat)—stained for calcitonin (58/59 positive), for beta-endorphin (25/31 positive), for ACTH (12/18 positive), and for somatostatin (9/19 positive); in some cases single cells appeared positive for all four; immune cross reactivity and peptide sequence in common were discussed
Nieuwenhuijzen Kruseman et al 1982	Anaplastic C cell carcinoma, 9/14 calcitonin positive
Mendelsohn et al 1980a	Anaplastic C cell carcinomas; value of calcitonin stains in differential diagnosis from lymphoma, giant cell carcinomas, etc. Some small cell carcinomas of thyroid are C cell carcinoma variants
Jolivet et al 1980	Case report of a medullary carcinoma associated with Cushing's syndrome; tumor cells stained for both calcitonin and ACTH (some lacunar cells contained calcitonin only); metastases largely lost ACTH reactivity
Kameda et al 1979	Nature of amyloid in medullary carcinoma, and "C cell reactive thyroglobulin"
Gibson et al 1981, 1982	C cell morphometry; concentrated about one third of the way down lateral lobes; numbers increase with age
Charpin et al 1982a	Bilateral medullary carcinoma (in a high risk family) with C cell hyperplasia; hyperplastic and tumorous C cells were calcitonin positive; tumor cells also reacted for ACTH and somatostatin
Charpin et al 1984	10 cases, with review of literature
Stjernholm et al 1980	C cell carcinoma in a two-year-old child
Mendelsohn et al 1980b	Both adrenal medullary cells and thyroid cells are neuroendocrine APUD cells but appear developmentally distinct
Ljungberg et al 1983	Compound follicular-parafollicular carcinoma of thyroid—common stem cell for follicular and "parafollicular" cells
Cooper et al 1980	Calcitonin(-like) reactivity in pituitary (human and rat) probably represents cross reactivity of related peptide precursors
Kameda & Ikeda 1980 } Kameda et al 1980 }	C cell development in fetus (dog)
Treilhou-Lahille et al 1979	Calcitonin in fetal mouse; best results with Bouin's fixative; claimed poor results with aldehyde fixatives, which does not appear to be a limiting factor in the later work of others
Dhillon et al 1982a	Hashimoto's disease stained for somatostatin, nonspecific enolase, calcitonin, and thyroglobulin (18 cases); enolase present in oxyphil cells of 4 cases; some cells apparently also contained somatostatin; speculated that somatostatin may inhibit release of thyroid hormone
Kameya et al 1983	Normal and neoplastic C cells produce both calcitonin- and gastrin-releasing polypeptide; the latter is the mammalian analogue of bombesin (see Chapter 7)
Geddie et al 1984	Value of calcitonin staining in fine needle aspirates
Kini et al 1984	"Specificity" of fine-needle biopsy improved markedly by staining for calcitonin
Saad et al 1984	Correlation of prognosis with extent of staining for calcitonin

well with thyroglobulin staining (Table 8–2).

The "main" cell adenomas consist of cells that cytologically are indistinguishable from cells of the normal thyroid gland. In most cases (especially types l.a and l.b) the immunohistologic staining pattern also parallels that of the normal thyroid in that cells forming larger follicles tend not to show immunostaining, and the intrafollicular colloid equally shows little staining, whereas the cuboidal epithelium constituting smaller follicles often shows quite marked positive staining with variable staining of colloid. These types of adenoma appear to be responsive to the normal controls for thyroglobulin production and behave in concert with the surrounding thyroid; on radioscanning they appear as cold or neutral nodules.

By contrast, the autonomous adenomas show intense staining for thyroglobulin (type l.c) within almost all of the cuboidal cells that comprise the numerous small-to-moderate–sized follicles that make up this tumor. Not much colloid is present, and it shows variable-to-slight staining. It is the intense staining of the cytoplasm that distinguishes this form of adenoma; it has some parallels with the hyperactive epithelium seen in the thyroid in Graves's disease.

The different types of adenomas that show specific cytologic differentiation give markedly differing patterns of immunocytochemical staining.

The oxyphilic adenoma, consisting of pale pink granular "oncocytes", shows almost no staining within these cells, though scattered within the tumor there may be follicular elements made up of more normal-appearing thyroid follicular cells, and these do show varying immunostaining for thyroglobulin.

The mitochondrion–rich cell adenoma may be related to the oxyphilic adenoma in that both cell types at electron microscopy are rich in mitochondria. A significant difference however is revealed by immunostaining, for the mitochondrion-rich cells show intense apical staining for thyroglobulin, in contrast with the almost total lack of staining of oxyphilic cells.

The gastroplasm–rich cell adenoma shows quite intense staining for thyroglobulin throughout the cytoplasm, with little evidence of colloid staining. On orthodox H&E section, these cells appear intensely eosinophilic and granular and are easily confused with the oxyphil adenoma; the immunocytologic staining is, however, totally different.

Clear cell adenomas in pure form are quite characteristic on routine sections, and on immunocytochemical preparations show diffuse peppery staining of the cytoplasm.

The so-called main cell adenomas comprise approximately 90 percent of all thyroid adenomas according to Böcker and colleagues (1981), the remaining 10 percent falling into the various types of adenomas with some evidence of specific cytologic differentiation. These authors lumped the papillary adenomas together with the papillary carcinomas, a common practice due to the difficulty of predicting benign versus malignant behavior of these tumors on the basis of morphology alone.

Thyroid Carcinomas

The great majority of thyroid carcinomas show positive immunohistochemical staining for thyroglobulin. Evidence suggests that carcinomas with a follicular pattern are almost always positive (Fig. 8–6), while more than 90 percent of papillary carcinomas show at least focal positivity (Fig. 8–7). It is important to emphasize that the number of positive cells within these neoplasms is quite variable and may range anywhere from 1 to 50 percent or more. In addition, the pattern of staining is uneven throughout the tumor, some follicles showing intense staining of the majority of the follicular lining cells, others showing only scattered positive cells or none.

In general terms, the less well-differentiated tumors show smaller numbers of thyroglobulin-positive cells. Anaplastic thyroid carcinomas may not show positive immunostaining within the anaplastic cells, but differentiated elements quite commonly may be found scattered throughout the tumor, and these typically do show positive immunostaining. Such differentiated components are more readily recognized in immunohistologic preparations than in straightforward hematoxylin and eosin sections.

A proportion of papillary carcinomas show areas of squamous differentiation; these areas do not show immunostaining, and, similarly, any psammoma bodies that are present do not contain detectable thyroglobulin.

Medullary carcinomas are consistently negative for thyroglobulin, although as described subsequently, they do show positive staining for calcitonin.

In conclusion, hyperfunctioning adenomas

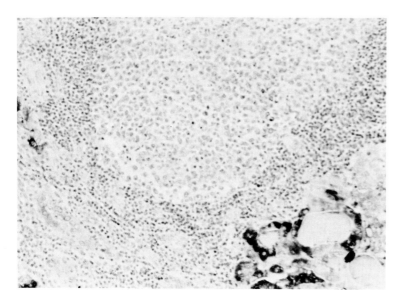

Figure 8–6. Metastatic carcinoma in lymph node showing intense positive staining (black) for thyroglobulin. Paraffin section, AEC with hematoxylin counterstain (×200).

that may be associated with, or responsible for, hyperthyroidism show distinctive immunocytochemical patterns, with the great majority of the tumor cells showing intense staining for thyroglobulin. Also, the majority of thyroid carcinomas do show detectable thyroglobulin, even when anaplastic in part, and thus the findings of thyroglobulin staining within a tumor effectively define its origin from the thyroid gland (with the very rare exception of thyroidlike epithelium within differentiated teratoma) (Table 8–2). Lack of positive staining for thyroglobulin within a tumor does not totally exclude an origin from thyroid but certainly weighs against such an interpretation.

It has been fashionable in the past for

pathologists to make statements as to active or inactive thyroid on the basis of the height of the epithelium lining the follicles or on the presence or absence of such other features as papillary folding, scalloping of the colloid, and the like. Immunocytochemical analysis reveals such distinctions to be rather crude and inaccurate and clearly demonstrates that if one wishes to assess thyroid function from a tissue section, then one should only do so after examination of an immunostain for thyroglobulin or thyroxin.

This section has emphasized the patterns of staining with antithyroglobulin antibodies. Antibodies against thyroxin (T4) give similar patterns both qualitatively and quantitatively. Antibodies against triiodothyronine (T3) have been described as giving some differences in distribution of positive cells, although reactivity still is confined to thyroid and its derivative tumors (Kawaoi et al, 1982). In one series anti-T3 marked 80 percent of approximately 100 thyroid tumors; anti-T4 stained 60 percent.

CEA and Keratin. Carcinoembryonic antigen (CEA) typically is present in the embryonic endoderm and in endodermally derived tissues and their malignant neoplasms in the adult. In this respect, follicular carcinomas of thyroid are somewhat unusual, since most investigators have reported lack of CEA reactivity in thyroid carcinomas, whether follicular, papillary, or anaplastic. Considerable variability has however been described, and overall CEA staining is of little value with reference to thyroid cancer, because inter-

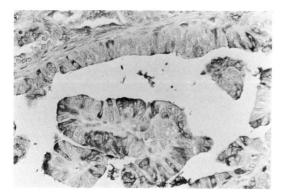

Figure 8–7. Papillary carcinoma of thyroid stained for thyroglobulin (brown-black). Note that only a proportion of the cancer cells are positive. Paraffin section, DAB with hematoxylin counterstain (×200). See color plate I–7.

pretation of the significance of positivity or the lack thereof is so uncertain.

Keratin is uniformly present in most papillary carcinomas but is inconsistently present in follicular carcinoma. Anaplastic carcinoma shows rare keratin-positive cells (see also Chapters 13 and 14).

Calcitonin

Calcitonin is a polypeptide with a molecular weight of 3500 and consists of 32 amino acids. Sensitive radioimmunoassay procedures are available for detection of calcitonin in human serum, the normal levels being less than 40 nanograms/100 ml in adult humans.

The composition of calcitonin in widely different species is sufficiently similar that antisera raised against calcitonin in one species will often significantly cross-react in other species. Any antiserum to be employed for calcitonin immunohistochemistry should be tested for quality of staining on sections of normal human thyroid prior to investigation of pathologic tissue. In staining normal thyroid, it should be noted that calcitonin-positive cells are sparsely distributed in much of the thyroid gland, being most numerous at the junctions of the middle and upper thirds.

The function of calcitonin in the normal adult is not clearly defined, though its source is known to be the so-called parafollicular C cells of the thyroid. The corresponding neoplasm, medullary carcinoma of the thyroid (parafollicular C cell carcinoma), is capable of producing the same hormone in large amounts. Production of hormone by normal, hyperplastic, or neoplastic tissues may be stimulated by infusion of calcium or gastrin; secondary C cell hyperplasia may occur in conditions of hypercalcemia or in association with hypergastrinemia as in the Zollinger-Ellison syndrome.

Medullary C cell carcinoma of the thyroid may occur in isolation or as part of multiple endocrine adenomatosis (type II, Sipple's syndrome, consisting of medullary thyroid carcinoma, pheochromocytoma, and parathyroid adenoma or hyperplasia).

The Parafollicular Cells of the Thyroid

Pearse (1968) has made major contributions to our understanding of the parafollicular cells of the thyroid. It has long been known that these cells were argyrophilic, and Pearse was among the first to show, utilizing immunofluorescence methods, that these cells contained calcitonin. From this demonstration Pearse and others went on to show that the parafollicular cells share many other characteristics with small clear cells scattered throughout the epithelium of the gastrointestinal tract and lung, namely, the amine precursor uptake and decarboxylation (APUD) cells. It is currently believed that many (or at least some) of these cells take their origins from the neural crest.

Immunohistologic methods have since considerably expanded our concepts of this system and have revealed that there exists a diverse population of neuroendocrine cells throughout the gastrointestinal tract (see Chapter 7) and also the lung (which of course is derived from the embryonic endoderm, in common with the gastrointestinal tract). It therefore is not surprising that the thyroid gland, derived as it is from the thyroglossal duct, an extension of the embryonic endoderm, should also contain neuroendocrine cells—in this instance, the parafollicular cells.

It is also worthy of notice that although the term *parafollicular* is well established by usage, it is no longer regarded as anatomically accurate. The parafollicular cells have been shown by DeLellis and Wolfe (1981) to be included within the basement membrane of the thyroid follicles, subjacent to the thyroid follicular epithelium (Table 8–3). They thus occupy a position in relation to the thyroid follicular epithelium exactly analogous to the position occupied by the neuroendocrine cells in relation to epithelium throughout the lung and gastrointestinal tract—that is, they lie between the basement membrane and the epithelial cell layer.

Distribution of Calcitonin in Normal Tissues

Calcitonin or calcitoninlike activity has also been described in a number of nonthyroid tissues, including thymus, parathyroid, adrenal medulla, and lung. Immunohistologic studies localizing the cellular source of calcitonin in these tissues are as yet scanty. KL Becker and colleagues (1981) have described immunoreactive calcitonin-positive cells in the lungs; these apparently correspond to the Kulchitsky's cells (the neuroendocrinal APUD cells of the bronchi and bronchioles), and calcitoninlike substances have been

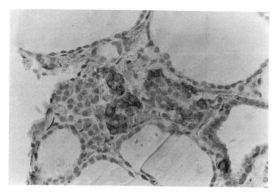

Figure 8–8. Thyroid stained for calcitonin. Positively stained (red-black) cells occur in the parafollicular area. Occasionally, cells in normal thyroid insinuate into the follicular epithelium (lower right). Paraffin section, AEC with hematoxylin counterstain (×320). See color plate I–8.

found in animal and human pituitary. Non-thyroidal neoplasms also may produce calcitonin, as described subsequently.

In the normal thyroid, the C cells are very difficult to distinguish from tangentially cut follicular cells in routine H&E sections. Histochemical stains based upon agyrophilia or metachromasia with toluidine blue have traditionally been used for recognition of C cells but are much less sensitive and much less specific than immunohistochemical methods, according to DeLellis and Wolfe (1981).

Calcitonin, being a polypeptide, belongs to that general class of antigens that are relatively resistant to the adverse effects of fixation and processing. Thus, calcitonin can usually be demonstrated readily in postmor-

tem tissues or in surgical tissues following fixation in buffered formalin and paraffin embedment. C cells are distributed unevenly in the normal adult thyroid, being concentrated in the deeper part of both lobes of the thyroid at approximately the junction of the upper and middle thirds. In the adult, C cells often tend to be spindle-shaped and to occur in small groups that rarely consist of more than three or four cells per group (Fig. 8–8), and of more than ten cells in adjacent high-power fields.

In the neonatal thyroid and in the young child, C cells are relatively plumper and more polygonal in shape and are considerably more numerous, occurring in groups of six to ten cells.

C Cell Hyperplasia

C cell hyperplasia occurs in two principal varieties. There is primary C cell hyperplasia that shows a high association with subsequent development of medullary C cell carcinoma, and there is secondary C cell hyperplasia in which the increased calcitonin production appears to represent a physiologic response to hypercalcemia or to hypergastrinemia (as in the Zollinger-Ellison syndrome). C cell hyperplasia cannot be assessed histologically in H&E sections, since calcitonin staining reveals that the hyperplastic C cells often occur in well-formed follicular structures indistinguishable from ordinary thyroid follicles in H&E sections (Fig. 8–9). Immunostaining is thus essential for this purpose.

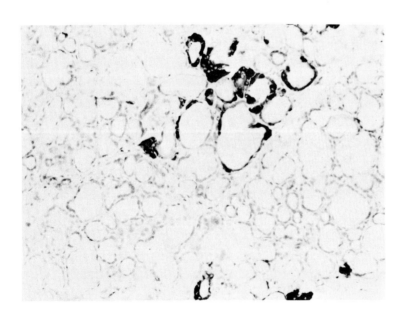

Figure 8–9. Thyroid stained for calcitonin showing marked C cell hyperplasia (black). Interestingly, the hyperplastic C cells are arranged in well-formed follicles that morphologically are not distinguishable from the remaining normal thyroid follicles. The importance of recognizing "C" cell hyperplasia is considered in the text. Paraffin section, AEC with hematoxylin counterstain (×125).

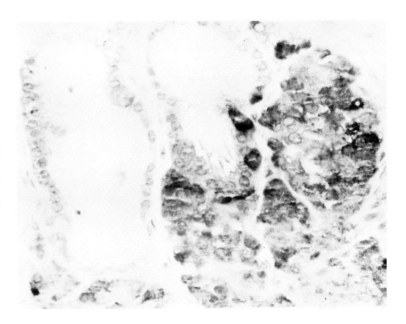

Figure 8–10. Two large thyroid follicles (upper left) plus large clusters of calcitonin-positive "C" cells in "noncancerous" thyroid from a case of familial medullary C cell carcinoma. Paraffin section, AEC with hematoxylin counterstain (×320). Large clusters of C cells are usually indicative of hyperplasia or carcinoma; when found in normal thyroid adjacent to a C cell carcinoma they indicate the "familial" nature of the case.

C cell hyperplasia occurring de novo represents part of a spectrum of disease extending from mild hyperplasia through to neoplasia, including frank invasive medullary C cell carcinoma. This form of hyperplasia is familial, as is the occurrence of medullary C cell carcinoma in these patients, and it may occur in association with other endocrine neoplasms as part of the multiple endocrine adenomatosis syndrome (Sipple's syndrome). DeLellis, Wolff, and colleagues have published extensively upon this topic (Table 8–3). They believe that the presence of C cell hyperplasia, whether diffuse or nodular, is of great diagnostic and prognostic significance in the recognition of familial cases of medullary C cell carcinoma (which is inherited as an autosomal dominant trait). According to these investigators, the presence of C cell hyperplasia in association with medullary C cell carcinoma identifies that carcinoma as of the familial type (Fig. 8–10) as opposed to the sporadic type, for in the latter, the numbers of C cells in residual thyroid are normal.

This distinction has important implications for clinician and pathologist. First, the diagnosis of a carcinoma as medullary C cell type can be accomplished with a high degree of certainty by immunostaining for calcitonin. Second, once this diagnosis is achieved, it is necessary to examine residual thyroid for the evidence of C cell hyperplasia. Third, if C cell hyperplasia is shown to be present, the case is identified as familial, and it is necessary to examine the patient's family. This is accomplished by assays of serum calcitonin levels and thyroid biopsy or thyroidectomy in patients in which the calcitonin level is raised. Assessment of the histologic features of such biopsy or thyroidectomy material in these cases demands immunostaining for calcitonin in order to assess distribution and numbers of C cells to determine whether the particular patient also suffers from the trait and whether the condition is still at the stage of hyperplasia or has progressed to neoplasia. This latter distinction may be very difficult morphologically, but in either event, the correct response is thyroidectomy.

Medullary C Cell Carcinoma of Thyroid

Classically, this neoplasm consists of small clear cells in irregular clusters, clumps, or nests in association with a pink matrix that shows the histochemical reactions of amyloid. As indicated above, the neoplastic cells themselves show staining for calcitonin, the intensity varying quite markedly from cell to cell in different cases, with some cells showing intense reactivity and others, weak reactivity or no detectable staining (Fig. 8–11). The amyloid material also shows staining for calcitonin, and this is thought to reflect the fact that the composition of amyloid includes fragments of the calcitonin polypeptide chain.

Although medullary C cell carcinoma was originally described as not showing a follicu-

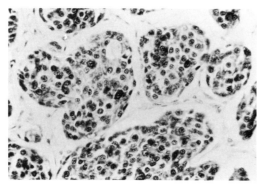

Figure 8–11. Medullary C cell carcinoma of thyroid showing positive cytoplasmic staining (brown-black) for calcitonin in approximately half of the tumor cells. Paraffin section, DAB with hematoxylin counterstain (×200). See color plate II–1.

lar pattern, it has since been recognized that some cases may show quite extensive follicle formation and may be mistakenly diagnosed as follicular carcinoma (Fig. 8–12). Differential diagnosis may be made apparent by staining for calcitonin and for thyroglobulin, medullary carcinoma giving positivity for calcitonin (Fig. 8–13) and follicular carcinomas giving positivity for thyroglobulin.

Medullary carcinomas, although they typically stain for calcitonin, may also show the presence of other polypeptide hormones, including somatostatin, VIP, ACTH, and corticotropic–releasing factorlike activity. Somatostatin is of particular interest because animal studies have revealed that many of the C cells contain both calcitonin and so-

matostatin, whereas some contain calcitonin alone. Similarly, medullary C cell carcinoma may contain both somatostatin and calcitonin, or calcitonin alone.

A recent extensive study of 44 cases of medullary carcinoma of the thyroid (Saad et al, 1984), provides some guidelines for current practice. The authors regard staining for calcitonin as essential in medullary carcinoma of thyroid: calcitonin-rich tumors (>75 percent positive cells) typically belonged to the multiple endocrine adenoma group and had a good prognosis, even if extensive; calcitonin-poor tumors (<25 percent positive cells) had a very poor prognosis.

Neuron specific enolase characteristically is present in neurons and the so-called neuroendocrine cells throughout the lung and gastrointestinal tract, and is also positive in C cells and in medullary C cell carcinoma.

Finally, as befits its embryologic origin from the endoderm, CEA may be present in medullary C cell carcinoma (up to 20 percent of cases). The presence of CEA is, however, not of great diagnostic value and cannot reliably be used to distinguish medullary C cell carcinoma from nodular C cell hyperplasia, since even cases of simple hyperplasia may show some CEA reactivity (this to some extent is analogous to the situation in colon in which hyperplastic colonic epithelium may also show increased expression of CEA, although CEA of course is most frequently and most intensely expressed by neoplastic colon, at least in the adult).

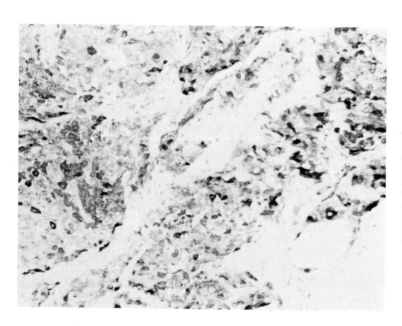

Figure 8–12. Medullary C cell carcinoma of thyroid showing variable staining of tumor cells for calcitonin. Some cells show intense positivity (black cytoplasm); others react moderately (shades of gray); and some contain no detectable calcitonin. The tumor was partially follicular (lower right). Paraffin section, AEC with hematoxylin counterstain (×125).

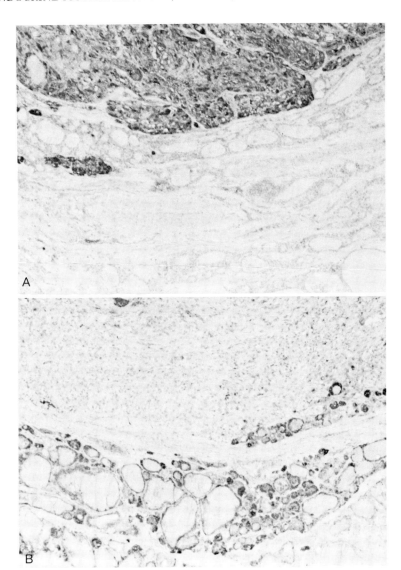

Figure 8–13. Medullary C cell carcinoma of thyroid abutting on residual normal thyroid. *A* shows staining for calcitonin in tumor cells. *B* shows staining for thyroglobulin in residual thyroid. Paraffin section, AEC with hematoxylin counterstain (×60).

Ectopic Calcitonin Production. As noted above, there is some evidence for the production of calcitonin by nonthyroidal tissues, and there is little doubt that it can be produced by a variety of nonthyroidal neoplasms, which include lung, pancreatic, and colonic tumors. Elevated calcitonin levels most particularly are associated with oat cell carcinoma of lung (again, this is in keeping with other recent knowledge pertaining to neuroendocrine origin of oat cell carcinoma).

PARATHYROID HORMONE

The recognition of parathyroid tissue and parathyroid neoplasms (particularly adenoma) has received little attention but may be achieved by staining with antibodies against parathormone. Parathormone appears relatively stable in fixed tissues and can readily be identified in frozen sections. The ability to demonstrate rapidly the presence of parathormone in small samples of frozen tissue is of particular value in facilitating tissue recognition during surgical procedures that attempt to identify parathyroid glands in cases of hyperparathyroidism. Both hyperplastic and neoplastic glands show positivity for parathormone to varying degrees.

It should be recognized that parathormone may also be produced "ectopically" by neoplasms that have originated in tissues other than the parathyroid proper. Thus, it has long been known that the clinical state of

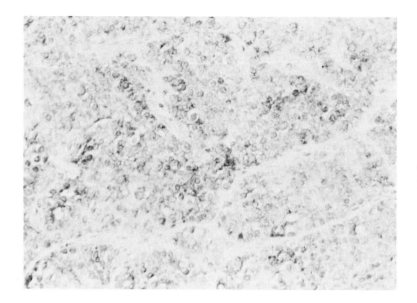

Figure 8–14. Frozen section of nodule from neck stained for parathormone; parathyroid adenoma. Frozen section, DAB, no counterstain (×125). This technique is of value in distinguishing parathyroid from thyroid tissue.

hyperproduction of parathyroidlike hormone may occur in association with lung tumors; such tumors may be shown to have immunohistologic reactivity with antibodies against parathormone, reflecting their production of the hormone. This type of staining may be of value in demonstrating that a particular neoplasm is indeed responsible for an associated clinical state of hyperparathyroidism.

Two of the more extensive reported studies of parathyroid adenomas are those of Dietel et al (1980) and Ordoñez et al (1983). The latter paper particularly points out the value of immunohistochemical staining for parathormone in the recognition of "nonfunctioning" carcinomas of the parathyroid gland, which though rare, are extremely difficult to distinguish from thyroid tumors or from metastases of other small cell carcinomas.

Immunostaining for parathormone may thus be attempted in tumors resected from patients with clinical evidence of parathormone hyperactivity, in an effort to establish that the resected tumor is indeed responsible for the increased levels of parathormone. One other indication for carrying out a stain for parathormone would be in thoracic surgery, during parathyroidectomy, to confirm that tissue removed is parathyroid. A rapid-frozen section can readily be stained for the presence of the hormone (Fig. 8–14); such a stain carried out using the 37° C incubation method may take only half an hour, which is consistent with the needs of the surgeon.

PITUITARY

Traditionally, the endocrine tissues of the pars anterior were considered to consist of three cell types according to their tinctorial properties. Nonstaining cells were termed chromophobes, others were termed eosinophils or basophils according to their predilection for eosin or the basic hematoxylin, and their reactions with "pituitary stains" such as PAS, orange-G, Herlant's tetrachrome, etc. Following the common principle that neoplastic cells mimic their normal counterparts, the corresponding pituitary adenomas were termed chromophobe adenomas, eosinophil adenomas, or basophil adenomas.

Normal pituitary chromophobe cells were observed to be small cells with cytoplasm containing no visible granules by light microscopy; they comprised approximately 50 percent of the cells of the anterior pituitary. Cells with eosinophil granules accounted for 40 percent, whereas basophils numbered 10 percent or less. These cell types were further subclassified by their reaction with other "special" stains, such as alcian blue, PAS, and orange-G, with or without oxidation and extraction by performic acid. By these means a complicated classification of cell types was devised, and attempts were made to relate this classification to the production of seven principal hormones and to the corresponding tumors and their proclivities for production or one or another of these hormones.

With the advent of immunohistologic methods, the potential for specifically iden-

Table 8–4. Selected Bibliography: Pituitary, Pituitary Adenoma

Charpin et al 1982c	Pituitary adenomas associated with Cushing's disease; all 13 contained ACTH-positive cells; 10 also showed positivity for beta-LPH/beta-MSH, and 8 for beta endorphin; two contained a few PRL-positive cells; all were negative for calcitonin
Kovacs et al 1980b	343 pituitary adenomas; 56 designated "null cell" adenomas with no evidence of hormone production clinically, biochemically or on immunostaining
Kovacs et al 1977	Initial immunohistologic classification into 8 types (based on 207 cases); later expanded to 10 types
Sternberger & Joseph 1979	Sequential double-stain method for pituitary hormones
Weindl & Sofroniew 1979	Review, including releasing factors, vasopressin, and oxytocin
Hassoun et al 1979	ACTH, beta-MSH, LPH, and endorphin demonstrated variable reactivity in basophilic adenomas (with Cushing's disease) and in chromphobe adenomas
Guy et al 1980	ACTH, gamma-endorphin
Kovacs et al 1980c	Survey of 152 unselected autopsies of individuals aged more than 80 years; 20 had "silent" adenomas, the majority being PRL-positive
Pelletier et al 1978	Immunoelectron microscopy for PRL, GH, FSH, LH, TSH, and ACTH: PAP method; good technique paper
Gross & Longer 1979	Relationship in developing fetus between somatostatin in hypothalamus and GH in pituitary (mouse)
Vandesande et al 1980	Hypothalamus, including staining for somatostatin; supported one hormone/neuron hypothesis (animals)
Childs & Ellison 1980	Review of use of PAP method in understanding pituitary function; two or three hormones in given single cells
Sofroniew et al 1981	Vasopressin, oxytocin, and neurophysin in hypothalamus and neurohypophysis by PAP method; also described neuronal projections to other neural target areas, including the amygdala and the nuclei of the vagus and tractus solitarius
Horvath et al 1981	15 acidophil adenomas (from a total of 347 surgically resected adenomas) positive both for GH and PRL
Dubois 1980	Long, detailed review of neuropeptide hormones (excluding pituitary but including hypothalamus); discussed releasing factors, beta-LPH, endorphins, VIP, CCK, substance P, etc.
Ito et al 1981	Transient presence of ACTH-like molecule in fetal adrenal medulla
Duello & Halmi 1979	EM, PAP method for GH and PRL; emphasized hazards of attempting cell recognition by morphology alone
Osamura et al 1980	ACTH and beta-endorphin(-like) immunoreactivity in adult, fetal, and pathologic pituitary (includes Crooke's hyaline change and adenomas with Cushing's disease)
Asa et al 1982	Prolactin cell hyperplasia in multiparous women
Li JY et al 1979	EM, PAP method, and ACTH localization in fetal pituitary
Urbanski et al 1982	Argyrophil granules (in Grimelius's silver method) show no correlation with specific hormonal products demonstrated by immunoperoxidase
Childs & Unabia 1982	ABC and PAP methods; excellent technique paper
Halmi 1982	Growth hormone and prolactin occurring together in adenomas
Horvath & Kovacs 1984	Gonadotroph adenomas
Kovacs & Horvath 1977	Initial immunohistologic classification of pituitary adenomas
Esiri et al 1983	Immunohistology and EM features of 118 adenomas, relationship to type of presentation
Asa et al 1984	Neuron-specific enolase in pituitary adenomas; also noted NSE positivity in two carcinomas (from breast + ovary)
Wahlström et al 1981a	hCG-like reactivity in normal pituitary and some chromophobe adenomas

tifying the type of cell producing a given hormone was realized. Initially, immunofluorescence techniques were applied and served to delineate hormone-producing cells quite clearly. However, it was difficult to refer back to orthodox histologic criteria using immunofluorescence techniques, and detailed comparisons with the special histochemical stains were not possible. In this area, immunoperoxidase staining of paraffin sections was to have a dramatic effect. Much of the work has been carried out on paraffin sections, but important contributions have been made upon epoxy resin–embedded thin sections and electron microscopic applications of immunoperoxidase techniques at the ultrastructural level. It is also of interest that immunohistologic studies of the pituitary represented one of the first areas in which double–staining immunoperoxidase techniques were widely utilized.

After extensive studies by many different investigators (Table 8–4), it has become apparent that essentially all of the pituitary hormones can be demonstrated in routinely processed paraffin sections. In fact, the pituitary hormones appear to be particularly resistant to the ravages of formalin, paraffin embedment, or storage, and autopsy tissues that have been fixed for long periods in formalin and stored for several years can be successfully employed in studies of the cellular localization of pituitary hormones by immunoperoxidase methods. In a research-oriented review, Kovaks, Horvath, and Ryan, major pioneers in this area, wrote:

Suffice it to say that the immunoperoxidase technique represents a real breakthrough in endocrine pathology, including pituitary research. . . . We are convinced that future immunoperoxidase techniques will be more widely used in pituitary studies, and will be introduced in every laboratory

that deals with problems related to the pathology of the pituitary gland. (See Kovaks et al, 1980a,b.)

Certainly by the evidence presently available, the basic special histochemical stains that were a source of contention and argument among the pituitary pathologists have proved to be obsolete, irrelevant, and sometimes misleading in terms of ascribing the production of particular hormones to particular individual cells.

At present it is fair to state that, if one is to assess the pituitary cell population for its potential to produce any particular hormone, the only satisfactory means of doing so is by immunocytochemical methods. A similar argument applies to pituitary tumors: the only way of reaching a definitive conclusion as to the hormone-producing potential of a particular tumor is to perform an immunoperoxidase stain with a panel of antisera directed against the pituitary hormones.

Finally, another hallowed concept has fallen by the wayside: the belief that individual pituitary cells are restricted to the production of a single pituitary hormone appears also to be false, for double-staining techniques have shown that individual normal cells may contain one or more hormones and that individual tumors may contain several.

Assessment of Pituitary Function

The tinctorial properties of cells on which special histochemical methods or hematoxylin and eosin stains are used do not correlate with their hormonal content. Numerous studies of animal and human pituitaries have given us certain insights into pituitary function (Tables 8–4 and 8–5). With the reservation that individual cells may have the

Table 8–5. Case Reports; the Pituitary

Tramu et al 1979	4 adenomas, nonreactive for ACTH but positive for beta-MSH and endorphins
Kovacs et al 1980a	A chromophobe adenoma positive for both FSH and LH
Cebelin et al 1981	A case of prolactin cell hyperplasia, with lymphocytic hypophysitis 14 months postpartum
Sherry et al 1982	A pituitary adenoma with 70% of cells positive for PRL and a separate, distinct 5% positive for ACTH (mixed adenoma?)
Kovacs et al 1982	Chromophobe adenoma positive for GH and TSH (nonreactive for PRL, ACTH, FSH, LH, endorphin); possibility of bi- or multihormonal clones discussed
Kovacs et al 1977	GH-positive acidophil adenoma with giant granules
Favre et al 1979	Mixed chromophobe/acidophil adenomas producing GH and PRL
Asa et al 1981a	Keratin positivity in squamous nests and cysts in both pituitary and craniopharyngiomas

Table 8–6. The Pituitary; Immunocytochemical Cell Types

1. Somatotrophs	Growth hormone	50%	Mainly lateral wings
2. Lacto(mammo)trophs	Prolactin	20%	Random
3. Corticotrophs	ACTH	20%	Medial and pars intermedia
	MSH		
	Beta-LPH and endorphins		
4. Gonadotrophs	FSH	10%	Medial and lateral
	LH		
5. Thyrotrophs	TSH	<5%	Medial
6. Null	0	?	

capacity to produce more than one hormone, it has been possible to distinguish five cell types within the anterior pituitary (Table 8–6).

Growth hormone–producing cells are most numerous in the normal pituitary, constituting approximately half of the secretory cells present (Fig. 8–15). They are scattered throughout the anterior pituitary with particular concentration in the lateral wings. Their number does not appear to change significantly with age or in response to different diseases; however, in chronic hyperthyroidism there appears to be some loss of granules among the growth hormone-producing cells.

Prolactin-containing cells are the next most numerous, constituting approximately 20 percent (Fig. 8–16). Again, they are randomly distributed with some concentration laterally. It should be emphasized that by conventional and special histochemical stains, it is difficult to distinguish these prolactin-containing cells from the growth hormone–containing cells; nonetheless, they appear

distinguishable by immunocytochemical methods. Unlike growth hormone–producing cells, the prolactin cells vary greatly in number with age and in response to certain disease processes. In the newborn, prolactin cells are numerous, possibly in response to the high levels of maternal estrogen. Subsequently, their numbers fall, but they increase remarkably in females during pregnancy and lactation. Kovaks et al (1980a) speculated that the numbers may change in response to usage of dopaminergic drugs and their antagonists, such as reserpine and chlorpromazine. Normal, nonpregnant females and males appear to show differences in numbers of prolactin-containing cells, but there is no consistent decrease in number with advancing age.

ACTH-containing cells are located particularly in the central part of the anterior pituitary and in the so-called pars intermedia, which may be difficult to discern in the human pituitary on the basis of morphology alone but is often clearly demarcated by immunostaining for ACTH. The ACTH cells also show positive reactivity for melanocyte-staining hormone. Most investigators believe that this reactivity represents the production of two hormones by a single cell type rather than two subsets within this cell population. ACTH-producing cells have also been reported to stain for beta-LPH and the endorphins. The number of ACTH-containing cells appears to be quite constant with age, although increasing numbers appear to stray into the posterior pituitary in the elderly. Kovaks and colleagues also discussed the nature of Crooke's hyaline change, which appears in Cushing's disease, in cases of ectopic ACTH production and in patients treated with steroids. These investigators pointed out that the hyaline material does not appear to stain for ACTH by immunocytochemical methods.

Gonadotroph cells comprise approximately

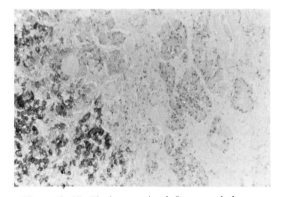

Figure 8–15. Pituitary stained for growth hormone showing positive (red-brown-black) cells in the pars anterior (left). Note absence of reactivity in pars intermedia and in neurohypophysis (right) Paraffin section, AEC with hematoxylin counterstain (×200). See color plate II–2.

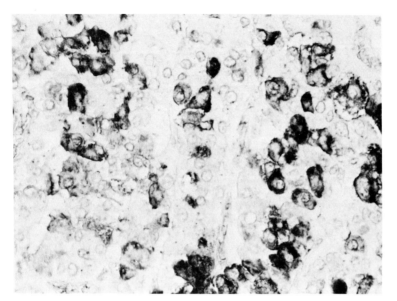

Figure 8–16. Anterior pituitary stained for prolactin (gray-black cytoplasm). Cells occur singly or in small clusters. Paraffin section, AEC with hematoxylin counterstain (×500).

10 percent of the anterior pituitary cells and are located in the central area. Individual gonadotroph cells may contain both follicle-stimulating hormone (FSH) and lutenizing hormone (LH), though some cells apparently contain either one or the other. Numbers of these cells appear to increase at the time of puberty; they may increase in both number and size following castration.

Thyroid-stimulating hormone (TSH)–containing cells appear to be the least numerous and particularly occur in a perivascular location in the anterior part of the pituitary. According to Phifer and Spicer (1973), TSH-containing cells account for less than 5 percent of the cells in the normal anterior pituitary. In the presence of inadequate function of the thyroid gland, with low levels of thyroglobulin, TSH cells become much more numerous. The PAS-positive cytoplasmic globules that appear in some atrophic TSH-containing cells do not show positive immunostaining for TSH. In analogy with Russell and Dutcher bodies, which show PAS positivity and do consist of immunoglobulin but often fail to immunostain with anti-immunoglobulin antibodies, this circumstance does not necessarily imply that the PAS-positive globues in thyrotrophs do not contain TSH.

Null cells, so designated by Kovacs and colleagues (Tables 8–4 and 8–6), contain no demonstrable hormone, are present in small but varying numbers on normal pituitary, and may produce corresponding null cell adenomas; these usually also are chromophobe.

Pituitary Adenomas

Positive immunostaining for one of the pituitary hormones confirms the pituitary origin of any tumor occurring in this anatomic region.

A lack of positive staining in the presence of adequate controls weighs as evidence against a pituitary tumor, though it does not totally exclude a pituitary origin, for a small portion of pituitary adenomas do appear to fail to stain even by the most sensitive immunohistologic methods (so-called null, or undifferentiated, cell adenomas). These cases still show positivity for neuron-specific enolase, which may be employed if the nature of the tissue is in doubt.

Pituitary adenomas formerly were classified as chromophobe, eosinophil, or basophil. The chromophobe adenomas were thought not to secrete any hormone; Kovacs et al

Table 8–7. Immunocytochemical Classification of Pituitary Adenomas*

1.	Growth hormone cell adenoma
2.	Prolactin cell adenoma
3.	Mixed growth hormone/prolactin cell adenoma
4.	Acidophil stem cell adenoma
5.	Corticotroph cell adenoma
6.	Thyrotroph cell adenoma
7.	Gonadotroph cell adenoma
8.	Undifferentiated (null) cell adenoma
9.	Oncocytoma
10.	Unclassified

*See Kovacs et al 1981.

(1981) used the term *null cell adenoma* (ie, no detectable hormone or immunohistologic staining) as a more precise designation for those chromophobe adenomas that do not produce hormone. The eosinophil adenomas were considered to produce principally growth hormones, and the basophil adenomas were believed to produce ACTH. These basic beliefs were erroneous, for there is now ample evidence that some chromophobe adenomas are capable of producing any of the pituitary hormones and that eosinophil adenomas produce not only growth hormone but also prolactin, whereas basophil adenomas may produce ACTH, beta-lipoprotein, or both, and the endorphins.

In addition, any of these three tinctorial types may fail to produce detectable hormones. Based on immunocytochemical studies, it has been proposed that pituitary adenomas can be classified into 10 separate types (Table 8–7). There do appear to be some subtle differences in the cellular morphology of these different neoplasms, in their special histochemical staining characteristics and in their electron microscopic characteristics. However, it seems pointless to present all of these differences here since in the final analysis the only reliable way of determining their hormone-production potential is to perform an immunohistologic stain; their other char-

acteristics are thus of academic interest only. The prolactin (PRL)-positive adenoma (Fig. 8–17) appears the most common variety both for these adenomas presenting pathologically and requiring surgery, and for those asymptomatic lesions discovered only at autopsy (in up to 12 percent in the 9th decade).

The so-called undifferentiated cell adenoma group includes those pituitary adenomas that are not accompanied by evidence of increased hormone secretion, either in terms of clinical manifestation or in terms of laboratory testing (Fig. 8–18). It is of interest that, immunocytochemically, it has been possible in some of these cases to detect hormones or hormone fragments such as beta-TSH or beta-FSH and that on electron microscopic examination the cells do appear to contain secretory granules, although the secretory product is at present unrecognized. Use of antisera versus the alpha or beta fragments may be expected to further clarify some of these issues.

Clearly, much remains to be discovered with reference to normal and neoplastic pituitary cells and their range of potentialities and function. The extensive bibliography that already exists documents considerable advances that have occurred and justifies consideration of the view that, henceforth, study of pituitary pathology cannot be real-

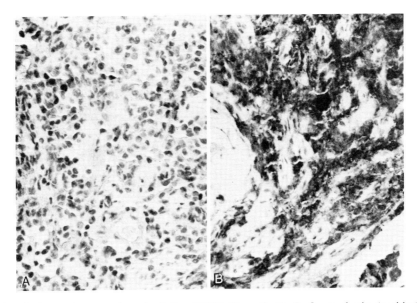

Figure 8–17. Pituitary adenoma, *A*, stained for ACTH ("negative"); *B*, for prolactin (positive). This was a pyroninophilic tumor of the base of the skull; the initial diagnosis was plasmacytoma. "Negative" staining for immunoglobulins led to staining for pituitary hormones and the correct diagnosis. Paraffin section, AEC with hematoxylin counterstain (×200).

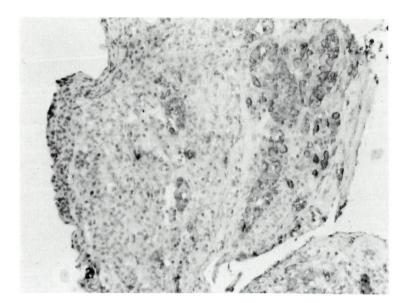

Figure 8–18. Wall of cystic lesion in sella turcica, stained for ACTH. Positive cells (gray-black cytoplasm) are arranged in clusters and cords (on the right). This was an aggressive locally invasive lesion. There was no clinical evidence of excessive ACTH production. Paraffin section, AEC with hematoxylin counterstain (×200).

istically accomplished without recourse to immunohistologic techniques. The fact that immunostaining kits are commercially available for most of the pituitary hormones places this method within reach of all pathology laboratories.

Finally, claims that other hormones may also be found in the pituitary gland (eg, calcitonin in dog or hCG in humans) (Table 8–4) require further investigation for possible relevance to human diseases of the pituitary.

9

TUMORS OF OVARY AND TESTIS

"Despite the apparent precision of morphologic definitions, the histopathologic diagnosis of neoplasia is at times hedged with uncertainty, owing in part to conceptual difficulties regarding the nature and origin of the neoplastic cells and also to a continuing lack of alternative methods of cell identification with which to validate the morphologic criteria employed."

TAYLOR ET AL, 1978

DEMONSTRATION OF STEROID HORMONES

The demonstration of steroid hormones by immunofluorescence or immunoenzyme techniques is governed by extremely complex and ill-understood rules, and interpretation of findings is difficult. Attempts to demonstrate steroid hormones by immunohistochemical methods have largely been restricted to two particular areas of need.

First, the demonstration of steroid hormones (specifically estrogen, progesterone, testosterone, and related substances) within cells has been employed in the study of ovarian and testicular neoplasms, with positive staining being presumptive of in situ synthesis of the respective steroid hormones. This type of staining has then been utilized in the investigation, diagnosis, and classification of ovarian and testicular neoplasms. The findings and the practical uses of these types of stains are discussed more fully in this chapter concerning ovarian and testicular neoplasms. There are three major obstacles to interpretation.

1. The antibodies employed are usually conventional antisera with specificity against one of the steroid sex hormones (eg, estradiol) but with measurable cross reactivity against one or more of the other steroid hormones or precursors (eg, cross reactivity with testosterone). To what extent low levels

of cross reactivity may produce detectable immunohistologic staining is difficult to assess. This problem has often been approached on a purely empirical basis—for example, in the demonstration that an anti-estradiol antibody produces obvious staining of granulosa or theca cells or both within the ovary but no obvious staining of interstitial cells of Leydig in the testis; this solution clearly is not science, but it does work.

2. It is somewhat surprising that steroid hormones are demonstrable to any extent in paraffin-fixed tissues, since such tissues have been processed extensively through organic solvents that might be expected to remove all of the steroid hormones. In this respect, it appears that fixation is to some extent "protective" and in some ill-understood way immobilizes at least part of the steroid hormone within a cell so it is not removed by organic solvents and remains immunologically reactive. The basis for this finding is a matter of conjecture; however, many investigators have reported the observation that antibodies with demonstrated specificity against particular steroid hormones are capable of producing immunocytochemical staining in the expected distribution within normal ovary and testis following adequate fixation in formalin and optimal processing and paraffin embedment (see Table 9–5).

3. The final problem in utilizing direct stains for steroid hormones in evaluation of

testicular and ovarian neoplasms is discussed more fully in the following pages; it relates to the need for cautious interpretation by the observer, particularly with reference to existing concepts as to which of the various potential hormone-producing cells of the ovary and testis produce which particular hormone. For example, antitestosterone antibodies not infrequently give positivity in ovarian tumors, whereas the converse may be observed with anti-estradiol antibodies.

The second major application of anti–steroid hormone antibodies, particularly antibodies against estrogen (estradiol), has been the attempted demonstration of estrogen receptor activity in carcinomas of the breast. This application is discussed in more detail in relation to breast carcinoma (Chapter 10). In principle, this approach depends upon the demonstration of estrogen within breast carcinoma cells as presumptive evidence of the expression of estrogen receptor activity by those cells, whether the estrogen was bound in vivo, or in vitro following addition of polymerized polyestradiol phosphate to the tissue prior to immunostaining. Positive results utilizing both techniques on frozen sections and even upon paraffin sections have been claimed. Proponents of the more usual methods of demonstrating estrogen receptor activity by preparing cytosols of fresh tumor tissue and deriving a quantitative value for steroid binding sites have, to state it bluntly, not given the immunohistologic techniques a very enthusiastic reception.

IMMUNOHISTOLOGIC TECHNIQUES FOR THE DIAGNOSIS OF OVARIAN AND TESTICULAR NEOPLASMS

"Tumors are classified like normal tissues on a histologic basis; the type of cells is the one important element in every tumor. From it the tumor should be named."

F. B. MALLORY, 1923

The concept advanced by Mallory is disarmingly simple but presupposes that one can confidently identify and reliably distinguish the various types of normal cells. As already described (Chapter 4), such a supposition is not justifiable with reference to recognition of the various lymphoid cells. Similarly, the keenest morphologist cannot

reliably identify the different germ cell and stromal cell derivatives found in the ovary and the testis.

Willis, in *Pathology of Tumors* (1948), prefaced the chapter pertaining to ovarian neoplasms with the following statement:

Several factors have combined to cause confusion in their [ovarian tumors] classification and nomenclature, namely, (1) uncertainties as to the histogenetic relationships of some of the tissues of the normal ovary, (2) uncertainties as to the derivation of particular tumours from particular ovarian tissues, (3) practical difficulties in some cases of distinguishing growths of ovarian origin from those of parovarian or tubal origin, and (4) the frequent mistaking of secondary for primary growths in the ovaries.

In his chapter on tumors of the testis, Willis encountered a similar veil of confusion.

Critical review of the literature reveals that with the passage of time a particular concept may attain popularity and may become so widely accepted that it is mistaken for fact. This circumstance has the desirable effect of inhibiting the formulation of further misleading hypotheses but at the price of sometimes suppressing the truth when it finally threatens to emerge. Much as in the area of malignant lymphomas, whenever many minds devote themselves to extensive studies of a particular group of neoplasms, differences of opinion develop and find expression in the form of diverse classifications varying in concept, nomenclature, and biologic relevance (see Chapter 4; Taylor 1980a, 1982b). Within the study of testicular and ovarian neoplasms, these difficulties are compounded by the lack of a firm scientific basis for the recognition and distinction of individual normal cells as well as their neoplastic counterparts.

It is often forgotten that normally proliferating cells of different cell lines may appear remarkably similar; tumors composed of a high proportion of proliferating cells may appear similar on this basis alone. Often pathologists distinguish such tumors not by the majority components, for these are quite similar, but by a minority population displaying some degree of differentiation along one or another cell line. In the final analysis, such distinctions, based as they are on subtle, subjective morphologic judgments, may be very difficult to make. To state the matter bluntly, the recognition and classification of many of the tumors of the ovary and testis depend solely upon morphologic interpretation; such interpretation is a matter of opinion, and opinions often differ.

Classification of Ovarian and Testicular Tumors

The basic classifications of ovarian and testicular neoplasms used within this chapter have been adopted on the basis of convenience and popularity.

The adoption of these classifications is not intended to convery support for their scientific rectitude or any preference for these schemata over those championed by other investigators (Taylor and Warner, 1982). The classification of testicular neoplasms (Table 9–1) is based on that used by Mostofi and Price (1973) in the Armed Forces Institute of Pathology (AFIP) *Atlas.* This in turn was founded upon the conceptual view advanced by Friedman and Moore that embryonal carcinomas, teratomas, and choriocarcinomas all originate from the pluripotent germ cells. Approximately 93 percent of the AFIP cases can then be considered to be of germ cell origin.

In Britain a somewhat different system applies: the British Testicular Tumour Panel (BTTP) classifies germ cell tumors as follows:
1. Seminoma
2. Malignant teratoma
   a. Differentiated
   b. Intermediate
   c. Undifferentiated
   d. Trophoblastic
and recognizes overlap between these groups.

Table 9–1. Classification of Testicular Neoplasms*

1. Germ cell tumors
   a. Single histologic type
      Seminoma
      Embryonal carcinoma
      Choriocarcinoma
      Teratoma
   b. More than one histologic type
      Any combination of types within *a.*
2. Gonadal stromal tumors
   Undifferentiated
   Leydig cell
   Serotoli (granulosa-theca) cell
   Combinations of these
3. Mixed germ cell and gonadal stromal tumors
4. Metastatic and other

*Modified from Mostofi and Price, 1973.

Table 9–2. Classification of Ovarian Neoplasms*

1. Germ cell tumors
   Dysgerminoma (seminomalike)
   (Embryonal carcinoma)†
   Choriocarcinoma
   Teratoma
   Endodermal sinus (yolk sac) tumor
   (Mixture of the above)†
2. Gonadal stromal tumors
   (Undifferentiated)†
   Sertoli-Leydig cell (androblastoma)
   Granulosa-theca cell
3. Mixed germ cell and gonadal stromal tumors
4. Tumors of ovarian surface epithelium
   Serous cystadenoma and carcinoma
   Mucinous cystadenoma and carcinoma
   Endometrioid carcinoma
   Undifferentiated carcinoma
5. Metastatic and other

*Modified from WHO–Sero et al, 1973.
†Parenthetical entries are relatively rare; they are included to maintain parallel with Table 9–1.

The simplified classification given for ovarian neoplasms (Table 9–2) is based upon the 1973 World Health Organization recommendations (Sero et al, 1973), somewhat condensed for the purposes of this discussion.

Clearly, many parallels exist between tumors of the ovary and tumors of the testis, as might be expected considering that the cellular composition of these two organs is identical in embryologic terms and differs only to the extent that the cells are subject to differing hormonal environments during embryologic differentiation and subsequent maturation.

It will be shown that immunohistologic techniques have given new insight into the origins and interrelationships of these tumors.

Immunostains for Ovary and Testis

Many antibodies are available, and some have been assembled in kit form. The latter are listed in Table 9–3; others, more experimental in nature, are described in the text.

The advantages of kits containing pretitered matched reagents plus all of the necessary substrate-chromogen systems may be considerable in terms of routine laboratory practice: they avoid the need for separate purchase, titration, and integration of a series of different reagents, but they may be more expensive, depending upon the degree of use. Those who prefer not to use the com-

Table 9–3. Commercially Available "Immunostains"*,†

Primary Tumors
    Human chorionic gonadotropin
    Pregnancy-specific beta$_1$-glycoprotein
    Human placental lactogen
    Estradiol
    Testosterone
    alpha-Fetoprotein
    Carcinoembryonic antigen

Metastases
    Prostate-specific antigen
    Acid phosphatase

*Modified from Taylor and Warner, 1982.
†Kits listed pertain particularly to the study of ovary and testis; as described elsewhere, more than 30 different immunostains are available for other purposes. Kits are available from Ortho (Immulok). Dako, Miles, Biomeda, BioGenex, Immunonucleonics Spectrum, etc., have also made available equivalent ranges of kits.

mercially available kits can purchase individual reagents from a wide variety of commercial sources or can prepare their own reagents, subject, of course, to the necessity for strict specificity controls. Even with the use of commercial kits, the pathologist should introduce specificity controls in the form of tissue sections known to contain the antigen in question (positive control), or known to lack it (negative control). The pattern and intensity of staining observed in the test section may then be judged against the pattern and intensity of staining observed in the positive and negative controls. Sections of normal ovary and testis processed in a manner identical to the test section, whether frozen or paraffin, provide excellent controls for staining with anti–steroid hormone antibodies. The distribution of positive staining in such sections serves as both intrinsic positive and negative controls (eg, antitestosterone—Leydig's cells positive; tubules, vessels, and the like—negative). Positive reactivity in the anticipated pattern confirms that the processing employed (including fixation and paraffin embedment) has not destroyed the antigen in question and demonstrates that the antibody gives a pattern of staining commensurate with the supposed specificity.

For the staining of paraffin sections, the procedure employed is basically as given in detail in Chapter 2. Direct and indirect conjugate methods have been employed; these have the advantage of simplicity but are considered by many to be less sensitive, thereby requiring the use of precious specific primary antibodies at higher concentrations. The PAP and biotin-avidin methods are therefore more widely utilized for the demonstration of steroid hormones.

If the tissue under study contains large amounts of "endogenous peroxidase" activity, it should be inactivated by pretreatment of the sections in 0.3% hydrogen peroxide in methanol for 20 minutes, otherwise the reaction of the endogenous peroxides with the chromogen may mask the sites of localization of the horseradish peroxidase label. Nonspecific binding of the reagents (antibodies) to charged components within tissue sections may also cause problems in interpretation but may be successfully combatted by pretreatment of sections with diluted serum of the bridge antibody species (Taylor, 1978b; see Chapters 2 and 3).

The chromogen most commonly used has been diaminobenzidine, with a hydrogen peroxide substrate. This produces a crisp, brown, reaction product that is alcohol-fast and will not be leached out during dehydration steps preparatory to mounting the section in a permanent mounting medium. The commercial kits include amino-ethyl carbazole (AEC) as the chromogen, for this is a noncarcinogen. The disadvantage of AEC is that it is alcohol-soluble, necessitating use of a water-miscible mounting medium.

The use of frozen sections has theoretical advantages in terms of avoiding the adverse effects of fixation and organic solvents (that might be expected to remove all lipid-soluble substances, including steroid hormones). In utilizing frozen sections, care should be taken to avoid fixation that damages or removes steroid molecules (eg, acetone). Paradoxically, fixation with formalin appears to stabilize at least some part of the steroid hormones in a manner that renders the molecules still accessible for detection by specific antisera.

Table 9–4 lists the principal types of testicular and ovarian neoplasms and the various immunostains that can be employed to assist in their discrimination from one another. It must be emphasized that in devising immunohistologic staining methods applicable to the testis and ovary the pathologist is not casting aside morphologic criteria but rather is taking advantage of the remarkable specific staining offered by immunologic techniques in order to validate, refine, and redefine if necessary the morphologic criteria upon which diagnosis is traditionally based.

Table 9–4. Immunostains of Ovarian and Testicular Neoplasms*

Tumor Category	hCG	SP1	AFP	Estradiol	Testosterone	Progesterone	CEA	Breast Antigens[1]	Other
Seminoma	(+)[2]			(+)[3]	(+)[3]				
Embryonal carcinoma	+ +	(+)[9]	+						
Choriocarcinoma	+ + +	+ +							
Teratoma									
With yolk sac differentiation			+ +						
With trophoblastic differentiation	+ + +	+ +							
With other secretory differentiation[4]							(+)[4]	(+)	+[4]
Endodermal sinus (yolk sac)	+	+	+ + +						
Leydig cell				+	+ + +	+			
Sertoli				+[3]	+	+			
Androblastoma (Sertoli-Leydig)				+[3]	+	+			
Granulosa-theca:									
Granulosa				+ +	+	+			
Luteinized theca				+ +	+	+ +			
Undifferentiated gonadal stromal				+ +	+ +	+			
Mucinous cystadenocarcinoma							+	+	
Metastatic and direct spread									
Colon (GI tract)							+ + +		
Breast	+[5]	+[5]		+[2,6]		+[3]		+ +	
Other	+[5]	+[5]	+[7]		(+)[6]				(+)[8]

*Modified from Taylor and Warner, 1982.

[1]Breast-associated antigens include "T antigen," mammary epithelial membrane antigen, and a variety of other antigens identifiable by use of monoclonal antibodies.

[2]Semiquantitative scoring, + to + + +; not every case, nor every cell of positive cases, will be positive. Parenthetical entries may or may not show positivity.

[3]Positivity of some cell elements, such as Sertoli's cells or even breast epithelial cells, for estradiol or other steroid hormones may reflect receptor binding of the hormone rather than intrinsic production.

[4]Rare teratomas containing "thyroid" elements will show immunostaining for thyroglobulin; teratomas with "gastrointestinal"-type epithelium may give a reaction for CEA; other epithelial elements may show other staining patterns according to product.

[5]Nontrophoblastic tumors sometimes contain hCG or SP1 (eg, carcinoma of breast) for reasons unknown.

[6]Nonovarian/testicular tumors may show positivity, presumably also owing to "receptor binding of steroid hormone;" breast tumor particularly is often positive for estradiol (Taylor et al, 1981); prostate tumor is sometimes positive for testosterone.

[7]Primary hepatocellular carcinomas typically stain strongly for AFP.

[8]Hormonally active tumors of many types may produce secondary deposits in the ovaries and, rarely, in the testes; immunostains are available against many of the hormones, and for many other cell products (Taylor and Kledzik, 1981). Other antigens detected include HbF, human placental lactogen, ferritin, alpha$_1$-antitrypsin, and keratin (see Tables 9–5 and 9–6 and also Chapter 14).

[9]Keratin is present in embryonal carcinomas, but absent in seminomas.

Observed Patterns of Staining: Germ Cell Tumors of Ovary and Testis

Note that the patterns described in the following paragraphs appear to also hold true for germ cell tumors occurring in extragonadal sites (Bjornsson et al, 1985—70 cranial tumors).

The Seminoma-Dysgerminoma Group

These tumors represent the most commonly encountered malignant tumors of germ cell origin. So-called pure examples of this group of tumors do not show staining either for human chorionic gonadotropin (hCG) or for alpha-fetoprotein (AFP), either in the majority of the tumor cells or in the associated tumor giant cells that may be present (Kurman and Scardino, 1981). However, some cases show the presence of large multinucleated giant cells that do give positive immunostaining for hCG (Fig. 9–1), but not for AFP; these cells are thought to represent isolated examples of syncytiotrophoblastic differentiation within a tumor that otherwise is pure seminoma (Table 9–5). Kurman and Scardino point out that prior to immunohistologic staining these cells had often been termed pseudotrophoblasts, and their relationship to functional, true syncytiotrophoblastic elements had not been appreciated. According to some investigators, hCG-positive cases have a worse prognosis (Roth et al, 1983; Morgan et al, 1982).

Seminomas may also show the presence of a minority of cells giving low-intensity staining reactions with anti-estradiol and anti-testosterone antisera, most likely representing the presence of the steroid hormone bound in vivo by active receptors or binding globulins. Two potentially useful seminoma markers exist. GK Jacobsen et al (1981) reported that most pure seminomas (14/16) are positive for antisera against ferritin (but are negative for AFP, hCG, alpha$_1$-antitrypsin, and carcinoembryonic antigen [CEA]). Cohen and colleagues (1984) describe all cases as ferritin-positive.

Also, placental alkaline phosphatase has been reported as present in more than 90 percent of seminomas, compared with 60 percent of other testicular tumors (Jacobsen GK and Nørgaard-Pedersen, 1984), with the use of monoclonal antibodies. Epenetos et al (1984) came up with somewhat different figures: one monoclonal antibody to placental alkaline phosphatase (H17E2) gave positivity in all seminomas and malignant teratomas; all other tumors with rare exceptions were nonreactive (exceptions included rare cases of ovarian, endometrial, and colonic cancers). The work of Sunderland et al (1984) is somewhat contradictory: with a different monoclonal antibody to placental alkaline phosphatase, these workers observed positivity in normal bronchus, fallopian tube, and thymus; no reactivity in normal testis, but positivity in most ovarian carcinomas (9/13 cystadenocarcinomas).

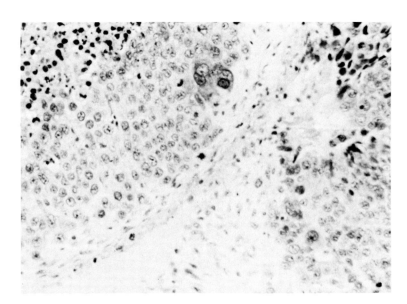

Figure 9–1. Germ cell tumor (seminoma) with rare hCG-positive giant cells not appreciated in H&E section. Paraffin section, AEC with hematoxylin counterstain (×200).

Table 9–5. Selected Bibliography: Testicular Tumors—AFP, hCG, SP1, Ferritin, and Alpha$_1$-Antitrypsin*

Alm et al 1984	Correlation of serum levels of hCG and AFP with staining of tumor sections—11 cases
Javadpour 1980b	Pregnancy-specific beta-1-glycoprotein in germ cell tumors; serum levels elevated in about 13 of 97 cases
Caillaud & Bellett 1981	90% of embryonic carcinomas positive for AFP or hCG; a small percentage of seminomas also positive for hCG (trophoblastic elements present)—study of 80 cases
Furumoto 1981	AFP, hCG, and SP1 (pregnancy-specific glycoprotein)—10 cases
Wittekind et al 1983	67 cases; distribution of AFP and hCG
Roth et al 1983	hCG and AFP in 32 nonseminomatous germ cell tumors; particularly noted hCG in mononuclear cells implied bad prognosis ("cryptocellular trophoblastic carcinoma")
Bosman et al 1980b	73 cases; stained for hCG and AFP; among embryonal carcinomas 83% positive for hCG, 75% for AFP
Javadpour et al 1980	AFP, hCG, and SP1 in 26 cases of germ cell tumors, 60% positive
Szymendera et al 1981	AFP, hCG, SP1, hPL (placental lactogen), and CEA; tumors could produce one or more (up to 5) markers
Shimatani et al 1980	AFP, hCG, SP1; distribution/significance
Jacobsen et al 1981	39 germ cell tumors; embryonal carcinoma positive for AFP in 9/16, for alpha$_1$-antitrypsin in 6/16, for ferritin in 14/16, and for CEA in 2/16; yolk sac tumors positive for AFP, alpha$_1$-antitrypsin, and ferritin in almost all cases and rarely for CEA; epithelium in teratomas showed variety of patterns
Jacobsen & Jacobsen 1983a	AFP and ferritin reactivity serves as evidence of "liver cell differentiation" in germ cell tumors; positive staining for albumin, prealbumin, transferrin, alpha$_1$-antitrypsin and hemoglobin F often also present in AFP-reactive cases (yolk sac differentiation)
Jacobsen & Jacobsen 1983b	Hemoglobin F in yolk sac tumors (common) and in embryonal carcinomas; yolk sac components appear to mimic fetal liver in this respect; elevated HbF levels in such patients may originate from tumor
Morinaga et al 1983	AFP and hCG both positive in the same tumors, but in separate cells
Cohen et al 1984	Positive ferritin reactivity in all seminomas, most staining intensely (used antisera against liver ferritin and myocardial ferritin; staining slightly higher with the former)
Morgan et al 1982	hCG-positive seminomas have a worse prognosis, compared with "typical" cases
Albrechtsen et al 1980	Hemoglobins A and F in normal yolk sac and endodermal sinus tumors
Engvall et al 1982	Monoclonals to SP1—effective in fixed tissues
Saigo et al 1981	Gastric choriocarcinoma (2 cases)—ectopic hCG
Mori H et al 1982	Adenocarcinomas of stomach with morphologic transition to hCG-positive choriocarcinoma (2 cases)
Bellett et al 1980	beta-hCG in nongonadal tumors (breast)
Wilson et al 1981	hCG in paraffin sections of lung tumors; 51/61 positive to some degree, especially large cell carcinomas
Inaba et al 1980	Production of SP1 (and other trophoblastic products, eg, PP5); common in nontrophoblastic malignancies (eg, SP1 positive in 50% of breast cancer and 40% of gastric cancer, although often only to minor extent)
Morgan et al 1982	hCG-containing seminomas have a worse prognosis
Caillaud et al 1979	beta-hCG in testicular tumors

*Reports relate principally to the testis; some ovarian tumors are included (see also Table 9–6).

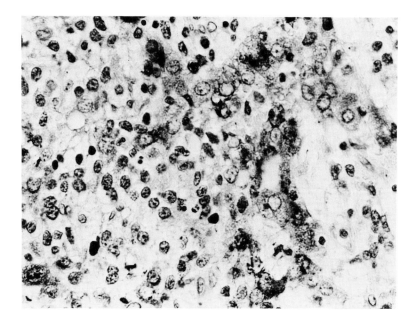

Figure 9–2. Germ cell tumor (embryonal carcinoma) with occasional areas of "yolk sac" differentiation, here stained for AFP, giving positive gray-black granules in the cytoplasm of "yolk sac" elements. Paraffin section, DAB with hematoxylin counterstain (×320). Morphologically these "yolk sac" areas were not recognized prior to immunostaining.

Embryonal Carcinomas

These tumors frequently contain syncytiotrophoblastic elements, emphasizing the close biologic relationship of germ cell–derived neoplasms. The embryonal carcinoma cells per se typically do not stain for hCG. However, syncytiotrophoblastic elements commonly present within these tumors do show a strong positive reaction. On the other hand, AFP staining is never observed within the syncytiotrophoblastic elements but may often be seen within an apparently pure embryonal carcinoma (Fig. 9–2), which apparently has functional differentiation even in the absence of histologic yolk sac differentiation (Kurman and Scardino, 1981). In different studies, 60 to 80 percent of embryonal carcinomas have been described as showing reactivity with hCG, AFP, or alpha$_1$-antitrypsin. Ferritin is detectable in almost all cases, and CEA rarely is present (Table 9–5). One useful feature is that embryonal carcinomas contain cytokeratin, but pure seminomas do not. With all antibodies the proportion of positive cells may be small, and positive cells may be widely scattered.

Choriocarcinomas

Choriocarcinomas, representing a malignant counterpart of the trophoblast, typically produce large amounts of hCG, and varying proportions of the tumor cells stain strongly with anti-hCG sera (Figs. 9–3 and 9–4). The normal trophoblast also produces pregnancy-specific beta$_1$-glycoprotein (SP1); choriocarcinoma also typically mimics this production. It should be emphasized that although the pattern of staining of choriocarcinomas for both hCG and SP1 is striking and characteristic of choriocarcinoma, the mere presence of staining with either of these antisera does not of itself define the tumor as of trophoblastic origin. For example, in addition to positivity in some seminomas, as many as 50 percent of cases of breast carcinoma have been observed to stain for hCG or for SP1 (Horne et al, 1976) or for both, and hCG

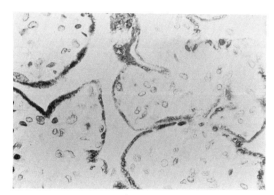

Figure 9–3. "Positive" control for hCG: normal placenta stained for hCG; positive staining (redbrown-black) is observed in the trophoblast. The villous stromal cells are nonreactive, affirming the specificity of the stain. Paraffin section, AEC with hematoxylin counterstain (×200). See color plate II-3.

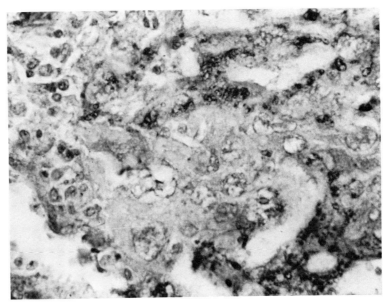

Figure 9–4. Bizarre anaplastic large cell tumor showing granular (black) reactivity with anti-hCG antibody. Positivity appears in individual small cells and in "syncytial" giant cells. Paraffin section, DAB with hematoxylin counterstain (×320). Serum hCG level subsequently became elevated; diagnosis choriocarcinoma.

staining has been reported less often in other tumors. A combination of trophoblastic giant cells and hCG (or SP1) positivity is highly suggestive of choriocarcinoma. The potential availability of monoclonal antibodies to cytotrophoblast (eg, Loke and Day, 1984) may provide an alternative means of recognition for trophoblastic tissue and tumors.

Teratomas

These neoplasms do not show positive staining for either hCG or AFP unless there is differentiation either toward trophoblastic elements or yolk sac elements (Jacobsen et al, 1981) within the teratoma. In such instances, the differentiated elements show the pattern of staining typical of trophoblast (Fig. 9–5) or yolk sac respectively. It should be remembered that teratomas may occasionally produce functional epithelial and glandular elements and that these may be stained for the appropriate cell product (eg, thyroglobulin within teratomatous thyroid (Fig. 9–6) or CEA within teratomatous gastrointestinal type epithelium).

GFAP has been described within glial elements of teratomas (Haugen and Taylor,

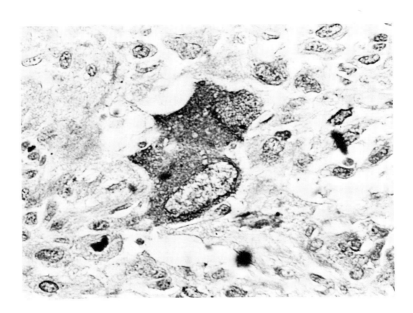

Figure 9–5. Germ cell tumor: malignant area within teratoma; giant cells show positivity for beta-hCG. Paraffin section, DAB with hematoxylin counterstain (×500).

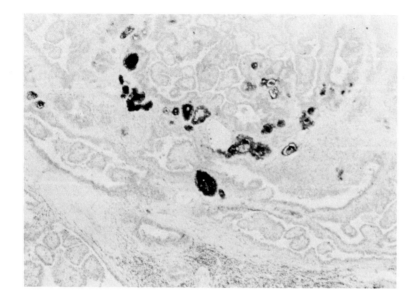

Figure 9–6. Papillary tumor within an ovarian teratoma showing focal, but definite, staining for thyroglobulin. There was no notable clinical effect of hypersecretion in this patient. Paraffin section, AEC with hematoxylin counterstain (×125).

1984) and AFP; alpha$_1$-antitrypsin, lysozyme, and so forth, within a variety of other differentiated elements (eg, Paneth's cells—lysozyme positive—Shousha and Miller, 1984). Finally, the presence of many of the cells of the APUD series, producing various "intestinal" polypeptide hormones (Bosman and Louwerens, 1981) or pituitary hormones (Fenoglio et al, 1982b), has been reported.

Endodermal Sinus (Yolk Sac) Tumors

These tumors show a typical pattern of staining regardless of the fine histologic subtypes. It is important to recognize that positivity for AFP may be distributed throughout the tumor or may occur only focally. Typically, morphologic elements in the tumor that

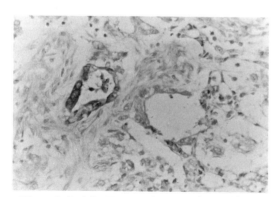

Figure 9–7. alpha-Fetoprotein (AFP) (brown-black cytoplasmic staining) in a yolk sac carcinoma. Paraffin section, DAB with hematoxylin counterstain (×200). See color plate II–4.

resemble yolk sacs show intense positive staining (Fig. 9–7). However, in other areas of the tumor or in other tumors that show no evidence of morphologic yolk sac differentiation, it usually is possible to demonstrate variable amounts of staining for AFP. Histologically, it has been shown that AFP staining correlates with intracellular and extracellular hyaline eosinophilic globules identifiable in routine H&E sections; however, immunostaining for AFP is a much more sensitive procedure. Many examples of tumors showing yolk sac differentiation will also stain for other liver cell products, such as transferrin, ferritin, and alpha$_1$-antitrypsin (Fig. 9–8). Positive immunoreactivity for hemoglobin F has also been described (Tables 9–5 and 9–6).

Positive staining for AFP can be used to identify an endodermal sinus, or yolk sac, tumor even when there is little evidence of morphologic yolk sac differentiation. Tumor yolk sac components appear functionally to mimic fetal liver (Jacobsen and Jacobsen, 1983b).

Steroid Hormones: Observed Patterns of Staining

Gonadal Stromal Cell Tumors

Immunostaining for the different steroid hormones has shed light upon the histogenesis and the histologic differentiation of hormonally active tumors within the ovary and testis. Previously, the nomenclature and clas-

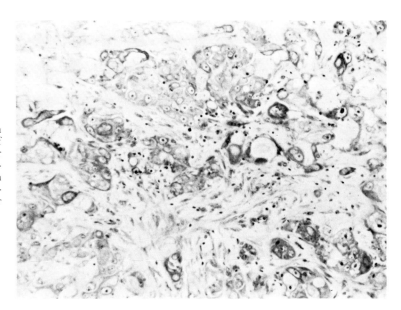

Figure 9–8. Yolk sac carcinoma showing staining of cytoplasm of majority of cells (gray-black) for alpha$_1$-antitrypsin. Paraffin section, AEC with hematoxylin counterstain (×125). Anti–alpha-fetoprotein antibody gave a similar pattern.

sification of these tumors have largely been dependent upon morphologic features coupled with clinical status and evidence of endocrine manifestations (Kurman et al, 1978, 1979, 1981a; Taylor et al, 1978a). The fact that these neoplasms often present variable patterns of hormone production and that the tumors themselves may display diverse histologic patterns has led to considerable difficulties in developing a consistent working hypothesis relating individual cell types to the production of particular hormones. The feasibility of preparing antisera against the different steroid hormones and of applying these antisera to the demonstration of these hormones in formalin-paraffin sections, as well as in frozen sections, promises to shed new light on this controversy.

Immunohistologic techniques have proved remarkably successful with some reservations, discussed in this paragraph. In general terms, staining for a particular steroid hormone within the cell cytoplasm is interpreted as evidence of intracellular synthesis, although the possibility of binding to various intracellular binding proteins or receptors is a real one. It has, for example, been recognized that Sertoli's cells contain receptors for various androgens, whereas granulosa cells apparently contain estrogen-binding proteins (Christensen et al, 1977; Schreiber et al, 1976). In addition, when using antisera to steroid hormones, one must be aware of the possibility of cross reactivity between the different antisera. In practical terms, this eventually can be controlled to some degree by

assessing the specificity of the antisera, one against another, in radioimmunoassay systems. With regard to immunohistologic studies, it is important also to include biologic controls, for example, in the intense staining of normal interstitial Leydig cells in testis with anti-testosterone serum (Fig. 9–9) and in the lesser degree of staining or absence of staining with anti-estradiol serum. Another potential problem is that in order to generate antisera against the steroid hormones, the hormones are first linked to some sort of carrier molecule. Bovine serum albumin (BSA) has often been used for this purpose; the resulting antiserum thus contains antibodies against the steroid moiety and also against the bovine serum albumin. These anti-albumin antibodies show varying degrees of cross reactivity with human albumin and can produce immunohistologic staining that may be confused with specific staining for anti-estradiol. For these reasons, antisera that are to be used for immunohistologic studies must, if coupled with BSA, be extensively absorbed with human albumin. A better course is to link the steroid hormone with keyhole-limpet hemocyanin (KLH) as a carrier, thus avoiding this particular form of cross reactivity.

The different patterns of staining anticipated among gonadal stromal tumors are illustrated in Table 9–4. Since the first clear recognition of this application of immunohistologic methods, more than 80 cases have been described in the literature (according to Okoye et al, 1985).

Table 9–6. Selected Bibliography: Ovarian Tumors—AFP, hCG, CEA, "Carcinoma" Antigens

Kurman 1984	Excellent review
Kramer et al 1984	14 children with yolk sac carcinoma; AFP, alpha$_1$-antitrypsin not of prognostic significance
Dictor 1982	Mixed mesodermal tumors of ovary; contain hyaline droplets that are negative for AFP, but positive for alpha$_1$-antitrypsin
Wagener et al 1981b	20 germ cell tumors stained for AFP: positive in embryonal carcinoma (9/16) and teratoma (2/7); positive in all tumors with morphologic yolk sac differentiation and in some "pure" embryonal cancers without morphologically recognizable yolk sac elements
Wilke & Harms 1979	160 tumors examined for AFP: positive in 5/6 endodermal sinus tumors, 19/40 teratomas, and 9/16 hepatomas; among various sarcomas all were negative except 1/15 rhabdomyosarcomas
Nørgaard-Pedersen et al 1979	AFP in childhood vaginal embryonal carcinoma (1 case)
Beilby et al 1979	AFP, alpha$_1$-antitrypsin and transferrin in 16 yolk sac tumors; absent in other tumors, except for transferrin positivity in an oat cell carcinoma
Takeda et al 1982	AFP and hCG in "embryoid" bodies of a polyembryoma (resembled normal 15-day embryo)
Hayata et al 1981	100 gynecologic tumors: 10% positive for hCG, 5% for CEA
Mohabeer et al 1983	hCG in 42% of ovarian cancers; no relation to prognosis
Kaplan & Hawley 1981	Case report: typical hCG-positive dysgerminoma; AFP, hCG in embryonal carcinomas and teratomas; CEA absent in embryonal carcinomas but sometimes present in teratomas
Obata et al 1980	AFP, hCG in embryonal carcinomas and teratomas; CEA absent in embryonal carcinomas but sometimes present in teratomas
Fenoglio et al 1981	CEA positive in most epithelial malignancies of ovary
Fenoglio et al 1982a	Good review of hCG reactivity in female genital tract lesions (456 patients): positive in germ cell tumors, 10% of ovarian carcinomas, and up to 20% of endometrial and cervical cancer; overall, less than 10% CEA-positive endometrial cancers and invasive cervical cancers
Fenoglio et al 1982b	Teratoma containing pituitary elements
Wahlström et al 1981a	Monoclonal antibody versus hCG: trophoblast positive, pituitary negative
Wahlström et al 1983	LH, FSH, and PRL receptors in human and rat testis; possible precedent for tests in human disease
Ettinger et al 1980	Histaminase in ovarian carcinomas
Ganjei et al 1983	Prekeratin in Brenner's tumor; other ovarian epithelial tumors were negative
Dietel 1983	CEA; benign and "borderline" lesions
Heald et al 1979	CEA of some value in separating benign and malignant lesions in ovary; mucinous tumors positive more often than serous tumors
Charpin et al 1982b	CEA positive in 60% of mucinous tumors (100% of carcinoma, 15% of benign neoplasms) but absent in serous tumors; 50% of mixed mesodermal tumors CEA-positive, plus 30% of endometrioid carcinomas, 14% of clear cell tumors, and 36% of Brenner's tumors; note that of colonic metastases to ovary more than 80% were CEA positive
Casper et al 1984	CEA in mucinous, endometrioid, and clear cell carcinomas; hPL (placental lactogen) present in endometrioid carcinoma only; AFP and hCG, in less than 10% of ovarian carcinomas
Bhattacharya et al 1984	GP48 human cancer antigen (monoclonal antibody) in ovarian cancer; also detected in some normal tissues (preliminary)
Negishi et al 1984	An absorbed antiserum with specificity for mucinous adenocarcinoma (preliminary)

Table 9–6. Selected Bibliography: Ovarian Tumors—AFP, hCG, CEA, "Carcinoma" Antigens *Continued*

Berkowitz et al 1985	Murine embryonic antigen (stage-specific) in trophoblastic tumors
Ma et al 1983	Ovarian mucin antigen (some resemblance to intestinal mucins)
Croghan et al 1984	Monoclonal antibody F36/22 recognizes 100% of ovarian carcinomas (30%–100% of cells positive) and only about 10% of benign lesions; mesothelial cells nonreactive; 12/12 ovarian metastases positive
Kabawat et al 1983	OC125 monoclonal antibody (anticelomic) reacts with Müllerian duct derivatives (fallopian tubes, endometrium, cervix) and mesothelial cells, plus corresponding tumors; more than 90% of other tumors nonreactive
Ferguson & Fox 1984a	Ca antigen of no discriminatory value for benign versus malignant lesions of ovary
De Ikonicoff 1979	hCG(-like) positivity in X cells of basal plate of full-term placenta
Knapp et al 1982 Sandhaus et al 1981	Primary embryonal carcinomas of mediastinum; giant cells hCG positive
Mirecka 1980	Review of immunohistologic localization of sex hormones
Crum & Fenoglio 1980	Review: demonstration of hormones, oncofetal antigens, enzymes, and viral antigens
Farley et al 1982	Estrogen immunostaining correlated with DCC receptor assay in endometrial and cervical cancer
Maurer et al 1980	Steroid hormones in extratesticular gonadal stromal cell tumor
Kurman et al 1979	Estrogen, progesterone, and testosterone in granulosa-theca cell tumors of ovary
Meuris et al 1980	Prolactinlike reactivity in decidual cells within endometrium
Lee JN et al 1981	Prolactin in trophoblastic tumors
Seppälä et al 1980	Presence of luteinizing hormone–releasing factor immunoreactivity in trophoblast and in trophoblastic tumors
Fields & Larkin 1981	Antirelaxin antibody stains cells in placental basal plate
Lojek et al 1980	ACTH immunoreactivity in small cell carcinoma of cervix
Kierszenbaum et al 1980	Immunostaining of an androgen-binding protein in Sertoli's cells
Valdiserri & Yunis 1981	68 sacral teratomas: 13% malignant, and all of these AFP-positive endodermal sinus tumor type
Irie et al 1982	Case report; mediastinal teratocarcinoma positive for AFP, CEA, and hCG
Pileri et al 1980a	Case report, endometrial endodermal sinus tumor
Nakagawa et al 1980	AFP-positive "endodermal sinus tumor" in IV ventricle
Heyderman et al 1981	Human placental lactogen is positive in giant cells of "syncytial endometritis" and is thus a marker of the trophoblastic origin of these cells and an indicator of an associated pregnancy
Whyte & Loke 1979	Heterologous antiserum with specificity for surface of trophoblast
Sunderland et al 1981	Monoclonal antibodies to surface of trophoblast (distinct from PAPP-A, SP1, hCG, lactogen, and alkaline phosphatase)
Searle et al 1981	Heteroantisera detecting different trophoblast-specific surface antigens
Saksela et al 1981	alpha$_2$-Macroglobulin in normal, but not in malignant, trophoblasts
Wahlström et al 1981b	PAPP-A (placenta-associated plasma protein-A) in formalin-paraffin sections; positive in all hydatidiform moles and 6/7 choriocarcinomas
Yamasaki et al 1981	Staining for hCG in paraffin sections of 52 squamous cell carcinomas of cervix; did not correlate with histology
Azer et al 1980	SP1 production by an ovarian cystadenocarcinoma (also hCG-positive)

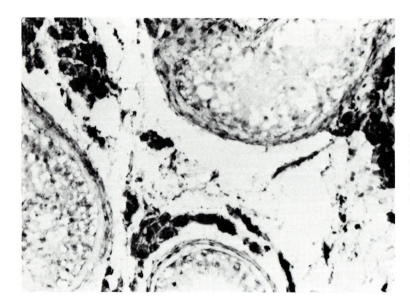

Figure 9–9. Testis with interstitial (Leydig) cells. Paraffin section, DAB with hematoxylin counterstain (×125). This tissue serves as an excellent "positive" control for the testosterone stain. Leydig cells appear black.

Leydig Cell Tumors and Sertoli-Leydig Cell Tumors (Androblastomas)

Characteristically, these tumors show intense staining for testosterone in the recognizable Leydig cell elements (Fig. 9–10). Leydig's cells may also show positive staining with antiserum to estradiol and less often with antiserum to progesterone. Occasionally, the recognizable Sertoli's cells, forming more or less well-organized tubules, also show staining for testosterone, estradiol, or both (Fig. 9–11).

Granulosa-Theca Cell Tumors

Quite commonly, these tumors are associated with clinical manifestations of hormone production. Classically, estrogen synthesis has been considered to be confined to theca cells, and the luteinized granulosa cells have been held responsible for progesterone production. These rigid definitions of cell type correlated to hormone production do not appear to hold true according to the evidence of immunoperoxidase staining. Granulosa cells have been observed to show positive

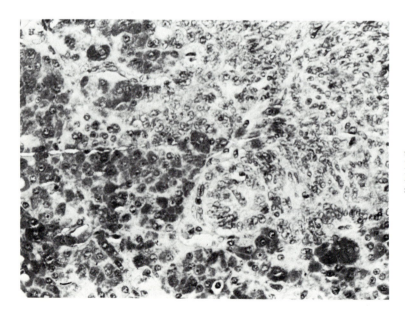

Figure 9–10. Large sheets of testosterone-positive cells in a Sertoli-Leydig cell tumor. Paraffin section, DAB with hematoxylin counterstain (×125).

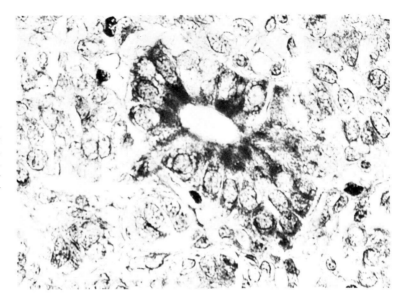

Figure 9–11. Positive cytoplasmic staining for testosterone in the cytoplasm of well-formed Sertoli's cells in a differentiated Sertoli-Leydig cell tumor. Paraffin section, DAB with hematoxylin counterstain (×320).

staining not only for estradiol, but also for progesterone and even for testosterone (Fig. 9–12). Similarly, luteinized theca cells may contain demonstrable progesterone but also may show staining for estradiol or testosterone.

These findings challenge the time-honored concept that individual morphologic cell types are responsible for, and restricted to, the production of single hormones: theca cells for estrogen, luteinized granulosa cells for progesterone, and Leydig's cells for testosterone. Immunoperoxidase studies suggest that the neoplastic counterparts of these cells certainly do not recognize these restric-

tions; there is increasing evidence that normal cells also break the accepted rules (Kurman et al, 1981a). In this respect, pathologists should be cautious in using observed positivity for testosterone or estrogen as evidence for the gonadal stromal cell origin of tumors elsewhere in the body, since it appears that testosterone positivity (reaction with antitestosterone antibodies) may be observed in other tumor types (eg, hepatoma—Wong LY et al, 1984), possibly due to absorption of testosterone by a specific receptor. This also, of course, occurs for estrogen in receptor-positive breast carcinomas.

Clearly, immunoperoxidase staining for

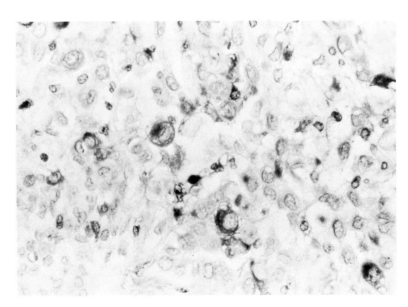

Figure 9–12. Granulosa theca cell tumor showing cytoplasmic staining for progesterone in a small proportion of cells (gray-black cytoplasm). Paraffin section, DAB with hematoxylin counterstain (×320).

these specific steroid hormones may be of diagnostic value but may also be expected to contribute to our understanding of the biology of these neoplasms. Such studies can be performed upon tissue biopsies in order to gain a more realistic assessment of the potential hormonal manifestations of individual tumors in individual patients, for it is clear that morphology alone is not a reliable indicator of the type of hormone produced by any individual morphologic type of neoplasm.

Undifferentiated Gonadal Stromal Cell Tumors

There has been another finding of real interest, namely the use of immunostaining in the recognition and differential diagnosis of undifferentiated gonadal stromal tumors. Morphologically, such tumors consist of highly undifferentiated "primitive"-appearing cells, reflecting the high proportion of cells in the S (synthesis) phase of cell cycle (see Chapter 14, Fig. 14–15). These neoplasms bear a close resemblance to other undifferentiated neoplasms that may be encountered in ovary and testis and, in our experience, have often been misdiagnosed as reticulum cell sarcoma (histiocytic lymphoma, including, in more modern terminology, immunoblastic sarcoma) of the testis. The staining of such tumors for steroid hormones—specifically, the demonstration of testosterone, estradiol, or both in the cyto-

plasm of the neoplastic cells—provides support for the diagnosis of a gonadal stromal neoplasm (Fig. 9–13) (Maurer et al, 1980).

Ovarian Carcinomas: Primary and Metastatic

There are two principal problems related to the histologic recognition of ovarian cancer: (1) the distinction of cancer from benign and borderline lesions, with assessment of the degree of malignancy and (2) the distinction of obvious carcinoma primary to ovary from metastases.

Staining for CEA has been advocated as of possible value in both respects. Certainly CEA staining (other than in scattered cells in cystadenomas or rare cells in differentiated teratomas) is rare in benign ovarian tumors and may be frequent and conspicuous in malignant tumors (Table 9–6; Fig. 9–14). For example, Charpin and colleagues (1982b) reported CEA positivity in 14 percent of clear cell carcinomas, 30 percent of endometrioid carcinomas, 36 percent of Brenner tumors, and 100 percent of mucinous carcinomas; by contrast only 15 percent of benign mucinous cystadenomas showed any positivity, and other benign lesions were negative. However, it should be noted that serous carcinomas mostly are CEA nonreactive; the absence of CEA does not guarantee a benign outcome.

One antigen potentially of real interest has

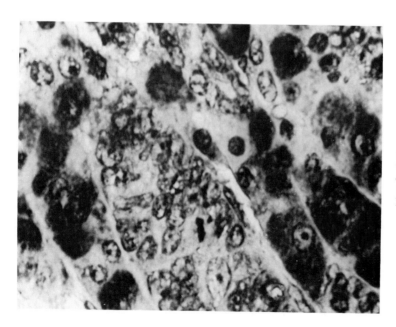

Figure 9–13. Testosterone reactivity (black) in the cytoplasm of "interstitial-type" cells in an "undifferentiated" tumor (see Maurer et al, 1980). Paraffin section, DAB with hematoxylin counterstain (×500).

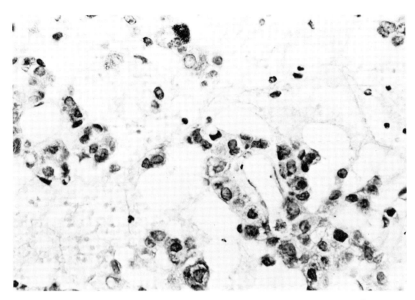

Figure 9–14. Widely invasive carcinoma of ovary (pseudomucinous) showing reactivity for CEA (carcinoembryonic antigen) in the majority of tumor cells. Paraffin section, DAB with hematoxylin counterstain (×500).

been described by Croghan et al (1984). The monoclonal antibody F36/22 appears to recognize 100 percent of ovarian carcinomas but only 10 percent of benign lesions. However, experience with this antibody is so limited that its general utility cannot be assessed at present. Likewise, the GP48 antigen (Bhattacharya et al, 1984) requires additional trials by other investigators. Claims for cancer specificity should be viewed with caution, as illustrated by increasing experience with the Ca antigen. Often called the Oxford antigen (whence it was first described), this antigen carried initial claims of great specificity for cancer. The experience of others has been less convincing, and it appears to be of little value with reference to ovarian tumors (Ferguson and Fox, 1984a).

In the matter of distinguishing primary ovarian carcinomas from metastases, there are two approaches: (1) to demonstrate the presence of an antigen restricted to ovary and (2) to demonstrate the presence of a non-ovarian antigen.

OC125 has definite value, being largely restricted to tumors occurring in tissues derived from the Müllerian ducts (ovarian epithelium, fallopian tubes, endometrium, and endocervix). Carcinomas of these tissues are positive; with rare exceptions other carcinomas are not (Kabawat et al, 1983). OC125 is sometimes called celomic antigen, since it is present on embryonic celom (from which the ovarian epithelium is derived); in the adult, mesothelial cells are positive. In our hands OC125 is consistently effective in frozen sections (Fig. 9–15), but we have not achieved satisfactory results in paraffin sections. Almost all nonmucinous carcinomas are OC125-positive; mucinous carcinomas tend to be nonreactive; CEA shows the opposite pattern. Other antigens that may be restricted to ovary have been described (Table 9–6), but experience is limited.

Staining for CEA is of limited value in defining a carcinoma as of ovarian or metastatic type, since, as noted above, 100 percent of mucinous carcinomas may be positive, whereas other ovarian tumors may be negative; approximately 80 percent of colonic carcinomas metastatic to ovary are CEA-positive (Charpin et al, 1982b).

Staining for keratin is of value, but interpretation is difficult because many different antikeratin antibodies are available, and the pattern of reactivity of most is not widely known. However, antibodies to "prekeratin" may be useful, since most ovarian carcinomas are nonreactive (Brenner's tumor provides an exception—Ganjei et al, 1983), whereas other adenocarcinomas contain low–molecular weight keratins and often also a variety of the higher molecular weight products and show variable positivity. Antibody to PAN keratin (low and high molecular weight) stains all ovarian carcinomas in frozen sections and a variable proportion in paraffin sections, according to the method employed

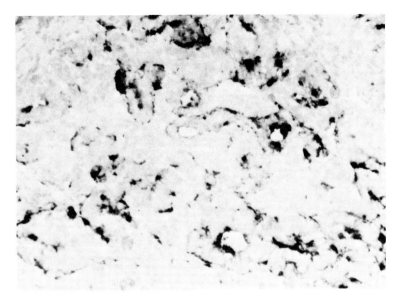

Figure 9–15. Frozen section of pelvic tumor treated with monoclonal antibody OC125 against "celomic antigen"; this is an example of endometrial carcinoma. Frozen section, AEC with light hematoxylin counterstain (×200).

(Nagle et al, 1983a): dysgerminomas are nonreactive for keratin.

Staining for keratin and other intermediate filaments is thus of use in the recognition of the various types of ovarian and uterine tumors, even in paraffin sections, if the patterns of reactivity of the antibodies are well defined, as demonstrated by Virtanen and colleagues (del Poggetto et al, 1983; Miettinen et al, 1983b).

Basically, the various carcinomas (serous, mucinous, endometrioid, and endometrial) show keratin positivity when various antibodies are used (available from Lab Systems Inc.; see Appendix 2) and do not stain for vimentin or desmin. Stromal sarcomas and leiomyosarcomas show the opposite pattern (Table 9–7), as do gonadal stromal (endocrine) tumors. Dysgerminomas (like seminomas) are keratin negative and vimentin positive: yolk sac carcinomas show a similar pattern. Teratomas with epithelial components, including so-called dermoid cysts, show keratin positivity. Embryonal carcinomas also are positive for keratin to varying degrees. In Brenner's tumor, the epithelial islands show strong central staining for keratin; the stroma stains for vimentin.

Clearly, demonstration of nonovarian antigens also is of value; for example, the pres-

Table 9–7. Intermediate Filament Expression in Gynecologic Tumors*

Tumor Type Carcinomas (Adenomas)	Keratin	Vimentin	Desmin
Serous	+	±	−
Mucinous	+	−	−
Endometrioid	+	−	−
Clear cell	+	−	−
Brenner's	+	− (+ stroma)	−
Endometrial	+	−	−
Cervical	+	−	−
Leiomyosarcoma	−	+	+
Stromal sarcoma	−	+	+
Granulosa/theca	−	+	+
Angioblastoma	−	+	+
Dysgerminoma (seminoma)	−	+	−
Yolk sac	−	+	−
Embryonal carcinoma	+	−	−
Teratoma	±	±	±

*Modified from del Poggetto et al (1983) and Miettinen et al (1983b). Occasional vimentin reactivity in serous adenocarcinomas may reflect the observation of both keratin and vimentin in the normal ovarian surface (celomic) epithelium. Note that the chart is based on reactivity in frozen sections: Whereas keratin may be stained in paraffin sections, vimentin and desmin are less readily demonstrated, and not with all antibodies.

ence of common leukocyte antigen clearly defines the tumor as leukocytic in origin (probably lymphoma), effectively excluding a poorly differentiated ovarian carcinoma. The same would be true of other cell- and tissue-specific antigens (eg, supposed breast or pancreas-specific antigens). The problem is that experience in using these antibodies is limited; for this purpose, strong staining for lactalbumin or casein is suggestive of metastatic breast tumor; but staining for milk fat–globule membrane antigen (or mammary epithelial membrane antigen) is less helpful, since it may also be seen in ovarian tumors. Likewise, staining for estrogen or estrogen receptor (see Chapter 10) cannot be used to separate primary ovarian carcinoma from breast metastases, since the former may show reactivity, albeit usually of a lesser degree than seen in positive breast cases. Staining for neuron-specific enolase or various hormones usually indicates a nonovarian tumor, but always remember that teratomas may produce any or several of these cell types and may develop the corresponding malignancies (Table 9–5).

TUMORS OF THE BREAST

10

"Histopathology, although part of the medical sciences curriculum, is viewed with some measure of scorn by practitioners of the 'pure' sciences, the micromolecular chemists, the cell physiologists, even the cellular immunologists and immunochemists, who regard histopathology as more akin to the collecting of butterflies than the splitting of the atom."

A reiteration of the sentiments of M. Bessis.
CR TAYLOR, 1983a

RECOGNITION OF SOLID TUMORS

The search for tumor-associated antigens within neoplasms of solid tissues has been most successful in hematopoietic malignant neoplasms. Our experience with lymphomas may serve as a model for the investigation of other tumors. By analogy with the multiplicity of lymphocyte antigens, we might expect to find tissue- (or cell-) restricted antigens in most tissues; also, fixed sections might be expected to show significant loss of many antigens in comparison to nonfixed cell preparations or frozen sections. Additional difficulties thus far encountered with solid tumors other than lymphomas may be due in part to the rather complex patterns in which the epithelial and mesenchymal cells are arranged within tissues and to the tendency for certain cell types, when neoplastic, to express characteristics more often associated with other tissues.

Also, attempts to develop antibodies to the cells of solid organs are preliminary compared with similar work on the leukocytes. This is a consequence of two principal factors: first, leukocytes conveniently present themselves in a readily purifiable form in the peripheral blood; second, early monoclonal antibody work was carried out by highly specialized immunologists whose interests principally covered the lymphoid system but not, for example, the prostate or kidney.

In recent years both of these factors have been subject to modification. Monoclonal antibodies are no longer the province of the "pure immunologist" but are legitimate tools at the disposal of tumor biologists interested in diverse tumor and normal cell types. Furthermore, attention has turned to developing screening techniques that to some extent obviate the need for careful purification of the immunizing cell type (ie, there is less need to purify the cells used for immunization in view of techniques available to screen for the antibody of interest against a wide spectrum of cell types).

Thus antibodies, both monoclonal and conventional, have been produced against tissue- or tumor-associated antigens or both in breast, colon, ovary, lung, pancreas, prostate, thyroid, melanoma, glioma, and several different types of sarcoma. The screening of many of these antibodies for their patterns of expression and specificity in normal and malignant tissue is still in the early stages; hence the usefulness of many of these reagents in the diagnosis and management of disease at this time cannot be fully evaluated. The realized and potential usefulness of many of these antibodies for the detection of malignant cells by immunoperoxidase techniques is discussed in this and succeeding chapters, first for particular categories of tumor and subsequently with reference to the diagnosis of anaplastic tumors of uncertain cellular derivation (the unknown primary).

Lymphomas

Many of the initial reports of immunoperoxidase methods were applied to routinely processed tissues from cases of lymphoma, and changes in diagnostic practice and concept resulted (Chapter 4). It is worth briefly reviewing the evolution of immunohistologic methods for the lymphomas, since it is reasonable to assume that similar principles apply to tumors of other cell types.

The early interest in lymphoma was partly circumstantial, contingent upon the availability of good antisera against antigens of interest (ie, anti-immunoglobulin antisera, anti-lysozyme, and the like). Recently, this interest in lymphomas has even been accentuated by the widespread production of monoclonal antibodies, many of which have specificity for leukocyte antigens (Chapter 4). A number of these antibodies of potential diagnostic interest are effective only in frozen sections. This limitation induced changes in practice, necessitating the preparation of frozen sections minimally fixed in acetone in parallel with paraffin sections. As a result, oncologists, surgeons, and pathologists were forced to coordinate their activities to make fresh tissues available to the pathology laboratory with minimal delay. Ideally, this should also occur for other types of neoplasms.

The availability of a large range of antibodies of potential interest also necessitated an additional strategy for the immunostaining of lymphomas, namely the development of a two-tier approach: screening the case initially for broad-spectrum cell markers (eg, panleukocyte, pan-T, pan-B) prior to further staining with antibodies specific to various cell subsets or differentiation phases (eg, OKT4, OKT8, OKT6, and the like). It is probable, as described later, that a similar approach will develop for other solid tumors (Chapter 14). In the lymphomas guidance as to which antibodies are most likely to yield useful results may be obtained by reference to the morphologic features of the lesion; this also is true of other tumor types.

If the diagnosis of lymphoma as opposed to other types of sarcoma or carcinoma is uncertain, it is wise to include antibody to common leukocyte antigen (CLA) in the initial screen; a positive result indicates the relationship of that cell to the lymphocytic, granulocytic, or monocytic series. Initially, this approach was possible only in frozen sections; however, antibodies to common leukocyte antigen that are effective on paraffin sections are now available. There is some indication that such antibodies may be the forerunners of a range of other monoclonal antibodies that effectively demonstrate leukocyte antigens in fixed paraffin sections (eg, LN1 and LN2 antibodies against follicular center B cells and B cell/monocytes respectively, developed by Epstein—Chapter 4). These antibodies have proved very effective in our laboratory and together with anti-CLA can be incorporated in schemes to investigate tumors of unknown origin, as described later (Chapter 14).

We may anticipate a similar course of events with reference to markers of other cell types and their derivative tumors, with the initial availability of reagents that are restricted to frozen sections but with an increasing discovery of antibodies that are effective in fixed tissues.

One other real possibility is the development of more effective fixatives that conserve antigens and cytologic features in response to the demonstrated need for immunohistochemical studies as part of tumor diagnosis.

Mammary Carcinomas

There are in excess of 100,000 new cases of breast carcinoma diagnosed annually in the United States alone. The most important prognostic factor is the extent of spread at diagnosis, which in turn relates to the importance of early histologic diagnosis. When the suspect nodule is removed, the distinction of carcinoma (necessitating some form of drastic intervention) from some form of hyperplasia (warranting some lesser form of clinical management) is fraught with difficulty. Morphology alone is remarkably successful in the recognition of established carcinoma; however, atypical hyperplastic lesions represent a major problem—whether or not to treat the lesion as pre-cancer or early cancer. In biopsy specimens this assessment is difficult; in aspiration cytology still more so, for in the latter instance, one no longer has the general architectural features to assist in the discrimination. Against this background the availability of immunohistologic stains that facilitate the recognition of actual or potential malignant cells would be a major breakthrough.

This approach may enhance not only the recognition and classification of tumors, but also the detection of small metastatic tumor

Table 10–1. Selected Bibliography: Breast Carcinoma, Lactalbumin, Casein, Pregnancy-Specific Glycoprotein, hCG

Clayton et al 1982	Lactalbumin positivity in 80% of ductal and 40% of lobular carcinomas; fibro-adenomas and normal breast also positive; other tissues and their tumors negative; 50% of metastatic breast cancer was positive
Bailey et al 1982	Found absence of lactalbumin in breast cancer;
Walker RA 1979	50% of breast cancers positive for lactalbumin; no correlation with differentiation
Le Doussal et al 1984	All lobular carcinomas and 75% of other types positive for lactalbumin; claimed positivity greatest in estrogen receptor-positive cases
Lee AK et al 1984	Lactalbumin detected in 67% of primary breast cancer and 62% of metastases; positivity in other tumors and tissues seen; some antibodies could be adsorbed; suggested some commercially available antisera contain cross-reactive antibodies
Inaba et al 1981	"Placenta-related proteins" in breast cancer
Kuhajda et al 1984	Pregnancy-specific glycoprotein in 40% of breast cancers; in some instances (especially in infiltrating ductal carcinoma) this presence indicated a poor prognosis
Wachner et al 1984b	hCG in 12% of breast cancers; only a small proportion of cells was positive in these cases
Ormerod & Sloane 1983	Casein and lactalbumin; believe that neither may be present in breast cancer and attribute staining to cross-reacting antibodies

foci in biopsy material and possibly the detection of steroid receptor expression.

A number of markers have been studied for their value in distinguishing malignant from normal mammary epithelial cells or breast cells (normal or malignant) from other cell types. Examples include the Thomsen-Friedenreich antigen, mammary tumor–associated glycoprotein, alpha-lactalbumin, casein, transferrin, or transferrin receptor. Antibodies to normal products of mammary epithelial cells, such as milk–fat globule membrane antigen (mammary epithelial membrane antigen), casein, and alpha-lactalbumin, have also been used as markers for breast cells (both normal or cancerous).

Lactalbumin, Casein, and Other Antigens

Both casein and lactalbumin appear to be of limited value, since their synthesis and secretion is very much dependent upon hormone stimulation during late pregnancy and lactation. Lactalbumin, for example, is detectable in only approximately 50 percent of breast cancers. It is perhaps surprising that the figure is this high in view of the lactational nature of this product in normal breast cells. Reference to the experience of different investigators reveals alarming discrepancies in the reported incidence of lactalbumin positivity in breast cancer (Table 10–1), ranging from absence of lactalbumin to its presence in 100 percent of lobular carcinomas and 75 percent of other types. Such large variations

almost certainly reflect the heterogeneity of the antisera employed. It is difficult to exclude the presence of cross-reactive components that may lead to positive staining. Indeed, Ormerod and Sloane (1983) speculate, on the basis of lack of evidence for lactalbumin production when using DNA probes to study breast tumors, that most of the "lactalbumin" activity reported is attributed to the presence of cross-reactive antibodies against a separate molecule that may show antigenic similarity to lactalbumin.

However, this is not to conclude that "antilactalbumin" antibodies have no value. When suitable positive controls are used to establish that reactivity is seen only in breast tissues, a positive stain may be taken as indicative of a breast origin even if the molecule stained is not actually lactalbumin. Thus, while a negative stain for lactalbumin (using antilactalbumin antiserum in the presence of good positive controls) does not exclude the possibility of breast origin for an anaplastic tumor, a positive stain is evidence in favor of derivation from breast (Fig. 10–1) in view of the lack of lactalbumin in other cell/tumor types as demonstrated with proper controls for the antiserum being used.

The rationale for use of antisera to casein is similar. Available antisera seem to differ widely in their patterns of reactivity, and careful in-house controls should be used prior to interpretation of staining patterns. Ormerod and Sloane (1983), noting the presence of epithelial membrane antigen in many casein preparations, have postulated that the observed staining with anticasein antibodies

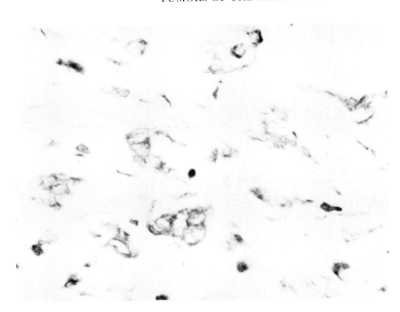

Figure 10–1. Scattered anaplastic cells in a pleural aspirate reactive for lactalbumin, suggestive of origin from breast. Necrotic debris also present, together with inflammatory cells (these show positivity for endogenous peroxidose which was not blocked). Acetone-fixed cytocentrifuge preparation, AEC with light hematoxylin counterstain (×200). Antilactoferrin antibody gave a similar pattern of reactivity.

is attributable to the presence of antibodies reactive with epithelial membrane antigens. Whether or not this is so, antisera may be used to provide information as to the mammary origin of tumors only if extensive positive and negative controls are used (ie, it must be demonstrated that the antiserum reacts only with breast tissues).

Staining for pregnancy-specific glycoprotein (SP1) (Fig. 10–2) and human chorionic gonadotopin (hCG) (Fig. 10–3) has also been reported in breast tumors (Table 10–1). However, although SP1 staining may have some adverse prognostic significance in infiltrating ductal carcinomas, its utility for recognition of breast tumors is limited. Likewise, hCG is quite widely distributed in different tumor types, staining a minor percentage of cells in germ cell, ovarian, endometrial, and breast tumor in addition to other types of carcinoma (eg, lung).

Transferrin, lactoferrin (Fig. 10–4), and various other molecules have also been observed in breast tissue and in breast cancer but have no diagnostic application (Mason and Taylor, 1978). There have been suggestions, however, that staining for transferrin or, better, for transferrin receptor (as with OKT9) may be of value in recognizing actively dividing breast cells, including of course cancer cells (Faulk et al, 1980, Rossiello et al, 1984). Transferrin receptor typically is expressed in dividing cells of many types; its presence is not unique to the breast,

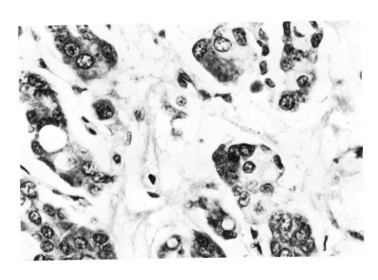

Figure 10–2. Infiltrating breast carcinoma showing reactivity with antibody to SP1 (pregnancy specific glycoprotein) in the majority of tumor cells. SP1 is quite commonly present in breast cancer but is not specific; it also occurs in endometrial and ovarian tumors.

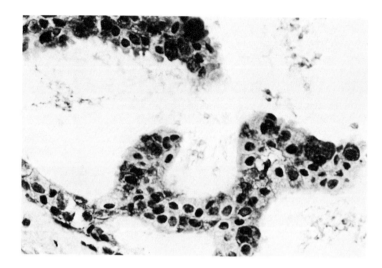

Figure 10–3. Intraductal breast carcinoma, cystic and papillary area showing presence of a small proportion of cells (black cytoplasm) reactive with an anti-hCG antibody. Paraffin section, DAB with hematoxylin counterstain (×200).

but rather is a reflection of an increased rate of cell division. Although there is some differential staining between breast cancer cells and normal breast and myoepithelial cells, it appears unlikely that this difference will be of sufficient degree to aid the histologist.

Milk–Fat Globule Membrane Antigen (Mammary Epithelial Membrane Antigen)

Milk–fat globule membrane (MFGM), or mammary epithelial membrane antigen (MEMA), is, in fact, not a single antigen but rather a group of overlapping epitopes on several different molecules that represent integral constituents of the apical plasma membrane of epithelial cells. They are widely distributed in the normal breast (even when nonlactating), and closely similar or cross-reacting antigens are present in various other epithelial tissues, especially those that contain secretory cells (eg, salivary gland and· pancreas). Antibodies to MFGM (MEMA) can be used to study the expression of this antigen group as a function of altered tissue architecture under various pathologic conditions (Table 10–2). Both polyclonal and monoclonal antibodies to MFGM have been raised and have been utilized to localize the corresponding antigens in breast and other tissues by immunoperoxidase methods. Although these antibodies are not totally specific for mammary epithelial cells, they can be useful in distinguishing adenocarcinoma from sarcoma, melanoma, and poorly differentiated lymphoma, in that positivity can be observed in many adenocarcinomas (Figs. 10–5 and

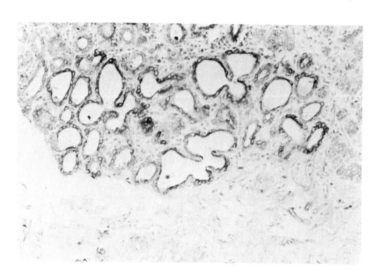

Figure 10–4. Lobule of "normal" lactating breast stained for lactoferrin. A small percentage of breast carcinomas are lactoferrin-positive. Paraffin section, DAB with hematoxylin counterstain (×60). This tissue would serve as a good positive control for lactoferrin.

Table 10–2. Selected Bibliography: Milk–Fat Globule Membrane Antigen (MFGMA), or Mammary Epithelial Membrane Antigen (MEMA)

Sloan & Ormerod 1981 Sloane et al 1983	Review of (M)EMA—generally distributed in different epithelial cells and carcinomas; a more reliable marker of epithelial derivation than prekeratin or CEA; 20/22 anaplastic carcinoma positive; effective in formalin paraffin sections; mesothelial cells positive
Sloane et al 1980	Value of EMA antiserum in detecting micrometastases
Imam & Tökés 1981 Imam et al 1984	Antibody to MFGM—one of several diverse glycoproteins widely distributed in epithelial cells; normal cells show apical distribution, but malignant cells show variable membrane and cytoplasmic staining that is distinctly different from normal
Hilkens et al 1984	Screened panel of 17 different anti-MFGM monoclonal antibodies; found at least 9 overlapping epitopes in at least 6 different molecules; some antibodies discriminated between carcinomas (positive) and sarcomas (negative); none were breast-specific
Wilkinson et al 1984	Two monoclonals to MFGM; possible value in relation to prognosis (loss of antigen-poor prognosis for breast cancer)
Berry et al 1985	Two monoclonals to MFGM; no relation to prognosis; patterns of reactivity in malignant tissue different from normal
Dearnaley et al 1981	Use of antiserum to EMA for detecting marrow metasases
Wells et al 1984	Detection of micrometastases with anti-EMA and antikeratin
Singer et al 1985	Monoclonal HMFG2 reacted with mesothelial cells in 50% of cases
Miettinen 1984	EMA in chordomas—indicative of epithelial derivation; noted mucinous carcinomas CEA⁺, EMA⁺; chordoma CEA⁻, EMA⁺
Delsol et al 1984b	Reported reactivity of several EMA antibodies with nonepithelial cells (lymphocytes, Reed-Sternberg cells)

10–6), whereas the other tumor types are nonreactive. Squamous carcinomas show weak or absent reactivity.

With polyclonal antisera to MFGM, specificity for breast adenocarcinoma as opposed to other types can be improved by extensive adsorption with extracts of either salivary gland or pancreas or both (Fig. 10–7). Absolute specificity for breast adenocarcinoma cannot however be achieved; similarly, monoclonal antibodies versus MFGM are not totally specific for breast adenocarcinoma (of

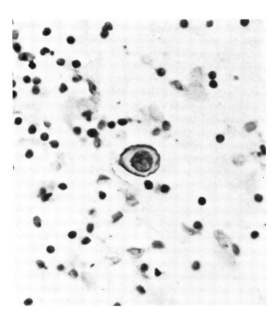

Figure 10–5. Solitary "suspicious" cell in a pleural effusion; positive surface staining for epithelial membrane antigen (black rim) provides support for a diagnosis of metastatic adenocarcinoma. The primary tumor was in the breast. Paraffin section, AEC with hematoxylin counterstain (×320).

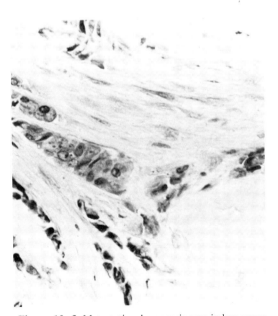

Figure 10–6. Metastatic adenocarcinoma in bone marrow with positive (gray) cytoplasmic reactivity for mammary epithelial membrane antigen (MEMA). The primary tumor was in the breast. Paraffin section, AEC with hematoxylin counterstain (×200).

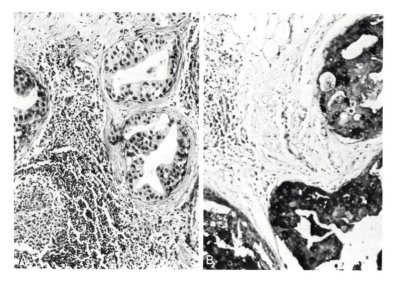

Figure 10–7. Metastatic adenocarcinoma in lymph node. *A* shows negative control (omitting primary antibody); *B* shows pattern of reactivity with an absorbed serum to mammary epithelial membrane antigen (MEMA, or milk fat globule membrane antigen). The primary tumor was in the breast. Paraffin section, AEC with hematoxylin counterstain (×125).

17 antibodies screened by Hilkens et al, 1984, none were breast-specific). Reactivity has been observed against renal tubules and some bronchial and alveolar cells. Normal sweat glands and sweat gland tumors are strongly positive—possibly an example of the occurrence of the identical antigen in sweat glands, which have a common embryologic origin with the breast.

With reference to the distinction of benign proliferations from carcinoma, antibodies to MFGM-GP70, a glycoprotein purified from MFGM, do reveal differences in the pattern of expression of this antigen in breast cancer as compared to normal breast cells (Table 10–2). In normal breast cells, this antigen is almost totally restricted to the apical membrane forming the lumenal surface of breast cells; in malignant breast cells, positivity may be observed at any point around the cell surface or even extensively within the cytoplasm (Fig. 10–8). These observations suggest that the morphologic disorientation of malignant cells observed in breast carcinoma is associated with failure of the normal process of insertion of structural glycoproteins into the breast epithelial cell membrane. This molecular disorientation, although typical of carcinoma cells, has also been observed in some hyperplasias with atypical features; the significance of this observation in terms of premalignancy is, however, not yet established.

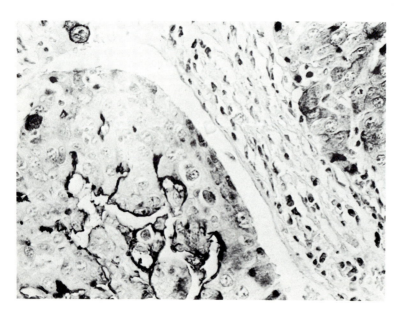

Figure 10–8. Carcinoma of breast showing characteristic staining pattern with antibody to milk fat globule membrane (MFGM) or mammary epithelial membrane antigen (MEMA). In the normal breast, only the apices of the cells stain. In carcinoma intense (black) apical staining may be seen in relation to rudimentary luminal structures; in addition, there is variable granular (gray) cytoplasmic staining. Paraffin section, DAB with hematoxylin counterstain (×320).

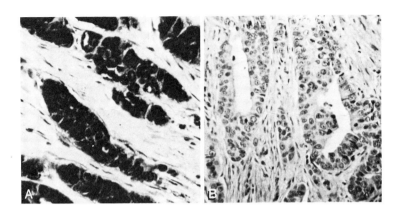

Figure 10–9. Breast carcinoma. *A* shows intense reactivity of breast carcinoma cells treated with an anti-T antibody (from normal human AB serum). *B* shows the "negative" control in which the anti-T antibody was omitted. Paraffin section, DAB with hematoxylin counterstain (×125) (from Howard and Taylor, 1979).

T Antigen and Other Cancer-Associated Antigens

T (Thomsen-Friedenreich) and Tn antigens are precursor antigens to the MN blood group system. They are masked in most normal adult tissues, and normal humans have anti-T and Tn antibodies evoked by cross-reactive antigens present in the intestinal flora. Both T and Tn may be revealed in tumor tissues (Fig. 10–9). This has been extensively explored in relation to breast cancer (Table 10–3), in which T and Tn antigens detected by normal human serum (containing anti-T and Tn activity, absorbed to re-move other unwanted antibodies) or by monoclonal antibodies have been shown to be present in most breast cancers, with lesser reactivity in "borderline" and benign lesions. Both T and Tn are detectable by immunostaining in most breast cancers, although some anaplastic lesions give weak reactivity or may be nonreactive.

T antigen has also been recognized in several other types of carcinoma (colon, bladder, lung, breast). Some claims have been made that the distribution may have prognostic significance. Generally, benign lesions are nonreactive (or weakly so); well-differentiated carcinomas give good staining of a high

Table 10–3. Selected Bibliography: T Antigen and Other Breast Cancer-Associated Antigens

Howard & Taylor 1979 } Howard & Batsakis 1980 }	Malignant breast lesions show increased expression of T antigen compared to benign tissues
Rahman & Longenecker 1982	Monoclonal antibody to T antigen
Springer et al 1985	Tn antigen and T antigen in breast cancer, monoclonal, and polyclonal antibodies; good literature resource on T antigen
Singer et al 1985	Ca antigen of value in detecting malignant cells in effusions (mesothelial cells negative)
Shah et al 1980	Antisera to antigen shared by breast carcinoma and trophoblasts
Yu et al 1980	Antiserum showing limited specificity to breast cancer
Nuti et al 1982 } Hand et al 1983 }	Range of antibreast monoclonals generated by Dr. Schlom
Brabon et al 1984	Monoclonal to a breast tumor–associated protein that is estrogen induced
Cardiff et al 1983	Report of 4 antibreast monoclonals developed by Dr. Schlom; good access to literature
Björklund et al 1982	TPA (tissue polypeptide antigen) positive in breast cancer
Clough et al 1984	Staining for Ca (Oxford antigen) seen more often in malignancy; however, false-negative rate was 70%, false-positive 56%. Ca 1 of little value
Simpson HW et al 1984	Ca 1 in all cancers, in 12/13 fibroadenomas, and in all normal breasts (focally): severe limitations to use
Croghan et al 1983	Monoclonal anti–breast cancer antibody
Mariani-Costantini et al 1984	Monoclonal breast cancer–associated antibody
Ellis IO et al 1984	Monoclonal anti–breast cancer antibody
Rowe & Beverely 1984	Leukocytic infiltrate in breast cancer (T & B cells)
Bhan & DesMarais 1983	Loss of HLA antigen in cancer cells; some cases Ia-positive
Shimokawara et al 1982	Reported T cell preponderance in lymphocytes around cancer cells

proportion of cells; anaplastic tumors show less intense or equivocal staining. Springer's group has concluded that staining for T and Tn may be of value in predicting the aggressiveness of the particular carcinoma (Springer et al, 1985).

A variety of other antibodies that show some evidence of detecting breast cancer-associated antigens have been described (Table 10–3). Some show promise (Brabon et al, 1984; Cardiff et al, 1983), but there are insufficient data to permit recommendation for diagnostic use (Fig. 10–10). Four of the murine antibodies developed by Jeffrey Schlom (B6.2, B50.4, B72.3, B38.1) were reviewed in a multicenter study (Cardiff et al, 1983). None of these antibodies was tissue-specific or cancer-specific; all reacted with at least some normal tissue components (eg, B6.2—normal sweat ducts and granulocytes), and all reacted with certain other carcinomas (eg, colon cancer). In addition, considerable heterogeneity of staining was seen within individual tumors and in different tumors. These antibodies were effective both in frozen and in paraffin sections, but many others react only with frozen sections (Table 10–3). If fixation is to be employed, many investigators have expressed a preference for methanol or B5 rather than formalin. Although a variety of immunogens have been used, including various fractions from primary tumors, metastases, and cell lines (eg, MCF7), many of the antibodies thus far described appear to show similar reactivity against sur-face-related antigens, including milk–fat globule membrane (see Table 10–2). Thus far none are specific for breast cancer; reactivity versus colon cancer has been observed most commonly.

Tissue polypeptide antigen (TPA) has been investigated extensively in Scandinavia; it shows some promise for facilitating the distinction of malignant from benign tissue and is not specific to tissue from the breast. Reactivity is distinct from CEA (Björklund et al, 1982).

Antibodies to actin and myosin have been used to demonstrate myoepithelial cells in cancer tissues rather than the cancer cells themselves. Although myoepithelial cells appear to be deficient in papillary, medullary, and lobular carcinoma, these findings do not have direct diagnostic application (Sugano et al, 1981; Bussolati et al, 1980b; Papotti et al, 1983).

Ca 1 antibody (against the so-called Oxford antigen) has also been investigated for possible utility in the distinction of malignant from normal and benign breast tissue. In spite of the fanfare with which this antibody was announced, it appears to have little utility in relation to breast cancer (Table 10–3), a fact that parallels its lack of cancer specificity reported for other tissues (Paradinas et al, 1984). H is present in both neoplastic and non-neoplastic lung tissue.

Murine mammary tumor virus antigen (MuMTV) has been shown by immunohistochemical methods to be present in breast

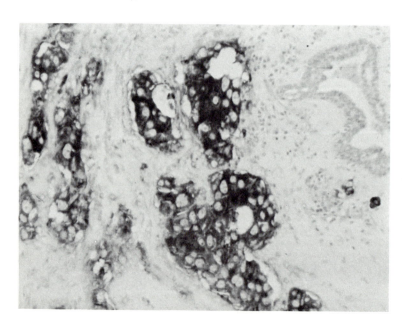

Figure 10–10. Breast carcinoma showing positive reactivity (black cytoplasm) with a monoclonal antibreast antibody prepared by Dr. J. Schlom (antibody 6.2). Note relative lack of staining of normal duct. Paraffin section, DAB with hematoxylin counterstain ($\times 200$).

cancer in mice (St. George et al, 1979), including spontaneous breast tumors of wild mice (Gardner et al, 1980). A 52,000 molecular–weight glycoprotein (GP52), similar or identical to that of MuMTV, has been described as widely distributed in human breast cancer (Hehlmann et al, 1981; Mitchell WM et al, 1980; Mesa-Tejada et al, 1979). The percentage of positive cases has been reported as approximately 45 percent, but there was no correlation for histologic type or prognosis.

Analyses of the subtypes of leukocytes, including proportions of T and B cells and helper and suppressor subtypes, have revealed little information of value (Table 10–3), although Shimokawara and colleagues (1982) did claim a dramatic increase in T lymphocytes in cancer tissue as compared to normal tissue. Tumor cells showed a tendency to lose HLA antigens from their surface. Some cases were positive for Ia-like antigen.

CEA

Carcinoembryonic antigen (CEA) is positive in breast tissue less often than in colon; the intensity of staining and the percentage of positively reacting cells also are less. Reported reactivity for CEA varies from 30 to 90 percent or more of cases (Table 10–4). In situ carcinoma and lobular carcinoma are rarely CEA-positive, whereas infiltrating ductal carcinoma is more often positive than not

(Fig. 10–11). Note that even in cases classified as positive, the percentage of positive cells is often low (10 to 30 percent). Discrepant findings among different investigators almost certainly reflect differences in antisera; as discussed elsewhere, CEA antisera frequently contain antibodies against NCA (nonspecific cross-reacting antigens) that are seen not only in certain cancers but also in normal tissues and granulocytes. Some studies have shown that adsorption of CEA antiserum to remove all NCA activity dramatically changes the observed patterns of immunostaining: eg, unadsorbed anti-CEA stained 85 percent of benign mastopathies, 66 percent of fibroadenomas, and 93 percent of breast cancers; following adsorption the percentages of positive cases were 0.0, 0.0, and 42 (Nap et al, 1984).

In our experience with anti-CEA antibodies (adsorbed for NCA, or monoclonal anti-CEA with no NCA activity), approximately 50 percent of breast cancers are positive, and definite positivity is suspect for malignancy. As a guide to the possible presence of NCA activity, the observer should look for evidence of staining of normal granulocytes in blood vessels; if positively stained granulocytes are present, it is likely that the anti-CEA antibody contains significant NCA reactivity, reducing its utility. The investigator should either adsorb the antibody with homogenized buffy coat (granulocytes) or obtain a better antibody (or antiserum). Note that some supposed anti-CEA monoclonal antibodies cross react with NCA; this activity

Table 10–4. Selected Bibliography: CEA in Breast Cancer

Walker RA 1980, 1982	CEA in 50% of breast cancers; also studied lactalbumin, IgA, "pregnancy proteins"
Halter et al 1984	CEA in 167 cases—no correlation overall; in disseminated disease, CEA-positive cases fared better
Barry et al 1984	CEA, lactalbumin, casein, secretory piece: rarely seen in normal breast; one or more markers present in cancer, but does not reflect differentiation or prognosis
Nap et al 1984	High reactivity of CEA antiserum to breast tissue attributed to presence of anti-NCA antibody
Wittekind et al 1982a	CEA in frozen, paraffin, and Paraplast tissues; all adequate
Wittekind et al 1982b	CEA in mastopathy not significantly related to development of cancer
Papotti et al 1983	CEA and actin (for myoepithelial cells) aided the diagnosis of papillary carcinoma, in which the myoepithelial layer is lacking
Kuhajda et al 1983a	70%–90% of duct carcinoma CEA-positive; in situ carcinoma and lobular carcinoma only 30% positive; benign breast tumor rarely positive
Mazoujian et al 1984	Paget's disease cells contain an apocrine antigen, are also CEA-positive and are negative for keratin (high molecular weight)
Kariniemi et al 1984a, b	Paget's disease cells contain apocrine antigen and CEA; sweat gland also commonly differentiates to produce apocrine antigen

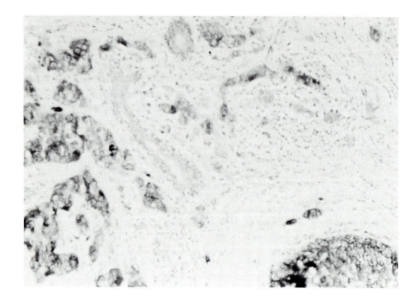

Figure 10–11. Carcinoembryonic antigen (CEA) reactivity within breast carcinoma. Paraffin section, AEC with hematoxylin counterstain (×125).

cannot be adsorbed out, because all antibody activity is then lost.

Human Monoclonal Antibodies

Recently, the generation of human monoclonal antibodies to mammary carcinoma cells has been reported by several investigators (Schlom et al, 1980; Teramoto et al, 1982; Imam et al, 1985a; Cote et al, 1983). It has been postulated that the development of these antibodies may reflect the host's capacity for recognizing malignant cells. In some cases these antibodies do appear to be able to distinguish malignant from normal epithelial cells, both quantitatively and qualitatively within the individual patient (Fig. 10–12). However, such antibodies appear not to be applicable or reproducible for recognition of carcinoma cells in a broader group of patients. Clearly, further study is necessary to establish whether these antibodies will have any role in immunohistologic diagnosis, in radioimmunolocalization, or in therapy. Also, because these are human antibodies, their utility with reference to immunohistologic studies of human tissues is limited by the difficulty in detecting human antibodies on human tissues, as described elsewhere.

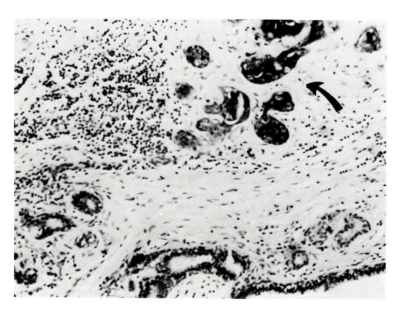

Figure 10–12. Section of breast showing carcinoma cells (arrow) reactive with a human monoclonal antibody, developed by Dr. Ashraf Imam at the University of Southern California, utilizing lymphocytes from a patient with breast cancer as one of the hybrid partners. There is differential staining of cancer cells (black cytoplasm) and normal breast elements (lower field—clear cytoplasm; the nuclei appear black due to the hematoxylin). Paraffin section, DAB with hematoxylin counterstain (×125).

Detection of "Steroid Hormone Receptors"

Evidence that the immunohistologic demonstration of steroid hormones within frozen and paraffin sections may be possible has resulted in attempts to demonstrate the corresponding receptors by evidence of cellular binding of steroid hormones. Such methods are in their infancy and are somewhat controversial; nonetheless, they do have some theoretic advantages over current procedures based on cytosol assays.

Cytosol-Based Assays

Receptors assays, as currently performed, require sufficient fresh biopsy material for preparation of a tissue homogenate, following which some form of competitive estrogen-binding assay is performed to obtain an overall numerical value for estrogen receptor activity. Such assays, if carefully controlled, are believed to detect only the specific estrogen receptor, excluding nonspecific estrogen-binding by other cell and tissue components. The technical procedure is relatively demanding and is not easily performed in "routine" diagnostic pathology laboratories. Receptor-binding activity is very labile and necessitates immediate and special handling techniques. In addition, the assay is performed upon a homogenate of the total tissue presented for analysis, without any precise knowledge of the number of tumor cells within the tissue relative to stromal cells, tissue fluids, and noncellular tissue components; this proportion remains a matter of guesswork based upon the presumption that the tissue assayed has a composition similar to histologic specimens of adjacent tissues. Finally, the cytosol-based assay gives a mean value of the receptor for the total tissue and provides no information for example as to whether all of the tumor cells show low levels of activity, or whether small percentages show high receptor activity, while the majority of cells do not express the receptor, or indeed whether the activity detected is a function of tumor cells or stromal cells.

Immunohistologic Assays

Theoretically, direct demonstration of receptor protein by immunohistologic techniques would obviate many of these difficulties. Detection of receptor in tissue sections could theoretically be achieved either by immunologic reactivity of the receptor protein (with an antireceptor antibody) or by utilizing the biologic binding activity of the receptor for the steroid then using antibody to the steroid molecule. Both methods would permit assay of receptor sites directly within the tumor cells; both the binding activity of any nontumor cell components and the exact proportion of tumor cells showing reactivity would be obvious. This clearly is of theoretical importance, because a tumor in which only 10 percent of the tumor cells are positive but strongly so would be expected to respond differently to hormonal manipulation than another tumor in which all of the tumor cells are weakly positive; both tumors, however, might show identical results on a cytosol-based assay.

The problem regarding the immunohistologic assays is that as yet both of these approaches remain unproven in terms of specific demonstration of the estrogen receptor.

The Use of Polymerized Estradiol. Initial attempts using the steroid–antisteroid antibody approach were pioneered by Pertshuk and colleagues (1980). Frozen sections were employed. The intention was to find the presence of estrogen receptor activity by adding polymerized estradiol phosphate (PEP) to the tissue section, followed by an immunostain (with anti-estradiol antibody) to localize the sites of binding of the estradiol phosphate. Immunofluorescence methods were used, but immunoperoxidase techniques have subsequently been shown to offer similar levels of specificity and sensitivity with improved morphologic resolution. With the use of these methods, binding of PEP to tumor cells can readily be demonstrated—the degree of binding varying both within individual tumors and in different cases—showing a broad correlation with cytosol-based assays performed on tissue from the same tumors. Subsequent studies by many investigators confirmed the validity of this technique on an anecdotal or empirical basis (Table 10–5).

Direct Staining with Anti-Estradiol Antibody. In the course of this work, it was also observed that direct staining of breast carcinoma with antibodies against estradiol (ie, without prior addition of PEP) produced patterns of reactivity similar to that observed when polymerized estradiol phosphate was used prior to the antisteroid antibody (Table 10–5: Taylor et al, 1981; Shimuzu et al,

Table 10–5. Selected Bibliography: Immunohistologic Methods for Steroids and Steroid Receptors in Breast Cancer

Mercer et al 1980	Detection of estrogen and progesterone; correlation with estrogen receptor activity
Taylor et al 1981	Direct detection of estrogen; 60% correlation with cytosol assays for estrogen receptor (paraffin sections)
Shimizu et al 1983	71% of 277 cases judged estrogen-positive (see Katayama et al: follow up)
Walker RH et al 1980	Immunohistologic method positive for all cases shown to have estrogen receptor by dextran charcoal method
Katayama et al 1984	82% correlation for staining endogenous estrogen and sucrose density gradient receptor assay. Clinically, 15/18 endogenous estrogen-positive cases responded to endocrine therapy, contrasted with only 1/9 responses in cases negative for endogenous estrogen
Underwood et al 1982	Doubtful validity of immunohistochemical methods for estrogen receptor
Chamness et al 1980	Great potential of immunohistochemical methods, not proved
Hanna et al 1982	Localization of estrogen-binding sites in breast cancer (52 cases)
Ciocca et al 1982	Monoclonal antibody to "estrogen-regulated proteins"
King WJ et al 1985 } Poulsen et al 1985	Monoclonal antibody to estrogen receptor protein used in frozen and paraffin sections; correlation with cytosol-based assays
Press & Greene 1984	Anti-estrogen receptor monoclonal in uterine tissues
Garancis et al 1983	Monoclonal antibody to estrogen receptor
Ioannidis et al 1982	Use of monoclonal antibody to glucocorticoid receptor; most carcinomas positive
Castro et al 1980b	Insulin in breast cancer cases
Woodard et al 1981	ACTH in breast cancer
Purnell et al 1982	Prolactin in breast cancer
Castro et al 1980a	hCG in breast cancer

1983). Intensity of staining was often less, but the qualitative interpretation was similar in terms of positive or negative cells.

It has been proposed that direct staining with anti-estradiol antibody may detect the presence of estradiol bound in vivo to estrogen receptor, whereas pretreatment with PEP followed by anti-estradiol antibody may detect the total amount of receptor present: both the free receptor, not bound to estrogen in vivo, and also the in vivo–bound receptors. Although there are little hard data to support these hypotheses, these immunohistologic stains do show considerable reproducibility and consistency from case to case, and give a positive correlation with cytosol-based assays performed upon tissues from the same tumors (Figs. 10–13, 10–14, and 10–15).

In addition to studies of frozen sections, it has also been shown that direct staining of

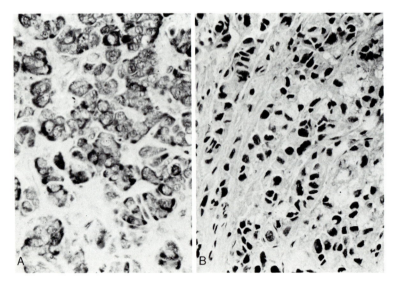

Figure 10–13. Breast carcinoma (**B**, H&E). Moderate cytoplasmic staining with antibody to estradiol is shown in **A**. Paraffin section, DAB with hematoxylin counterstain (×320).

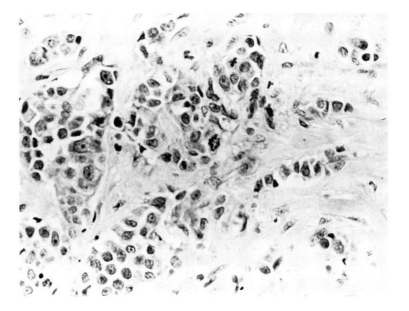

Figure 10–14. Estrogen-poor breast carcinoma showing lack of cytoplasmic or nuclear reactivity with anti-estradiol antibody. Paraffin section, DAB with hematoxylin counterstain (×320). Cytosol assay gave estrogen receptor value less than 10 femtomoles.

paraffin sections with anti-estradiol antibodies gives a pattern of staining similar to that observed by direct anti-estradiol staining of frozen sections and again correlates at the 80 percent level with cytosol-based assays (Table 10–5). All of these demonstrations fall short of scientific proof that the immunohistologic method either with or without prior treatment with polymerized estradiol phosphate detects the specific receptor; it may be that a significant part or all of the observed binding is attributable to binding of estrogen to globulins or other tissue components, or even to nonspecific binding of the anti-estradiol antibody. In unfixed frozen sections, there appears to be significant loss of receptor protein into the incubation medium; following fixation some receptor protein is immobilized and retained, and some is lost (acetone is particularly damaging). Either approach represents some compromise; in the final analysis, the method must be judged by the results.

Precautions concerning the specificity control of the anti-estradiol antibodies used in attempts to detect estrogen receptor protein are of course equally rigorous compared with the methods for detecting synthesized estro-

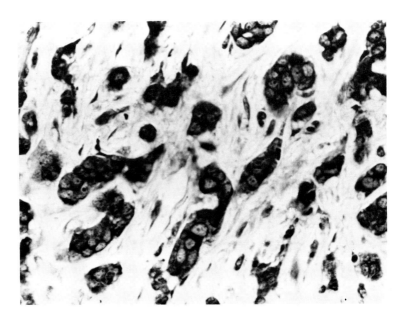

Figure 10–15. Estrogen-rich breast carcinoma showing intense black cytoplasmic reactivity, plus scattered nuclear staining. DAB with hematoxylin counterstain (×320). Cytosol assay gave estrogen receptor value >200 femtomoles.

gen as described in Chapter 9. Cross reactivity of anti-estradiol antisera with albumin is a particular problem and may render attempts to demonstrate estrogen or estrogen receptor invalid, since degenerating tumor cells frequently contain imbibed albumin that may show reactivity with any anti-albumin antibodies contaminating the anti-estradiol antisera. Antisera made against KLH-linked steroid molecules theoretically avoid this pitfall.

A number of attempts have been made to improve the level of confidence in immunohistologic assays of estrogen receptor.

First, if an immunohistologic technique is to be employed, whether or not use of polymerized estradiol phosphate is a preliminary step and whether frozen or paraffin sections are used, it is important to emphasize that interpretation of the staining pattern is a matter of the experience of the histopathologist. Just as the histopathologist needs to spend considerable time acquiring experience in straightforward morphologic interpretation of normal versus neoplastic cells in the breast, so he or she must devote a comparable effort to learning interpretation of immunohistologic staining patterns. This experience clearly requires that cytosol-based assays should be performed in parallel in order to provide a reference point for the histopathologist. Interpretation of the immunohistologic staining pattern, whether negative or positive for estrogen receptor activity, should be performed by the histopathologist on a blind basis, but should always be compared later to cytosol-based assays. Staining of breast tumor cell cytoplasm or nuclei may represent specific staining for estrogen.

The degree of staining does correlate with cytosol-based assays. The staining of very small proportions of tumor cells (less than 10 percent) is invariably associated with low-level or negative cytosol-based assays; the higher the proportion of positively stained tumor cells, the higher the level of steroid receptor in the cytosol-based assay within a broad correlation. On this basis, almost all cases described as negative (ie, no positive cells) on the basis of the immunohistologic technique would also be negative on the basis of the cytosol-based assay. However, discrepancies are observed in about 20 percent of cases overall. Most discrepancies relate to cases in which small proportions of cells are considered to show significant positive staining in immunohistologic preparations (10 percent

or less positive cells), but the corresponding cytosol-based assay levels fall below the critical value considered significant by the performing laboratory. The result may reflect false positivity by immunostaining or may alternatively reflect the presence of relatively small numbers of positive tumor cells within a much larger population of negative cells; the cytosol value will be the mean value of all tumor cells present and may be low if only a few cells express the receptor. This problem is particularly observed in histologic sections in which tumor cells are sparsely distributed among residual normal breast cells, reactive inflammatory cells, and connective tissue. This eventuality emphasizes the need for developing a broad base of experience involving cases in which both immunohistologic and cytosol-based assays are available for comparison.

The clinical response should be the ultimate measure of validity of the immunohistologic methods; comparison with the cytosol method, which itself may be flawed, should be only an interim step. In this context the study of Katayama and colleagues (1984) is particularly interesting. They stained directly for endogenous estrogen: of 18 positive cases, 15 showed an excellent clinical response to endocrine therapy, in contrast with a good clinical response in only 1 of 9 cases judged negative by this method. Whether the method detects the "true receptor" or not, it appears to give the clinician the information required for therapy.

Use of Antibody to Estrogen Receptor. A second, theoretically more rigorous approach, designed to avoid uncertainty as to whether estrogen detected within the tissue by immunohistologic methods is bound to the specific receptor or to nonspecific tissue components, has been to develop antibodies against the estrogen receptor protein itself. This method has been attempted in a number of laboratories with varying success (Table 10–5), and some investigators have developed monoclonal antibodies believed to be specific for estrogen receptor protein. These antibodies are not widely available; however, various commercial organizations have shown intense interest in the monoclonal antibodies, suggesting that progress may be rapid (Abbott has recently released a kit containing one of these antibodies). The pattern of staining observed in frozen and paraffin sections when such antibodies are employed compares rather closely with that observed when utilizing staining with anti-estradiol an-

Figure 10–16. Staining of estrogen-rich breast cancer (intraductal) with monoclonal antibody to estrogen receptor (estrophilin). The staining is mostly intranuclear, the majority of tumor cells showing detectable staining (black nuclei). Frozen section, DAB with no counterstain (***A***, ×200; ***B***, ×320). (Courtesy of Abbott Laboratories; note that in using this reagent the procedure given by Abbott must be strictly followed.)

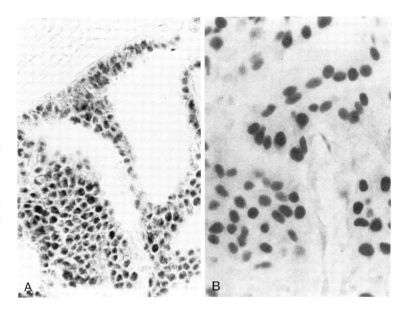

tibody, except that in frozen sections the staining observed is almost entirely intranuclear (Fig. 10–16). Preliminary publications outlining the findings obtained (WJ King et al, 1985; Poulsen et al, 1985) and discussing the remaining problems have appeared. At present frozen sections are recommended: following sectioning, these are treated sequentially with 3.7% formaldehyde, methanol, and acetone, each for five minutes or less. Slides are then maintained in PBS prior to staining (Abbott procedure). Some investigators believe that it is essential to develop antibodies against the "native-bound receptor" prior to achieving a successful immunohistologic assay system. So far this has not been reported.

Finally, other investigators are working to combine the histologic precision of the tissue section approach with the biologic specificity of the competitive cytosol-based assays. In this method, standardized frozen sections of breast tumor are incubated with tritiated estradiol. The relative amount of binding of the labelled estradiol in the tissue section compared with that remaining in the incubation medium provides the basis for calculation of the amount of specific estrogen receptor within the tissue; histologic examination of the adjacent tissue section permits inclusion of a factor reflecting the number of tumor cells in the section. This assay is perhaps too cumbersome for a general immunohistologic use but certainly would be an excellent approach for developing comparative studies between immunohistologic methods and cytosol-based assays.

In conclusion, immunohistologic techniques offer the advantages of rapidity (available within a few hours), correlation of positivity with tumor cell numbers, and tumor cell morphology. The encouragement given by studies to date must be tempered by recognition of the preliminary nature of many of these studies and the lack of detailed correlations with cytosol-based assays that currently form the basis for therapy. It should also be realized that the basis for the validity of immunohistologic procedures is not a comparison with the cytosol-based technique but rather a correlation with the results of therapy by hormonal manipulations. Such studies are in hand; clearly it will take some time to accumulate and analyze the data. Preliminary results are, however, encouraging, and the immunohistologic assessment of estrogen receptor does appear to be predictive of the results of hormonal manipulation and may have prognostic significance for tumor recurrence.

11

LUNG, PANCREAS, COLON AND RECTUM, STOMACH, LIVER

"Liver n. *A large red organ thoughtfully provided by nature to be bilious with . . . . It was at one time considered the seat of life; hence its name—liver, the thing we live with.*"

AMBROSE BIERCE, 1842–1914
The Devil's Dictionary

"*Do you ever ponder the advisability of not making a diagnosis and thereby avoiding a death sentence?*"

MARLIN H. FISCHER, 1879–1962

LUNG TUMORS

In the lungs, as in other organs, tumors should ideally be classified according to the normal, presumed progenitor, cell type that the neoplastic cells most closely resemble. In the lungs, however, this has posed a considerable problem, even in such a simple matter as determining the origin of peripheral adenocarcinoma, whereas oat cell carcinoma and the large anaplastic carcinomas have been the subjects of acrimonious debate.

The problem has been compounded by the discovery of neuroendocrine cells in normal lung, leading to speculation as to the relationship of these cells to bronchial adenomas, carcinoid tumors, and oat cell carcinoma.

Immunohistochemistry has been of value in unraveling at least the question of the neuroendocrine tumors (vide infra). It would be a mistake, however, to assume that the concept of neuroendocrine cells is clear, for it is not. The term *neuroendocrine* is used in this book to describe cells that secrete, or at least contain, one or more of the various neurotransmitter type of products. Although some of these cells, in certain organs, are accepted as being of neural crest origin, oth-

ers almost certainly are not (eg, some neuroendocrine carcinomas, oat cell carcinomas, and carcinoids react with antikeratin antibodies, evidence that would seem to weigh against a neural crest origin). The tables included in relation to the hormone-producing cells of the gastrointestinal tract (Chapter 7) thus serve as a general framework, which it is hoped will approximate the truth as, and if, it emerges.

Keratin

Pankeratin antibodies stain almost all lung tumors. Antibodies against "squamous" or high molecular weight keratins particularly stain well-differentiated squamous carcinomas, but they also give less uniform reactivity in poorly differentiated squamous tumors and in some of the large cell anaplastic carcinomas (Fig. 11–1) that presumably represent the least differentiated variety of recognizable squamous carcinoma. Antibodies against low molecular weight keratins stain lung adenocarcinomas much the same as adenocarcinomas of other organs, but also show variable reactivity for squamous carcinomas. Oat cell carcinomas also are frequently posi-

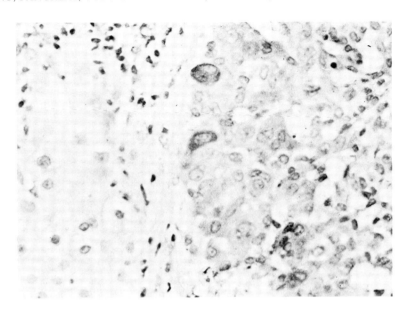

Figure 11–1. Large cell anaplastic tumor of lung (right) showing occasional cells with cytoplasmic reactivity for high molecular weight keratin. Low molecular weight keratin was present more extensively. Bronchial cartilage is seen on the left side of the field. Paraffin section, AEC with hematoxylin counterstain (×320). For discussion of keratins see Chapters 13 and 14.

tive. For example, Battifora and Kopinski (1985), using an antikeratin antibody designated AE1, which is reactive against low and intermediate molecular weight keratins (molecular weight 40 to 56kd), have reported that all squamous carcinomas of lung are positive, as are all adenocarcinomas and about 50 percent of carcinoids. Staining may be patchy or focal in some cases; these nonetheless are considered positive. Doctors Said, Banks-Schlegel, and others (Table 11–1) have provided good evidence that differential staining with antikeratin monoclonal antibodies, having specificity against different keratin subsets, will prove to be of value in separating the different histologic types of lung cancer. However, more experience is needed, and the adverse effects of fixation require clarification. In our hands, antibodies against "squamous" and "nonsquamous" keratin do provide useful, if not absolute, discrimination in paraffin sections, and monoclonal antibodies against squamous carcinoma, adenocarcinoma, and small cell carcinoma hold great promise, not only for immunohistology but also for radio-immunologic studies.

CEA and Epithelial (Milk–Fat Globule) Membrane Antigen

CEA reactivity has been reported in 30 to 100 percent of lung carcinomas; staining is more intense in adenocarcinomas, but weaker reactivity has been described in up to 100 percent of squamous tumors. Reactivity

for CEA cannot be used to distinguish primary lung adenocarcinoma from metastatic deposits, nor can it be used to separate squamous tumor from adenocarcinoma or either of these from small cell carcinoma, which also may be positive, albeit less frequently (Table 11–1). Again, care must be taken to use CEA antibodies that are free of NCA activity. Limitations also exist for the use of milk–fat globule membrane antibodies for the distinction of metastatic breast carcinoma from primary lung adenocarcinoma. Many of the antisera to milk–fat globule membrane antibody show significant cross reactivity with normal lung and therefore may be expected to show reactivity against primary lung adenocarcinoma (Fig. 11–2). Following extensive absorption, the specificity of these antibodies to breast can be enhanced, but absolute specificity probably cannot be achieved. Antibody to epithelial membrane antigen is best considered as a broad spectrum antibody reactive against many types of adenocarcinoma and cannot be used to differentiate the different glandular organs of origin.

Other antibodies explored, but of limited utility for diagnostic purposes, include antibodies to lactoferrin, alpha$_1$-antitrypsin, pregnancy-specific glycoprotein (SP1), human placental lactogen (HPL), hCG, calcitonin, IgA, and secretory piece (Table 11–1). SP1 has been detected in up to 80 percent of lung cancers, and HPL in 20 percent. Neither appear to have diagnostic value. Similarly hCG, although found in 10 to 40 percent of tumors of lung (Fig. 11–3), has no known significance. Calcitonin reactivity may

Table 11–1. Selected Bibliography: Lung Carcinomas

Harach et al 1983	Study of 101 lung cancers: positivity for CEA in 70%, pregnancy-specific glycoprotein in 68%, hCG in 36%, placental lactogen in 20%, and calcitonin in 14%; no correlation with histology
Singh et al 1984	Used surfactant apoprotein as marker of type II pneumocytes; approximately 25% of 100 lung adenocarcinomas positive; paraffin sections
Singh et al 1981	Included EM study of surfactant immunostaining
Dairaku et al 1983	Surfactant staining of normal type II pneumocytes; other lung cells negative; 50% of 55 bronchiolo-alveolar carcinomas positive
Espinoza et al 1984a	Keratin, surfactant, IgA, and CEA were positive in bronchiolo-alveolar carcinoma; hCG and AFP, negative
Eckert 1983	Alpha$_1$-antitrypsin in 75% of bronchial carcinomas
Bowes et al 1981	Lactoferrin in bronchial glands
Bhagavan et al 1982	Factor VIII antigen defining a sclerosing epithelioid angiosarcoma of lung
Brooks & Ernst 1984	Secretory piece positive in 40% of lung cancers (also 50% of breast and 90% of colon cancers); no staining of ovarian, prostatic, biliary, pancreatic or gastric carcinomas
Sehested et al 1981	CEA in small cell carcinoma
Sappino et al 1983	Keratin in 20% of small cell carcinomas; no prognostic significance
Sun NC et al 1983	CEA and NCA in 130 lung cancers; reported some correlation with histologic type
Okamura et al 1984	CEA in 90% of adenocarcinomas, 100% of squamous carcinomas, and a minority of large cell and small cell carcinomas; staining was weak in squamous cases but strong in adenocarcinomas
Said et al 1983	Keratins in lung tumors; squamous carcinoma stained for both low and high MW keratin; adenocarcinomas for low MW keratin only; mesotheliomas (and mesothelial cells) were strongly positive for high MW keratin
Gusterson et al 1982	Antisera to whole (callus) keratin positive in all squamous carcinomas, 80% of adenocarcinomas, 50% of large cell and 10% of small cell carcinomas
Banks-Schlegel et al 1984	"Keratin profiles"—a distinctive 44-kd MW keratin in squamous tumors; poorly differentiated tumors showed lesser amounts
Kasai et al 1981	Lung cancer–associated membrane antigen
DeSchryver-Kecskemeti et al 1979	"Oat cell" plasma membrane antigen appears to be marker for neurosecretory granules: positive in 12/17 oat cell carcinomas
Sikora & Wright 1981	Human monoclonals to lung cancer-associated antigens
Veltri et al 1980	Lung squamous carcinoma–associated antigen
Mazauric et al 1982	Panel of monoclonals to lung cancer antigens, cross reactivity to other tumors and various normal tissues
De Leij et al 1984	"Anti–small cell carcinoma" antibodies—7 monoclonals
Mulshine et al 1983	"Anti–small cell carcinoma" antibodies
Broers et al 1985	Small cell carcinomas contain cytokeratin
Cuttitta et al 1978 ⎱ Minna et al 1981 ⎰	Production of anti–lung cancer antibodies
Bunn et al 1985	Natural killer antibody (NK1, Leu 7) positive in 80% of small cell carcinomas
Wachner et al 1984a	CEA, hCG, keratin, and SP1 (pregnancy-specific glycoprotein) in 129 cases of lung cancer; keratin only in squamous cancer; CEA positive in 80% overall, hCG in 10%
Tsutsumi et al 1983	Calcitonin and "gastrin-releasing peptide" (bombesinlike) in bronchial cells
Nathrath et al 1985	Tissue polypeptide antigen (TPA) in almost all simple and stratified epithelia but not in epidermis, renal tubules, myoepithelial cells, hepatocytes, or glandular acini

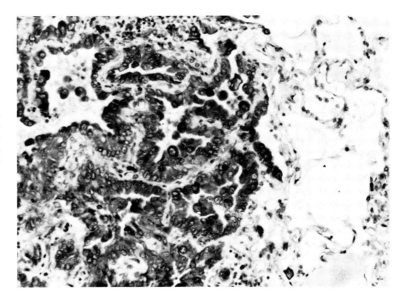

Figure 11–2. Adenocarcinoma in lung (primary) showing reactivity with a broad-specificity antibody to epithelial membrane antigen (EMA). Paraffin section, AEC with hematoxylin counterstain (×200).

correlate with the neuroendocrine group (discussed later). Reactivity for IgA is not uncommon in glandular epithelium, its presence being related to the production of secretory piece (component) for the transport of IgA across epithelial surfaces (particularly respiratory tract, breast, and colon). Staining for secretory piece is thus of interest, being present in 40 percent of lung cancers, 50 percent of breast cancers, and 90 percent of colon cancers (Brooks and Ernst, 1984); ovarian, prostatic, biliary, pancreatic and gastric cancers are negative. Alpha$_1$-antitrypsin reactivity is typical of yolk sac tumors and hepatomas; however, Eckert (1983) reported 75

percent of bronchial carcinomas as positive (we have seen a much lower incidence). Carcinoid and neurogenic tumors were described as negative.

Lung-Specific Antibodies

Nonetheless, some progress has been made toward the development of lung-specific antibodies. Several investigators have reported the production of monoclonal antibodies to lung or lung tumor–associated antigens (Fig. 11–4); (Table 11–1). Recently, a panel of monoclonal antibodies has been shown to have some specificity for non–small cell car-

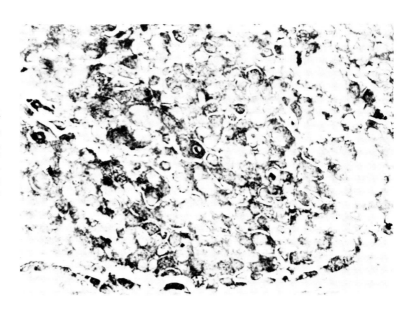

Figure 11–3. Oat cell carcinoma (small cell carcinoma) of lung. This tumor gave positive reactivity for NSE, bombesin, and hCG. Figure shows reactivity with an anti–beta-hCG antibody. Paraffin section, AEC with light hematoxylin counterstain (×320).

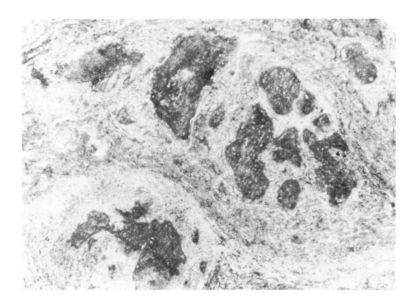

Figure 11–4. Adenocarcinoma of lung treated with a monoclonal antibody that shows reactivity with a panel of primary adenocarcinomas of lung. Positive nests of cells have gray-black cytoplasm. Frozen section, AEC with hematoxylin counterstain (×60). (Antibody from Dr. Pawel Kowski, University of Southern California.)

cinomas as distinct from small cell carcinomas of lung (Mulshine et al, 1983). Other antibodies have been described for squamous cell carcinoma of lung (Veltri et al, 1980), and as discussed above, antikeratin antibodies have been used extensively in an attempt to discriminate between squamous and adenocarcinomas, although this can only be achieved by the selection of antikeratin antibodies with defined reactivity against the different molecular subspecies of keratin (eg, 40kd vs 56kd vs 63kd, etc).

The Ca 1 antibody (so-called cancer 1 antibody), first described by investigators in Oxford (Ashall et al, 1982; McGee et al, 1982), appears to be of relatively little value in recognizing lung malignancy, since although positivity was observed in all tumors,

the antigen also was present on normal alveolar cells (type II pneumocytes—Paradinas et al, 1984). This is a disappointment, because early reports of this antibody were optimistic concerning its value in distinguishing carcinoma cells from normal cells (Fig. 11–5), stating that "Ca 1 does not react with any benign tumour," and also that the "only normal tissues that react are the epithelia of the fallopian tube and the urinary tract." Subsequent studies have reported activity in various other cell types (Table 11–2).

The production and use of antibodies to surfactant apoprotein is of interest (Table 11–1). In normal lung, only the type II pneumocytes are positive, the remaining alveolar and bronchial cells being nonreactive. Among lung cancers, only adenocarcinomas

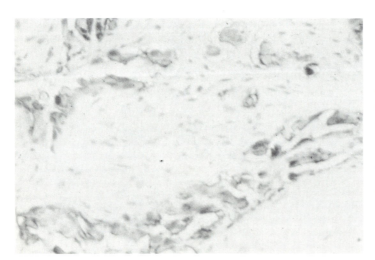

Figure 11–5. Section of bone marrow biopsy showing moderate positivity for Ca 1 antigen within clusters of cells. Although staining for Ca 1 is of limited value in some tissues because of its presence in normal cells, it is of more value in lymph node and marrow, which normally lack Ca 1 positive cells. Paraffin section, AEC with hematoxylin counterstain (×125).

Table 11–2. Selected Bibliography Ca 1 Antigen

Ashall et al 1982 ⎫ Woods et al 1982 ⎬ McGee et al 1982 ⎭	The three initial "new cancer antigen" papers from the Oxford group
Ferguson & Fox 1984a	Ca 1 of no value in discriminating between benign and malignant lesions of ovary
Ferguson & Fox 1984b	Ca 1 of no value in discriminating between benign and malignant endometrium
Bramwell et al 1983	Description of the Ca 1 antigen
Singer et al 1985	Ca 1 in pleural and ascitic fluids; stained 51 of 57 known "malignant" effusions; cells in 7 effusions without conclusive evidence of malignancy were also positive (possible false-positives)
Shabana et al 1983	Ca 1 not sufficiently specific for cancer to be of value in diagnosis of malignancy of oral mucosa
Ghosh et al 1983a, b	Pleural and peritoneal effusions stained with several monoclonal antibodies, including CEA, milk–fat globule membrane, Ca 1, and common leukocyte antigen; noted Ca 1 positivity in some mesothelial cells
Lloyd JM et al 1984b	Ca 1 detected in normal, dysplastic, and neoplastic cervix

are positive, and only a minority (25 to 50 percent) of these. This circumstance has led to speculation that some types of adenocarcinomas are derived from the type II pneumocyte, whereas other types have a different origin (or have lost the antigen). The stain is of diagnostic use, since successful results may be achieved in paraffin sections.

Neuron-Associated Antigens: NSE-HNK1, Bombesin

The role of antibodies versus neuron-associated antigens is somewhat uncertain, but they may be of value in distinguishing so-called neuroendocrine small cell tumors from other lung tumors. Antibodies to bombesin (gastrin-releasing polypeptide in man), neuron-specific enolase, neurofilament antigen,

and neurosecretory granules have all been exploited in this fashion (eg, DeSchryver-Kecskemeti et al, 1979). In our experience, staining for bombesin cannot be reproducibly elicited in formalin paraffin sections unless fixation is optimal and carefully controlled (Fig. 11–6). Good antibodies to bombesin are not widely available. We have had more success in staining for neuron-specific enolase, for which there are a number of sources of antibody. Staining for NSE may be elicited in fixed paraffin sections (Fig. 11–7), although the intensity of staining again is greatly influenced by tissue processing and may be reduced by prolonged exposure to formalin. It is therefore important to utilize positive control tissues exposed to an identical fixation and processing method. An excellent positive control tissue is pancreas (see Fig. 7–1), of which the islets of Langerhans

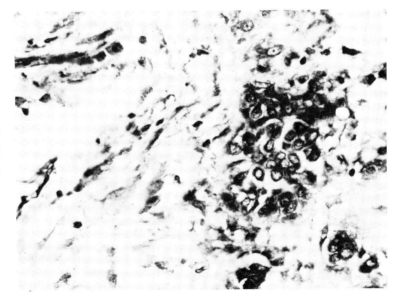

Figure 11–6. Small cell carcinoma in lung showing positivity for bombesin; parathormone also was positive. Paraffin section, DAB with hematoxylin counterstain (×320).

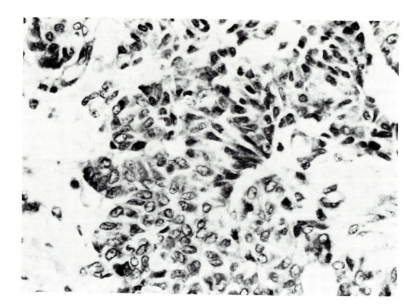

Figure 11–7. Small cell carcinoma of lung showing variable cytoplasmic staining (gray-black) for neuron specific enolase (NSE). Paraffin section, DAB with hematoxylin counterstain (×200).

show excellent staining for NSE, even in autopsy specimens in which considerable autolysis of the exocrine pancreas may be apparent. Similarly, pancreas, specifically the islets of Langerhans, may be used as a control for antibodies to neurosecretory granules. Oat cell carcinoma and carcinoids are typically positive, with antibodies to neuron-specific enolase, and this fact serves as an excellent distinguishing feature from lymphomas and other small cell tumors that occur in this area.

Other possibilities include the use of one of the monoclonal antibodies against natural killer cells (HNK1 or Leu 7), that in paraffin sections appears to react with neuroendocrine cells and their tumors, including oat cell carcinoma (Bunn et al, 1985). Of 20 small cell carcinomas examined by Bunn, 80 percent showed reactivity with Leu 7, usually within excess of 50 percent of cells staining. Only 20 percent of non–small cell carcinomas were positive; and in those cases, only isolated cells or small cell clusters reacted. Other natural killer antibodies (eg, Leu 11) stained about 30 percent of small cell carcinomas.

Finally, staining for histaminase appears to serve as a good marker of small cell carcinoma (Mendelsohn, 1981). The method is effective in paraffin sections, giving staining of cytoplasm in a varying proportion of tumor cells. Medullary C cell carcinoma of thyroid was also reported as giving similar staining.

Nonepithelial tumors may occur as primary lesions within lung or as metastatic deposits. The recognition of lymphomas is described at length elsewhere. Otherwise, anaplastic tumors that show no evidence of reactivity with antikeratin antibodies or with anti-CEA should be suspected as metastatic sarcomas or as melanoma. The positive recognition of these diverse types of tumors is described elsewhere (see Chapter 14, concerning anaplastic tumors of unknown origin).

LUNG CANCER—MESOTHELIOMA, MESOTHELIAL CELLS

Pathologists particularly are faced with the problems of identifying malignant cells in pleural (or peritoneal) effusions and then separating the different kinds of malignancy that can be found in the pleural space: the primary differential diagnosis rests among malignant mesothelioma, lung adenocarcinoma, and metastatic adenocarcinoma.

In fine-needle aspirates or cytologic preparations from pleural effusions, it may be difficult or impossible to recognize with certainty the occasional cancer cell among a population of reactive mesothelial cells. Immunostaining may then be of particular value (Fig. 11–8). In theory cytologic preparations are more suitable for immunohistologic studies than formalin-fixed paraffin sections, since the antigens have been subjected to less abuse. Immunostains for CEA and keratin

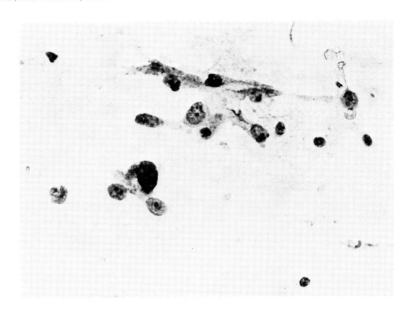

Figure 11–8. Malignant cells in pleural effusion showing variable cytoplasmic reactivity (gray) with monoclonal antibody to low molecular weight ("nonsquamous") keratin. Antibody to high molecular weight ("squamous") keratin gave no detectable staining. Diagnosis: probable adenocarcinoma, since both squamous carcinoma and mesothelial cells would stain strongly for high molecular weight keratin (see Chapter 13). Alcohol-fixed cell smear, AEC with hematoxylin counterstain (×320).

have been utilized for this purpose; they are effective in air-dried or ethanol-fixed cytopreparations and in formalin-fixed paraffin sections of cell blocks. Minor disagreements among different investigators almost certainly reflect either the fixation or processing employed, or the exact specificity of the antibodies used (eg, with anti-CEA, whether or not anti-NCA activity has been removed). Most investigators agree that CEA staining is helpful (Table 11–3). Some reports have described CEA reactivity as restricted to adenocarcinoma, with mesothelioma and reactive mesothelial cells totally negative; others have described weak reactivity for CEA in mesothelioma.

Keratin, especially high molecular weight (63kd) keratin, stains intensely in mesothelioma (reactive or malignant) but is not present in adenocarcinoma (low molecular weight [MW] keratins are present, and broad–spectrum antikeratin antisera are not helpful in

Table 11–3. Selected Bibliography: Pleural Effusions—Mesothelial Cells Versus Cancer-Mesothelioma

Whitaker D et al 1982	CEA positive in most (adeno)carcinomas, negative in mesothelioma
Corson & Pinkus 1982	Mesotheliomas strongly keratin-positive, CEA-negative (in 11 cases), or weak (in 8 cases); adenocarcinoma showed strong CEA and weak keratin; keratin in mesothelioma cells was diffuse, in adenocarcinoma cells peripheral
Marshall RJ et al 1984	CEA present in 22 of 27 carcinomas, absent in 16 mesotheliomas, absent in reactive mesothelium; antibodies to milk–fat globule membrane (HMFG1 and 2) were positive in most carcinomas and some mesotheliomas but not in reactive mesothelium
Walts et al 1983	Fine-needle aspirates; reactive mesothelium strongly keratin-positive, weak or negative CEA
Walts et al 1984	Mesothelial cells, high MW keratin; adenocarcinoma cells, low MW keratin
Kahn et al 1982	Prekeratin in mesothelial cells (peripheral pattern) also positive in adenocarcinoma (arborizing pattern)
Kyrkou et al 1985	Peritoneal fluid cells: lysozyme-positive, CEA-negative usually indicated nonmalignant process
Loosli & Hurlimann 1984	CEA, keratin, milk–fat globule membrane antigen and factor VIII antigen: CEA usually weak or negative in mesothelioma but keratin positive
Orell & Dowling 1983	CEA, AFP, SP1, placental alkaline phosphatase: negative in nonmalignant effusions, negative in mesothelioma, positive in 60% of carcinomas; CEA was best indicator of malignancy
Holden J & Churg 1984	CEA in adenocarcinoma; negative or weak in mesothelioma; keratin positive in about 50% of each tumor type
Kabawat et al 1983	OC125 antibody versus celomic cells (mesothelium, plus Mullerian duct derivatives)
Epenetos et al 1982	Detection of carcinoma cells in pleural effusions

this respect). Different patterns of keratin reactivity, whether homogeneous or diffuse, have been described by some investigators but findings are contradictory (Table 11–3). This circumstance may be due to differences in fixation or differences in antibody.

The most useful antibody for recognizing mesothelium would appear to be the monoclonal antibody OC125, against the so-called celomic antigen (Kabawat et al, 1983). Mesothelial cells stain positively; adenocarcinomas (with the notable exception of many ovarian adenocarcinomas) are nonreactive. The antibody is available commercially but is not effective in paraffin sections.

PANCREATIC CARCINOMAS

The tumors of the islet cells of the pancreas, like their normal counterparts, often produce hormones and are logically included under the broad designation of neuroendocrine tumors (Chapter 8). Immunostaining to determine the nature and patterns of production of these hormones, which include insulin, glucagon, somatostatin, gastrin, and vasointestinal polypeptide can be diagnostically useful and may contribute to planned management. This application is true not only for pancreatic islet cell neoplasms but also for other neuroendocrine cell–derived neoplasms in the intestine, and it is discussed more extensively elsewhere (see Chapter 8). Examples include the demonstration of gastrin-producing neoplasms within the pan-

creas in relation to recurrent peptic ulcer (Zollinger-Ellison syndrome). Occasionally, these tumors behave as true carcinomas; even so, their neuroendocrine origin is usually identifiable by the presence upon immunostaining of a small number of cells producing one or another of the "islet cell hormones." These tumors are thus distinguishable from those of the exocrine pancreas.

The histologic diagnosis of pancreatic carcinoma often occurs too late for effective surgical intervention, the disease having extended beyond resectable margins prior to surgical exploration and biopsy. Fine-needle aspiration of suspected pancreatic masses might advance the time of diagnosis but is cytologically difficult. As described below, immunocytochemical stains for tumor-associated antigens may be helpful in distinguishing atypical epithelium in inflammatory lesions from carcinoma. CEA positivity is encountered much more often in carcinoma (Fig. 11–9) and is more intense in carcinoma compared to inflamed epithelium. However, not all carcinomas of the pancreas are CEA-positive. Ca 1 (cancer 1) antibody might also be expected to be positive in pancreatic carcinoma and negative in normal pancreas, but in view of the increasing numbers of reports describing Ca 1 in normal tissues (eg, breast and lung), some reservations must be retained concerning the use of this antibody in pancreas carcinoma.

Ascribing a metastasis of unknown origin to a primary site in the pancreas is a different problem for which there is at this time no

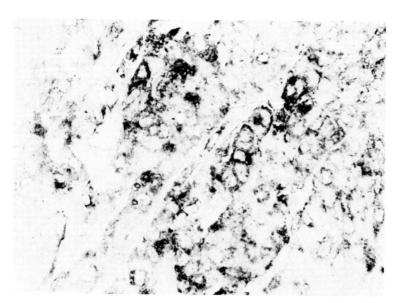

Figure 11–9. Anaplastic tumor showing reactivity for CEA. Paraffin section, AEC, counterstain omitted to display relatively sparse staining more effectively in a black and white medium (×320). This was a pancreatic carcinoma.

Table 11–4. Selected Bibliography: Pancreas-Specific Antigens and Tumor Antigens

Loor et al 1981	Isolated a pancreas-specific antigen from saline extract, prepared antibody, and showed immunohistochemical localization in acinar cells
Metzgar et al 1982	Utilized monoclonal antibodies reactive with pancreatic carcinoma cells; some showed reactivity with fetal tissues
Klavins 1981	CEA and AFP produced by some pancreatic cancers; pancreatic oncofetal antigen is produced by the majority of pancreatic cancers and cross-reacts with some other carcinomas (serologic study)
Schmiegel et al 1981	Oncofetal pancreatic cancer–associated antigen MW 40,000 (detected in pancreatic juice and serum); serum positive in 80% of sera of pancreatic carcinoma patients; not CEA or NCA
Shimano et al 1981	Pancreatic cancer–associated antigen, MW 1,000,000, located in ductal epithelial cells and found elevated in serum of 70% of patients with pancreatic cancer (25% of other cancers also positive)
Oguchi et al 1984	Serum assays of a pancreatic oncofetal antigen
Sindelar et al 1983	Antiserum to hamster pancreas cross-reacts with normal pancreas and pancreatic cancer (but not with other cancers)
Borowitz et al 1984	Antibody versus pancreatic cancer also reacts with carcinomas of gall bladder and stomach but not of other sites
Tsutsumi et al 1984	NCA (nonspecific cross-reacting antigen) present in ducts of normal pancreas; CEA not detectable in normals but present in cancers; monoclonal and conventional antibodies
Horie et al 1984	Serum CEA levels and pancreatic cancer; in most cases levels not elevated
Murao et al 1983	Staining for amylase and alpha$_1$-antitrypsin to confirm pancreatic origin
Amouric et al 1982	Kallikrein in acinar cells (immunoperoxidase and protein A-immunogold methods)
Aho et al 1983	Altered distribution of trypsin in pancreatitis

final solution. Although pancreas-specific antigens have been reported (Table 11–4), both their availability and our experience with them are limited. CEA is positive in most pancreatic carcinomas to some degree, but this reaction does not facilitate distinction between carcinoma of pancreatic origin and that from colon, stomach, breast, lung, and other organs. Likewise, all pancreatic carcinomas are positive with antibodies to low molecular weight keratin, certainly separating potential pancreatic carcinoma from lymphomas or sarcomas but not further specifying among the adenocarcinomas.

There have been reports of pancreatic tumor–associated antigens. The exact identity of the antigens described (Table 11–4) is still unclear, nor have there been detailed studies of the distribution of many of these antigens in other tissues of the body. At least some of the reported antibodies show cross reactivity with fetal pancreas; thus they may be considered oncofetal antigens similar to, but distinct from, CEA and alpha-fetoprotein (AFP), and also separate from NCA. With increased utilization, some of these antibodies may prove to be of value in assigning a pancreatic origin to a poorly differentiated metastatic tumor; however, at least one of the antibodies (Shimano et al, 1981) is found in other cancers (lung, colon, breast) with sufficient frequency to render it useless for this purpose. The

possibility of serologic assays for antigen released into serum has also been explored, and there have even been reports of use of these reagents for therapy.

Pancreatic carcinomas may express CEA (in up to 50 percent of cases) (Fig. 11–9) and less often AFP. The extent of CEA reactivity is usually considerably less than is seen in colonic or gastric carcinomas. CEA is said not to be present in normal pancreas; however, NCA is present, and because many antisera to CEA also react with NCA, this presence may lead to erroneous interpretation. Epithelial membrane antigen (see Chapter 10) is also expressed in pancreatic carcinoma cells, and many antisera to milk–fat globule membrane (mammary epithelial membrane antigen) cross react with pancreas. Finally, antibodies to low molecular weight keratin (so-called nonsquamous keratin—Chapter 13) show extensive reactivity with pancreatic cancer cells. Staining for kallikrein, amylase, alpha$_1$-antitrypsin, and trypsin has also been reported (Table 11–4), but is of limited utility. The demonstration of laminin (Haglund et al, 1984) has been advanced as of potential value in distinguishing pancreatitis from carcinoma: in the former the laminin of the basement membrane is intact, in the latter it is disrupted. A similar approach has been advocated for other tumors, but interpretation is difficult.

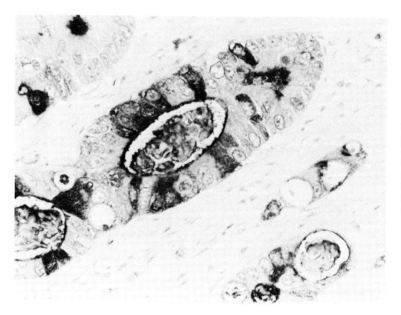

Figure 11–10. Well-differentiated colon cancer showing a minority of cells with intense reactivity for CEA throughout the cytoplasm. Other cells show apical staining, and the luminal secretions appear positive. Paraffin section, DAB with hematoxylin counterstain (×500).

COLORECTAL AND GASTRIC CARCINOMAS

CEA

The presence of carcinoembryonic antigen (CEA) in colonic cancer has long been recognized. There was initial optimism that measurement of serum levels of serum CEA might be of value in early detection of carcinoma of colon. This hope proved largely unfounded, since elevated serum CEA levels were detected in patients with other tumors and in a number of non-neoplastic conditions. Immunohistologic studies have since revealed the presence of CEA in many tissues developed from the embryonic endoderm, including derivative neoplasms. Serum CEA levels correlate with histochemical reactivity; the level of serum CEA, reflects the degree of production by individual tumor cells, the proportion of tumor cells secreting CEA, and the total tumor bulk (cell number). Invasion and tumor cell necrosis may produce higher levels for some positive tumors. Within tumor tissue, immunohistochemical methods are

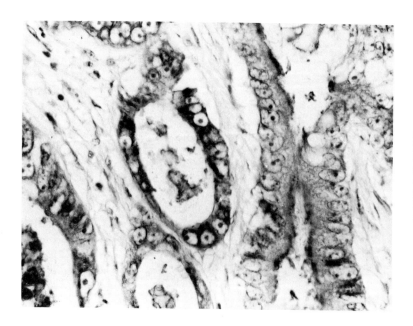

Figure 11–11. Carcinoma of stomach stained for CEA. A positive reaction (black) is observed in the cytoplasm of some cells and at the luminal surface of others. Some carcinoma cells appear negative. Paraffin section, DAB with hematoxylin counterstain (×320).

able to detect CEA at levels below 3 μg/gm of tumor tissue; theoretically, one positive cell among several hundred thousand is detectable. Staining is effective in formalin paraffin sections, although the distribution and intensity of staining may differ from that seen in frozen sections. Fixation in ethanol seems to emphasize cytoplasmic staining.

Foremost among positive tumors is colon cancer (Fig. 11–10), but carcinomas of pancreas (Fig. 11–9), stomach (Fig. 11–11), and lung also commonly show varying degrees of positivity (Table 11–5). Up to one third of breast cancers have also been described as

Table 11–5. Percentage of Malignant Tumors Showing CEA Positivity*

Tumor	Location	CEA Positive (%)
Squamous carcinoma	Skin	0
	Cervix	50–70
	Lung	50–80
	Esophagus	0
Mesothelioma		0
Adenocarcinoma	Stomach	50–100
	Colorectal	80–100
	Pancreas	30–100
	Small intestine	80–100
	Lung (adeno)	70–100
	Breast	30–60
	Prostate	0–10
	Hepatoma	0–10
	Ovary	
	mucinous	80–100
	serous	0–30
	Endocervix	30–80
	Endometrium	20–80
	Thyroid	
	Medullary	up to 100
	Follicular	0–20
Transitional carcinoma	Bladder	Occasional
Teratomas	Testis/ovary	Occasional in differentiated elements
Myoblastoma		100
Chordomas		Occasional (weak)
Gliomas		0
Lymphomas		0
Other sarcomas (muscle, liposarcoma, fibrosarcoma, etc)		0
Melanomas		0

*From the literature. Note that some of these figures probably are falsely high due to NCA reactivity in the anti-CEA antibodies employed. This possibility may also account for the broad range. Note that the benign counterparts of these lesions usually contain much less or no detectable CEA (eg, mucinous cystadenoma of ovary—about 20%–30% positive), but this is not always true (eg, in C cell hyperplasia of thyroid CEA [or NCA] often is positive).

positive by immunocytochemical methods. The intensity of staining for CEA and the proportion and distribution of positive cells may be of value in distinguishing malignant colon from normal colon, but the distinction is less than absolute, for proliferating non-neoplastic colon also shows scattered positive cells. Thus attempts to determine the malignant potential of colonic polyps by the extent of CEA staining have met with variable success in the hands of different investigators (Ahnen et al, 1982; Wagener et al, 1981a; Neffen et al, 1980—Table 11–6).

The net result is that staining of a colonic or rectal biopsy for CEA is of strictly limited value in the diagnosis of carcinoma. Although it is true that intense reactivity for CEA in the cytoplasm of all cells would be highly suggestive of malignancy, such a finding should only serve to support a diagnosis that is tenable on a cytologic basis. In the opposite situation, lack of reactivity for CEA is not proof of the benign nature of a lesion. Isaacson and Le Vann (1976) had earlier reached the conclusion that CEA positivity indicates malignancy, in situ carcinoma, or premalignancy.

Likewise, the typical "polar" distribution of CEA in non-neoplastic colon cells typically is lost in cancer, but gradations exist and are difficult to assess reliably (Fig. 11–10). Hasleton et al (1980) thought that definite CEA staining in a polyp represents "functional malignancy" prior to histologic evidence; loss of polar distribution of staining would reinforce this view.

CEA staining does have value in certain defined situations. First, it may be very helpful in searching resected lymph nodes for rare, well-differentiated carcinoma cells in that it is abnormal to find CEA-positive cells in lymph nodes. Similarly, staining for CEA is helpful in evaluating bone marrow smears, aspirate sections, or trephine biopsies. Second, in tumors of unknown origin, whether situated in the abdomen or elsewhere, strong CEA reactivity should prompt a careful study of the GI tract, especially the colon. Lung or breast cancers are not excluded; ovarian and endometrial cancers remain possibilities. Sarcomas, including lymphomas, are effectively excluded, as are melanomas. Prostatic carcinoma is typically CEA-negative; rare, weakly reactive cases have been described.

Absence of CEA reactivity in a lesion makes origin from colon highly unlikely (in the presence of appropriate controls). In our

Table 11–6. Selected Bibliography Carcinoembryonic Antigen (CEA)—Colorectal Tumors

Primus et al 1981	Excellent comprehensive review of immunohistology of CEA
Wiley et al 1981	CEA in 41 colonic carcinomas plus 15 metastases; also stained for blood group antigens
Ahnen et al 1982	CEA at light and EM levels within goblet cells of small intestine and columnar and goblet cells of colon; polar distribution, seen on normal epithelium, is lost in cancer
Heidl 1982	CEA (or CEA-like substance) at high levels in colon cancer, slightly less in stomach cancer; little if any in melanoma, prostatic cancer, basal cell carcinoma, and various sarcomas
Miwa et al 1980	CEA in colorectal neoplasms in Japan
Lascano et al 1979	CEA in colorectal neoplasms in Argentina
Sharkey et al 1980	Compared indirect conjugate with bridge method for detecting CEA; preferred the former
O'Brien et al 1980	CEA and epithelial membrane antigen in pleural and peritoneal fluid; compared to cytologic criteria
Pascal & Slovin 1980	Glomerular immune complexes in a patient with gastric cancer contain CEA
Harrowe & Taylor 1981	CEA in adenocarcinoma of colon in routinely processed blocks stored up to 40 years
Avagnina et al 1980	CEA in benign and malignant colonic tumors
Wagener et al 1981a	CEA staining reflects proliferative activity of colonic epithelial cells; high in carcinoma, in epithelium adjacent to carcinoma, and in ulcerative colitis
Goslin et al 1981	Gland-forming or signet cell colorectal carcinomas most often CEA-positive; serum CEA levels can then be used to monitor therapy and relapse
Gray et al 1984	CEA in recognition of metastases in bone marrow trephine biopsies
Friedman & Mills 1983	CEA not useful in assessing degree of dysplasia in ulcerative colitis
O'Brien et al 1981	Assessment of diagnostic value of CEA in colorectal tissue—valuable in recognizing cancer cells
Neffen et al 1980	CEA in glycocalyx in normal colon and benign polyps; poorly differentiated carcinoma often shows loss of glycocalyceal CEA with cytoplasmic positivity; absence of CEA in a metastatic adenocarcinoma makes origin from colon unlikely
Hasleton et al 1980	CEA staining in polyps reveals "functional malignancy" before histologic evidence of malignancy is found
Au et al 1984	CEA in all colorectal cancers; could not be used to distinguish prognostic groups
Hamada et al 1985	CEA tissue and serum levels, correlations
Hedin et al 1982	8 CEA monoclonals: 2 reacted also with NCA; recognized at least 6 different CEA epitopes
Colcher et al 1983	5 CEA monoclonals vs different epitopes: suggested some differential staining of different types of cancer
Wagener et al 1984	5 CEA monoclonals: binding to several tumor types; cross reactivity (NCA) present (granulocytes positive)

experience staining may be evident in only a small proportion of tumor cells, and reactivity may vary in different areas of the tumor. Definite positive cells at a frequency of 5 percent or even less are, in our experience, significant.

One caveat with CEA staining, referred to elsewhere, relates to the specificity of the antibody for CEA. Antisera (containing polyclonal antibodies) to CEA frequently contain activity against NCA, a cross-reacting antigen present in normal tissues. This is difficult to adsorb out (repeated adsorption with granulocytes, which contain NCA, may be effective). Even monoclonal antibodies, thought to be CEA-specific, may react with NCA (Table 11–6). On a practical level, NCA reactivity in a CEA reagent may be suspected if the granulocytes appear strongly reactive (Fig. 11–12; Pattengale et al, 1980). Interpretation of a CEA stain under such circumstances must be cautious, for NCA activity is widely distributed, not only in many tumor types but also in normal tissues.

Carcinoembryonic antigen activity has also been utilized in the differential diagnosis of tumors of skin adnexae: sweat gland tumors may be positive (like breast tumors); other adnexal tumors are nonreactive. In the differential diagnosis of carcinoma of the endometrium from carcinoma of the cervix, the situation is less straightforward, with conflicting reports as described in relation to uterine tumors. In brief, invasive squamous carcinomas may show scattered positivity (30 percent overall); 80 to 100 percent of endocervical carcinomas are positive, and in endometrial carcinomas positivity is patchy, 10 to 30 percent of cases showing some reactivity. As might be expected for the "first" possible cancer-specific marker, there is a very extensive literature pertaining to CEA; some of

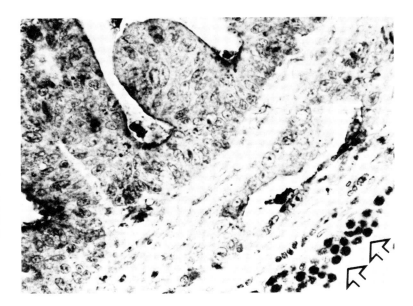

Figure 11–12. Pattern of staining in a colonic carcinoma treated with an antiserum to carcinoembryonic antigen (CEA). Staining of apex of tumor cells plus irregular positivity in the cytoplasm is typical for CEA in colon cancer. However, staining of granulocytes in an acutely inflamed vessel (arrows) strongly suggests that this anti-CEA antiserum also contains significant antibody to NCA (normal cross-reacting antigen) (see text). Paraffin section, AEC with hematoxylin counterstain (×320).

the more recent immunohistologic studies are listed in Tables 11–6 and 11–7.

Other Intestinal Antigens

Colorectal carcinoma has been extensively studied for potential markers. Several antigens of potential interest have been described; some may distinguish malignant from normal colonic epithelial cells (eg, Herlyn M et al, 1979; Atkinson et al, 1982; and Table 11–8). One of the better characterized markers is the so-called GI tract carcinoma antigen (GICA; Table 11–8). This marker is a monosialoganglioside that has some struc-

Table 11–7. Selected Bibliography: CEA in Gastric Carcinoma and Tumors Other Than Colorectal Cancer

Janunger et al 1979	CEA in gastric biopsy specimens: present much more frequently in malignant and premalignant biopsies (70%) than in non-neoplastic states (10%)
Wurster & Rapp 1979	Emphasized use of "immunoadsorbed" CEA in marking dysplastic gastric epithelium
Nishida 1983	CEA in 80% of gastric cancers: cytoplasmic and apical staining; loss of apical stain in poorly differentiated lesions
Kojimao O et al 1984a	70/162 gastric cancers strongly CEA positive; these had worse prognosis than negative or weakly positive cases (independent of histology)
Kojimao O et al 1984b	Colorectal cancer shows more intense CEA staining than gastric cancer
Higgins et al 1984	Antibody to fetal tissue (antigen undefined) reacts with gastric dysplasia and cancer
Hockey et al 1984	CEA positivity in 90% of primary gastric cancer and 80% of metastases
Nielsen K & Teglbjaerg 1982	Different CEA patterns correlated with histologic subtypes of gastric cancer
Seifert & Caselitz 1983	CEA and keratins in parotid tumors
De Boer et al 1981	Glandular metaplasia of gallbladder represents a form of intestinal metaplasia, is CEA positive, and should be considered premalignant; also stained for large and small intestinal mucin antigens
Albores-Saavedra et al 1983	Gall bladder cancer CEA-positive (lesser positivity in normal gall bladder); all "in situ" carcinomas also CEA positive
Wahlström et al 1980	Use of CEA for differential diagnosis of adenocarcinoma of uterus and carcinoma of cervix
Shevchuk et al 1980	CEA in Brenner tumors taken as evidence of transitional cell nature
Robertson et al 1981	Malignant granular cell tumor (myoblastoma) positive for CEA
Shevchuk et al 1981	CEA positive in transitional epithelium and at reduced levels in transitional cell carcinoma
Nielsen K et al 1983	CEA in granular cell myoblastoma
Penneys et al 1981, 1982a	CEA in eccrine sweat glands and in sweat gland carcinomas; identifies these lesions as derived from eccrine or apocrine adnexal epithelium
Caselitz et al 1981b	CEA in acinar and intercalated duct cells of parotid

Table 11–8. Selected Bibliography: Cancer-Associated Antigens (Other Than CEA) in Colorectal and Gastric Cancer

Skinner & Whitehead 1982	Analysis of gastric carcinoma, atrophic gastritis, and intestinal metaplasia; found "colon-specific antigen" and SP1 were closely linked to cancer bu also were present in the metaplastic cells in cancer cases; also examined CEA, AFP, transferrin, hCG, placental lactogen, and ferritin
Sato & Spicer 1982	Utilized peanut–lectin-peroxidase in EM study of glycoproteins in gastric epithelium
Kumpulainen 1979	Demonstration of carbonic anhydrase localization
Sato et al 1980	Ultrastructural localization of carbonic anhydrase in gastric parietal cells (role in acid production)
Rapp & Wurster 1981	Antibody to "chief cell esterase" revealed alterations of numbers of chief cells in gastritis and cancer
Tahara et al 1982	Detected immunostaining for lysozyme in 40% of 171 gastric cancers; most of positive cases were mucin-producing adenocarcinomas (including signet ring cases); lysozyme-positive case showed poor prognosis
Skinner & Whitehead 1981	Placental alkaline phosphatase detected in slightly less than half of the cases of gastric cancer (and colon and rectal cancer); statistical difference between positivity in cancer cases and in normal tissues but not sufficient to serve as a reliable histologic indicator of malignancy
Uchida et al 1981	Placental alkaline phosphatase in a case of gastric cancer; tumor also produced hCG and was CEA-positive
Ma et al 1982	Normal colon contains "large intestinal mucin antigen" (LIMA), also present in some nonmucinous cancers of colon; normal colon does not contain "small intestinal mucin antigen" (SIMA), present in the adult only in duodenum and jejunum; mucinous colon cancer positive for SIMA; CEA present in the nonmucinous cases; concluded that colon cancer developed in areas of metaplastic change
Gold 1981	Discussed role of "colonic mucoprotein antigen" as a marker for colon cancer; 60% of colon cancers were positive; gastric, pancreatic, and lung cancers were negative, as were 4 out of 5 ovarian cystadenocarcinomas
Finan et al 1982	Used immunohistochemical method for initial screening of antibodies versus colonic epithelium
MacLean et al 1982	Some monoclonal antibodies with anti-Ia activity show reactivity against colon cancer cell lines
Yachi et al 1983	Monoclonal reactive with normal stomach and with gastric and colonic cancer (not CEA)
Atkinson et al 1982	Monoclonal to monosialoganglioside antigen; effective in paraffin sections (59% colonic, 80% pancreatic, 89% gastric cancers)
Arends et al 1983b	Monoclonal (116NS19–9) to monosialoganglioside antigen (GICA—gastrointestinal cancer–associated antigen); reacts with tumor and colon adjacent to tumor, not normal colon; some in stomach; some reaction with normal endocervix, pancreas, and gall bladder
Olding et al 1984	Monoclonal (S19–9) versus GICA in fetal small intestine and bronchus, not colon
Raux et al 1983	Reported GICA in fetal GI tract and biliary and pancreatic ducts only
Arends et al 1984	Of 311 colorectal cancers, 11% were uniformly GICA positive; these tended to behave more aggressively than negative tumors (36% of total) or focally reactive tumors (53%)
Daar & Fabre 1983	Heterogeneity of staining of colorectal tumors with monoclonal antibodies; including anti-HLA–DR (Ia-like) antigens
Selby et al 1983	HLA-DR (Ia) in normal colon; decreased in inflammatory states (Crohn's and ulcerative colitis)
Zweibaum et al 1984	Monoclonal antibodies to small intestinal brush border hydrolases
Slocombe et al 1980	Blood groups A and B and H antigens in gastric cancer; no clear relationship to differentiation
Nardelli J et al 1983	3 monoclonals distinguish goblet cells in different parts of gut
Kittas et al 1982	Lysozyme, alpha$_1$-antitrypsin, and alpha$_1$-antichymotrypsin in gastric cancer but not in colon cancer
Capella et al 1984	Lysozyme in 35% of gastric cancers
Wiley et al 1981	Blood group substances in 30% of colon cancer
Orntoft et al 1985	T antigen in 72% of colon cancers
Hsu & Raine 1982	Peanut lectin (T antigen) staining in colon cancer
Allen et al 1985	Progressive loss of "secretory component" in dysplasia and cancer of stomach
Sumiyoshi et al 1984	Loss of "secretory component" in poorly differentiated gastric carcinomas; weak staining in well-differentiated cases
Togo et al 1981	"Secretory component" in 45% of gastric cancers; especially intense in signet ring cases
Isaacson P 1982 a,b	Dysplasia and cancer showed reduced secretory component

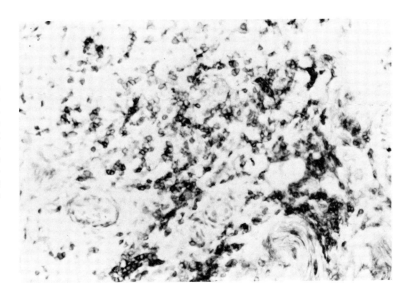

Figure 11–13. Antibody to Ia antigen identifies leukocytes infiltrating mesentery in an area invaded by colonic carcinoma. Occasional carcinoma cells show weak reactivity; such stains are sometimes difficult to interpret due to the excessive numbers of Ia-positive histiocytes and lymphocytes present. Frozen section, AEC with hematoxylin counterstain ($\times 200$).

tural similarity to the Lewis blood group antigens. Recognized by a monoclonal antibody, the antigen has been found on pancreatic and gastric tumors in addition to colon carcinoma. Approximately 60 percent of colon cancers are positive; normal colon is nonreactive, but positivity may be seen adjacent to tumors. Mucin and mucoprotein antigens have also been described and may be of value as "tissue recognition" markers that are present in colon but absent in other tissues. For example, the mucoprotein antigen described by Gold (1981) was detectable in most colon cancers but not in lung, pancreatic, or ovarian cancer (one case of ovarian cancer proved an exception). LIMA (large intestinal mucin antigen—Ma et al, 1982) is found in normal colon and some colon cancers; SIMA (small intestinal mucin antigen) is reported in normal small intestine, not colon, but is present in mucinous colon cancer, offering some potential for distinguishing benign from malignant (premalignant) colon. Reagents such as these are promising and justify further investigation. As yet, experience is insufficient for clinical utility.

Skinner and Whitehead (1981, 1982) described two studies of gastric cancer in which the presence of "colon-specific antigen" and SP1 correlated with the diagnosis of cancer. Also, placental alkaline phosphatase was detected in about half of the cases of gastric cancer studied (plus some colorectal cancers); however, it did not serve as a reliable histologic indicator of malignancy. Other antigens studied were not helpful (including CEA, AFP, and transferrin).

It is noteworthy that Ia-like antigens have been observed in cell lines (of colon cancer—MacLean et al, 1982) and in some fresh tumors (Fig. 11–13); this brings into question the practice recommended by some investigators of using Ia positivity as evidence for identifying lymphoma, as opposed to carcinoma (see Chapter 6).

LIVER: HEPATOMA, HEPATITIS

Immunohistologic techniques have found application within three more or less separate aspects of the interpretation of liver biopsies:
(1) Recognition of primary hepatocellular carcinoma or carcinoma metastatic to liver
(2) Detection of alpha$_1$-antitrypsin deficiency
(3) Detection of hepatitis B virus antigen.

Recognition of Primary Hepatoma and Metastatic Adenocarcinoma

Primary hepatomas (hepatocellular carcinomas) clinically are considered to be positive for alpha-fetoprotein (AFP); typically, they have elevated levels of AFP in the serum and show immunoreactive AFP within tumor cells.

Alpha-fetoprotein is a so-called oncofetal antigen, normally expressed in fetal tissues (liver) (Fig. 11–14), normally absent in adult tissues, but prone to be reexpressed in neoplasms of the adult tissue corresponding to the site of fetal production (principally liver).

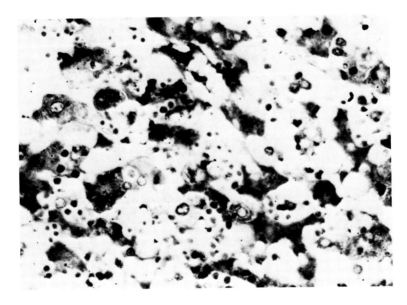

Figure 11–14. Fetal liver displaying intense reactivity for alpha-fetoprotein (AFP). This tissue serves as a good "positive biological control" for AFP staining in germ cell tumors or hepatoma. Paraffin section, AEC with hematoxylin counterstain (×200).

Table 11–9. Selected Bibliography: Liver Hepatoma—Alpha-Fetoprotein (AFP), Alpha₁-Antitrypsin (APT)

Kojiro et al 1981	AFP positive in 70%–90% of hepatocellular carcinomas (the lower percentage based on autopsy cases); albumin also present, inversely related to AFP; AFP not detected in non-neoplastic liver cells
Kuhlmann & Kuhlmann 1982	AFP in regenerating liver cells in experimental animals
Uchino et al 1981	AFP in liver cells (including giant cells) of neonatal hepatis and biliary atresia
Nemoto et al 1982	Pattern of AFP staining in human embryos and fetuses
LeBouton & Masse 1980	Studies of factors influencing distribution of albumin staining in an experimental system
Nakagawara et al 1982	Hepatoblastoma in a 1-year-old; AFP and hCG positive; separate cell populations
Butenandt et al 1980	Hepatoblastoma with hCG positivity
Courtoy et al 1981	Sites of production of fibrinogen, alpha₂-macroglobulin and haptoglobulin in experimental animal
Wolfe & Palmer 1981	Excellent review of AAT in deficiency states, in hepatoma, germ cell tumors, and other cancer
Cohen et al 1982a	AAT in about 50% of hepatomas (with neoplastic cells); South African series
Totović & Kron 1980	AAT in paraffin sections; 10 of 339 cases of cirrhosis positive (correlated with PAS–diastase resistant granules)
Ordóñez & Manning 1984	19/33 hepatomas positive for AAT(in neoplastic cells); 33/33 cases positive for alpha₁-antichymotrypsin
Vecchio et al 1983	AAT in needle biopsies as marker for AAT deficiency
Kelly et al 1979	AAT positive globules in AAT deficiency
Reintoft & Hägerstrand 1979	AAT positive globules indicate carrier state of AAT Z gene; increased incidence in liver cell carcinoma (note Cohen et al 1982—see above—found no correlation of AAT deficiency with carcinoma in South Africa)
Rubel et al 1982	AAT globules in residual normal hepatocytes in patients with hepatoma
Clausen et al 1984	Good review—60 needle biopsies; concluded AAT-positive globules larger than 3 μ reliably indicate the presence of the Pi Z allele; however, only about 50% of Pi Z carriers are detected by this method; the remainder have granules approximately 1 μ diameter, as may occur in other conditions
Bonetti et al 1983	Cholangiocarcinoma positive for epithelial membrane antigen, hepatoma negative
Goodman et al 1985	Cholangiocarcinoma positive for keratin, negative for AFP; hepatoma, the reverse. Both could show CEA and AAT; "combined" tumors showed mixed features
Stromeyer et al 1980	Ground-glass cells in hepatoma stain for fibrinogen
Leader & Jass 1984	Immunostaining for AFP in a primary ileal carcinoma
Espinoza et al 1984b	AFP positive in 3/10 hepatomas, HBsAG in 4/10, and CEA in 3/10 (CEA variable, often more marked in surrounding cirrhotic areas)
Aroni et al 1984	AAT, alpha₁-antichymotrypsin, and lysozyme in adenocarcinoma of gall bladder; variable expression unrelated to histologic type

Figure 11–15. Liver biopsy containing anaplastic tumor cells; staining for AFP (alpha-fetoprotein) shows intense staining of some of the larger cells, with lesser degrees of reactivity in other cells. Paraffin section, AEC with hematoxylin counterstain (×320).

Sections of fetal liver therefore provide excellent "positive controls" for this stain. Alpha-fetoprotein is readily demonstrable by immunoperoxidase methods in paraffin sections with most fixatives. Staining is cytoplasmic with a granular appearance. Conventional and monoclonal antibodies are available. Apart from hepatomas, AFP is occasionally expressed by other tumors, most notably germ cell tumors of ovary, testis, or extragonadal sites (yolk sac carcinomas—with a functional correspondence to the embryonic yolk sac, the primordium of the liver).

Among hepatomas 70 to 90 percent are reported as AFP positive in most series (Table 11–9). Among positive cases, the frequency of individual AFP-positive cells varies from 5 up to 50 percent or more (Figs. 11–15 and 11–16). In some cases positive cells are confined to small focal areas of the tumor. Some studies have reported that AFP positivity is confined to the tumor cells and that nonneoplastic liver tissue is nonreactive for AFP. This pattern is not our experience nor is it the experience of others. With sensitive techniques and specific antisera, AFP reactivity may be seen in regenerating liver cells in hepatitis or in cirrhosis or in the liver cells

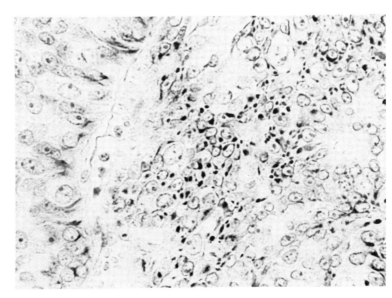

Figure 11–16. Pleomorphic liver tumor; globules (black) of material reactive with antibody to AFP (alpha-fetoprotein) support a diagnosis of primary hepatocellular carcinoma. Paraffin section, AEC with hematoxylin counterstain (×200).

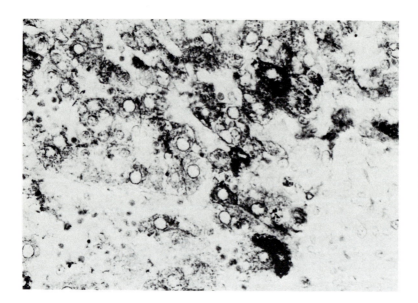

Figure 11–17. Ferritin demonstrated within a moderately differentiated hepatoma. Antibodies to ferritin also react positively with histiocytes (depending upon level of iron storage) and some germ cell tumors. Paraffin section, AEC with hematoxylin counterstain (×320). Staining for alpha$_1$-antitrypsin or antichymotrypsin shows similar appearances in many cases.

around a hepatoma. Such staining is, however, typically much less intense than that encountered in hepatomas. With regard to the distinction of hepatoma from adenocarcinoma metastatic to liver, strong AFP positivity effectively confirms hepatoma and excludes metastasis. Primary cholangiocarcinoma is AFP-negative.

Alpha-fetoprotein positivity also has been reported in hepatoblastomas of childhood; these may also show reactivity for hCG.

Certain other "markers" may be of value in discriminating between primary hepatomas and other types of carcinoma. Hepatomas typically show a proportion of cells staining for albumin, ferritin (Fig. 11–17), alpha$_1$-antitrypsin (Fig. 11–18), and alpha$_1$-antichymotrypsin (Table 11–9). Alpha$_1$-antichymotrypsin is perhaps most commonly present; in one series, Ordóñez and Manning (1984) detected alpha$_1$-antichymotrypsin in 33/33 cases of hepatoma and alpha$_1$-antitrypsin in 33/33 cases. Apart from germ cell tumors, which are usually not easily confused with hepatomas, these antigens are found only rarely in other tumor types (pancreas, lung, colon, breast). Alpha$_1$-antichymotrypsin has been advocated as a possible marker of certain types of histiocytic tumor (Chapter 6). Again, these are not easily confused with hepatoma, and AFP will be lacking.

Positive staining for CEA is, of itself, not of great value since, although carcinomas metastatic to liver (usually from the GI tract)

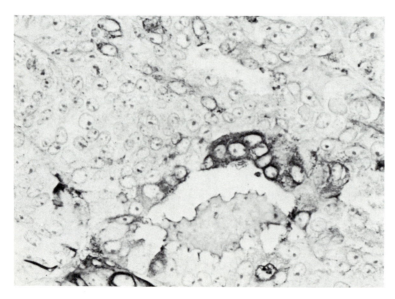

Figure 11–18. Alpha$_1$-antitrypsin within a hepatoma, positive cells (gray-black cytoplasm) are present singly and in clusters. Paraffin section, AEC with hematoxylin counterstain (×200).

are usually strongly reactive for CEA, hepatomas may show some staining of tumor cells or surrounding proliferating bile ducts. CEA staining of hepatomas does, however, have an unusual distribution, tending to concentrate at the surface aspect of those cells forming small bile canaliculi. This pattern, when seen, is quite distinctive.

As epithelial neoplasms, hepatomas do contain keratin; however, they contain only a narrow band of the total spectrum of different molecular weight keratins, and some antikeratin antibodies fail to detect liver keratin. Note that in liver, as in other tissues, staining for keratin is most readily achieved in frozen tissues; if formalin in paraffin sections are utilized, staining is compromised and proteolytic digestion (trypsin—see Chapter 2) is almost essential. Some polyclonal antikeratin antibodies usually show some staining of normal hepatocytes, variable staining of hepatomas, and strong staining of bile ducts; others do not stain hepatocytes (eg, Schlegel et al, 1980a, b). Battifora (1984) reports that in his studies with Dr. Sun, the antikeratin antibody designated AE3 (against high-MW keratin) does stain normal hepatocytes, whereas AE1 (versus low-MW keratin) does not, although the latter may stain hepatomas, which presumably express a different keratin profile. In our tests, Nagle's K4 antikeratin monoclonal antibody fails to react with normal liver or with hepatoma in paraffin sections; cholangiocarcinoma by contrast reacts intensely, as do normal bile ducts. By contrast the anti–"nonsquamous keratin" monoclonal reagent (35 β H11) produced by Gown and Vogel (1984) stains normal hepatocytes and hepatomas (not surprisingly since it was made using the hepatoma line Hep 3.3 as the immunogen), while their "anti–squamous keratin" antibody (34 β E12) does not react with hepatocytes. Both stain bile ducts.

In passing it should be mentioned that Mallory bodies, considered to represent accumulations of abnormal intermediate filaments, react poorly with many antikeratin antibodies; AE1, however, stains them intensely (Battifora, 1984).

In practical terms this variety of staining patterns with different reagents emphasizes the need for an investigator to run some in-house controls on normal and tumor tissues prior to lauching into the investigation of a series of "unknown tumors."

Cholangiocarcinomas typically are strongly positive for keratin (with most if not all antikeratin antibodies); whereas hepatomas may be positive or negative depending upon the choice of primary antibody. Cholangiocarcinomas also are said to be positive for epithelial membrane antigen (Table 11–9), whereas hepatocellular carcinomas react weakly or not at all. Hepatomas may contain AFP and alpha$_1$-antichymotrypsin; cholangiocarcinomas do not; both tumor types may contain CEA, alpha$_1$-antitrypsin, fibrinogen, and immunoglobulins (Goodman et al, 1985).

Worth mentioning also is one relatively rare liver tumor, considered by some to be a variant of hepatocellular carcinoma, the so-called fibrolamellar carcinoma. Typically, it contains little AFP and reacts poorly or not at all with alpha$_1$-antitrypsin, and the like. Positivity for neurotensin has however been reported, leading to the suggestion that this may be a neuroendocrine tumor derived from the neuroendocrine cells distributed in the bile ducts. As such a tumor, it can be considered analogous to "carcinoids," for which it has some morphologic resemblance.

Hepatomas have also been reported frequently to show positive immunostaining for hepatitis B antigens, especially HBsAg (surface antigen) and to a lesser degree HBcAg (core antigen). However, the frequency of positive reactions for HBsAg varies enormously in different populations in different parts of the world (Table 11–10). From 5 to 80 percent or more of cases are described as positive. The term *positive* must also be defined. In most instances the cells that show a positive staining reaction for HBsAg are not neoplastic cells but are residual non-neoplastic hepatocytes surrounding the tumor; this particularly is true if cirrhosis coexists (Fig. 11–19). In some cases a positive reaction is observed in a minority of tumor cells.

Hepatitis—HbsAg

Staining for HBsAg has also been utilized in the investigation of hepatitis and the HBsAg cancer state. In chronic hepatitis up to 30 percent of cases have shown positive reactivity for HBsAg in hepatocytes (Table 11–10); in cirrhosis 5 percent were positive (Thomsen and Clausen, 1983) (Fig. 11–19), whereas 10 percent of livers with minimal changes showed positivity. This study was performed in Denmark; rates vary greatly in

Table 11–10. Selected Bibliography: Hepatitis B Surface Antigen (HBsAg), Hepatocellular Carcinoma (Hepatoma), Hepatitis

Burns 1975	HBsAg, paraffin sections
Afroudakis et al 1976	HBsAg in paraffin sections and Araldite; more sensitive than orcein
Huang 1975	HBsAg in paraffin sections and immuno-EM
Clausen & Thomsen 1978	HBsAg by immunoperoxidase; more sensitive than orcein
Huang & Neurath 1979	HBsAg and HBcAg (core) in paraffin sections, includes EM, and an immunoferritin method
Isaacson C et al 1979	Two South African series of hepatoma cases: Baragwanuth series 4/17 positive for HBsAg; series of black mineworkers 16/22 positive
Omata et al 1980	Artifactual binding of peroxidase to HBsAg
Hsu et al 1983	284 cases of hepatoma from Taiwan; HBsAg detected in residual nontumorous liver in 86%
Thomsen & Clausen 1983	HBsAg–positive staining in 28% of chronic hepatitis, 5% of cirrhotics, and 10% of minimal change liver (Denmark)
Theodoropoulos et al 1979	In seropositive cirrhosis 84% showed positive HBsAg staining of cells; in seropositive hepatoma 94% gave positive staining (chiefly in non-neoplastic cells); seronegative cases showed no positive staining for HBsAg; orcein staining gave some false-positives and some false-negatives
Kew et al 1980	South African hepatoma cases: 68% seropositive, 41% gave tissue staining, mostly in nontumor cells; scattered tumor cells were positive (in 12% overall only tumor cells were positive)
Al Adnani & Ali 1984	HBsAg detectable in 30% of chronic hepatitis and 30% of cirrhosis (in Kuwait)
Yamada et al 1980	Evidence that HBsAg is expressed at the cell membrane as well as in cytoplasm
Ilardi et al 1980	15/18 hepatoma cases in China showed HBsAg positive
Blum et al 1984	In situ hybridization of hepatitis B virus DNA
Shimizu YK et al 1982	Hepatitis A antigen detected within cytoplasmic vesicles by immunoperoxidase method
Romet-Lemonne et al 1982	Transformation of liver cells by hepatitis B virus produces a tumor-related antigen
Swenson et al 1980	HBsAg in 33% of hepatomas with cirrhosis but in none of 16 hepatomas without cirrhosis (Zenker-fixed tissues)
Sarno et al 1984	HBsAg and HBcAg in paraffin sections of 3% (approximately) of acute hepatitis
Dormeyer et al 1981	HBcAg (core) in intranuclear location in chronic hepatitis
Wang WL et al 1980	HBcAg in hepatoma cases
Clausen et al 1983	HBsAg, different fixatives including frozen sections; formalin gave some loss of staining after 7 hours; could be restored by proteolytic digestion; approximately 40% of seropositive cases showed positive tissue staining for HBsAg
Thung & Gerber 1983	Delta antigen in paraffin sections—chronic active hepatitis
Govindarajan et al 1984	Delta antigen in Araldite sections (after sodium ethoxide treatment)

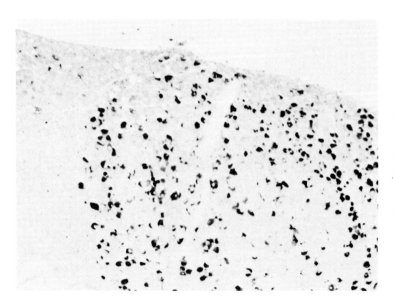

Figure 11–19. Liver biopsy; large numbers of cells show cytoplasmic reactivity (black) with antibody to HBsAg (hepatitis B surface antigen). Chinese patient with hepatoma; section is from noncancerous liver adjacent to tumor. Paraffin section, AEC with hematoxylin counterstain (×60). In some cases hepatoma cells also contain detectable HbsAg.

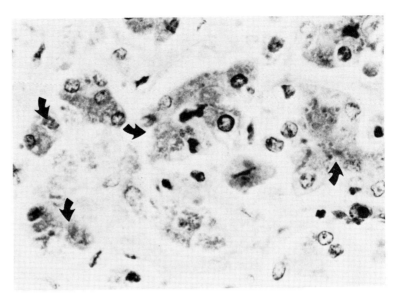

Figure 11–20. Alpha₁-antitrypsin (AAT) -positive granules within hepatocytes in a case of AAT deficiency. Conglomerations greater than 3 μm in diameter (arrows) are typical of the disease. Paraffin section, AEC with hematoxylin counterstain (×320).

different parts of the world and in different types of cirrhosis according to the prevalence of hepatitis B virus as an etiologic factor. Perhaps most useful is the knowledge that immunostaining of liver biopsies may detect the presence of antigen in 80 percent or more of cases with serum positivity (for HBsAg); rarely, one may find specific immunostaining of liver cells for HBsAg in a seronegative case. The presence of HBsAg and HBcAg (core antigen) in asymptomatic patients was reported by Dormeyer and colleagues (1981); significance and prognostic factors were discussed; most cases did not progress to chronic liver disease. HbsAg is cytoplasmic; HBcAg is demonstrable within the nuclei of hepatocytes.

Alpha₁-Antitrypsin Deficiency and Cirrhosis

With the recognition of alpha₁-antitrypsin (AAT) deficiency and its association with emphysema, there has been considerable interest in concurrent liver abnormalities in this condition. In the homozygous deficiency state, serum levels of AAT are very low, and 70 percent or more of the patients have serious emphysema; in the heterozygous state the levels are less depressed, and the risk of emphysema is mainly confined to smokers. In the population of the United States and Europe, the heterozygote frequency is approximately 3 percent; the homozygote is about one hundred times less common. There are many different alleles contributing to the varying expression of the disease.

Alpha₁-antitrypsin is manufactured by the liver; in deficiency, although the serum levels are depressed (in some variants of the disease there may be no detectable AAT in serum), the hepatocytes do contain immunoreactive AAT distributed as discrete globules. These globules vary in size from less than 1 micron diameter to 3 microns or more; they are clearly revealed by immunoperoxidase staining for AAT (Fig. 11–20), but also may be seen as PAS–diastase resistant granules (Table 11–9). They are most numerous and largest in the homozygous state. In heterozygotes they are smaller and less numerous but are readily detectable.

In the homozygote the liver disease varies from neonatal hepatitis to childhood cirrhosis to no significant clinical effect. Heterozygotes are subject to less risk, the exact degree being controversial (Table 11–9). Clausen and colleagues (1984) concluded that the presence of AAT-positive globules of diameter greater than 3 microns was a reliable indication of the deficiency (carrier) state; about 50 percent of cases were detectable by this approach; the remaining cases contained smaller granules that may also be observed in other states. The AAT deficiency state has been implicated in cryptogenic cirrhosis and as a possible etiologic factor in hepatoma (Table 11–9).

12

PROSTATE, BLADDER, KIDNEY, CERVIX, UTERUS

"Diagnosis is a system of more or less accurate guessing, in which the endpoint achieved is a name. These names applied to disease come to assume the importance of specific entities, whereas they are for the most part no more than insecure and therefore temporary conceptions."

SIR THOMAS LEWIS
Lancet 1:619, 1944

PROSTATE AND PROSTATIC CARCINOMA

Two commonly used markers for prostatic carcinoma are prostate-specific acid phosphatase (PSAP) and prostate-specific epithclial antigen (PSEA); both are detectable by immunoperoxidase staining methods in paraffin sections. The normal prostate epithelial cells contain relatively more PSAP than do their malignant counterparts. Raised serum levels of PSAP in prostatic carcinoma may reflect either an increase in cell number (tumor mass) or a rapid release of PSAP by dying tumor cells. Prostate-specific acid phosphatase has been reported to be present in almost all primary and secondary prostatic cancer and has not been detected in other carcinomas (Naritoku, 1982; Nadji et al, 1980). The purpose of staining with PSAP is not to distinguish normal from malignant cells but to identify poorly differentiated carcinoma cells of unknown origin as prostatic carcinoma. Prostate-specific epithelial antigen, purified from semen, has a similar distribution, and the antibody to it can be utilized in a similar manner (Kuriyama et al, 1982; Frankel et al, 1982). In addition, various monoclonal antibodies have been reported to recognize antigens on primary or metastatic prostatic carcinoma (Table 12–1): the usefulness of these antibodies in the immunoperoxidase method has yet to be established.

The principal problems facing the surgical

pathologist in relationship to the prostate gland are as follows:

1. Given a piece of tissue from the prostate, is it malignant?
2. Given a piece of malignant tissue, is it derived from prostate?
3. Given a known malignancy of prostate (carcinoma), will it respond to hormonal manipulation?

At present the surgical pathologist attempts to answer these questions on morphologic grounds utilizing quite detailed histologic criteria, subclassifications of prostatic carcinomas (eg, Gleason), and correlations with known patterns of clinical behavior.

In the past, staining for acid mucopolysaccharide has been used by some investigators as a possible indicator of malignancy because sulfomucins and sialomucins may be seen in the majority of prostatic adenocarcinomas but are usually not present in normal prostatic epithelium. Stains that are effective in routinely processed paraffin sections have been developed for acid mucopolysaccharides but have not achieved widespread utilization due in part to difficulties in standardization and interpretation. Immunohistochemistry has not yet achieved any striking advance in identifying malignant change; this fact reflects the lack of a well-characterized antibody against a prostatic carcinoma–associated antigen. Thus, although some antigens have been observed to show increased expression in prostatic carcinoma (including T antigen, Ca 1 antigen, and less often

Table 12–1. Selected Bibliography: Prostate-Specific Acid Phosphatase (PSAP), Prostate-Specific Epithelial Antigen (PSEA), and Other Antigens

Jöbsis et al 1981	Survey of activity of antiserum vs PSAP on 200 prostatic cancers—193 positive (96.5%); of control tissues (nonprostatic), 98% were negative; some positivity was observed in 6/10 insulinomas and 1/10 carcinoids; this antiserum also stained beta cells of normal islets; study also used a television quantitation system for assessing staining
Lillehoj et al 1982	Described 8 monoclonal antibodies vs 3 nonoverlapping determinants in the prostatic acid phosphatase molecule
Nadji et al 1980 ⎫ Nadji & Morales 1982 ⎬	Review of prostatic acid phosphatase immunohistochemistry; all prostatic tumors positive; no evidence of positivity in nonprostatic tumors
Lee CL et al 1982	Described 4 monoclonal antibodies vs 3 different determinants on the acid phosphatase molecule; two antibodies also reacted with nonprostatic acid phosphatase
Clarke et al 1982	Described monoclonal antibodies vs a prostatic epithelial acinar cell antigen distinct from PSAP or PSEA; effective in formalin-fixed tissues
Bentz et al 1982	Use of PSAP antibodies for determining prostatic origin of metastases; found little difference among grades
Kuriyama et al 1982	PSAP and PSEA
Witorsch 1979	Use of immunoperoxidase to detect prolactin-binding sites in human prostate
Romas et al 1979	Review of serum PSAP, antigenically distinct from other acid phosphatases
Lee P et al 1981	Labelled antigen method for detection of PSAP
Winkler et al 1981	Orbital metastasis of prostatic cancer
Ordóñez et al 1982	Carcinoma of prostate with sarcomatoid change
El Etreby & Mahrous 1979	Detection of growth hormone and prolactin target sites in prostate
Mahan et al 1980	Acid phosphatase staining of prostate before and after radiotherapy—well maintained
Li CY et al 1980	20 of 20 prostatic metastases were positive for PSAP; metastases from all other sites were negative with exception of weak staining in some breast cancers of women
Javadpour 1980a	Review of tumor markers in urologic disease; includes prostate
Stegehuis et al 1979	Utilized indirect peroxidase on paraffin and paraplast sections with success in 56 prostatic tumors, primary and secondary
Bates et al 1982	Correlation of tumor grade with acid phosphatase staining; well-differentiated tumors stained most intensely; great variation was seen in poorly differentiated tumors
Frankel et al 1982	Described 3 monoclonal antibodies to prostate epithelial antigens defining 2 non–cross-reacting sites: these antibodies appeared to react with cytoplasmic, not surface, components
Ware et al 1982 ⎫ Webb et al 1984 ⎬	Monoclonal to "prostatic carcinoma antigen," also stains blood vessel endothelium
Wright GL Jr et al 1983	Prostatic carcinoma–associated antigens: 2 monoclonals, heterogeneous staining; normal prostate and other normal tissues negative (except proximal tubule of kidney); some other cancers showed reactivity—about 70% of prostate cancers (primary and secondary) were positive
Shevchuk et al 1983	In 39 cases stained for PSAP, found positivity in 70%–83% with different antisera but only 59% positive with a monoclonal antibody; poorly differentiated tumors showed least positivity
Keshgegian & Kline 1984	Aspiration biopsy cytology: 44/46 cases positive for PSAP in standard Papanicolaou stained slides; observed rare positive cells in breast cancer; otherwise, 22 other cancers were negative
Ghazizadeh et al 1984a	T antigen present in about 50% of prostatic cancers and 10% of benign prostatic epithelium (myoepithelial cells were positive); used peanut lectin to detect T antigen
Takeuchi et al 1983	Serum levels of PSEA—valuable
Kuhajda et al 1984	Papillary carcinoma of prostate positive for PSAP
Walker AN et al 1982	"Endometrial" carcinoma of prostatic urethra positive for PSAP, therefore probably not of Mullerian origin
Purnell et al 1984	CEA rarely positive in prostatic cancer; however, NCA found in 40% (most reported CEA staining may be due to cross–reactive NCA antibodies); 10% hCG positive
Bentz et al 1984	Reported good results with commercial kits for PSAP and PSEA
Ghazizadeh et al 1984b	Reported CEA in almost 90% of carcinoma—rare in benign prostate (note: may be NCA cross reactivity)
Pollen & Dreilinger 1984	PSAP and PSEA in periurethral glands of female
Ellis DW et al 1984	Prostatic carcinoma positive for PSAP in 58/60, for PSEA in 59/60, for CEA in 4/60; hCG and AFP negative; epithelial membrane antigen weak
Ghazizadeh et al 1984c	All primary and metastatic prostate cancers positive for PSEA (30 cases); other types of cancer negative
Ansari et al 1981	Carcinoidlike tumor, PSAP-positive
Azumi et al 1984	Carcinoid tumor (argyrophil), PSAP- and PSEA-positive
Almagro 1985	Review of prostatic "carcinoids"
Schron et al 1984	Small cell carcinoma of prostate PSAP positive

CEA—Table 12–1), none of these have as yet been incorporated into the decision of benign versus malignant within the prostate. The two monoclonal antibodies described by GL Wright and colleagues (1983) do show promise in that there appears to be differential staining between malignant and normal prostate; of other normal tissues, only renal tubules show reactivity. Antibody D83-21 reacted only with prostate and bladder cancer; antibody P6-2 reacted in addition with cancers of lung, breast, and pancreas.

With regard to the second problem, the recognition of metastatic adenocarcinoma as of prostatic origin, immunohistochemistry has made major progress. Within the prostate, two separate antigens have been identified that have a highly restricted tissue distribution confined totally (or almost totally) to normal or malignant prostatic epithelial tissues. The first of these antigens is prostatic acid phosphatase, and the second is prostate-specific epithelial antigen.

Prostatic Acid Phosphatase

Prostatic acid phosphatase is secreted by the columnar epithelium of the prostatic acini. It is present in semen and blood, in the latter in considerably elevated amounts in many cases of invasive prostatic carcinoma. Prostatic acid phosphatase may also be directly demonstrated within frozen sections of prostate and distinguished from other acid phosphatase by reaction with its specific substrate, phosphorylcholine. Although the biologic activity of this prostate enzyme is to some extent resistant to fixation in formalin, results are much less reliable in routinely processed paraffin-embedded tissues. This is at least partly attributed to the inhibition by alcohol (used as part of the embedding procedure) and its destruction during decalcification methods in bone biopsies, and so forth.

However, although the enzymatic activity of prostatic acid phosphatase is compromised by routine processing of tissues, its antigenic integrity is largely preserved. Thus, antisera raised against prostatic acid phosphatase will readily detect the presence of the molecule within routinely processed tissues (Fig. 12–1), following decalcification with most decalcification solutions or EDTA (Fig. 12–2). Zenker's fixative has, however, been described as having adverse effects. Aspiration cytology Papanicolaou-stained specimens also give excellent results (Keshgegian and Kline, 1984).

Thus immunohistochemical techniques can be utilized to detect the presence of prostatic acid phosphatase in routinely processed tissues including bone biopsies, providing the surgical pathologist with a ready staining method for prostatic tissues. As with most immunostaining procedures, an observed lack of staining is of less value in interpretation than a clear-cut positive stain, for the latter allows the pathologist to conclude with a high degree of certainty that the tissue in question is derived from the prostate (which

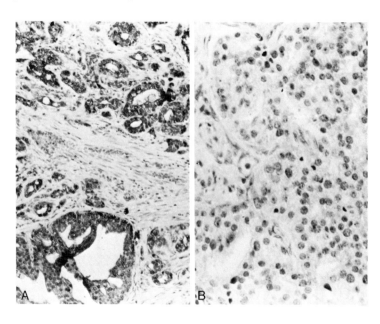

Figure 12–1. "Biologic controls'" for prostatic acid phosphatase. In *A* (positive control), there is positive black staining of the cytoplasm in a case of prostatic carcinoma treated with anti–prostatic acid phosphatase antibody in the PAP method. The fact that connective tissue cells do not stain suggests specificity. *B* is the negative control, treated in an identical manner except that the anti–prostatic acid phosphatase antibody has been omitted. The lack of cytoplasmic staining of tumor cells suggests that the staining seen in the positive control is due to the anti–acid phosphatase antibody. Both are formalin paraffin sections processed in an identical manner (from the same block). AEC with hematoxylin counterstain (×125 *A*; ×300 *B*).

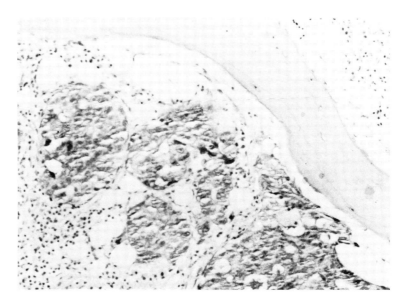

Figure 12–2. Bone marrow containing PSAP (prostate–specific acid phosphatase)-positive tumor (gray cytoplasm). Diagnosis: metastatic prostatic carcinoma. Paraffin section, AEC with hematoxylin counterstain (×125).

in the case of a malignant tumor means metastatic prostatic carcinoma).

However, in spite of the uniform reliability of the method, there are certain pitfalls for the unwary.

First, of course, the specificity of the anti–prostatic acid phosphatase antiserum is critical. Specificity of any antiserum utilized should be demonstrated not only by radioimmunoassay techniques but also by immunostaining of nonprostatic tissues and screening against a wide variety of glandular tissues other than prostate. Such "negative" screening should include representative tissues from colon, small intestine, pancreas, kidney, and salivary gland. If the antiserum under consideration shows no evidence of reactivity in these tissues but is clearly positive in normal prostatic epithelium, then it has diagnostic utility for the purpose under discussion.

The same requirements must also be met by any monoclonal antibody prior to utilization for immunostaining of prostatic acid phosphatase.

If the antiserum is to be used upon routinely processed tissues, then clearly, the specificity screening described above must also be carried out on routinely processed tissues, processed in a manner identical to that of the test specimens (ie, same fixation, same fixation time, same processing schedule). Many conventional antisera against prostatic acid phosphatase function very well on routinely processed tissues, but the same is not necessarily true of monoclonal antibodies. For example, of a series of more than 70 monoclonal antibodies shown to have specificity against prostatic acid phosphatase by radioimmunoassay, only 9 produced consistent reactivity in formalin-fixed, paraffin-embedded sections of prostate, although all of them gave consistent staining in frozen sections (Naritoku and Taylor, 1982; Naritoku, PhD dissertation, 1982; see Fig. 1–22). Those monoclonal antibodies giving positive reactivity were not necessarily those of highest titer or highest affinity. The logical explanation seems to be that an individual monoclonal antibody recognizes only one of several determinants on the acid phosphatase molecule, and that fixation and processing may so alter many of these determinants that they are no longer detectable by the corresponding antibody; only those monoclonal antibodies that happen to react with determinants that survive fixation will prove effective when applied to routinely processed tissues. With conventional antisera, consisting of an immunologic cocktail of many different antibodies of differing affinities to different determinants on the molecule, the chance that some of the component antibodies will recognize a determinant that survives fixation is much enhanced. The study of Shevchuk et al (1983), which reported approximately 80 percent positivity with a conventional antiserum versus only 60 percent with a monoclonal antibody, may be interpreted in similar fashion.

Manley and colleagues (1981) have nicely summarized the effects of different fixatives on the preservation of acid phosphatase im-

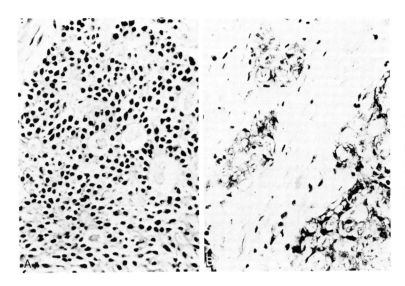

Figure 12–3. Area of obvious cancer in the breast of a 70-year-old male on estrogen therapy for prostatic cancer (**A**, H&E). Staining for prostatic acid phosphatase shows intense positivity in the cytoplasm (**B**), betraying a prostatic origin. Diagnosis: metastatic prostatic carcinoma. Paraffin section, DAB with hematoxylin counterstain (×200).

munoreactivity, noting excellent results with neutral buffered formalin, Bouin's, or B5. Carnoy's and Helly's fixatives also gave good staining, as did Zenker's (note that this latter result is a discrepancy from the findings of Jöbsis [1983]). Again, discrepancies here may reflect differences in composition of the fixative, in fixation time, or in the antisera used in the studies. Similarly, the efficacy of trypsinization has varied in different laboratories, and in our experience trypsinization has been of minimal benefit for prostatic acid phosphatase. Staining for prostatic acid phosphatase is effective after embedding in paraffin and paraplast, with some fall-off in reactivity in methacrylate and epon (in the latter after etching with NaOH). In frozen sections staining, of course, is uniformly intense.

Taken together, the reported experience of staining for prostatic acid phosphatase in prostatic adenocarcinoma exceeds 500 cases with an overall rate of positivity in excess of 90 percent. Almost all of the well-differentiated tumors appear positive, although a few of the poorly differentiated tumors believed to be of prostatic orgin have been reported as showing no detectable positivity. In interpretation of staining for prostatic acid phosphatase, it is important to review as large an area of tumor as possible, since the proportion of positive cells within the tumor population may very enormously—from 70 to 80 percent down to less than 5 percent. Metastases also show a similar high incidence of positivity (Figs. 12–3 and 12–4), which persists with perhaps a slight fall-off in post-radiation specimens.

Of an extensive range of nonprostatic tissues (both normal and neoplastic) tested, all have been uniformly negative with the possible exception of beta cells in the islets of Langerhans and some beta cell–derived tumors (this latter observation is by no means generally accepted; we certainly have not seen it, and it may reflect differences in staining reactivity of antisera from different sources). For example, Manley et al (1981) found no evidence of staining in normal pancreas, pancreatic carcinoma, or islet cell tumors and noted only that levels of prostatic acid phosphatase had been detected by radioimmunoassay in pancreatic extracts. In particular, Manley and colleagues noted that adenocarcinomas from thyroid, salivary

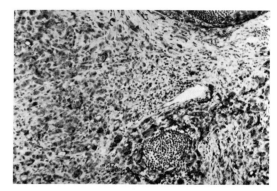

Figure 12–4. Lymph node partially replaced by anaplastic tumor. Tumor cells show positive cytoplasmic staining (red-black) for prostatic acid phosphatase; this is metastatic prostatic carcinoma. Paraffin section, AEC with hematoxylin counterstain (×125). See color plate II–5.

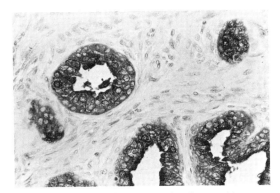

Figure 12–5. Normal prostate showing positive cytoplasmic staining (brown-black) of epithelial cells by antibody to prostate-specific epithelial antigen. Paraffin section, DAB with hematoxylin counterstain (×320).See color plate II–6.

glands, breast, lung, stomach, biliary tract, small bowel, pancreas, and kidneys, and from transitional cell carcinoma of the bladder all were uniformly negative. Vas deferens, epididymis, and seminiferous tubules were also nonreactive, which has been our experience, too.

Prostate-Specific Epithelial Antigen

Although present in semen along with prostatic acid phosphatase, prostate-specific epithelial antigen is a distinct molecule, and antisera (antibodies) against it do not react with prostatic acid phosphatase. Prostate-specific epithelial antigen, like prostatic acid phosphatase, is normally confined to the prostate gland and is not found in other normal tissues. It also is present in the vast majority of prostatic carcinomas (in excess of 95 percent) and has not been detected in other adenocarcinomas.

Conventional and monoclonal antibodies against prostate-specific epithelial antigen are widely available and readily detect it in routinely processed tissues (Figs. 12–5, 12–6, and 12–7). The antigen survives most decalcification procedures. A combination of staining of unknown tissues with both prostate-specific epithelial antigen and prostatic acid phosphatase increases the threshold for recognition of a tumor as of prostatic origin to the order of 98 to 99 percent. We have occasionally observed tumors positive for prostatic acid phosphatase but negative for prostate-specific epithelial antigen and the reverse.

Overall these two antibodies are extremely reliable for the recognition of prostatic tissue, including metastatic epithelial neoplasms derived from prostate. The only exceptions, in our experience, to the presence of either of these antigens in nonprostatic tumors is their detection within some epithelial cells in a minority of cases of well-differentiated teratoma, which thus seem to display the ability to differentiate toward a prostatic type of epithelium as well as many other epithelial types. This circumstance does not represent a diagnostic problem.

In addition to giving reliable results on frozen and routinely processed tissues, stains for prostatic acid phosphatase and prostate-

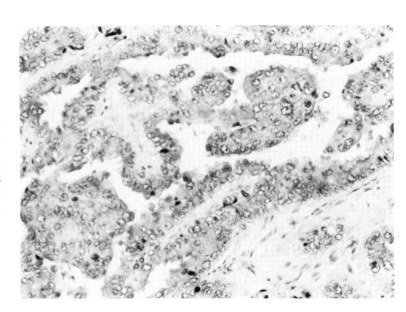

Figure 12–6. Solitary lung tumor of debatable origin, resolved by demonstration of prostate-specific epithelial antigen within tumor cell cytoplasm, particularly at the apical margins (shades of gray). Paraffin section, AEC with hematoxylin counterstain (×300).

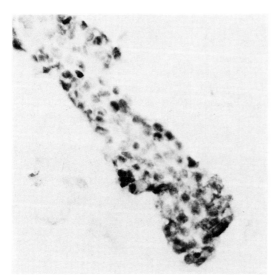

Figure 12–7. Needle biopsy of pelvic mass showing positive cytoplasmic staining with antibody to prostate-specific epithelial antigen. Diagnosis: metastatic prostatic carcinoma. Paraffin section, AEC with light hematoxylin counterstain (×200).

specific epithelial antigen are equally applicable to cell smears or other cytology preparations; Papanicolaou-stained aspiration cytology preparations give good results in our experience.

Staining for prostate-specific epithelial antigen or prostatic acid phosphatase has not been shown to correlate in any useful way with the responsiveness of prostatic carcinomas to hormonal manipulation. Attempts have been made to demonstrate the presence of estrogen receptor, testosterone receptor, or both in sections of prostatic tissue, somewhat in analogy to studies made in reference to breast cancer. However, for prostatic tumors the results are even less conclusive than they are for breast tumors, and immunostaining methods for the presence of testosterone, estrogen, or both (including staining for estrogen following addition of exogenous estrogen to the section) have not yet progressed beyond early research studies. The development of monoclonal antibodies against estrogen (or testosterone) receptor protein itself may, of course, change the situation dramatically in the near future.

CEA and Other Antigens

The proportion of prostatic carcinomas staining for CEA varies enormously in dif-

ferent studies—from less than 10 percent to 80 percent or more (Table 12–1). It appears likely that these discrepancies are explicable on the basis of whether or not the anti-CEA antibody (antiserum) contains activity against NCA (normal cross-reacting cancer antigen). The study of Purnell et al (1984) describing NCA activity in approximately 40 percent of cases, mostly in the absence of CEA activity, would support this interpretation. If NCA activity is present, normal tissues also frequently show positivity; if it is absent, then true CEA activity is a good indicator of malignancy. Note, however, that a strongly CEA-positive tumor in this region of the body is much more likely to be an extension of a primary tumor of the colon than of the prostate. As noted elsewhere, a crude guide to the presence of NCA activity in an "anti-CEA" antiserum may be obtained by examining normal granulocytes in vessels distant from tumor: if granulocytes are positive, this suggests NCA activity (Pattengale et al, 1980).

T antigen (described in relation to breast cancer—Chapter 10) is detectable within the malignant cells in up to 50 percent of prostatic cancer (Ghazizadeh et al, 1984a). It is rarely present in normal prostatic epithelium but is often present in the normal myoepithelial cells of the prostate (as in the breast).

Human chorionic gonadotropin is present in 0 to 10 percent of prostatic cancers but is absent in normal prostate. As in other tissues (breast, lung), the presence of Ca 1 antigen is not a reliable guide to malignancy.

Carcinoid Tumors of the Prostate

A minority of carcinomas of the prostate are of the small cell type. Often termed carcinoid tumors of prostate, they closely reproduce the morphologic features of carcinoid tumors elsewhere and may even show distinctive silver stain (argyrophil). There has been debate concerning their origin (Table 12–1). Immunohistologic methods have not supported the relationship of these small cell prostatic tumors to carcinoid tumors (neuroendocrine tumors) but, on the contrary, have shown that such cases are frequently positive for prostatic acid phosphatase (Fig. 12–8), prostatic epithelial antigen, or both; they are thus best regarded as small cell anaplastic variants of prostatic carcinoma.

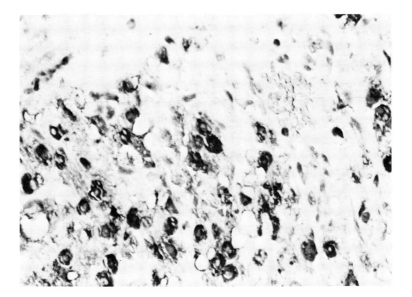

Figure 12–8. Anaplastic "small cell" tumor in pelvis; positive cytoplasmic staining for prostate-specific acid phosphatase. Diagnosis: small cell prostatic carcinoma (gray-black cytoplasm). Paraffin section, AEC with hematoxylin counterstain (×500).

Their resemblance to carcinoids is coincidental, their silver staining unexplained.

BLADDER CANCER

Screening for bladder cancer may be carried out by microscopic examination of the cellular sediment in urine or bladder washes. Cystoscopic examination provides the opportunity to assess gross morphologic appearances of lesions within the bladder and permits the surgeon to biopsy visible lesions.

Papillomas within the bladder are grossly recognizable. A major problem relates to prediction of the clinical course, or the invasive capacity, of individual tumors. Whether or not the tumor is invasive influences clinical management, governing the decisions for surgical intervention and the extent of surgical resection. During radical resection multiple lymph nodes are sampled as frozen sections; the detection of tumor cells in frozen sections is time-consuming for the surgical pathologist and really is only possible for metastases consisting of several cohesive cells. Immunohistologic methods may facilitate not only the recognition of invasive carcinoma but also the detection of single cell metastases.

Blood Group Antigens

The presence of blood group antigens in urothelium and bladder cancer was initially demonstrated utilizing red cell adherence methods. With such methods it was possible to detect some loss of blood group antigens in bladder cancer, compared with normal urothelium.

With the availability of monoclonal antibodies to the ABO(H) antigens, it became possible to demonstrate A, B antigens in paraffin sections by immunoperoxidase methods. The sensitivity of detection of blood group antigens was thereby enhanced, and morphologic detail was much improved (Table 12–2). The method works well in Groups A, B, and AB patients; some difficulties are still encountered in Group O patients (tumors appear as false negatives) due to low expression of the O(H) antigen. In spite of overall similarities in technique, results and conclusions do vary among different investigators.

Using monoclonal antibodies in paraffin sections, Ernst and colleagues (1984) detected A, B antigens in normal epithelium of bladder, stomach, pancreas, and proximal (but not distal) colon; others have reported ABO(H) antigens in the epithelia of esophagus, gall bladder, kidneys, fallopian tubes, and cervix. Ernst observed loss of antigen in carcinomas of bladder, colon, stomach (50 percent of cases showed loss), and pancreas (only 13 percent showed loss). Interestingly, distal colon, which normally is ABO(H) antigen–negative, in cancer frequently (85 percent) became positive.

In bladder cancer most, but not all, investigators have found that loss of ABO(H)

Table 12–2. Selected Bibliography: Bladder (Urothelium)

Javadpour 1980a	Tumor markers in urologic cancer—review
Flanigan et al 1983	Immunoperoxidase method of detecting blood group antigens is more specific than the red cell adherence method and improves morphologic detail; invasive tumors tend to show antigen loss
Chapman et al 1983	Monoclonal antibodies to A and B antigens; normal urothelium (5 cases) and noninvasive transitional cell carcinoma (12 cases) positive; 8/12 invasive carcinomas negative
Coon & Weinstein 1981	Loss of ABO(H) antigen correlates with invasive course in bladder cancer; effective in paraffin sections
Giraldo et al 1983	Blood group antigen detectable in 80% of low-grade, and 40% of high-grade, carcinomas of bladder
Ernst et al 1984	Monoclonal antibodies to A and B antigens in paraffin sections; detectable in normal bladder, stomach, pancreas, and proximal (not distal) colon; lost in 50% of carcinomas of stomach and proximal colon and in 13% of pancreatic cancer; distal colon negative but cancer of distal colon positive
King CT et al 1983	Concluded testing for AB antigens not clinically useful in transitional cell carcinoma
Nakatsu et al 1984	ABO(H) antigens not of prognostic value, but CEA has prognostic significance
Holmberg et al 1984	65% of malignant cells CEA positive; only 24% of benign cells positive; with increasing malignancy there was more CEA
Jautzke & Altenaeher 1982	Overall, 57% of transitional cell carcinomas showed some CEA positivity (scattered cells); 24% of grade I, 72% of grade II, and 76% of grade III; none of grade I cases contained more than 20% malignant cells
Wiley et al 1982	Found that CEA did not correlate with prognosis but loss of ABO(H) antigen did (48 cases studied)
Vafier et al 1984	T antigen is expressed in bladder cancer but not of prognostic value; loss of ABO(H) antigens is useful for prognosis
McAlpine et al 1984	Loss of T antigen in high-grade malignancy
Coon et al 1982	Normal bladder and low-grade tumors have cryptic T antigen; higher grade tumors have no cryptic T antigen but may or may not express overt T antigen
Neal et al 1985	Monoclonal antibody to epidermal growth factor (EGF) positive in 21/24 invasive tumors but in only 7/24 superficial tumors
Nathrath et al 1982	Urothelium-specific antiserum made by using calf bladder epithelium as antigen, followed by multiple adsorptions
Fradet et al 1984	2 monoclonals, one of which reacts preferentially with noninvasive bladder cancer (URO 9); the second reacts principally with invasive cancer (URO 10)

antigen is of prognostic significance. Normal urothelium and well-differentiated (noninvasive) transitional cell carcinomas show positivity; poorly differentiated (high grade—invasive) carcinomas are more often nonreactive. According to Giraldo et al (1983), 80 percent of low-grade, but only 40 percent of high-grade carcinomas are positive, whereas Chapman and colleagues (1983) found all well-differentiated tumors positive and almost 70 percent of invasive carcinomas negative.

It should however be noted that other investigators have reported contrary results, and some have concluded the demonstration of ABO(H) antigen has no prognostic significance in bladder cancer (Table 12–2). These discrepancies are likely to be technical in nature, reflecting differences in specificity of antibodies or variations in methodology. In spite of the lack of prognostic significance recorded by some investigators, the positive correlations obtained by others suggest that this approach has merit and, when coupled with other evidence (vide infra), may aid the surgeon in selection of the appropriate procedure.

CEA, URO 9 and 10

Carcinoembryonic antigen is positive in some transitional carcinomas. The proportion of positive cases is considerably less than for the colon; also, the percentage of positive cells is lower, and individual cells usually stain much less intensely. Jautzke and Altenaehr (1982) reported that, overall, 57 percent of transitional cell carcinomas showed scattered CEA-positive cells. The incidence of CEA positivity appears to increase in parallel with increasing malignancy: 24 percent of grade I tumors, 76 percent of grade III tumors. Also, the high-grade tumors tend to contain more CEA-positive cells; in the low-grade tumors, even those called positive contain less than 10 percent of CEA-reactive cells. In essence, the more CEA, the more malignant the tumor. Hence CEA positivity coupled with demonstrable lack of ABO(H) antigen strongly indicates invasive carcinoma.

As with staining for CEA in other tissues, the investigator should select the anti-CEA antibody with care and establish a "track record" of the reactivity of the method by staining several known low- and high-grade bladder tumors in order to prove the method (in house). The same approach should be adopted for establishing the in-house reliability of the ABO(H) system.

More recently, two monoclonal antibodies (dubbed URO 9 and URO 10) have become available (Fradet et al, 1984). Preliminary data (personal communication, Dr. C. Cordon-Cardo) suggests that these antibodies are of great value in distinguishing between normal urothelium, well-differentiated noninvasive bladder carcinoma, and invasive carcinoma. URO 9 stains only the well-differentiated tumors (and normal urothelium); URO 10 stains only invasive tumors (Fig. 12–9). Focal URO 10–positive areas may be seen in predominantly URO 9–positive tumors and presumably represent progression to a more aggressive mode of behavior. It should be emphasized that data is still limited. However, the antibodies are available commercially (for research use only—Ortho Diagnostics) and provide the pathologist with an opportunity for direct evaluation of their utility. Currently, Ortho recommends that URO 9 and URO 10 be used in frozen sections (fixed briefly in buffered formalin); little data is available for paraffin sections. In our hands, these reagents also show potential for immunocytochemical staining of cells obtained in bladder

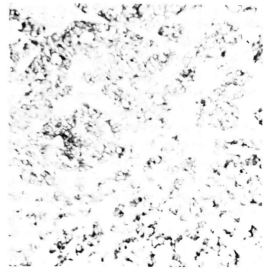

Figure 12–9. Invasive carcinoma of bladder wall showing reactivity with monoclonal antibody URO10, which shows preferential binding for invasive carcinoma of bladder rather than noninvasive papillomas. (Antibody courtesy of Ortho Diagnostics). Frozen section, AEC with light hematoxylin counterstain (×60).

washes (in which fixation can be carefully controlled), the presence of URO 10–positive cells correlating with invasive carcinoma.

Other Antigens

Three other possible markers of invasive malignancy have been described for bladder cancer. Staining for OKT9 (transferrin re-

Figure 12–10. Moderately differentiated bladder carcinoma treated with an anti-T antibody (provided by Dr. G. Springer), showing intense reactivity in a minority of cells and weak positivity in the remainder. Breast carcinomas typically are T antigen positive (see Chapter 10). Paraffin section, AEC with hematoxylin counterstain (×200).

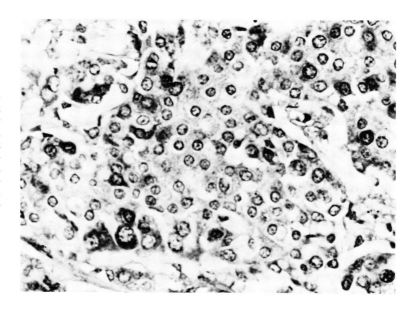

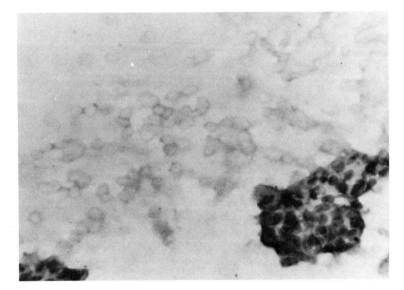

Figure 12–11. Fine-needle aspirate showing cluster of cells with positive (gray) cytoplasmic staining for pan-keratin; bladder carcinoma. DAB with hematoxylin counterstain ($\times 200$).

ceptor) has yielded encouraging results in bladder as it has in other tissues (eg, carcinoma of cervix–Table 12–2) but little published data. T (Thomsen-Friedenreich) antigen is present (after neuraminidase stripping) on well-differentiated papillomas but is usually absent on high-grade tumors. There is some controversy here since others (Table 12–2) have reported that some invasive tumors lack T antigen, whereas others express it in easily detectable form (Fig. 12–10), in contrast with low-grade tumors and normal urothelium in which it is present in "cryptic form" (ie, detectable only after treatment with neuraminidase). Finally, Neal and colleagues (1985) found that a monoclonal antibody believed to be specific for epidermal growth factor reacted with 21/24 invasive tumors but only 7/24 superficial (low-grade) tumors.

The recognition of single cell metastases of bladder cancer is greatly facilitated by staining for keratin, preferably with a "pankeratin" antibody (Fig. 12–11), since the more malignant tumors show irregular expression of the different subtypes of keratin. Staining for CEA also is useful, but some malignant cells will be overlooked if this procedure is used alone.

KIDNEY

Immunohistochemical studies of the kidney have concentrated upon two entirely separate aspects of renal pathology: (1) tumors and (2) the various forms of glomerulonephritis.

Tumors

Tumors of the renal pelvis (urothelium) have the same general characteristics as those of ureter and bladder and show similar immunohistochemical reactions. They are strongly keratin-positive. With regard to renal cell carcinoma, the problem is less the recognition of malignancy than the determination of a renal origin for a metastatic deposit.

Renal carcinomas are said not to be keratin-positive (Nagle et al, 1983b), as befits the embryologic origin of the tubules from the mesonephros (mesoderm). Monoclonal antibodies against nonsquamous keratins have however been shown to react with renal tubules and with renal cell carcinoma (Gown and Vogel, 1984). Staining with the appropriate antikeratin antibody may therefore be of value in distinguishing anaplastic clear cell carcinoma of the kidney from sarcomas (including lymphomas). It however is not useful in separating carcinoma of the kidney from carcinomas of the colon, stomach, pancreas, and so forth. One other observation of possible utility comes from the work of Holthöfer et al (1983), who reported that 60 percent of renal carcinomas contain both cytokeratin and vimentin, whereas, overall, 93 percent reacted to keratin. That this was a frozen section study may account for some of the differences from the findings of others.

The panel of monoclonal antibodies produced by the Sloane-Kettering group (Cordon-Cardo et al, 1984; Finstad et al, 1985) and marketed by Ortho Diagnostics (URO 1

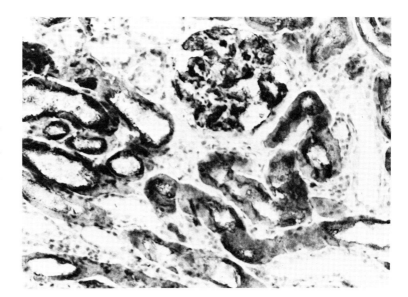

Figure 12–12. Normal kidney displaying pattern of reactivity for URO2, proximal tubular cells and glomeruli show positive-staining (black cytoplasm). Frozen section, AEC with hematoxylin counterstain (×200).

Table 12–3. Reactivity of URO Series of Monoclonal Antibodies with the Nephron

	Glomerulus	Proximal Tubule	Loop of Henle	Distal Tubule	Collecting Duct	Ureter Bladder
URO 1	←----→					
URO 2	←--------------→					
URO 3		←------→				
URO 4		←----------→				
URO 5			←------------------------------→			
URO 8			←----→			
URO 9*						←----→
URO 10†		←------→				←••••••→

*URO 9 reacts with normal urothelium and low-grade malignancy.

†URO 10 reacts with high-grade (invasive) carcinoma, not with normal urothelium.

Note: URO antibodies, although showing remarkable differential specificity within the nephron, nonetheless show significant reactivity with a wide variety of other tissues (eg, URO 1–skin, cervix, thyroid; URO 4–gut, prostate, placenta; URO 10–skin, esophagus, cervix).

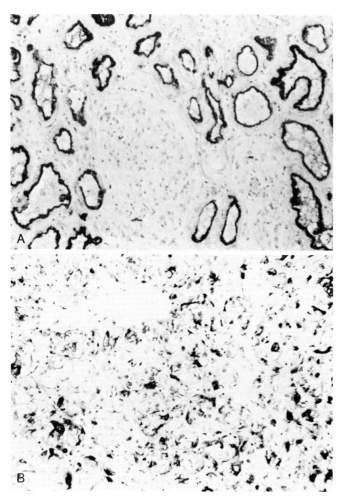

Figure 12–13. Pattern of staining with antibody to proximal tubular cells of kidney; this is conventional absorbed antiserum prepared at the University of Southern California by Dr. S. Yoshida. The monoclonal antibodies URO3 and URO4 give a similar pattern but are effective only on frozen sections. *A* shows staining of proximal tubules in a normal kidney; distal tubules and glomerulus are nonreactive. *B* shows a solitary tumor resected from lung; intense reactivity of a proportion of tumor cells with this antibody betrays a renal origin. Diagnosis: renal cell adenocarcinoma. Paraffin sections, DAB with hematoxylin counterstain (×125).

through 10) may be of value here. These antibodies show remarkable differential specificity for different parts of the nephron (Fig. 12–12; Table 12–3) and, in frozen sections, will identify carcinomas as of renal (proximal tubule) origin with great reliability. Ortho recommends use on cryostat sections of snap-frozen (liquid nitrogen) blocks with brief prefixation in buffered formalin. These antibodies appear not to be reliable on paraffin sections. It is possible, however, to produce "polyclonal" antisera with specificity to the renal proximal tubules that are effective in paraffin sections (Figure 12–13—antibody prepared at USC by Dr. S. Yoshida). This antibody reacts with primary and metastatic deposits of most renal cell carcinomas, the percentage of positive cells varying from 10 to 60 percent or more. A positive stain in a tumor deposit permits one to ascribe a renal origin with confidence; a negative stain is of lesser value.

The URO series has enormous potential for the study of the embryology of the kidney and assessment of degenerative diseases of the nephron. Preliminary studies are exciting (Cordon-Cardo et al, 1984), but much remains to be accomplished. That the nephron can be dissected by phenotype suggests that the same may be possible for other tissues, providing the histologist with new tools of remarkable potential.

While on the topic of renal cell carcinoma, it should be noted that about 50 percent contain renin (or a reninlike molecule), although clinical effects of renin hyperactivity are not usually observed. Rare cases of renin-producing tumors appear to be benign (Table 12–4).

Glomerulonephritis

The immunohistology of glomerulonephritis is sufficiently complex to warrant a book

Table 12–4. Selected Bibliography: Kidney

Kemény et al 1983	Found that trypsin-immunoperoxidase method gave good results on paraffin sections
Tubbs et al 1980c	127 renal biopsies examined using immunoperoxidase method on frozen sections for IgG, IgA, IgM, and C3; counterstain was PAS; superior to fluorescence in many ways
MacIver et al 1979 MacIver & Mepham 1980, 1982	Description of technique for immunoperoxidase studies of formalin-fixed renal biopsies; utilized PAP method and controlled trypsinization (1982 paper is most comprehensive)
Bolen et al 1983	Immunoperoxidase of needle biopsies from renal allografts
Sisson & Vernier 1980	Good technical paper evaluating different methods of fixation and tissue preparation for light and EM studies of kidney (rat)
Vieira et al 1979	50 renal biopsies studied; immunoperoxidase judged superior to fluorescence
Carlo et al 1981	Use of peroxidase-labelled immune complexes linked with C3 to detect presence of C3 receptors in human glomeruli
Dyck et al 1980	Amyloid "P" proteinlike molecule in normal renal glomerulus
Lindop & Fleming 1984	7/19 renal carcinomas contained renin but gave no clinical evidence of secretion
Tetu et al 1984	Case of renin secreting tumor (hamartoma) with clinical effects
Cordon-Cardo et al 1984	Several monoclonal antibodies (the URO series) that react specifically with different parts of the nephron
Finstad et al 1985	Reactivity of subsets of renal carcinoma with URO series of monoclonal antibodies
Naruse et al 1982	Angiotensins I and II in JG cells
Zaki et al 1982	Renin in JG cells (animal study: rats, mice, monkeys)
Camilleri et al 1984	3 renin-secreting JG tumors; at least one appears to be a hamartoma
Piscioli et al 1984	"Sarcomatoid carcinoma" of renal pelvis—keratin and epithelial membrane antigen positive
Wick et al 1985	"Sarcomatoid carcinoma" keratin-positive; also expressed T antigen (peanut lectin) and blood group antigens
Sens et al 1984	Myosin positivity in areas of skeletal muscle formation in a Wilms's tumor
Holthöfr et al 1983	Use of intermediate filament antibodies to assess origin of renal cell carcinomas; keratin and vimentin positive, plus positive for brush border antigen

of its own; indeed, such texts exist but are based almost entirely on immunofluorescence studies, sometimes coupled with ultrastructural analysis by electron microscopy.

Immunofluorescence techniques on frozen sections of renal biopsies certainly seem to have satisfied most investigators; the demonstration of linear staining is usually obvious, and the assignment of granular deposits to the mesangium or to "lumps and bumps" on the glomerular membrane is also usually straightforward. Nonetheless, the pathologist is dealing with "darkfield" microscopy; the standard morphologic criteria for cell recognition are not directly available for assessment, and the tradition of correlating the immunofluorescence findings (often recorded as photomicrographs) with the EM findings (also recorded as photomicrographs) has developed.

It would seem obvious that immunoperoxidase techniques, providing the potential for direct correlation of the pattern of immunologic staining with detailed light microscopy, should be adapted to renal biopsies.

Indeed, recent studies have concluded that immunoperoxidase is superior to immunofluorescence for the study of renal biopsies in frozen sections (Tubbs et al, 1980a; Vieira et al, 1979—Table 12–4). Morphologic detail in thin frozen sections was much more readily appreciated by the immunoperoxidase method; Tubbs used a PAS counterstain to highlight the basement membrane. Preparations are permanent; maintenance of a photographic record is a matter of choice, not necessity.

The practical utility of immunoperoxidase staining of paraffin sections of renal biopsies in glomerulonephritis is much more controversial. Many investigators have tried, and failed, to demonstrate immunoglobulin or complement deposits in fixed paraffin sections of renal biopsies. The prize, of course, is superb morphology coupled with the additional convenience of dispensing with the need for splitting samples several ways (frozen section immunohistology, EM, light microscopy). Successful immunostaining of thin paraffin sections would theoretically permit assessment of all of the essential diagnostic criteria for the glomerulonephritides in a single set of preparations (stained for IgG, IgA, and complement). Angus MacIver (MacIver and Mepham, 1982—Table 12–4) appears to have come closest to the prize. He advocates controlled trypsinization to facilitate detection of the immunoglobulin deposits in paraffin sections (this is the same ill-understood "unmasking" process that is described in detail for lymphomas). We have followed MacIver's protocol exactly, with good results; it is recommended that others do the same. Kemény et al (1983) used a similar approach with success.

Finally, amyloid is demonstrable in renal biopsies not only by the traditional (but inexact) congo red or methyl violet method but also by immunostaining with antibodies to amyloid components (eg, Dyck et al, 1980—P component; see also Chapter 5).

CARCINOMAS OF THE CERVIX AND UTERUS

Here surgical pathology and cytopathology are closely interwoven, and rightly so. Immunohistologic methods have, however, been explored more extensively for tissue utilization than for application to Pap smears. The demonstration of antigens in paraffin sections of uterus and cervix is subject to the same limitations of antigen preservation that apply to other tissues. Theoretically, the demonstration of antigens in Pap smears (whether treated and stained by the classic Papanicolaou method or not) avoids most of these problems, since the antigens are exposed to minimal abuse.

In reading the following chapter, one should recognize that any antigen demonstrable in paraffin sections can be stained with equal or greater facility in cervical smear preparations. Also, some antigens that require the use of frozen sections may readily be stained in alcohol-fixed smears. The use of immunostaining as an adjunct to the cytologic interpretation of cervical smears is a rapidly growing area; the availability of specific cell markers will enormously reinforce the reliability of diagnoses, which otherwise are based upon fine cytologic criteria that are subjective. The first area to find application in cervical smears has involved recognition of infectious agents, as discussed later.

The principal problems in this anatomic region are, as always, the distinction of normal tissues from malignant neoplasms and the recognition of the site of origin of anaplastic tumors. To these may be added the perceived need for receptor assays and the new ability to recognize the presence of potentially infectious agents by their antigenicity.

CEA

There have been many studies of CEA reactivity in the cervix and uterus (Table 12–5). As with immunohistologic studies of CEA in other tissues, there are some major discrepancies among different investigators, probably attributable in large part to the different anti-CEA antibodies used and their degrees of cross reactivity with NCA. There is one other caveat: cervical and endometrial epithelium does contain an endogenous peroxidase that under certain conditions may produce "false-positive" staining. The presence of such activity will be revealed by the "negative" controls (which will show some positivity); exposure of sections to methanol and hydrogen peroxide (Chapter 3) will effectively suppress this endogenous activity.

The general consensus is that CEA is detectable in most cases of squamous carcinoma of cervix, regardless of invasiveness and differentiation, including carcinoma in situ. Severe dysplasia also is positive in 80 percent or more of cases, whereas the proportion of cases of moderate dysplasia that are classified as positive falls to 30 percent or so. In positive cases staining is mainly cytoplasmic, and the proportion of positive cells is quite variable; most investigators require more than 5 to 10 percent positive cells before categorizing any particular case as positive. Mild dysplasia may also show scattered positively reacting cells, but such cells are rare in the normal cervix. In essence, the higher the proportion of CEA-reactive cells and the greater the intensity of staining, the more confident one is of a diagnosis of carcinoma, but there is no absolute distinction between normal (benign) and malignant.

With regard to adenocarcinoma of the (endo)cervix and uterus, the situation is a little different. Most authorities hold that staining for CEA is of little value in separating endometrial hyperplasia from carcinoma, since it is uncommon for either to show significant positivity; the exception is adenosquamous carcinoma of the endometrium, which usually is positive.

CEA staining is, however, of more value in endocervical adenocarcinoma, which usually is positive (80 percent), whereas normal endocervical glands are negative. That endo-

Table 12–5. Selected Bibliography: Carcinomas of the Uterus and Cervix

Crum & Fenoglio 1980	Review of immunoperoxidase application to diseases of female genital tract; included CEA, AFP, viral antigens, hCG, peptide hormones, hormone receptors
Van Nagell et al 1979	CEA positive in 60% of 241 cases of cervical cancer (correlated well with serum level)
Cohen et al 1982b	CEA positive in 100% of endocervical cancer, either cytoplasmic cell surface or cell secretion, and only 50% of endometrial cancer (most of these stained only lightly)
McDicken & Rainey 1983	CEA in 80% invasive squamous carcinoma of cervix, and in 80% of severe dysplasias and carcinomas in situ; in 30% of moderate dysplasias; normal squamous epithelium and mild dysplasia negative (formalin-paraffin sections)
Wahlström et al 1979, 1980	CEA in adenocarcinomas of cervix and uterus: cervix 80% positive (except mesonephroid carcinoma–negative); endometrium, all negative except adenosquamous cancers, which were positive
Fenoglio et al 1981	CEA does not assist discrimination of endometrial hyperplasia versus carcinoma
Fray et al 1984	Monoclonal antibodies to milk–fat globule membrane (HFMG 1 and 2), Ca 1, and CEA: paraffin sections: none specific for carcinoma of cervix; all found to some degree in metaplasia
Ferguson & Fox 1984b	Ca 1 no value in discriminating between hyperplastic and neoplastic endometrium
Lloyd JM et al 1984b	Ca 1 found in normal, dysplastic, and neoplastic tissues
Valkova et al 1984	Epithelial membrane antigen (milk-fat globule), monoclonal antibodies less sensitive than conventional antiserum; positive in cancer and dysplasia, negative in normal cervix, rare positive cells in metaplasia; cervical smears
Hayata et al 1981	Study of 180 gynecologic disorders for CEA and hCG
Hurlimann & Gloor 1984	CEA, keratin, milk–fat globule membrane antigen (MFGM), and secretory component (SC) in adenocarcinomas of cervix; positive for CEA 77%, for MFGM 77%, for SC 49%, for keratin 90%
Okudaira et al 1984	CEA posiive in 9/37 endometrial cancers and 19/23 cervical adenocarcinomas
Ueda et al 1984b	CEA positive in 16/41 endometrial cancers and 22/23 cervical adenocarcinomas; hCG in 3/41 and 1/23 respectively
Crum et al 1983	Staining for Ig facilitates recognition of endometritis (plasma cells)
Arends et al 1983a	Secretory component (of IgA); weak focal staining in endometrial hyperplasia, strongly positive in well-differentiated carcinoma, largely negative in poorly differentiated carcinoma
Press et al 1984	Monoclonal antibodies to estrogen receptor: frozen sections revealed positivity in nuclei of epithelial and stromal cells in proliferative phase; much less in secretory phase; postmenopausal tissue strongly positive; nuclei of myometrium also positive
Farley et al 1982	Positive correlation of direct estrogen staining with estrogen receptor assays
Lloyd JM et al 1984a	Transferrin receptor (OKT 9) positivity in all cervical carcinoma and in severe dysplasia; negative in normal and mildly dysplastic epithelium (except rare cells in the basal layer)
Ueda et al 1984a	Antibody to a cervical squamous cell carcinoma—associated antigen (TA4) positive in squamous carcinoma and less so in adenocarcinoma; normal squamous epithelium also positive
Mattes et al 1984	5 antigens detectable by monoclonal antibodies antibodies in endometrial and ovarian cancers; some cross reactivity with other cancers; some antibodies react with normal tissues
Jha et al 1984	5 monoclonals against 3 different antigens "failed to discriminate between benign and neoplastic conditions of cervix"
Ueda et al 1980	Calcitonin in endometrial carcinomas (with and without argyrophil cells)
Yamasaki et al 1984	Argyrophil–small cell carcinomas of cervix; 2/5 positive for gastrin
Inoue M et al 1984	Scattered argyrophil cells in 43/68 endometrial cancers; somatostatin and gastrin in rare cases
Lojek et al 1980	Small cell carcinoma of cervix positive for ACTH
Nørgaard-Pedersen et al 1979	AFP in infantile vaginal embryonal carcinoma

cervical adenocarcinomas are usually positive for CEA whereas endometrial carcinomas are usually negative has been used as an aid to distinguish the two lesions. Two exceptions exist: mesonephroid endocervical cancer is negative (not positive), and adenosquamous endometrial carcinoma is positive (not negative).

Other Antigens

Other immunohistologic stains may also be helpful (Table 12–5). Several investigators have reported that epithelial membrane antigen (or milk–fat globule membrane antigen) is expressed occasionally or not at all on normal cervix but is usually present in carcinoma; note that some investigators describe scattered positive cells in metaplasia and mild dysplasia. Ca 1 (cancer 1 antigen), which initially was claimed to be quite specific for cancer of various types (McGee et al, 1982), appears to be of little value for recognition of cervical cancer (Fray et al, 1984) and was said by Ferguson and Fox (1984b) to have no value in discrimination between endometrial hyperplasia and endometrial cancer. For the latter purpose, the presence of strong staining for secretory component (of IgA—Arends et al, 1983b) is suggestive of cancer, since normal endometrium stains only focally and lightly; however, only well-differentiated cancers show strong staining, and the distinction is, in our experience, less than absolute.

With regard to carcinoma of the cervix, staining for transferrin receptor (with OKT9 monoclonal antibody—Lloyd et al, 1984a) shows promise. All carcinomas and severely dysplastic epithelia stained strongly; normal and mildly dysplastic epithelium did not stain, except for occasional presumptive "stem" cells in the basal layer. Results were most clear-cut in tissue sections (frozen) of biopsies (145 cases), but the technique may also prove helpful in cytocentrifuge (and smear) preparations (50 cases). The method is limited by the requirement for frozen sections (Lloyd used tissues snap-frozen in liquid nitrogen; the cytocentrifuge preparations were stored at $-80°$ C prior to immunostaining). Application of the method to routine Pap smears needs further study. Both immunoperoxidase and immunofluorescence methods were used in Lloyd's study; the former was preferred because of superior morphology.

Transferrin receptor, demonstrated by OKT9 and initially described as an early thymocyte marker, is now recognized as a common phenotypic expression of the proliferative state in many tissues, whether normal cell replacement or neoplastic proliferation. In this respect, an "index" of proliferating cells (judged by an OKT9-positive phenotype) might prove helpful in evaluating "cytologic atypia" in Pap smears.

Relatively few monoclonal antibodies have been prepared against cervical and endometrical cancer (Fig. 12–14); to date none

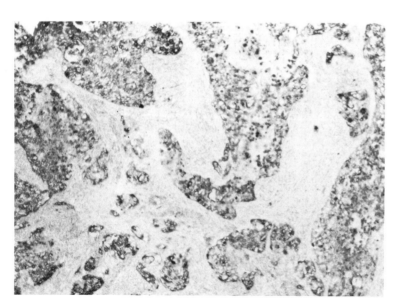

Figure 12–14. Invasive carcinoma of the cervix stained with a murine monoclonal antibody that shows preferential staining for malignant cells as compared with a normal cervix. Frozen section, AEC with hematoxylin in counterstain (×125). Antibody prepared at the University of Southern California by Dr. A. Imam using a mouse tolerized for normal human squamous epithelium prior to immunization with cervical carcinoma cells, as the lymphocyte donor for hybridoma production.

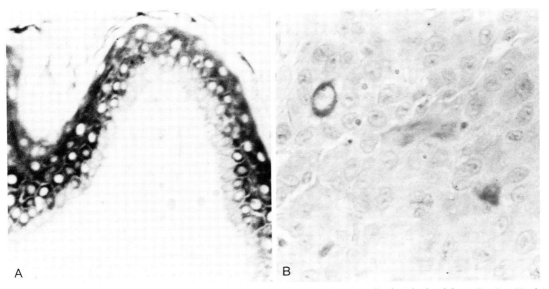

Figure 12–15. *A* shows the "positive" control for a "pankeratin" monoclonal antibody (obtained from Dr. Ray Nagle), with positive staining in the superficial layers. *B* shows a poorly differentiated carcinoma of cervix with rare keratin-positive cells betraying a squamous origin. Paraffin section, AEC with light hematoxylin counterstain (× 320).

have an accepted clinical role (Table 12–5). Of the five antigens identified by Mattes et al (1984), one (dubbed MF116) shows some promise, being present in ovarian, uterine, bladder, and other cancers, but absent in normal tissues. Some of the antibreast monoclonal antibodies (eg, 6.2 and 72.3) developed by Schlom and collaborators (Chapter 10) show reactivity not only in breast cancer, but also in uterine and cervical cancer. However, at this point the clinical utility, if any, is not apparent.

With regard to keratins, as might be anticipated, adenocarcinomas of the endometrium and endocervix show reactivity principally with monoclonal antibodies to low MW keratins (cytokeratin, nonsquamous keratin), whereas squamous carcinomas of the cervix show strong staining, albeit focal and patchy, for high MW keratin (squamous keratin; Figs. 12–15 and 12–16). Disorganized patterns of keratinization also are valuable in evaluating dysplasia in tissue sections (low MW keratins near surface, high MW keratins near basal layer, which is the reverse of normal), and it is anticipated that keratin profiles may prove valuable in assessing dysplasia in Pap smears.

Figure 12–16. Focal deposit of tumor cells within the perineal muscles in the lateral vaginal wall; differential diagnosis of sarcoma or carcinoma resolved by demonstration of a positive reaction for keratin. The primary tumor was a moderately well-differentiated squamous carcinoma of cervix; most of the cells in both primary and metastatic tumors were keratin positive. Paraffin section, AEC with light hematoxylin counterstain (× 125).

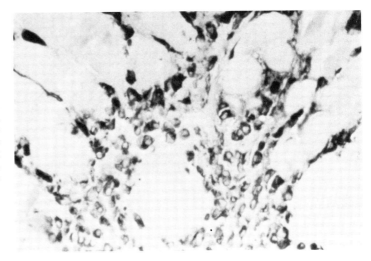

Small Cell Carcinoma (Carcinoids)

Small cell carcinomas of the uterus or cervix may represent anaplastic small cell variants of squamous or adenocarcinomas, metastases, or neuroendocrine tumors derived from normal neuroendocrine cells that are scattered within the epithelium of the cervix and uterus, much as they are in other epithelial tissues (Chapter 7).

In the past these cells and tumors have been recognized by the argyrophil reaction. More recently, specific polypeptides have been demonstrated, including calcitonin, gastrin, and somatostatin (Table 12–5). The cell population as a whole may be recognized by positivity for neuron specific enolase or HNK1 (Leu 7), both of which are demonstrable in paraffin sections (Chapter 7).

Estrogen Receptor

Assessment of estrogen receptor activity is almost mandatory for proper management of breast cancer. With respect to uterine cancer, the situation is less clear. As with breast cancer, the usual method is based upon a biochemical binding assay performed upon a cytosol; with regard to uterine tissue, there is even greater difficulty in determining the degree to which the assay measures the receptor in tumor cells, stromal cells, or myometrium. An immunohistologic method would offer the distinct advantage of direct visualization of the cell type that shows positivity for estrogen receptor.

Several approaches have been explored, including direct staining for estrogen, treatment with polymerized estradiol phosphatase followed by staining for estrogen, and staining for the estrogen receptor protein (estrophilin). Principles and practice are exactly as described for breast, with similar criticisms and pitfalls (see Chapter 10).

Direct staining with anti-estradiol antibody has shown a good correlation with cytosol-based assays (Farley et al, 1982); there is, however, no guarantee that the stained product represents the "true" receptor. Also, correlation with the cytosol-based assay, which itself may be seriously flawed, is not the ultimate test; rather, a clinical correlation is required. Similarly, the immunohistologic assay (stain) for estrophilin (estrogen receptor protein) must be evaluated by the clinical results, not simply by comparison with existing assays.

Staining for estradiol has been carried out both on frozen and on formalin paraffin sections. As pointed out earlier (Chapter 10), frozen sections suffer the risk of loss of estradiol (or receptor or both) by diffusion or other means; formalin-paraffin sections risk denaturation of the antigen. Satisfactory results have been claimed by both approaches.

With regard to staining for estrogen receptor, the monoclonal antibody employed (Press et al, 1984) produces convincing staining in frozen sections; the stain is restricted to nuclei—unlike estradiol staining in formalin paraffin sections, which may be both nuclear and cytoplasmic. Staining for estrogen receptor also has been seen in formalin paraffin sections; currently, however, the sole commercial source of the antibody (Abbott) recommends use of frozen sections (for research purposes only), noting inconsistent findings in fixed tissue. It may be that with increasing experience and utilization by other investigators, data may accumulate to permit utlization of the stain in paraffin sections. At present the method requires overnight incubation. Positive nuclear staining is seen in endometrial epithelium, stromal cells, and myometrium. Staining is maximal in the proliferative phase of the normal cycle, less in the secretory phase, and quite pronounced in the postmenopausal endometrium. With the availability of the antibody in kit form, experience with this method may be expected to increase rapidly.

Papillomavirus, Herpesvirus, and CMV

An extensive bibliography describing the immunohistologic demonstration of various viral antigens in cervix and uterus has developed. Most attention has focused upon the demonstration of herpesvirus and papillomavirus antigens.

Herpesvirus

Several commercial methods have become available for detection of herpes infection. Some methods involve short-term culture on a specially prepared monolayer followed by immunoperoxidase staining for the presence

Table 12–6. Selected Bibliography: Viral Antigens in Cancer of the Female Genital Tract—Herpesvirus

Cabral et al 1982	Staining with an antibody to herpesvirus (HSV2) revealed positivity for an early nonstructural polypeptide and for an envelope glycoprotein in cases of severe dysplasia and cancer, whereas condylomata and vulvitis were nonreactive; virus was not detectable by EM or by antibodies to capsid proteins
McDougall et al 1982	Immunoperoxidase method for herpesvirus–specific RNA positive in cervical cancer
Schmidt NJ et al 1983	Comparison of techniques showed direct immunoperoxidase staining for herpes simplex is specific and sensitive, detecting 82% of cases in which virus was isolated
Moseley et al 1981	Immunoperoxidase technique showed good correlation with virus isolation in genital herpes (76 cases); may detect some cases that are culture-negative (used commercial kits)
Adams et al 1984	Herpes antigen in routine cervical smears; agreed with isolation results in 47 of 50 cases; advocated use of technique as accurate and rapid

of virus antigen in the monolayer, as an early indicator of the presence of replicating virus. This method has become well established and shows an excellent correlation with virus isolation results (Table 12–6).

Of more direct interest to the surgical pathologist or cytologist is the possibility of directly detecting herpesvirus antigen in tissue sections or in cell smears such as routine Pap smears. In this respect the study of Adams and colleagues (1984) is particularly helpful. A total of 158 patients were studied: 84 had clinically suspected herpes; 72 were clinically normal. The results of direct immunostaining of smears agreed with virus isolation results in 47 out of 50 cases in which isolation was attempted. Of the 158 patients, 26 showed positive staining for HSV2 antigen (this included 9 cases from the clinically normal group); virus isolation confirmed the staining in those cases in which it was performed.

Staining for HSV2 is predominantly cytoplasmic, but some apparent nuclear reactivity is seen. It should be noted that in "positive smears" only 5 to 15 percent of cells show positivity, and these cells are mainly of the intermediate squamous variety.

Adams explored several different fixatives, including acetone, methanol, formalin, Bouin's, and Sprayfix; acetone and methanol were best; formalin gave poor results. A few tissue sections were also studied. In frozen sections, positive staining for HSV2 was within endocervical glands. Controls should be employed; Adams and colleagues used HSV1- and HSV2-infected cultures. They noted that anti-HSV2 cross-reacted weakly with HSV1 antigen, and vice versa.

Clearly, this approach to the detection of herpesvirus is within the compass of "routine" pathology practice. It is inexpensive, rapid, and reliable; the sensitivity of the method is enormously greater than that achieved by cytologic interpretations alone. In Adams's series, none of the 26 positive patients were detected by evaluation of cytologic criteria; it seems fair to conclude that the cytologic criteria are of little value.

Herpesvirus has been implicated in chronic cervicitis and in cervical carcinoma. Application of immunostaining may permit more rapid evaluation of the role of the virus in these conditions.

Immunostaining for herpes antigen also has been used successfully in the study of tracheobronchitis.

Papillomavirus Antigen

Like herpesvirus, papillomavirus has also been implicated in the etiology of cancer. There is much evidence linking HSV2 infection to an increased incidence of carcinoma of the cervix. More recently, papillomavirus antigen has been found in association with atypical proliferations of squamous epithelium at several sites in the body, including the skin (warts, bowenoid papillomatosis), the oral mucosa (squamous papilloma and condylomata), and the female genital tract (vulval and cervical condylomata).

Much of this evidence has been garnered from immunoperoxidase studies demonstrating the presence of papillomavirus antigen in cell smears and tissue sections (Table 12–7).

The most comprehensive studies are those of Kurman et al (1983), Syrjänen et al (1983b), Crum and colleagues (1982a),

Table 12–7. Selected Bibliography: Viral Antigens in Cancer of the Female Genital
Tract—Papillomavirus

Jenson et al 1982a	Papillomavirus antigens demonstrable in 18/29 warts, and 3/5 condylomata; 28 keratoacanthomas were nonreactive; positivity was intranuclear
Kurman et al 1981b	Found papillomavirus antigen in 20/40 genital warts and 24/50 cases of cervical dysplasia
Lutzner et al 1982	Papillomavirus antigens in oral condylomata
Jablonska 1982	Review of various types of papillomavirus producing different warts; especially associated with diminished immunity; possible role in neoplasia discussed
Crum et al 1982a	Positive staining for papillomavirus of value in distinguishing condylomata (positive) from carcinoma (usually negative)
Ferenczy et al 1981	Papilloma antigen in 48 of 97 cervical condylomata; positivity mainly in nuclei of koilocytic cells
Morin et al 1981	Papillomavirus infection most commonly present as inconspicuous flat lesion; not deteced in dysplasia or carcinoma
Lack et al 1980	5 serotypes of papillomavirus cause different warts with different features; laryngeal papillomas also positive with papillomavirus common antigen; immunoperoxidase more rapid and more effective than EM
Quick et al 1980	Human papillomavirus 2 in laryngeal papillomas correlated with presence of maternal condylomata at parturition; suggested possibility of cesarean section if condylomata present
Woodruff et al 1980	Broad antipapillomavirus antibody positive in 50% of condylomata to intranuclear staining, especially of superficial cells
Meisels et al 1981	Value of staining for papillomavirus antigen in distinguishing atypical condylomata (positive), about 19% of which progress to more advanced lesions
Syrjänen & Pyrhönen 1982a, b	Staining of condylomata with antipapillomavirus antibody
Crum et al 1982b	Utilized staining with antipapillomavirus antibody as part of the criteria for distinguishing atypical condylomata from carcinoma
Syrjänen et al 1983b	Examined 110 dysplastic cervices; in 79, various condylomata present; more than 70% of these had positive papillomavirus antigen; of the 31 noncondylomatous lesions (dysplasia and carcinoma in situ), all were negative
Dyson et al 1984	Koilocyte (cell with perinuclear halo) carries papillomavirus antigen in the nucleus
Winkler et al 1984a	Study of papillomavirus induced atypia and the presence of abnormal mitotic figures
Reid et al 1984	Role of papillomavirus in cervical neoplasia; decreased expression of papillomavirus antigen in neoplastic states.
Gupta et al 1983	Correlation of staining for papillomavirus antigen in smears and in sections; noted that morphology not a good predictor of antigen positivity
Pilotti et al 1984	Carcinoma in situ of vulva: 64% positive for papillomavirus antigen (resembles bowenoid carcinoma); verrucous carcinomas were negative
Kurman et al 1983	322 cases of cervical dysplasia: papillomavirus positive in 43% of mild dysplasia, 10% of moderate and severe dysplasia, and 10% of carcinoma in situ; noted that in the high-grade lesions the antigen usually not in the neoplastic cells but in surrounding tissue (formalin-paraffin sections)
Mariuzzi et al 1983	37% of condylomata positive for papillomavirus antigen
Syrjänen et al 1984	191 oral tumors: 75% of condylomata positive for papillomavirus antigen, 41% of squamous papillomas also positive
Fu et al 1983	DNA quantitation study of papillomavirus positive lesions

Winkler et al (1984a), and Reid et al (1983). Immunostaining for PVA may be reliably accomplished in formalin-fixed paraffin sections and in cell smears. The most useful information has been derived from studies of tissue section relating to the presence of PVA in condylomata, dysplasia, and carcinoma.

As a general rule, condylomata are usually positive (including the inconspicuous flat variety) (Fig. 12–17) and carcinomas are usually negative, although PVA-positive cells are fre-

quently seen in the epithelium adjacent to severely dysplastic epithelium or carcinoma in situ. Some pathologists have gone so far as to advocate the use of PVA staining as an aid to distinguishing atypical condylomata (positive) from severe dysplasias and carcinomas in situ (negative). Positive staining, when present, is intranuclear. Typical koilocytes (cells with clear perinuclear halos) are positive, but some investigators have stated that staining does not correlate well with such cytologic features; the most reliable guide to

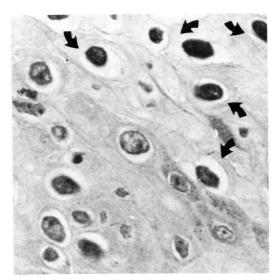

Figure 12–17. Typical appearances in a flat condyloma of cervix showing presence of scattered cells with a positive nuclear reaction (deep black nuclei—arrows) with anti-PVA (anti-papillomavirus) antibody. Paraffin section, DAB with hematoxylin counterstain (×500).

the presence of papillomavirus is staining for PVA.

Because of the role of papillomavirus in the causation of laryngeal papilloma, it has been recommended that pregnancies complicated by the presence of papillomavirus infection of the cervix should be managed by elective cesarean sections.

Other Infectious Agents

The recognition of the high frequency of infections with *Chlamydia* generated interest in developing immunohistologic stains for chlamydial antigens. As with herpes- and papillomavirus infections, the cervicitis that occurs with chlamydial infection is also associated with an increased incidence of carcinoma of the cervix. However, it is not clear whether the presence of *Chlamydia* is causal or coincidental. One study, by Mitao et al (1984), detected staining for chlamydial antigen in 16 percent of severely inflamed cervices (mildly inflamed cervices were nonreactive). In the severely inflamed cases, *Chlamydia* was detected in 20 percent of simple inflammation, in 25 percent of condylomatous inflammation, and in only 8 percent of biopsies containing carcinoma.

The same investigators (Winkler et al, 1984b) identified chlamydial antigen in 4 percent of cases of chronic endometritis and noted that the stain should be performed in the postabortal state, in chronic pelvic inflammatory disease, and in infertility.

One other useful application of immunoperoxidase techniques has emerged in relation to gynecologic pathology, namely the identification of *Trichomonas*. The morphologic recognition of *Trichomonas* is not difficult when intact organisms are present and when the disease is suspected, so that the pathologist is alert to the possibility. However, trichomonads are very fragile and stain poorly; in many instances they are not seen.

Bennett and colleagues (1980; O'Hara et al, 1980) identified *Trichomonas* in smears and in formalin-paraffin sections with a sensitivity that exceeded cytologic or histologic evaluations.

Other infectious agents (eg, cytomegalovirus [CMV]) that may be found elsewhere in the body but on occasion in the female genital tract are described in Chapter 15.

13

IMMUNOHISTOLOGY OF THE SKIN: MELANOMA, INTERMEDIATE FILAMENT

"The world thinks of the man of science as one who pulls out his watch and exclaims, 'Ha! half an hour to spare before dinner: I will just step down to my laboratory and make a discovery.' "

SIR RONALD ROSS, 1857–1932

The histopathology of the skin is a matter of great complexity and esoteric lore, justifying large texts devoted exclusively to the portrayal of its mysteries. Clearly, at some time the "immunohistology of the skin" will form a major part of such texts or will justify volumes of its own. That time is not yet. Although there have been several reviews (notably Jordon, 1980, and Wright, 1983) of the contribution of immunohistology to the understanding of skin disease, the subject still is in its infancy. Studies of skin diseases with monoclonal antibodies, which gave such great impetus to the study of tumors in general and lymphomas in particular, have been relatively few and far between. This is partly attributable to the fact that skin biopsies tend of necessity to be small, and by tradition all of the tissue obtained is committed to a fixative (Bouin's, formalin, or others). Displaying the distribution of immunoglobulins within the epidermis for the differential diagnosis of pemphigus and pemphigoid utilized cryostat sections, paving the way for studies with monoclonal antibodies, many of which have an absolute requirement for frozen sections.

Three areas have proven of particular interest for the surgical pathologist:

(1) The recognition of malignant melanoma and its distinction from other tumors

(2) The analysis of the various keratins, leading to characterization of other intermediate filaments and their roles in tumor classification in the skin and elsewhere

(3) Studies of immunoglobulin deposition and leukocyte populations in the diagnosis of inflammatory and neoplastic skin diseases. These areas are considered in the order listed.

MELANOMA

Melanomas constitute one of the commonest types of malignant neoplasms in humans. Many melanomas are recognized at an early stage, while only a few millimeters thick, and usually are curable by excision. Established malignant melanoma is difficult to treat, though recurring reports of "immune" regressions foster optimism.

The problems that confront the pathologist in this area are twofold. First, the benign must be distinguished from the malignant and, more difficult, from the premalignant. Complex histologic criteria have been developed, and the incidence of malignant change is well understood in various types of nevi; though in any particular lesion, the decision may be difficult. Now there is optimism that monoclonal antibodies may be developed to facilitate this distinction.

Second, the pathologist faces the problem of recognizing anaplastic varieties of melanoma in metastatic sites, positively distinguishing such lesions from poorly differentiated carcinomas, lymphomas, and the like. This discrimination may be difficult or impossible in some cases; pigment frequently is absent, and EM is relatively insensitive and time-consuming. Staining for melanoma-associated antigens may provide a convenient solution to the problem.

Melanoma cells do not react with anti-keratin antibodies, with anti-CEA, or with antibodies to epithelial membrane antigen. However, such "negative" staining is of little value in immunohistologic diagnosis, since the possibility of an artifactual "false-negative" due to technical error or, more importantly, to adverse handling of the tissue cannot easily be excluded. Melanomas have been reported to react with antivimentin antibodies (Miettinen et al, 1983c) but not with antineurofilament antibody, a matter of developmental interest, because neural crest derivatives are neurofilament- and keratin-negative.

S100 Protein

For these reasons, staining for S100 protein has found a place in the recognition of anaplastic melanomas, in spite of its relative lack of specificity for melanoma cells (Tables 13–1 and 13–2). S100 is an acidic protein that is relatively resistant to the adverse effects of fixation and paraffin embedment. It

Table 13–1. Pattern of S100 Reactivity

S100-Positive Cells	Corresponding Tumors
Glial cells, Schwann cells	Gliomas, schwannomas, neurofibromas
Neurons, neuroblasts	Neuroblastomas
Melanocytes	Various nevi, malignant melanomas
Myoepithelial and duct cells Salivary glands Sweat glands	"Mixed" tumors, pleomorphic adenomas
Chondrocytes	Chondromas, Chondrosarcomas
Langerhans's cells	Histiocytosis X
Some histiocytes (macrophages)	Malignant histiocytosis
?	Granular cell myoblastomas
?	Some liposarcomas
?	Chordomas

Other cell types are negative, including hepatocytes, Kupffers cells, epithelial cells of various types, endothelium and muscle cells, and lymphocytes. Negative tumors include all (almost all) carcinomas, lymphomas, muscle cell sarcomas, and the like.

can be successfully demonstrated in sections from paraffin blocks aged 10 or more years.

S100 typically is present in neural cells (glial cells and Schwann cells) and their corresponding tumors (gliomas and schwannomas, and others; see Chapter 16). Melanoma

Table 13–2. Selected Bibliography: S100

Nakazato et al 1982a	S100 and GFAP in pleomorphic adenoma of salivary glands; both stained minor subpopulations of apparent tumor cells; S100 was also present in some cells of normal parotid; GFAP was not
Stefansson et al 1982b	S100 in chondrocytes
Stefansson et al 1982a	S100 in Schwann cells (thought to be restricted to those cells outside CNS); S100 positive in tumors from Schwann cells and melanocytes; neurofibromas, melanomas, nevi, granular cell myoblastomas, and so forth, also positive; oat cell and medullary cell carcinomas, neuroblastomas, and paragglionomas, negative
Takahaski K et al 1981	S100 in interdigitating reticulum cells of "T cell zone" of lymph nodes; EM showed it to be present in nuclear and cytoplasmic membranes, suggesting in situ synthesis
Nakajima et al 1982b	S100 positive in 44 of 47 melanomas, including amelanotic melanomas; intradermal nevi and juvenile melanomas also strongly positive; blue nevi weakly positive
Nakazato et al 1982b	S100 in granular cell myoblastomas
Lauriola et al 1984	S100 in interdigitating cells of thymus and in thymomas
Cochran et al 1982	S100 in melanoma
Wen et al 1983	S100 in melanoma
Kahn et al 1983	S100, distribution and utility
Weiss SW et al 1983b	S100 in soft tissue tumors and schwannomas
Watanabe et al 1983	S100 in malignant histiocytosis and Letterer-Siwe disease
Kahn et al 1984a	S100 in melanocytes, Langerhans's cells, interdigitating reticulum cells (in T zones of lymph nodes), sweat glands, and Schwann cells; also in nevi, melanomas, histiocytosis X, mixed sweat gland tumors, and chondrosarcomas
Hood et al 1984	S100 in needle aspirates of schwannomas
Isobe T et al 1984	Alpha subunit of S100 in melanoma but not in schwannoma

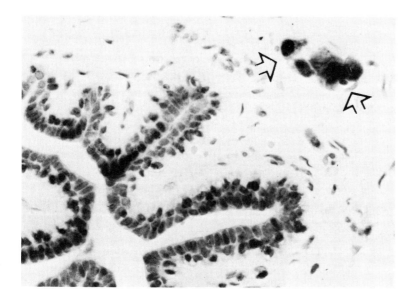

Figure 13–1. Breast biopsy containing normal breast elements (lower left) plus two or three small clusters of obviously malignant cells (arrow) within lymphatics. Diagnosis: presumptive breast carcinoma. Immunohistologic stains failed to detect lactalbumin, MEMA, CEA, or keratins, effectively excluding a diagnosis of breast, or indeed any other, carcinoma. Anti-S100 antibody revealed intense positivity. Subsequent studies revealed the presence of melanoma-associated antigens. Paraffin section, AEC with hematoxylin counterstain (×320).

cells, nevus cells, and melanocytes also are positive: staining for S100 is thus of little value in attempting to distinguish benign from malignant. Various other nonneural cells have been described as showing positivity (Table 13–1).

Most studies (Table 13–2) have reported S100 positivity in all (or almost all) melanomas, both primary and metastatic (Fig. 13–1). The staining is cytoplasmic, the proportion of positive cells varying from 10 to 70 per cent or more. Usually, focal nuclear staining is also present in a minority of cells. Almost all nevi also contain positive cells, including junctional and compound nevi, intradermal and blue nevi, and spitz tumor. Ocular melanomas also are positive.

Because of its conservation in paraffin sections, S100 staining has proved to be of particular value for the recognition of anaplastic melanomas. It is positive in practically 100 percent of amelanotic melanomas. We utilize it in conjunction with anti-HNK1 (or Leu 7—see Caillaud et al, 1984, and Mackie et al, 1984), which also stains melanomas in paraffin sections: most of the monoclonal antibodies to melanoma-associated antigens are effective only on frozen sections or cell smears (vide infra).

Melanoma-Associated Antigens

The production of monoclonal antibodies to melanoma-associated antigens has roused many investigators to a frenzy, resulting in the development of numerous antibodies with esoteric codings, so that only the experts of the field are easily able to translate from one manuscript to another. Many of these antibodies are similar or identical. A recent workshop resulted in the sharing and cross-testing of antibodies from several different investigators (Table 13–3). It appears that at least eleven different antigens are recognized by these antibodies; several are assayed on the cell surface; some are cytoplasmic (Fig. 13–2).

Among malignant neoplasms not one of these antibodies is totally restricted to staining melanoma, but some give "preferential" staining. Equally, although some appear to stain malignant cells more intensely, none can yet be relied upon to distinguish benign from malignant proliferations of melanocytes. Also, in our experience many of these antibodies do produce variable, often weak reactivity with other cell types, particularly endothelial cells, which undermines one's confidence of their utility for cell recognition. For example, the monoclonal antibodies against P97, a glycoprotein with an apparent molecular weight of 97 kd (Brown et al, 1981a and b; Stuhlmiller et al, 1982), react with both melanoma and nevus cells. However, only 50 percent of melanomas tested showed detectable binding with the antibody, and myoepithelial cells and sweat glands also displayed some reactivity. Other monoclonal antibodies recognize a proteoglycan with an apparent molecular weight of 200 kd: this antibody has been reported to be a very

Table 13–3. Selected Bibliography: Malignant Melanoma

Wilson BS et al 1984	Two monoclonals to melanoma associated antigens
Reisfeld 1982	Workshop: 24 monoclonal antibodies recognizing at least 11 different antigens
Hellström et al 1982	Report of 30 "workshop" monoclonal antibodies against cell surface antigens of human melanoma: p97 recognized by several antibodies
Carrel et al 1982	Report of 30 workshop monoclonal antibodies on panels of cell lines; none restricted to melanoma, several cross-reacted with neuroblastoma and glioma
Harper et al 1982	Workshop antibodies against tumor and normal cell lines, preferential reaction with melanoma
Natali et al 1983, 1984	Melanomas show loss of HLA-A, B, and C antigens and appearance of Ia antigens, plus a variety of high–molecular weight melanoma associated antigens
Herlyn M et al 1982	24 to 30 workshop monoclonal antibodies bound to most, but not all, melanoma lines; cross reactivity with various carcinomas and with fetal cells
Chee et al 1982	Antimelanoma monoclonal reacted with most carcinomas but not with benign nevus (preliminary study)
Dippold et al 1980	Surface antigens on human melanomas
Thompson et al 1982	Monoclonal antibody reacting with melanoma and dysplastic nevus but not normal skin or benign nevi; other antibodies showed different pattern
Heaney-Kieras & Bystryn 1982	75,000 MW antigen common to most melanomas; absent or low levels in other malignant cells and normal cells
Herlyn D et al 1983	Production of monoclonal antibodies by grafting mice with melanomas
van Duinen et al 1984a	Immunoelectron microscopy using NK1 as antimelanomas antibody
Mackie et al 1984	NK1 antibody positive in 100% of melanoma and most intradermal, junctional, compound, and dysplastic nevi; also some reactivity with carcinomas (breast and prostate); effective in paraffin sections
van Duinen et al 1984b	NK1 in paraffin sections: positive in 25/34 melanomas and only 2/58 carcinomas; 10/20 neuroendocrine tumors positive
Tilgen et al 1983	Light and EM study of intracellular distribution of P97 antigen
Garrigues et al 1982	P97 antigen in most melanomas and compound nevi; some staining of sweat glands; other tissues said to be nonreactive
Folberg et al 1983	Ocular melanoma reactive with antibody 149 2A-17 in paraffin sections
Mitchell et al 1981	Monoclonal NU 4B, antimelanoma
Morgan AC et al 1981	Monoclonal to melanoma-specific glycoproteins
Brown JP et al 1981a	P97 antigen and antibody
Brown JP et al 1981b	Distribution of P97 in normal and neoplastic tissues
Stuhlmiller et al 1982	Assays of antimelanoma monoclonals
Pukel et al 1982	Ganglioside antigen in melanomas
Houghton et al 1982	Melanocytes and melanoma-associated antigens
Imam et al 1985b	Human antimelanoma antibodies
Houghton et al 1983	Human antimelanoma antibodies
Katano et al 1983	Human antibodies to melanomas, neuroblastomas, and gliomas

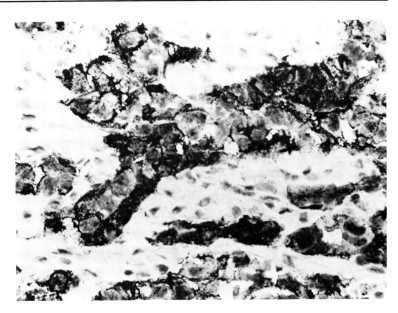

Figure 13–2. Malignant melanoma showing surface and cytoplasmic staining with a monoclonal antibody to a melanoma-associated antigen (antibody courtesy of Xoma Corporation). Frozen section, AEC with hematoxylin counterstain (×320).

sensitive marker for melanoma, but it also is occasionally expressed on nonmelanoma tumors (Morgan AC et al, 1981; Wilson BS et al, 1984). The monoclonal antibody termed 691-15-NU4B, directed against a four-chain glycoprotein, was reported to be expressed only on malignant melanoma but not on nevus cells on normal melanocytes in frozen tissue sections (Mitchell KF et al, 1981; Thompson et al, 1982). It does, however, react with astrocytomas (Morgan AC et al, 1981), and the distinction of benign from malignant cells with the microscope is less clear than one would hope: negative staining does not guarantee benignity, and weak positivity does not of itself provide grounds for embarking upon radical therapy.

Of the MEL series of 5 antimelanoma monoclonal antibodies (Ortho), MEL 1 (antiganglioside) and MEL 3 react also with nevi and normal melanocytes; MEL 4 and 5 react only with subsets of melanoma, and MEL 3 is an anti–Ia-like reagent. MEL 2, 3 and 4 show extensive reactivity against normal tissues, especially endothelial cells. Only MEL 5 is effective in paraffin sections.

For routine practice the surgical pathologist requires an antibody that can reliably distinguish malignant melanoma from nevus cells, especially in borderline or difficult cases, in routinely processed tissues as well as in frozen sections. Such a reagent is not yet available, or at least there is not yet one of proven value.

The distinction of melanoma from other anaplastic malignancies is a more practical proposition. Several monoclonal antibodies, although not absolutely specific, do have potential value in this respect (Table 13–3). Because of the lability of corresponding antigens, most of the antibodies so far described are of use only in frozen sections (or optimally fixed cell preparations from fine-needle aspirates). For example, the MEL series of 5 monoclonals marketed by Ortho (MEL 1, 2, 3, 4, and 5) is recommended for use on frozen sections (blocks snap-frozen in liquid nitrogen): only MEL 5 gives satisfactory results in paraffin. Since pathologists cling to paraffin sections, with which the traditional morphologic approach to diagnosis is most secure, the majority of monoclonals to melanoma-associated antigens are excluded from practical consideration. At least one commercial concern has marketed a melanoma monoclonal antibody claiming effectiveness in paraffin sections, a claim that in our hands could not be substantiated even after prolonged incubation. By contrast MEL 5 (Ortho) monoclonal against a 75,000-kd molecule does react in paraffin sections and does not react with (most) carcinomas and sarcomas; however, it stains only a proportion of melanomas—unfortunately and principally, those containing pigment granules that already are recognizable with the microscope—and it does react with nevus cells and normal melanocytes.

A Practical Approach: Staining for S100 and HNK1 (Leu 7)

At present, therefore, the best approach to the distinction of melanoma from other tumors in paraffin sections is to stain with HNK1 (Leu 7) and S100, both of which produce staining of almost all melanomas—including amelanotic forms—in routinely processed tissue. Other monoclonals should be reserved for confirmatory stains on frozen sections if deemed necessary. For the recognition of malignancy per se in paraffin sections, none of the antibodies currently available meet the task. However, Ia-like antigens appear to be expressed preferentially on malignant melanomas, compared with nevus cells. For example, MEL 3 reacts against Ia-like antigens and shows differential staining between melanoma cells and normal melanocytes; it is not melanoma-specific, since several other tumors are positive (Ia-positive). Several monoclonal antibodies are available that detect Ia-like antigens on paraffin sections.

Human antibodies to human malignant melanomas also have been produced by several laboratories. Some, in our experience, appear to show greater specificity for melanoma than is observed with murine monoclonals and may discriminate between melanoma cells and nevus cells (Imam A et al, 1985b). However, being human antibodies, they are of little use for immunohistologic studies of human tissue, at least by sandwich techniques (Chapters 2 and 3).

INTERMEDIATE FILAMENTS: KERATIN, VIMENTIN, DESMIN

Recent studies have demonstrated that most cells of the body contain cytoskeletal elements, or intermediate filaments, charac-

Table 13–4. Distribution of Intermediate Filaments* in Different Cell Types

Cell Types	Intermediate Filaments
Epithelial	"Keratins" (family of 19 or more proteins, MW 40–68 kd)
Mesenchymal	Vimentin (MW 55 kd)
Muscle	Desmin (MW 53 kd)
Glial-astrocytes	GFAP (glial fibrillary acidic protein, MW 55 kd)
Neurons (most)	Neurofilament proteins (MW 68–100 kd)
Embryonic	No intermediate filament

*Filament types are distinguishable antigenically.

teristic of the cell type. Although similar in structure at electron microscopy, these filaments, midway in size between microfilaments and microtubules, are divisible into several types on the bases of antigenicity and biochemical analysis (Table 13–4).

True epithelia contain cytokeratin, mesenchymal cells contain vimentin, and cells with myogenic differentiation contain in addition desmin (also known as skeletin). Astrocytes contain glial fibrillary acidic protein filaments (GFAP), and most neurons contain neurofilament antigen (Chapter 16). Most normal adult cells contain only one type of intermediate filament (exceptions include some muscle cells—vimentin and desmin—and possibly epithelial cells in the salivary glands and kidneys—vimentin and keratin).

The restricted cellular distribution of these different intermediate filaments lends itself to attempts to identify cells and their derivative tumors on the basis of the type of intermediate filament present. The availability of conventional (polyclonal) antisera and monoclonal antibodies to each of these intermediate filament types facilitates this process and offers the pathologist an approach to immunohistologic classification of neoplasms.

Keratin is the most complex of the intermediate filaments and is not so much a single species of molecule as a whole family of related proteins that vary in molecular weight from about 44 to 68 kd and are coded by a complex set of genes. Immunologic and biochemical analysis reveals at least 19 different proteins within the keratin family. Polyclonal and monoclonal antibodies react with one or several of these molecular subspecies of keratin (Figs. 13–3 and 13–4).

As noted above, all epithelial cells contain keratins, but the different types of epithelium contain different keratin profiles (Tables 13–5 and 13–6). In practical terms these different epithelia (and the corresponding neoplasms) may therefore be distinguishable by judicious application of selected antibodies that react only with well-defined groups of keratin molecules. The ability to make such fine discriminations is still in its infancy, but preliminary studies utilizing monoclonal antibodies show great promise for the recognition of certain types of epithelial neoplasms (see Chapter 14).

In simple terms, stratified squamous epithelium contains mainly complex, high–molecular weight keratins, whereas simple epi-

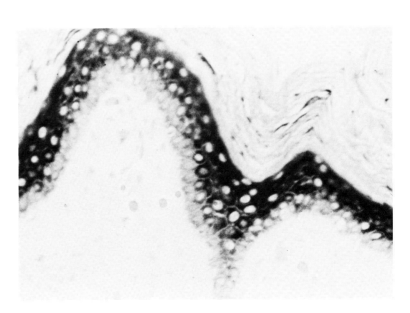

Figure 13–3. Squamous epithelium stained with a pankeratin antibody; positivity is greatest in the suprabasal layers. Paraffin section, AEC with hematoxylin counterstain (×320). This tissue serves as the "biologic positive control" for staining of the bone marrow biopsy shown in Figure 13–4.

Table 13–5. Selected Bibliography: Intermediate Filaments in Tissue and Tumor Typing

Osborn & Weber 1983	The definitive study to date; comprehensive review of intermediate filaments and tissue distribution
Bejui-Thivolet et al 1982	Found keratin-positive staining in squamous carcinomas, weak in primary lung adenocarcinoma, and negative in oat cell, carcinoids and undifferentiated lung tumors
Löning & Burkhardt 1982	Dyskeratosis and keratin distribution: used antibodies against "small" and "large" keratin; small keratins found in all layers of epidermis; large keratins found only in suprabasal layers in normal tissue, but randomly distributed in dyskeratosis and malignancy
Thivolet et al 1980	Antikeratin antisera versus different keratin bands in polyacrylamide gel; anti-P1 and anti-P2 antibodies versus antigens (MW 67,00 and 62,000 respectively) reacted only with upper malpighian layers (not basal layers); anti-whole keratin antibody reacted with all layers as did anti-P3 (MW 55,000).
Gomes et al 1981	Used Thivolet's antibodies in a study of keratinization in lichen planus
Schlegel et al 1980a, b	Use of keratin antibodies in studies of histogenesis and carcinogenesis. In paraffin sections, glandular acinar cells, plus muscle, blood, and lymphoid cells were keratin-negative; breast and lung cancer gave variable staining; colon, renal, and prostate carcinomas were negative; squamous epithelium and ducts of epithelium-derived glands plus respiratory and urinary tract epithelium were positive
Caselitz et al 1981a	Again used Thivolet's antibodies, in this instance to study parotid glands; duct cells were positive, acinar cells negative, and myoepithelial cells positive (antibody versus actin also stained ducts and myoepithelial cells); in pleomorphic adenomas ductlike structures and spindle cells were keratin- and actin-positive
Carbone & Micheau 1982	Four cases of nasopharyngeal carcinoma confused with lymphoma; staining for keratin faciliated the proper diagnosis
Miettinen et al 1982b	Eight nasopharyngeal carcinomas: keratin-positive
Madri & Barwick 1982	Forty cases of nasopharyngeal neoplasia; all squamous carcinomas stained for keratin whether or not they were termed keratinizing or non-keratinizing by conventional methods
Asa et al 1981a	Fifteen craniopharyngiomas positive for keratin; pituitary tumors nonreactive
Azar et al 1982	Used EM and immunoperoxidase to increase diagnostic precision in "anaplastic" large cell tumors
Shi et al 1984a, b	Keratin antibodies, utility for diagnosis of head and neck tumors
Corson & Pinkus 1982	Keratin and CEA in mesotheliomas and adenocarcinomas; mesotheliomas strongly keratin-positive but CEA-negative (with rare equivocal exceptions); adenocarcinomas—CEA-positive, keratin weak or negative; used rabbit antiserum (Banks-Schlegel)
Rosai & Pinkus 1982	Tibial adamantinomas are keratin-positive and factor VIII–negative therefore are probably epithelial in origin
Viac et al 1982	Utilizing antisera against extracted keratins suggested that different cell types show different pathways of keratinization (epidermis is distinct from mucosa)
Weiss RA et al 1983a	Monoclonal antikeratin antibody (designated AE1) showed selective staining of basal cells in normal epidermis and different patterns in various dyskeratotic diseases (psoriasis, seborrheic keratosis, actinic keratosis, verruca, Bowen's disease, and carcinoma)
Viac et al 1983	Monoclonal antikeratin antibody (designated KL1) stained predominantly upper layers of skin; used frozen sections and trypsinized paraffin sections
Warhol et al 1983	Lower molecular weight keratin in basal layers (individual tonofilament), high–molecular weight keratins in upper layers (web of tonofibrils)
Kuhajda et al 1983b	Esophageal cancer positive for keratin, including "sarcomatous" areas
Espinoza & Azar 1982	Rabbit antiserum to keratin; Epithelial tumors keratin-positive; keratin-negative group included nevi, melanomas, lymphomas, carcinoid tumors, various sarcomas
Gown & Vogel 1984	Three monoclonal antikeratin antibodies with different patterns. One, nonsquamous, reacts with glandular type epithelia; a second, squamous, gives intense staining of squamous epithelium (available commercially—see Appendix 2)
Morton et al 1980	Antisera to Mallory's body protein (keratin)
Kahn et al 1984b	Antibody to Mallory's body cytokeratin stained a variety of anaplastic tumors of epithelial derivation but not lymphomas, melanomas, etc.
Gown & Vogel 1982	Monoclonals to vimentin and keratins, description of patterns of tissue reactivity

Table 13–5. Selected Bibliography: Intermediate Filaments in Tissue and Tumor Typing
Continued

Nagel 1983b	Antiserum to keratin, frozen section tissues, and tumor distribution
Nelson et al 1984	Monoclonals to keratin (AE1 and AE3 antibodies)
Nagle 1983a	Antiserum to keratin, distribution in ovarian tumors
Mitchell & Gusterson 1982	Combined keratin and mucin stain for lung cancer
Larker & Sun, 1982	Different cell types in basal layer of epidermis
Miettinen et al 1983d	"Synovial" sarcomas are keratin-positive, vimentin-negative (normal synovium is the reverse), suggesting an epithelial origin for these tumors, which are named because of their appearances
Miettinen & Virtanen 1984	Extensive study of synovial sarcoma; concluded epithelial origin; included keratin, vimentin and reactions
Van Muijen et al 1984	Three antibodies against different subsets of keratin; differential staining of normal tissues and tumors
Debus et al 1984	Monoclonal antibodies of keratin subsets: differential staining of tumors
Chase et al 1984	Epithelioid sarcomas contain both keratin and vimentin
Walts et al 1983	Keratin and CEA in fine needle aspirates and pleural fluids; emphasis on distinguishing mesothelial cells from cancer cells; noted keratin more readily demonstrated in cytocentrifuge preparations than in paraffin sections
Gabbiani et al 1981	Cytokeratin, vimentin, and desmin in neoplastic cells
Miettinen et al 1983e	Keratin and vimentin in ovarian tumors
del Poggetto et al 1983	Keratin and vimentin in ovarian tumors
Holthöfer et al 1983	Keratin, vimentin, and desmin in renal carcinoma
Miettinen et al 1983b	Chordomas, ependymomas, and chondromas; keratin, desmin, vimentin and GFAP. Chordomas keratin-positive, but vimentin-and GFAP–negative (note also S100 protein, positive)
Miettinen et al 1982a	Vimentin, keratin, and desmin in soft tissue tumors
Osborn & Weber 1983	Differential diagnosis of tumors using antibodies to keratin, vimentin, and desmin
Miettinen et al 1983c	Merkel cell tumor positive for neurofilament antigens, negative for vimentin and keratin
Lehto et al 1984	Bronchial carcinomas positive for neurofilament antigens but negative for keratin, vimentin, and GFAP

Table 13–6. Patterns of Reactivity with Two Antikeratin Antibodies

Normal Tissue Type	Squamous (34BE12)[1]	Nonsquamous (35BH11)[1]
Muscle, fibrous tissue, bone, cartilage, lymphoid tissue, melanocytes, etc.	−	−
Squamous epithelium	+	−
Sweat gland acini	−	+
Sweat gland ducts	+	±
Mesothelium	+	+
Lung alveolar cells	+/−	+
Bronchial epithelium	+	+
Liver hepatocytes	−	+
Liver bile ducts	+	±
Kidney—collecting tubules	+	+
—proximal tubules	−	+
Bladder	+	+
Pancreas—acini	−	+
—ducts	+	±
Breast—acini	−	+
—ducts	+	±
Thyroid (follicular epithelium)	+/−	+
Gut epithelium and glands	+/−	+

[1]Antibodies of Gown and Vogel (1984).
Plus (+) indicates consistent strong staining; minus (−) indicates trace or nonreactivity; ± indicates weak variable staining; +/− indicates a mixture of positive and nonreactive cells.

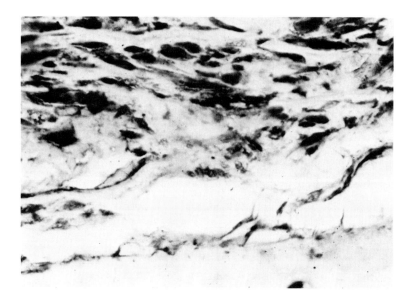

Figure 13–4. Antikeratin antibodies are very useful for screening tissues (lymph nodes, marrow) for the presence of keratin-positive cells, which in these sites are presumptive carcinoma cells. Anaplastic spindle cells in bone marrow stained with pankeratin antibody. Tumor cells show intense cytoplasmic staining. Paraffin section, AEC with hematoxylin counterstain (×320).

thelium and glandular epithelium contain a preponderance of low–molecular weight keratins. A conventional (polyclonal) antiserum made in rabbit using human callus, which contains much high–molecular weight keratin, may therefore react intensely with squamous epithelium and to a lesser degree (or if suitably diluted, not at all) with glandular epithelium or liver cells. Clearly, different antisera, each composed of a "cocktail" of different antibodies of varying affinity and specificity, depending upon the exact source of keratin(s) used as the immunogen, may vary greatly in their pattern of reactivity with normal tissue. This variance may account for some of the discordant findings in the literature.

The method of fixation and processing of tissue is also important. Keratins (and other intermediate filament antigens) are most readily and most consistently demonstrable in cryostat sections of snap-frozen tissue. Following formalin fixation and paraffin embedment, findings are less reproducible; many investigators advocate trypsinization as a means of enhancing the immunoreactivity of keratins under these conditions. As with trypsinization for staining of immunoglobulins (Chapter 4), the proteolytic process needs to be carefully managed and must be adjusted to provide optimal results with paraffin tissues in each separate laboratory (selection of appropriate concentration of trypsin and

time of incubation). Whether or not trypsin digestion was employed also affects the findings reported in the literature. Some investigators have utilized paraffin sections of tissues fixed in Carnoy's solution for detection of intermediate filaments with much greater success (Gown and Vogel, 1984). Ethanol fixation also is clearly superior to formalin for this purpose (Fig. 13–5).

The use of monoclonal antibodies offers the prospect of greater reproducibility among different investigators than was possible using polyclonal antisera. With time the patterns of tissue reactivity with certain monoclonal antibodies will become well recognized, and the discriminatory function provided by these antibodies will thus become available to all. Many different antikeratin monoclonal antibodies have been produced (Table 13–5), some with broad spectrum activity (pankeratin), others with more restricted specificity for different high– or low–molecular weight keratins (Figs. 13–6, 13–7). The accompanying table (Table 13–6) illustrates the patterns of staining that may be obtained with selected reagents. Those antibodies illustrated are here dubbed squamous (mainly versus high-MW keratins) or nonsquamous (mainly versus low-MW keratins) (Fig 13–8). The reagents prepared by Gown and Vogel (1982, 1984) typify those that are available. These antibodies are not unique; many others have been described of

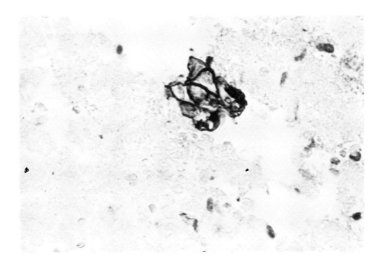

Figure 13–5. Fine-needle aspirate of cerebral mass; positivity with antibody to low MW ("nonsquamous") keratin supports a diagnosis of metastatic carcinoma. AEC with hematoxylin counterstain (×200). Fine-needle aspirates, producing cell smears that may be fixed briefly in ethanol, acetone, or paraformaldehyde provide an excellent basis for immunostaining, since fixation can be carefully controlled by the pathologist.

equal or greater utility. They are simply the reagents, together with Ray Nagle's K-4 antibody, with which we personally have had the most extensive experience. Table 13–6 illustrates the expected pattern of distribution in normal tissues (frozen sections, Carnoy's fixed tissues, or trypsinized formalin-fixed tissues). K-4 is more of a pankeratin antibody although some epithelial cells escape staining in paraffin sections.

Although studies using polyclonal antibodies are included in the literature listing, I have not attempted to summarize the findings reported with such antisera since no two antisera are exactly the same and each new antiserum produced in rabbit must be characterized anew.

The pattern of reactivity of tumor tissue (Fig. 13–9) is largely predictable from the normal cell types shown in the table (see Chapter 14). It should be noted that sometimes tumors express profiles that differ from the normal tissues, especially if the tumor is poorly differentiated. One example is hepatoma; normal hepatocytes do not react with AE1 (versus low-MW keratins), whereas hepatoma cells show positivity; other antikeratins react with both (see Table 13–6). Thus, although normal tissue cultures provide a legitimate guide, anomalies will be encountered. Typical tumor keratin profiles are given in Table 14–3, which summarizes the use of these antibodies in the differential diagnosis of anaplastic tumors. Further dis-

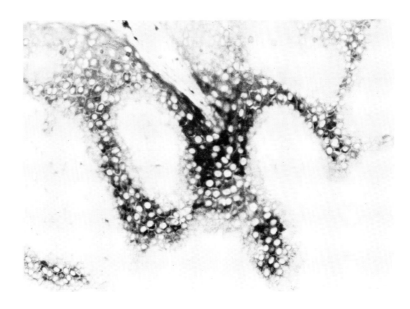

Figure 13–6. Skin showing pattern of reactivity with a monoclonal antibody to high molecular weight keratin (so-called "squamous keratin"). Staining is most intense in the stratum spinosum and the stratum granulosum. The stratum germinativum (basal layer) shows variable weak reactivity. Compare with Figure 13–7. Paraffin section, AEC, counterstain was omitted in order more clearly to depict positive reaction in black and white medium (×200).

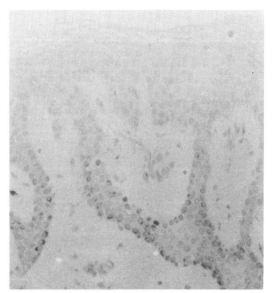

Figure 13–7. Skin showing pattern of reactivity with a monoclonal antibody to low MW keratin (so-called "nonsquamous keratin"). The basal layer shows traces of granular (black) staining in some cells; the more superficial layers show no reactivity. Compare with Figure 13–6. Paraffin section, AEC with hematoxylin counterstain to render epidermis visible (×200).

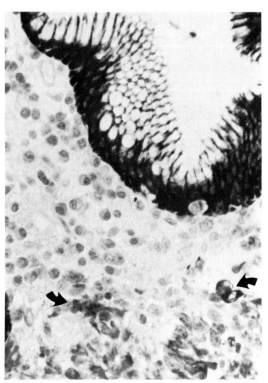

Figure 13–9. Section of stomach wall showing epithelium staining intensely (black) with antibody to low MW keratin ("nonsquamous"). Underlying plasma cells show no evidence of staining, but clusters of malignant cells deeper within the lamina propria are positive (arrows). These initially were thought to be lymphoma cells; positivity for keratin indicates carcinoma. Paraffin section, AEC with hematoxylin counterstain (×200). Compare with Figure 13–8.

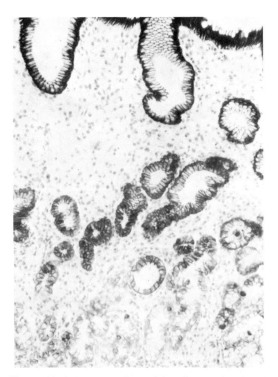

Figure 13–8. Patterns of reactivity of monoclonal antibody to low MW keratin ("nonsquamous") within stomach wall. The epithelial cells show moderate to intense reactivity (gray-black cytoplasm). Paraffin section, AEC with hematoxylin counterstain (×125).

cussion of keratin staining of individual tumor types is given in appropriate chapters (eg, ovarian tumors—Chapter 9).

Other monoclonal antikeratin antibodies also provide useful differential staining patterns; the interested pathologist intending to use these reagents should refer directly to the appropriate original report. These antibodies include Sun's AE1 and AE3 (low-, intermediate-, and high-MW keratins—see, Nelson et al, 1984; Battifora, 1984); CK1–CK4 (versus cytokeratin 18 and K_G8–13) (pankeratins) of Debus et al (1984); and clones 77, 78, and 80 (versus squamous epithelium and pankeratin) of van Muijen et al (1984). References to other reagents are listed in Table 13–5. It should be noted that it may be possible to subdivide epithelial tumors to an even greater degree by attending to 9 subspecies of keratins (Osborn and Weber, 1983). It is not yet established, however, that such detailed profiles remain constant across large numbers of tumors within any individual histologic type.

Vimentin

Just as keratin is the intermediate filament of epithelial cells, so vimentin characterizes mesenchymal cells (Table 13–5). Vimentin, also known as fibroblast intermediate filament (FIF) is, unlike keratin, composed of a single type of subunit with a molecular weight of approximately 55 kd. Vimentin is not present in normal epithelial cells "in vivo," although it has been described in epithelial cells in culture and may rarely appear within the tumor cells of epithelial neoplasms (carcinoma); vimentin of course is almost always present within tissue sections of carcinomas but is usually confined to blood vessels and supporting stromal elements (fibroblasts and the like).

Vimentin can be demonstrated within cells by immunohistologic methods and can readily be shown in frozen sections and in Carnoy's fixed paraffin sections. Following formalin fixation, staining is much reduced and is inconsistent from case to case. Conventional antisera to vimentin may be prepared using vimentin extracted from SV40 transformed human fibroblasts (eg, Gabbiani et al, 1981; del Poggetto et al, 1983). In addition, several investigators have prepared monoclonal antibodies (Gown and Vogel, 1982 and 1984—antibody 43B-E8). Some antivimentin antibodies are available commercially. It

Table 13–7. Vimentin-Positive Cell Types by Tissue Location

All tissues	Blood vessels—smooth muscle, fibrocytes, etc.—endothelium, connective tissue (fibroblasts), fat cells (variable)
Lungs	Alveolar histiocytes
Liver	Sinus lining cells
Spleen/lymph nodes	Lymphocytes, dendritic cells, histiocytes
Kidneys	Glomerular endothelium, occasional tubular cells
Muscles	Fibroblasts, etc., variable muscle cells
Skin	Nevus cells (melanocytes)
Skeletal system	Chondrocytes, osteocytes
CNS	Rare astrocytes, ependymal cells, dural cells

Compiled from the literature, combining conventional and monoclonal antibodies. Note that not all antibodies react with all these cell types; in spite of the known presence of vimentin in lymphocytes, the monoclonal antibodies of Gown and Vogal (1984) fail to react positively, although other cell types are well stained.

should be noted that whereas "good" keratin antisera and most antikeratin monoclonals do not react with vimentin, the converse is less true; antisera versus vimentin must be carefully tested to demonstrate lack of reactivity with epithelial cells (Fig. 13–10); likewise, even some monoclonals with reactivity to vimentin have been shown to react with some of the intermediate MW cytokeratins.

The patterns of reactivity in normal tissues are shown, somewhat tentatively, in Table 13–7. For malignant tumors it is a general

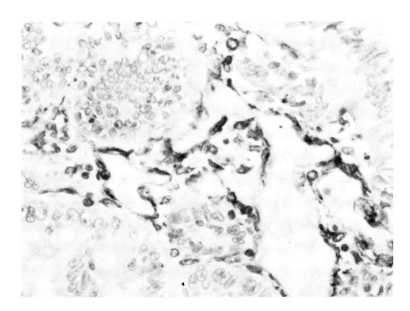

Figure 13–10. Vimentin reactivity (black) within the cytoplasm of endothelial and connective tissue cells present as part of the stroma of a carcinoma of colon. The carcinoma (epithelial) cells are negative, providing some evidence for lack of cross reactivity of this antibody with keratins. Paraffin section, AEC with hematoxylin counterstain (×200).

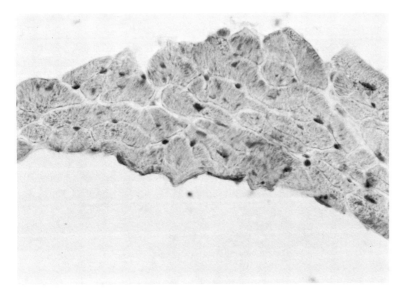

Figure 13–11. Needle biopsy of myocardium showing typical bands or stripes of desmin-positive material. Striated muscle will show similar positivity. Paraffin section, AEC with hematoxylin counterstain (×200).

rule that sarcomas stain but carcinomas do not, with a few exceptions (see Tables 14–2, 14–3, and 14–4).

Desmin

Desmin is a relatively simple intermediate filament, which, like vimentin, is composed of a single type of repeating unit (MW 50 kd). Although desmin appears to have some amino acid homology with vimentin (and keratin), antibodies can be prepared that will effectively discriminate between these filament types. In the normal human adult, desmin is found only in muscle cells, in the Z disc of skeletal and cardiac muscle (Fig. 13–11), and to a variable degree in smooth muscle cells; uterus and gastrointestinal tract smooth muscles usually stain well, vascular smooth muscle shows variable reactivity (references, Table 13–5). Note that myoepithelial cells are keratin-positive and nonreactive for desmin.

Among the neoplasms, carcinomas do not react with antidesmin antibodies, leiomyosarcomas and rhabdomyosarcomas are positive, and other sarcomas (with some exceptions) are negative (see Table 14–4).

Glial Fibrillary Acidic Protein and Neurofilament Protein

Full discussion of these intermediate filaments is given in the chapter pertaining to the central nervous system (Chapter 16). In brief, GFAP is found only within astrocytes (Fig. 13–12), some ependymal cells, and the corresponding tumors. Neurofilament proteins are found in most neurons (axons, dendrites and cell bodies) and neuroendocrine cells; neuroblastomas, ganglioneuromas, pheochromocytomas, and neuroendocrine tumors react positively in at least some cases, although data are limited.

CLASSIFICATION OF SKIN TUMORS

Tumors of the skin, like those of other tissues, are generally classified with reference

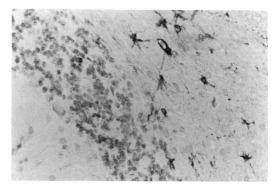

Figure 13–12. Normal brain tissue showing staining of astrocytes for GFAP (glial fibrillary acidic protein); positive cells have red (black) cytoplasm. Paraffin section, AEC with hematoxylin counterstain (×200). See color plate II–7.

to the nature of the supposed progenitor cell. Broadly speaking, there are tumors of the epidermis (squamous epithelium), the skin appendages (ductular epithelium, glandular epithelium), the connective tissue elements (vessels, fibroblasts, leukocytes, and so forth), and the melanocytes (nevi and melanomas, discussed earlier).

As indicated earlier, the variety of supposedly separate morphologic lesions produced from these elements is staggering, but classification of these skin tumors is subjective, and discrepancies among separately trained observers are probably of the same order of magnitude as seen in the classification of the lymphomas (Chapter 4) in which the level of disagreement exceeds 50 percent in some instances. As with the lymphomas, attempts have been made to exploit the specific recognition that immunohistology (potentially) offers to achieve a more objective method of cell, and thereby tumor, recognition. As with the lymphomas, a beginning has been made, but it is only a beginning. Within paraffin sections, we are restricted to the study of only those few antigens that survive the abuses of fixation and processing. For the much more discriminating studies possible with monoclonal antibodies, we are limited to the use of cryostat sections, preferably of snap-frozen tissues, and the routine collection of such tissue is a matter that seems to require a greater measure of leisure and coordination than is available to most of us. Nevertheless, the preliminary studies that have been performed indicate, as with the lymphomas, that the information to be gained may be of real clinical utility, and this possibility may force the general adoption of frozen tissue samples or at least exploration of less abusive fixation techniques.

Paraffin Sections

A number of antigens, demonstrable in paraffin sections to some degree, are of proven value; these include immunoglobulins, lysozyme, alpha$_1$-antitrypsin, S100 protein, CEA, epithelial membrane antigen, keratin, involucrin, and collagen (type IV). With regard to keratin (and immunoglobulins), trypsinization is considered necessary for optimal staining of formalin-fixed tissues.

Keratins

Carcinomas of the epidermis (a squamous epithelium) typically stain strongly for keratin (Fig. 13–13), albeit with some variation from cell to cell and tumor to tumor. The higher molecular weight keratins typically are present, and pankeratin antibodies produce positive staining. As indicated in the preceding pages, these complex keratins may be stained quite specifically using antibodies to squamous keratins; antibody to nonsquamous keratins (cytokeratin) stains only cells in the basal layer of normal skin (Figs. 13–6 and 13–7) and reacts with relatively few cells of squamous carcinomas (the positive cells are mainly distributed around the periphery of the squamous nests). Basal cell carcinomas,

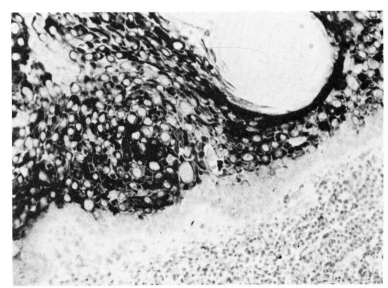

Figure 13–13. Well-differentiated squamous carcinoma showing pattern of reactivity with antibody to high MW keratin (squamous keratin). The peripheral "basal" type cells stain only weakly and the lymphocytes not at all. Paraffin section, AEC with hematoxylin counterstain (×200).

by contrast, are positive with cytokeratin (low-MW) antibodies (and therefore to some degree with many keratin antisera) but are nonreactive with squamous keratin antibodies (versus high-MW keratin). Bowen's disease shows some differences from squamous carcinoma in the exaggerated presence of high-MW keratins and marked abnormalities in the normal maturation sequence (dyskeratosis; Tables 13–8 and 13–9).

Tumors of the skin appendages also show differential staining with the different anti-keratin antibodies (Figs. 13–14 and 13–15); carcinomas of the glandular components (of sweat and sebaceous glands) stain with nonsquamous keratin (but not with squamous keratin), whereas those tumors of ductal origin show a mixed picture (Fig. 13–16). It is worth noting that tumors of sweat glands show many staining patterns in common with breast cancer, including frequent reactivity for CEA, mammary epithelial membrane antigen (epithelial membrane antigen or milk–fat globule membrane antigen) and apocrine

Table 13–8. Differential Diagnosis of Malignant Tumor in Skin[1]

Antibody Versus	Conclusion: Positivity Consistent with
Pankeratin[3]	Epithelial-derived neoplasm, includes synovial sarcoma
Squamous keratin (high-MW)[3]	Squamous carcinoma, Bowen's disease
Nonsquamous keratin (low-MW)[3]	Adenocarcinoma, basal cell carcinoma
Vimentin[2]	Sarcoma (various types)
Desmin[2]	Rhabdo- and leiomyosarcomas
Myoglobin	Rhabdomyosarcoma
CEA	Squamous and adenocarcinoma (BCC[4]-negative) Paget's disease
Involucrin	Squamous carcinoma (BCC[4]-negative)
Immunoglobulin[3]	Monoclonal: lymphoma and plasmacytoma
Enolase	Merkel tumor, melanoma
S100	Melanoma, histiocytic tumor, schwannoma
F VIII Ag	Kaposi's sarcoma, angiosarcomas
Lysozyme, alpha₁-antitrypsin, alpha₁-antichymotrypsin	Malignant fibrous histiocytoma, malignant histiocytosis, histiocytosis X, granulocytic sarcoma, lysozyme in some apocrine tumors
T and B cell monoclonals	Lymphomas, mycosis fungoides/Sezary's syndrome, inflammatory infiltrate
Viruses	Herpes, papilloma virus/warts, some carcinomas
Others	Reagents versus particular tumor types applied as necessary (eg, anti-prostatic acid phosphatase)

[1]Lists major reaction patterns discussed in detail in text or in Chapter 14.
[2]These reagents are less effective in formalin paraffin sections; frozen sections give good results. Carnoy's fixed paraffin sections also are satisfactory.
[3]Trypsinization improves results in formalin paraffin sections.
[4]BCC = basal cell carcinoma.

cyst antigen (see Table 13–9 and Chapter 10 pertaining to the breast). Antibody to apocrine cyst fluid particularly stains breast and apocrine carcinomas. It should be noted that some antibodies to mammary epithelial membrane antigen show staining that is not restricted to sweat gland tumors but extends to several tumor types, including sebaceous and squamous carcinomas (Table 13–9).

Other Antigens

Two other antibodies have been reported to have possible value in distinguishing squamous from basal cell carcinoma (Table 13–8). Antibody to involucrin, a complex cross-linked molecule, is found almost exclusively in squamous carcinomas and not in basal cell carcinomas or adenocarcinomas except when squamous change occurs (eg, adenocarcinoma of uterus; Warhol et al, 1984). Antibody to CEA also commonly stains squamous carcinomas but rarely stains basal cell carcinomas. As indicated previously, adenocarcinomas of the skin appendages frequently are positive for CEA. Blood group antigens (ABO [H]) are detectable in normal skin in all layers of epidermis but are partly lost in squamous carcinoma, Bowen's disease, and solar keratosis (Schaumburg-Lever et al, 1984).

Paget's disease of the nipple (and other sites) is considered in relation to the breast (Chapter 10): in brief, the large pale cells of Paget's disease typically express apocrine cyst (epithelial) antigen and CEA and react preferentially with antibodies to low–molecular weight (nonsquamous) keratin.

Merkel or neuroendocrine cell carcinoma is positive for neuron-specific enolase and neurofilament antigens but negative for cytokeratin and vimentin. Anti-Leu 7 (HNK1-versus natural killer cells) also appears to show positivity similar to that seen for other neuroendocrine tumors (Chapter 7). Anti-Leu 7 is effective in paraffin sections. Saurat et al (1983) described a monoclonal antibody that appeared to react with Merkel cells but has not yet been fully characterized. Morphologically and immunohistologically, Merkel cell tumors show a close resemblance to carcinoid tumors of the gut.

Another monoclonal antibody of potential utility reacts with the Psi 3 antigen (Strefling et al, 1985): this antibody shows positivity in some squamous carcinomas and condylomata but not in basal cell carcinomas. Strefling

Table 13–9. Selected Bibliography: Immunohistology of the Skin*

Sun TT et al 1983	Distribution of different keratins in epidermis
McArdle et al 1984	Type IV collagen stain showed focal loss of basement membrane in carcinoma
Said et al 1984	Involucrin—a precursor of cross-linked envelope protein in the stratum corneum—not detected in basal cell carcinoma (except in cysts), strongly positive in squamous carcinoma and Bowen's disease; dyskeratosis accentuated
Murphy et al 1984	Involucrin nonreactive in basal cell carcinoma, positive in squamous carcinoma except for invasive areas (negative)
Jordon 1980	Excellent review of handling of skin biopsies and staining processes
Scurry and de Boer 1983	CEA absent in normal postnatal skin, positive in squamous carcinoma (10/10), solar keratosis, Bowen's disease, and keratoacanthoma; rarely positive in basal carcinoma (1/10), negative in seborrheic keratosis
Heyderman et al 1984	CEA and EMA (epithelial membrane antigen); CEA positive in 12/15 squamous carcinoma and focally in sebaceous carcinomas; negative in basal cell carcinoma and malignant eccrine poroma; only basal cell carcinoma lacked EMA
Wright JE 1983	Review of immunoglobulins, FVIII, CEA, virus, monoclonal antibodies
Kuwano et al 1985	Staining for keratin distinguishes spindle cell carcinoma from five "atypical" fibroxanthomas (keratin-negative)
Syrjänen et al 1983a	Papilloma virus antigen in oral squamous carcinomas, especially the papillomatous type (for other references, see Uterus, Chapter 12)
Inoue A et al 1984	Lysozyme (or muramidase—MX), alpha$_1$-antitrypsin (AAT), fibronectin (FN), and immunoglobulin to distinguish subtypes of malignant fibrous histiocytoma
Modlin et al 1984c	Frozen section, monclonal antibodies used to subtype leukocytes in granuloma annulare
Modlin et al 1984a	Interleukin 2 in granulomas (frozen sections)
Modlin et al 1984b	Monoclonal antibodies to subtype leukocytes in leprosy
Kanitakis et al 1984	Monoclonal antibodies in the dermatofibromas: Ia- and OKM1-positive cells consistent with histiocytes, OKT6 negative
Gatter et al 1984b	Excellent study of skin tumors with a panel of 9 monoclonal antibodies, including keratin, CEA, Ia, S100, and milk–fat globule membrane antigen (frozen sections)
Trost et al 1980b	Pemphigus/pemphigoid using protein A method at EM
Holubar et al 1975	Immunoglobulins in pemphigoid (frozen section)
Maciejewski et al 1979	Pemphigoid, immunoglobulin, and complement (EM)
McMillan et al 1981	T cell subsets (Leu 1, 2, 3; OKT3, 4, 6, 8) in lichen planus
Chu and MacDonald 1979	Antiserum to T cells in mycosis fungoides
Nelson et al 1984	Keratin subtypes in squamous neoplasms
Miettinen et al 1982a	Vimentin and desmin for diagnosis of soft tissue sarcomas
Miettinen et al 1983c	Neurofilament antigen in neuroendocrine (Merkel) cell carcinoma of skin
Kariniemi et al 1984b	CEA and AEA (apocrine epithelial antigen) in sweat gland tumors (32/33 CEA positive)
Kariniemi et al 1984c	Paget's disease, extramammary: CEA and apocrine antigen (gross cystic disease fluid) positive but keratin negative (with this particular antibody)
Thomas P et al 1982	Keratin profile in squamous and basal carcinoma and Bowen's disease
Thivolet et al 1980	Distribution of staining of different keratin antisera in epidermis
Nadji et al 1982	Paget's disease: 7 cases mammary, 16 extramammary, CEA positive
Penneys et al 1981	CEA in apocrine and eccrine glands
Penneys et al 1982a	CEA in benign sweat gland tumors
Penneys et al 1982b	CEA in sweat gland carcinomas
Viac et al 1982	Distribution of keratins in squamous and basal cell carcinomas (used antisera raised in animals versus different keratin fractions)
Warhol et al 1983	Low-MW keratin in basal layer, high MW keratin in upper layers
Weiss RA et al 1983a	AE1 antibody (antikeratin, low MW) in keratoses and neoplasms; in Bowen's disease, disorganized; in squamous carcinoma, patchy; in basal cell carcinoma, diffuse, homogeneous; in normal skin staining in mainly of basal layer
Hoefler et al 1984	Neuroendocrine (Merkel) carcinoma; all positive for NSE (neuron-specific enolase), neurofilament antigen, and cytokeratin; all negative for S100, actin, and specific neuropeptides; similarities to carcinoids noted
Strefling et al 1985	Psi 3 antigen (monoclonal antibody) stains keratinocytes in psoriasis but not in normal skin; positive in 35/36 case of psoriasis; also positive in some squamous carcinomas and condylomas but not in basal cell carcinoma nor in ichthyosis
Schaumburg-Lever et al 1984	ABO(H) blood groups in skin; Group O has H antigen, Group A A + H, and Group B B + H throughout the epidermis; ABO(H) lost in Bowen's disease, squamous carcinoma, and irregularly in solar keratosis; warts still contained ABO(H) but in upper layers only
Mogollon et al 1984	Myelin basic protein in a schwannoma

*For general intermediate filament references, see Table 13–5.

297

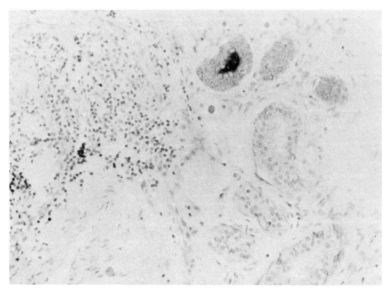

Figure 13–14. Normal sweat gland and duct demonstrating pattern of reactivity with monoclonal antibody to "squamous" keratin. Only the duct lining cells stain, lightly in the cytoplasm, intensely at the apices. The epithelial cells of the gland proper are nonreactive. Paraffin section, AEC with hematoxylin counterstain (×200). The corresponding tumors show similar keratin profiles. Compare with same antibody in Figure 13–6; and with Figure 13–15.

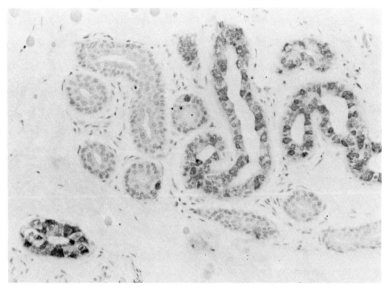

Figure 13–15. Normal sweat gland and duct demonstrating pattern of reactivity with monoclonal antibody to "nonsquamous" low MW keratin. Duct cells react weakly or not at all; glandular epithelium shows variable to intense reactivity typical of glandular epithelium throughout the body. Paraffin section, AEC with hematoxylin counterstain (×200). Compare with same antibody in Figure 13–7; and with Figure 13–14.

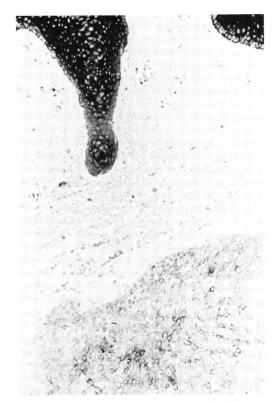

Figure 13–16. Normal skin (top) and underlying neoplasm. The epidermis displays intense reactivity with antibody versus "squamous" keratin (note the relative sparing of the basal layer, which contains mainly low MW keratin). The tumor shows weak to moderate reactivity in most cells with intense staining in a minority. This was an aggressive tumor—eccrine carcinoma. Paraffin section, AEC with hematoxylin counterstain (×125).

showed that 35 of 36 cases of psoriasis were positive for Psi 3 but normal skin was nonreactive. This monoclonal antibody gives optimal results in frozen tissue.

Finally, OKT6 (monoclonal antibody) recognizes not only early thymocytes but also Langerhans's cells in the skin (Fig. 13–17) and histiocytosis X, believed to be the derivative neoplasm (Chu et al, 1982; Beckstead et al, 1984). OKT6 is not reliable in paraffin sections; frozen sections are preferred. Immunostaining with OKT6 antibody has also been used to study the number of Langerhans's cells in different skin diseases; specific diagnostic features have not been forthcoming (Rowden, 1980 and 1981; Modlin et al, 1984b; Czernielewski et al, 1983; McMillan et al, 1981).

Other stains may be applied to paraffin sections for the diagnosis of particular tumor types, including melanomas (considered separately), metastatic tumors, lymphomas, and various soft tissue tumors. To fully exploit the power of immunohistology with regard to tumor diagnosis, it will also be necessary to resort to frozen sections for successful utilization of many monoclonal antibodies (eg, in lymphomas, soft tissue sarcomas, and others). In general, the antibodies that may be utilized are those employed for the differential diagnosis of anaplastic tumors in general. These are fully discussed in the next chapter. A brief listing is given here (Table 13–8).

Figure 13–17. Skin with underlying tuberculosis granuloma. Increased numbers of reticulate OKT6-positive (Langerhans's) cells are seen in the epidermis; a few OKT6-positive "reticulum cells" are present on the periphery of a granuloma in the dermis. Frozen section, AEC with light hematoxylin counterstain (×200).

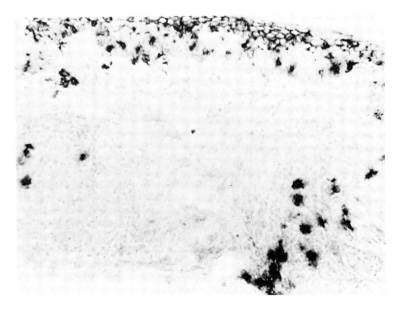

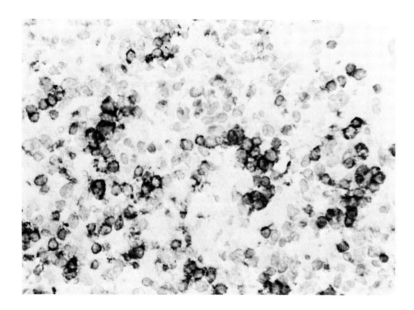

Figure 13–18. Cutaneous T cell lymphoma in dermis, stained for OKT9 (transferrin receptor). Admixture of large cells resulted in a designation as immunoblastic sarcoma of T cell type. Frozen section, AEC with hematoxylin counterstain ($\times 200$).

Frozen Sections

Basically, those antibodies applicable to paraffin sections also may be utilized with frozen sections fixed in ethanol, acetone, or buffered formol acetone. In addition, a broad range of monoclonal antibodies may be applied to frozen sections; many of these antibodies are important for recognition of anaplastic tumors as summarized in Table 13–8 and discussed more fully in Chapter 14.

Various leukocyte antigens have been studied quite extensively in frozen sections of skin diseases. In chronic inflammatory conditions, T cells predominate over B cells. The B cells show polyclonal SIg, and the T cells show a mixture of helper and suppressor phenotypes with a predominance of the helper phenotype within a very broad "normal" range ("normal" here implying only that the lymphoid cells are non-neoplastic) in different inflammatory conditions (lichen planus, psoriasis, and so forth); disease-specific changes have not been recognized. Thus, of the numerous leukocyte antigens studied (Table 13–9; see also Chapter 4), few have any use in diagnosis of skin diseases today.

The most common lymphoma encountered in skin is "cutaneous T cell lymphoma"

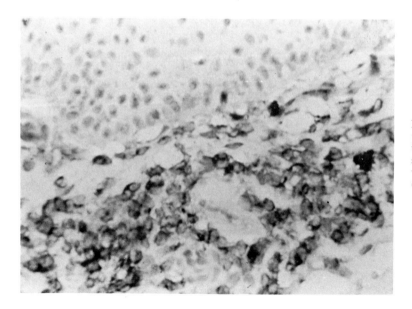

Figure 13–19. OKT4 (helper phenotype)-positive cells infiltrating the dermis in Sezary's syndrome. Frozen section, AEC with hematoxylin counterstain ($\times 320$).

Table 13–10. Immunoglobulin Distribution in Bullous Disease of the Skin

Disease	Tissue Distribution of Immunoglobulins
Pemphigoid	$IgG + C_3$—linear pattern on basement membrane[1]
Pemphigus (all types)[2]	$IgG + C_3$—outlining individual cells in epidermis: "normal" skin also positive
Dermatitis herpetiformis	$IgA \pm C_3$ granular deposits; at deep aspect of basement membrane, "normal" skin also is positive
Herpes gestationis	Similar to pemphigoid
IgA pemphigoid	IgA linear deposits on basement membrane
SLE	IgG, IgM, C_3—patchy on basement membrane and in vessels, also in "normal" skin
Erythema multiforme	IgM—in vessels
Vasculitides[3]	IgG, IgM, $IgA \pm C_3$

[1]Properdin, factor B, Cly, and C_4 also present (activation of alternate pathway).
[2]Similar patterns (and serum antibodies) may be seen in patients with burns and drug rashes (eg, penicillin).
[3]Includes Henoch-Schönlein purpura, necrotizing vasculitis, and rheumatoid vasculitis.

(Fig. 13–18), including the defined entities of mycosis fungoides and Sézary's syndrome. In these conditions T cells (by phenotype) may comprise 95 percent or more of lymphoid cells, and helper cells (by phenotype) 80 percent or more (Fig. 13–19); however, the suppressor phenotype occasionally predominates, or cells may "double" mark. These aspects are discussed more fully in relation to the lymphomas (Chapter 4). Monoclonal cytoplasmic or surface immunoglobulin in paraffin or frozen sections is indicative of plasmacytoma, deposits of myeloma, plasmacytoid lymphocytic lymphoma, immunoblastic sarcoma (B cell type), or follicular center cell lymphoma of large cell type. The small cell lymphomas (B CLL, lymphocytic lymphomas, small cell follicular center cell lymphomas, and some plasmacytoid lymphocytic lymphomas) typically possess SIg detectable only in frozen sections of skin. The detection of immunoglobulins and its significance is discussed in Chapters 4 and 5.

IMMUNOGLOBULIN DEPOSITION IN INFLAMMATORY DISEASE

Examination of skin biopsies for evidence of deposition of immunoglobulin or complement is of value with reference to the recognition and distinction of pemphigus, pemphigoid, dermatitis herpetiformis, and systemic lupus erythematosus (SLE/DLE) (Table 13–10). Traditionally, immunostaining has been performed using immunofluorescence techniques and frozen sections (see Jordon, 1980 for an excellent detailed review). If skin biopsies cannot be frozen immediately, they can be placed in a "holding" or "transport" medium (Michel solution) prior to freezing. The pH of the Michel solution is critical (7.0–7.4), and specimens must be washed prior to freezing. Michel solution contains the following: 3.12 M $(NH_4)_2SO_4$, 0.0005 M $MgSO_4$, 0.0005 M N-ethylmaleimide, and 0.025 M citrate. The

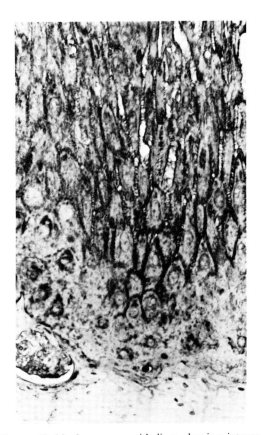

Figure 13–20. Squamous epithelium showing intense black staining of "prickles" for IgG in a case of pemphigus with incipient acantholysis. Paraffin section, DAB with hematoxylin counterstain (×320).

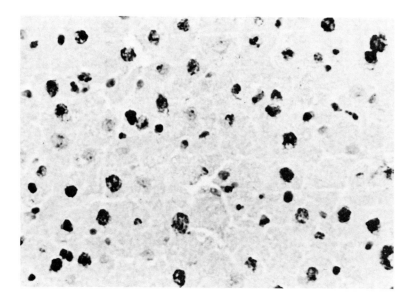

Figure 13–21. Rat liver frozen section showing speckled staining patterns typical of an antinuclear antibody as found in SLE, Sjögren's syndrome, and mixed connective tissue disease. AEC, no counterstain (×320). The "test" serum is added to the frozen section, followed by an antihuman immunoglobulin antibody and a suitable labelling system designed to detect human Ig. Permanent preparations are obtained. The sensitivity is similar to that of immunofluorescence methods.

washing solution is basically a citrate buffer: 2.5 ml of 1 M potassium citrate buffer (pH 7.0) plus 5.0 ml of 0.1 M MgSO$_4$ plus 87.5 ml of H$_2$O, pH adjusted to 7.0 with 7 M KOH.

For staining of immunoglobulin, the results obtained with rapid liquid nitrogen frozen tissue and tissue held in Michel solution are closely similar; this is not, however, true for all of the leukocyte cell surface antigens detected by monoclonal antibodies.

Immunofluorescence has generally been considered satisfactory for the purposes of demonstrating Ig deposition in frozen sections: morphology is not at a premium, only a general tissue distribution is required; precise cell recognition is not even attempted. Immunoperoxidase staining (by the direct or indirect conjugate, PAP, or ABC methods) serves equally well, with the advantage of permanent preparations and more precise morphology when utilized in frozen sections. In formalin-fixed paraffin sections, results are less consistent, and no general recommendation can be given. The situation is best summarized as follows: a positive characteristic staining pattern for Ig deposition in a trypsinized paraffin section is a reliable indication of that particular disease (Fig. 13–20); a negative result is of little value, and there will be a variable proportion of false negatives when compared with frozen sections. Thus, for these purposes frozen sections are to be preferred; if they are not available, paraffin sections may be used with reservations; rebiopsy should be considered if the findings are negative but the index of suspicion is high.

Perhaps the most sensitive means of demonstrating Ig deposition in skin is to resort to immunoelectron microscopy using either the procedure of Trost et al, 1980b (a protein A-peroxidase method) or Holubar et al, 1975 (a PAP method). Such procedures are, however, beyond the compass of most routine laboratories.

Note that for the inverse procedure, the detection of "auto-antibodies" in serum of patients with suspected pemphigus/pemphigoid, SLE and the like, either immunofluorescence or immunoperoxidase may be used, employing rhesus monkey esophagus or rat liver frozen sections as substrate (Fig. 13–21).

14

APPROACH TO THE "UNKNOWN PRIMARY"— ANAPLASTIC TUMORS

"An expert is a person who tells you a simple thing in a confused way, in such a fashion as to make you think the confusion is your own fault."

W. D. CASTLE
Harvard Medical Bulletin, 1955

"It is an old maxim of mine that when you have excluded the impossible, whatever remains, however improbable, must be the truth."

Sherlock Holmes,
in SIR ARTHUR CONAN DOYLE,
1859–1930
"A Study in Scarlet"

Perhaps the most challenging aspect of diagnostic surgical pathology is the determination of the site of origin of poorly differentiated metastatic tumor deposits, wherever they may occur; in approaching this problem, the pathologist must seek and utilize whatever clues are available.

One of the most convincing demonstrations of the fallibility of orthodox morphologic diagnosis and the value of immunohistologic studies is a study emanating from Dr. Mason's laboratory in Oxford (Gatter et al, 1985). The study encompassed 120 consecutive cases of malignancy in which the precise diagnosis was difficult; morphologically, 53 were thought to be lymphomas and 43 carcinomas; 24 were unclassifiable. Following application of a panel of antibodies (including antibodies to keratin, CEA, and common leukocyte antigen), 80 were diagnosed as lymphoma (including 29 cases formerly classified as carcinoma!) and 27 as carcinoma (including 9 cases formerly called lymphoma but only one quarter of the cases originally diagnosed as carcinoma). Only 13 cases (11 percent of the total) remained unclassified.

Our own experience at the University of Southern California, which now covers more than 2500 referred cases, demonstrates an equally alarming disparity between the initial morphologic diagnosis and the revised final diagnosis following immunohistologic studies. Clearly, morphology alone may suffice for some "well-differentiated," "absolutely typical" tumors (although we have seen striking revisions of diagnosis even here, as with a pyroninophilic plasmacytoma of the base of the skull that contained prolactin, in reality a pituitary adenoma). However, for poorly differentiated and anaplastic tumors, morphology alone is wrong so frequently (almost 50 percent of cases overall) that it is difficult to defend either ethically or legally a failure to perform immunohistologic studies.

From immunohistology we have learned that "primitive" "undifferentiated" tumor cells look like primitive undifferentiated tumor cells, whatever their ultimate cell of origin. The surgical pathologist is accustomed to seeking fine morphologic clues as evidence of differentiation upon which to base a decision as to the cell of origin and hence the likely primary organ site within the body. These morphologic clues may be so subtle as to defy recognition by other "experts" or even by the same expert on a subsequent occasion.

The Traditional Approach

Faced with an anaplastic tumor, the sensible pathologist resorts to one of several options: he or she discusses the case with the clinicians to see what they think it is, requests another biopsy, does some special stains, orders electron microscopic studies, consults immediate colleagues, sends the case out to a consultant pathologist, or any combination of these options.

Circumstantial evidence, such as the known presence of tumor elsewhere, or a social or family history, or even statistical incidence of tumor types at the site in question, is admissible; but in reaching a diagnosis such evidence should be considered last rather than first. If orthodox light microscopy alone does not permit a confident diagnosis, then the pathologist may search for microstructural clues, such as the presence of "prickles or intracellular bridges" (presumptive squamous carcinoma) or intracellular striations or fibrils (presumptive rhabdomyosarcoma), recognizing that faith and imagination fired by circumstantial evidence play large parts in determining whether or not these features are perceived by a particular pathologist in a particular tumor. Electron microscopy may of course be of value in providing ultrastructural evidence of squamous differentiation, muscle cell differentiation, or glandular differentiation, but often the pathologist does not have material available for electron microscopic studies; even if material is available, the time necessary for processing and examination produces, in most institutions, an inordinate delay in reaching a final diagnosis, and it is expensive.

Histochemical stains have proved of value in some instances, such as in the demonstration of PAS-positive material or mucins in suspected adenocarcinomas, the use of "melanin" stains in suspected melanoma, and evidence of pyroninophilia in putative B cell lymphomas or plasmacytomas. However, these types of histochemical stains lack true specificity in terms of defining particular cell or tumor types and can do no more than sway the pathologist in one direction or another; the last may be particularly misleading in that pyroninophilia is characteristic of any protein-producing cell (cytoplasmic RNA), including of course many rapidly dividing cells other than B cells or plasma cells.

The Immunohistologic Approach

The advent of immunocytochemistry promises tangible advantages in the precise definition of cell types that escape morphologic recognition. It must be admitted that the range of antibodies currently available is inadequate for the purpose in hand and that, in the use of immunohistochemical methods for classification of tumors, we stand at the beginning, but it is a beginning full of promise.

Table 14–1 lists many of the antigens that have been stained in paraffin sections by immunohistochemical methods. The antigens included are those for which there is reasonable evidence in the literature concerning the reproducibility of staining. The possible diagnostic utility of some of these antigens is self-evident and well documented. Other antibodies of equal or greater potential value (eg, anti-pancreatic cancer antigen, antilung cancer antigens) have been described, but data relating to their usefulness are nonexistent, limited, or subject to such controversy that no recommendation can at present be given. Finally, some of the antigens demonstrated do not, and may not ever, have practical application except for the purposes of histologic research.

The practical utilization of antibodies against many of these antigens, with respect to particular cell or tumor types, has been described elsewhere in this text. This chapter considers only those antibodies that may be of value for the express purpose of determining the cellular origin, and thus the likely tissue (organ) of origin, of anaplastic tumors.

Selection of Antibodies for Immunohistologic Staining

The fact that many different antibodies are available poses certain logistic problems. It is neither sensible nor practical to test all unknown tumors with a panel of 30 to 40 antibodies, 1 or 2 of which might provide useful positive information; note that a specific positive stain for a particular antigen is more reliable and more valuable than a negative stain, for a negative reaction might

Table 14–1. Antigens of Value for Analysis of Anaplastic Tumors

Antigens	Tumor Type
Keratins CEA MEMA (MFGM)	Epithelial tumors only (carcinomas)
Vimentin	Mesenchymal tumors (sarcomas)
Desmin Actin Myosin Myoglobin	Muscle cell tumors
Lactoferrin Lactalbumin Casein MEMA ER	Breast tumors
Ferritin AFP Alpha$_1$-AT	Liver and germ cell tumors
Lysozyme Alpha$_1$-AT Alpha$_1$-CT Leu M1 Ia CLA S100	Histiocytic tumors
HBA HBF Erythroid Ags	Erythroleukemias
CLA LN1, LN2 Ia B and T cell Ags CALLA	Lymphomas, leukemias
NSE Leu 7 (HNK1) Endocrine granule Ag Bombesin	Endocrine and neuroendocrine tumors
PSAP PSEA	Prostatic cancer only
F VIII Ag	Angiosarcomas
Blood Group Ags	Bladder cancer
S100 Leu 7 Melanoma Ags	Melanoma
Specific hormones (see Table 1–1)	Specific endocrine tumors, ectopic production
Specific tissue Ags (eg, lung, pancreatic, colonic,celomic)	Specific tumor types

result from a fixation or processing artifact, inadequate staining technique, or mutational loss of antigen by poorly differentiated tumor cells. Lack of positivity may also represent a "true negative" reaction, indicative of a cell lineage that does not express the antigen. It should also be emphasized that controls are, as always, essential, including known positive and known negative (nonreactive) tissues for every antibody employed. Thus, one is faced, not only with staining 60 sections of the tumor for 60 different antibodies, but also with performing 200 or so controls. The investigator must therefore attempt to "focus" the staining along a particular probability pathway or according to some form of algorithm. There are two possible approaches that may be combined to some degree.

Morphologic examination of the tumor

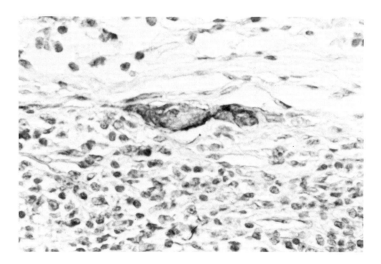

Figure 14–1. Isolated cluster of carcinoma cells within the marginal sinus of a lymph node, readily detected by intense reactivity with antibody to CEA; by the same token, CEA positivity excludes sarcoma, lymphoma, melanoma, and the like. Paraffin section, AEC with hematoxylin counterstain (× 200).

coupled with evidence from the patient's history and various histochemical stains (PAS and so forth) is a prerequisite leading to some form of differential diagnosis that may suggest a particular group of stains as a starting point. In this approach "stains" (antibodies) are then selected to address the list of differential diagnoses, ideally seeking a specific positive confirmation (eg, demonstration of prostatic acid phosphatase in a tumor within an inguinal lymph node). It should be recognized that many of the currently available immunostains (eg, CEA) give less specific information, since the antigen in question occurs in more than one cell or tumor. Even these relatively "broad spectrum" stains serve to reduce the number of differential diagnoses by excluding certain possibilities (eg,

positive staining for CEA virtually excludes liposarcoma, lymphoma, and the like (Fig. 14–1).

If a confident "final" diagnosis has not been made following interpretation of this first group of stains, then it may be necessary to proceed sequentially with other stains in an attempt to confirm or deny the remaining possibilities (Table 14–1).

As an alternative to the preceding approach, the pathologist may choose to proceed via a pathway according to a working algorithm (Table 14–2 and Fig. 14–2). This may be made as simple or as complex as suits the pathologist's clinical need, intellectual appetite, and pocketbook. The schemes of greatest complexity will be the most comprehensive, including the majority of known

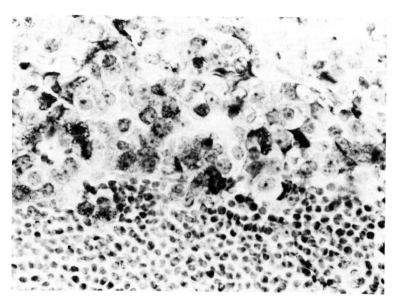

Figure 14–2. Following initial screening for keratins (positive), CEA (negative), and vimentin (negative), this anaplastic large cell tumor was thought possibly to be an adenocarcinoma (Table 14–3). Additional stains were carried out in an attempt at a precise diagnosis; positivity was observed with antibody to prostate epithelial antigen. Diagnosis was metastatic prostatic carcinoma. Paraffin section, AEC with hematoxylin counterstain (× 320).

Table 14–2. Use of Keratins, CEA, and Vimentin in Anaplastic
Malignancies

Initial Stain Panel

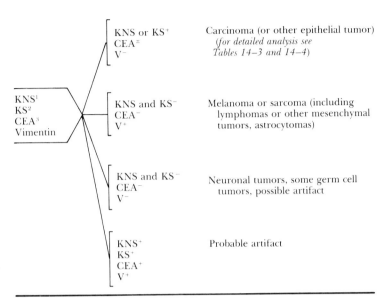

KNS[1]
KS[2]
CEA[3]
Vimentin

KNS or KS+ CEA± V−	Carcinoma (or other epithelial tumor) *(for detailed analysis see Tables 14–3 and 14–4)*
KNS and KS− CEA− V+	Melanoma or sarcoma (including lymphomas or other mesenchymal tumors, astrocytomas)
KNS and KS− CEA− V−	Neuronal tumors, some germ cell tumors, possible artifact
KNS+ KS+ CEA+ V+	Probable artifact

[1]KNS - keratin nonsquamous (low MW)
[2]KS - keratin squamous (high MW)
[3]Antibody to milk–fat globule membrane may be used in addition to, or instead
of, CEA; it marks many adenocarcinomas.

antibodies with clinical utility and embracing both paraffin and frozen sections; the simplest schemes will of necessity include only selected antibodies and possibly only paraffin sections. Either option may be expected to lead to a definitive diagnosis in some cases, more in the comprehensive scheme, less with the simpler approach. The algorithm given here is designed to follow the middle road: the more commonly available and better characterized antibodies are included, and an attempt is made to address those problems of differential diagnosis that are encountered most frequently.

Although the following material is written with the tissue section in mind, the principles are equally applicable to the recognition of cells in cell preparations from body fluids (eg, pleural effusions), Pap smears of the cervix, bronchial brushings, or fine-needle aspirates (Fig. 14–3). Indeed, in many respects such cell "preparations" are superior to tissue sections for immunologic staining, since the antigens can be treated with minimal fixation (a few seconds in alcohol, acetone, or buffered formol acetone).

Staining for Keratins, CEA and Vimentin

The first step in the algorithm is to stain serial sections of the tumor, with the appropriate controls, for keratins and vimentin; antibody to CEA may be utilized at this juncture or may be deferred until the result of the keratin-vimentin staining is known. CEA reactivity is of some value in analyzing the keratin-positive tumors. Some investigators would advocate the use of antibody to milk–fat globule membrane antigen (Fig. 14–4) in addition to, or instead of, CEA; we do not do this routinely since we feel that it does not add much if antibodies to both squamous and nonsquamous keratin are used, as described later.

This approach presupposes that frozen tissue is available, since in our hands staining for vimentin (with different antibodies) cannot be achieved reproducibly in paraffin sections unless the sections are fixed in Carnoy's solution or Methacarn fixative: 60% methanol, 30% chloroform, 10% glacial acetic acid (Gown and Vogel, 1984). Also, keratin is less

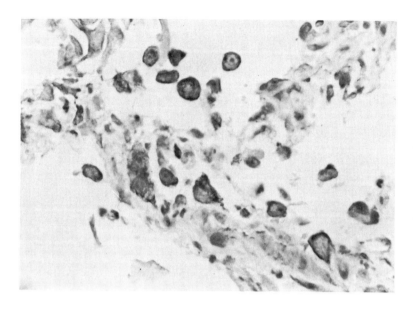

Figure 14–3. Fine-needle pleural biopsy; positivity with antibody to low MW (nonsquamous) keratin is suggestive of adenocarcinoma; lack of reactivity for squamous keratin in a parallel section virtually excludes presence of mesothelial cells or squamous carcinoma cells. Paraffin section, AEC with hematoxylin counterstain (× 200).

readily stained in formalin paraffin sections than in frozen sections, and trypsinization should be employed routinely. If only formalin paraffin sections are available, then we would strongly advocate staining for both CEA and keratin, since antivimentin is less reliable (Fig. 14–5),* and one must rely upon a negative CEA and keratin to exclude carcinoma without the benefit of a positive vimentin to indicate sarcoma. Of course, a "negative" stain is far less reliable for this purpose than a specific positive reaction;

staining for keratin may be unsuccessful in tissues subjected to prolonged fixation, whereas CEA may still be detectable.

With regard to the choice of antikeratin antibody, there are two approaches, either to use a pankeratin antibody or to begin by staining with both "squamous" and "nonsquamous" keratin antibodies as shown in the algorithm. These, together with antibodies to vimentin (or CEA or both), may be used as an initial panel of stains. This approach can save time, permitting the distinction of most squamous carcinomas and adenocarcinomas and their separation from sarcomas at the initial stage (Table 14–2).

Tables 14–3 and 14–4 portray in more detail some of the conclusions that may be

---

*Recently there have been claims for antivimentin antibodies giving reproducible results in routine paraffin sections (Miles); insufficient data is at hand to permit a recommendation (see Fig. 14–5).

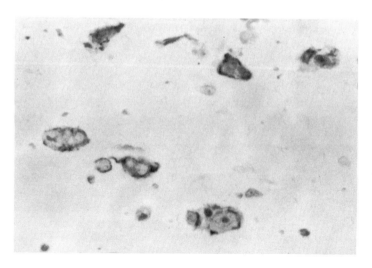

Figure 14–4. Reactivity for epithelial membrane antigen in an ascites preparation; metastatic adenocarcinoma; definite positivity weighs against sarcoma, melanoma, or mesothelioma. AEC with hematoxylin counterstain (× 320).

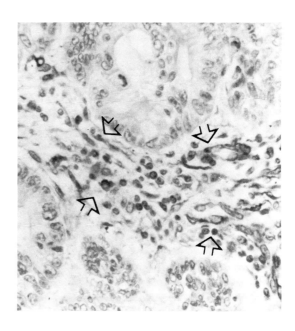

Figure 14–5. Vimentin-positive cells (black—arrows) within an area involved in invasive carcinoma of colon. The carcinoma cells are not positive; residual connective tissue elements do show staining. Paraffin section, AEC with hematoxylin counterstain (× 200). Note that all tumors will contain some vimentin-positive cells, but vimentin occurs within tumor cells only in the sarcomas.

Table 14–3. Keratins, CEA, Vimentin: the Epithelial Tumors

STEP I				Confirmatory—Step II[2]; Comments	Described in Chapter
Keratin + Vimentin − Group (carcinomas)	KS −[3] KNS + CEA − V −	Adeno-carcinoma	Endometrium Thyroid (follicle) Kidney Embryonal	OC125, ER Thyroglobulin, thyroxin Renal tubular antigen, UR01, UR02 AFP, hCG	12 8 12 9
	KS − KNS + CEA ± V −	Adeno-carcinoma	Prostate Liver Endometrium Parotid Lung	PSAP, PSEA AFP, alpha$_1$-antitrypsin, alpha$_1$-antichymotrypsin OC125, ER Lung antigen, surfactant protein	12 11 12 11
	KS − KNS + CEA + V −	Adeno-carcinoma	Colon GI tract Thyroid (medullary)	Colonic antigen, various mucin antigens Various mucin antigens Calcitonin	11 11 8
	KS − KNS ± CEA ± V −	Adeno-carcinoma	Germ cell tumors Choriocarcinoma Carcinoids Oat cell carcinoma Pituitary adenoma Parathyroid adenoma/carcinoma Chordoma	AFP, hCG hCG, pregnancy-specific glycoprotein, placental lactogen NSE, Leu 7, specific polypeptides NSE, Leu 7, bombesin Specific hormones Parathormone Usually K+/CEA−/S100+	9 9 7 7,11 8 8 8
KNS[1] KS[1] CEA Vimentin	KS + KNS + CEA ± V −	Adeno-carcinoma	Sweat glands Breast Pancreas Cholangiocarcinoma Bladder (urethra)	MEMA, apocrine cyst fluid MEMA (MFGM—not specific), casein∓, lactabumin±, ER± Pancreatic antigen URO9, URO10, blood group antigens	10,12 10 11 12
	KS ± KNS ± CEA − V −	Adeno-carcinoma	Thyroid (follicle) Basal cell carcinoma Synovial sarcoma Mesothelioma	Thyroxin, thyroglobulin, patchy K staining Usually KNS predominates, but KS may be positive Variable but definite keratin positivity OC125, strongly keratin-positive; V ±	8 13 11 11
	KS + KNS − CEA ± V −	Squamous carcinoma	Lung Skin Nasopharynx Esophagus Cervix	Lung cancer antigens Involucrin Involucrin Involucrin KNS may also be positive, human papilloma virus	11 13 12
Keratin − Vimentin + Group- (Sarcomas)	KS − KNS − CEA − V +		Melanomas Lymphomas Sarcomas Others	(see Table 14–4)	
Kertin − Vimentin − Group	KS − KNS − CEA − V −		Gliomas Neuroblastomas Germ cell tumors Others	(see Table 14–4)	

[1]Initial panel of four antibodies—KNS (monoclonal versus nonsquamous low molecular weight keratin); KS (versus squamous high molecular weight keratins): CEA (carcinoembryonic antigen); V (vimentin)

[2]Details of antibodies and patterns of reactivity are given in text with reference to particular types of tumors.

[3]The patterns of reactivity given are those usually ascribed to the particular tumor type; most examples of each tumor type will give the anticipated pattern of staining. When great variation is encountered, a single tumor type may appear under more than one category (eg, oat cell carcinoma may or may not be keratin-positive).

Table 14–4. Keratins, CEA, Vimentin: Mesenchymal Tumors

Step I[1]	Step II[2]					Confirmatory—Step III[3]; Comments	Described in Chapter
Keratin + Vimentin − Group	KS	±	KNS	+		Carcinoma and other epithelial tumors	See Table 14–3	4, 5, 6
	CEA	±	V	−				
Keratin − Vimentin + Group					CLA +	Lymphoma	Surface Ig, cytoplasmic Ig, T & B cell antigens, LN1, LN2, etc, Ia	6
						Histiocytic (true)	Lysozyme ±, alpha₁-antitrypsin ±, OKM1, S100 ±, Leu M1	6
						Histiocytosis X	OKT6 + (Langerhans's cells), Lysozyme +, S100 ±	6
						Granulocytic sarcoma	Lysozyme	6
KNS[1] KS[1] CEA Vimentin	KS	−	KNS	−	S100 +	Melanoma	Leu 7, melanoma antigens, MEL.5, Ia	13
	CEA	−	V	+		Schwannoma, neurilemmoma	Myelin basic protein	13
						Neurofibroma		13
						Histiocytosis	CLA + (see above)	6
					Desmin +	Rhabdomyosarcoma Leiomyosarcoma	Myoglobin	14 14
					GFAP +	Glioma/astrocytoma Ependymoma	Some types are vimentin −	16 16
					Factor VIII +	Kaposi's and angiosarcoma		14
						Other tumors	Ewing's sarcoma, chondrosarcoma, fibrosarcoma, gonadal stromal tumors	
Keratin − Vimentin − Group	KS	−	KNS	−	Neurofilament antigen	Merkel cell carcinoma	NSE (neuron specific enolase), Leu 7	13
	CEA	−	V	−		Neuroblastoma	NSE, neuroblast antigen, cathepsin D	16
						Ganglioneuroma	NSE	16
						Oat cell tumors	NSE; note some are keratin-positive	11
						Pheochromocytoma	Endocrine granule antigen	8
						Yolk sac carcinoma	AFP, alpha₁-antitrypsin, HBF; some cases vimentin +	9
						Seminoma/dysgerminoma	Ferritin (most); some cases vimentin +	9
	KS	+	KNS	+		Probably technical artifact	No useful conclusion	
	CEA	+	V	+		Rare tumors: both KS+ and V+	Some renal cell carcinomas, Wilm's tumor	12
							Chordoma	13
							Synovial sarcoma	13
							Epithelioid sarcoma	13

[1]Initial panel of four antibodies—KNS (monoclonal versus nonsquamous low molecular weight keratin); KS (versus squamous high molecular weight keratins); CEA (carcinoembryonic antigen); V (vimentin)

[2]Patterns of reactivity with individual antibodies are described in the text with reference to particular tumor types.

[3]The patterns given are those most commonly encountered; some tumors appear in more than one category.

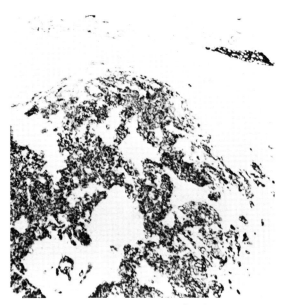

Figure 14–6. Anaplastic tumor in the mesentery, stained for low and high MW keratins (pankeratin). Frozen section, AEC, no counterstain (× 60). The extent of invasion by carcinoma is clearly depicted, the counterstain was omitted for purposes of photography. This technique is applicable to the rapid screening of frozen sections for carcinomatous involvement during radical lymph node resection procedures.

drawn from examination of the staining pattern observed with the initial four antibodies. Additional antibodies may then be used further to focus the diagnosis, or as confirmatory stains (Steps II and III); these antibodies are discussed in detail in the appropriate chapters.

Keratin-Positive Group

Positive staining of tumor cells with antibody to any of the keratin components is considered strong evidence of the epithelial origin of the tumor although mesotheliomas (epithelial type) typically fall into this category (Chapter 11). Antibodies to squamous (high molecular weight) keratins and nonsquamous (intermediate to low molecular weight) keratins provide additional information, as shown in Table 14–3. Squamous (epidermoid) carcinomas usually react with antibody to high molecular weight keratin (KS, keratin squamous; Figs. 14–6 to 14–8) and are weakly reactive or nonreactive with antibodies to low molecular weight keratins (KNS, keratin nonsquamous). In many adenocarcinomas the converse is observed (Figs. 14–9 and 14–10), while in other adenocarcinomas (usually those of ductal origin) both squamous and nonsquamous keratins may be detectable (Fig. 14–11). Mesotheliomas contain a predominance of high molecular weight keratins. Typically, the staining of cells within an individual anaplastic tumor is heterogeneous; definite specific staining of 5 percent or more of morphologically recognizable tumor cells constitutes a positive reaction. This number admittedly is an arbitrary cutoff, but it does serve to focus the attention of the observer upon the need to ascertain that the staining reaction is related to the tumor cells and is specific as judged from examination of both positive and negative controls. It should be noted that scattered vimentin-positive cells (fibroblasts,

Figure 14–7. Isolated cluster of mononuclear and polyploid cells within a cervical lymph node; coexistence of eosinophils and fibrosis resulted in a diagnosis of Hodgkin's disease. Cytoplasmic staining (gray) in the Reed-Sternberg lacunarlike cells with antibody to keratin suggested a diagnosis of metastatic carcinoma. Nasopharyngeal carcinoma was diagnosed and later confirmed at autopsy. Paraffin section, DAB with hematoxylin counterstain (× 320). This was a nontrypsinized formalin paraffin section; trypsin digestion enhanced staining but at a loss of morphologic detail.

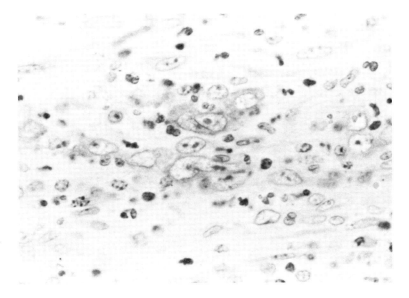

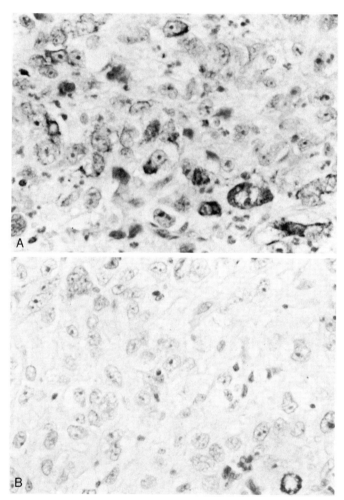

Figure 14–8. Anaplastic tumor: *A* shows (positive) staining with antibody to high MW "squamous" keratin; *B* shows minimal (negative) staining for low MW "nonsquamous" keratin. This is metastatic squamous carcinoma. Paraffin section, AEC with hematoxylin counterstain (× 320).

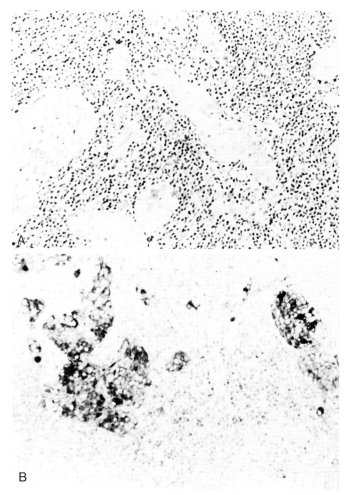

Figure 14–9. *A* shows metastatic adenocarcinoma in a lymph node; with antibody to high MW "squamous" keratin, there is little staining. *B* shows the same case treated with antibody to low MW "nonsquamous" keratin; there is strong positivity. Paraffin section, AEC with hematoxylin counterstain (× 125).

endothelial cells, and so forth) will be observed in all tumors (Fig. 14–5), whereas the tumor cells may or may not show reactivity. Staining may also vary dramatically in different areas of a single tumor or between primary tumor and metastasis.

The patterns shown in Tables 14–2 and 14–3 are those usually ascribed to the tumor types listed; we have occasionally observed exceptional tumors in almost every category that fail to give the anticipated pattern of reactivity. In many instances these discrepancies are attributable to technical factors, particularly in instances of "false negatives" resulting from the adverse effects of fixation or processing. In cases in which the results are equivocal, repetition of the stain with a fresh batch of reagents may produce an interpretable result.

CEA-Positive Group

Staining for CEA is particularly difficult to predict for any particular tumor type, since the intensity of reactivity and the proportion of positive cells may vary enormously within a single class of tumors, or even within different areas of a single tumor. One feature, however—the positive reactivity of colonic carcinoma—is constant to such an extent that a "negative" stain for CEA in the presence of the appropriate controls should cast doubts upon the diagnosis. The presence of specific CEA reactivity also effectively excludes all mesenchymal tumors (Fig. 14–12). One other practical application of antibodies to CEA has been in the examination of pleural effusions (or ascites): CEA-positive cells are presumptive adenocarcinoma cells;

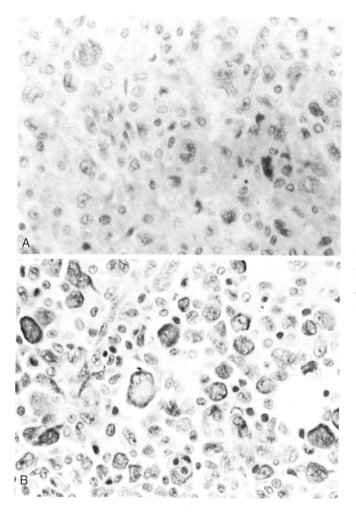

Figure 14–10. Anaplastic tumor in lymph node treated with monoclonal antibody to high MW keratin (**A,** "squamous") and low MW keratin (**B,** "nonsquamous"). Reactivity for "nonsquamous" keratin only (**B,** positive cells show gray-black cytoplasm) is consistent with carcinoma of the kidney, endometrium, or GI tract (Table 14–3). Paraffin section, AEC with hematoxylin counterstain (× 320).

Figure 14–11. Adenocarcinoma cells in lymph node showing variable to intense cytoplasmic staining with monoclonal antibody to low MW "nonsquamous" keratin. Paraffin section, DAB with hematoxylin counterstain (× 200). Antibody to high MW keratin also gave patchy staining; this was a carcinoma of the pancreas.

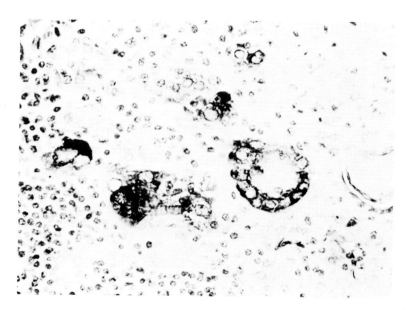

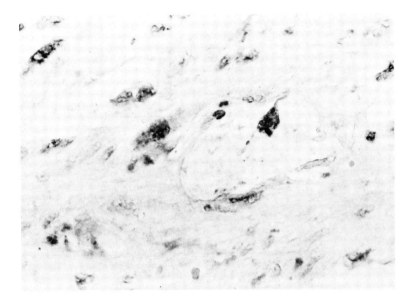

Figure 14–12. Initial histologic diagnosis was liposarcoma. Section shows scattered large cells within retroperitoneal tissue; positive granular staining for CEA excludes a diagnosis of liposarcoma and favors metastatic adenocarcinoma. Paraffin section, AEC with hematoxylin counterstain (× 320).

mesothelial cells are CEA-negative, and mesothelioma usually is CEA-negative. Controversial viewpoints are discussed in Chapter 11.

Keratin- and CEA-Negative Group

Keratin-negative and CEA-negative tumors are presumptive sarcomas. The observation of positive staining for vimentin is, however, a more reliable route to the same conclusion. These tumors are dissected in Table 14–4, again using antibodies that are widely available and quite well characterized.

Vimentin-Positive Group

The vimentin-positive group (Fig. 14–13) is rather diverse, and there is no logical approach to a final diagnosis. We therefore employ one or more of a battery of secondary antibodies (Step II, Table 14–4) selected according to the morphologic differential diagnosis and the clinical indications (eg, Figs. 14–14 and 14–15). Note that while epithelial mesotheliomas are keratin-positive and vimentin-negative, "fibrous" mesotheliomas are vimentin-positive (Blobel et al, 1985).

CLA and S100. Antibodies to common leukocyte antigen and S100 are particularly

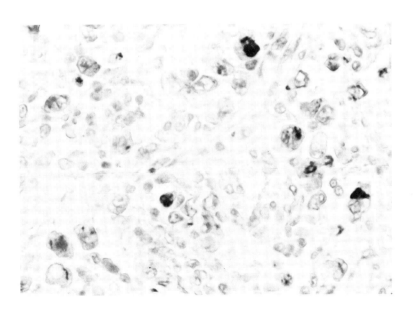

Figure 14–13. Anaplastic large cell tumor showing a pattern of reactivity with antibody to vimentin; there is variable cytoplasmic staining (gray), with intense blocks of positively stained material in some cells (black). This is a sarcoma, not a carcinoma (see Tables 14–2 to 14–4). Paraffin section, AEC with hematoxylin counterstain (× 200).

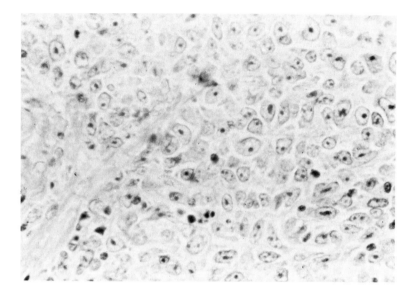

Figure 14–14. "Undifferentiated gonadal stromal cell tumor" showing morphology of the cells; initially classified as reticulum cell sarcoma, it was pyroninophilic and was termed immunoblastic sarcoma by more modern hematopathologists. Such cases reveal that "primitive undifferentiated" tumor cells look like "primitive undifferentiated" tumor cells! Demonstration of testosterone provided the true diagnosis (see Fig. 14–15). Paraffin section, H&E (× 320).

valuable, since both work on paraffin sections (Figs. 14–16 to 14–19) and both show a characteristic pattern of reactivity that quite definitely excludes some tumor types. Indeed, if either malignant lymphoma or melanoma is strongly suspected, then both CLA and S100 will be included in our initial screen, and CEA and vimentin will be omitted if necessary.

Further detailed characterization of lymphomas and melanomas is given in the appropriate chapters (4 and 13). For lymphomas a plethora of antibodies is available for use on frozen sections (Fig. 14–20), and the enthusiastic or unwary pathologist may cheerfully become lost in the maze of different patterns obtained. On paraffin sections, LN1, LN2 and anti-immunoglobulin antibod-

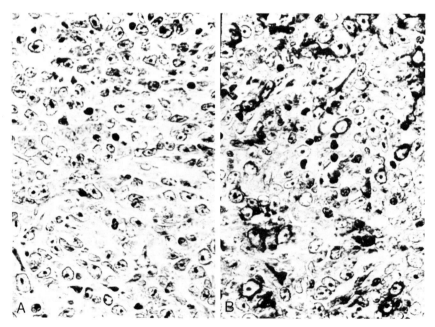

Figure 14–15. Anaplastic tumor of testis, originally classified as "reticulum cell sarcoma," showing negative control (**A,** omitting primary antibody, hematoxylin only) and section stained with antitestosterone (**B,** positive [black] staining of cytoplasm of a proportion of cells). Paraffin section, DAB with hematoxylin counterstain (× 200). Final diagnosis: "undifferentiated" gonadal stromal cell tumor (see Chapter 9).

Figure 14–16. Gastric wall containing anaplastic large cell tumor; tumor cells show variable reactivity (gray to black cytoplasm) with antibody to S100 protein. Eventual diagnosis was melanoma, confirmed on frozen sections with antibodies to melanoma-associated antigens. S100 stains other cell types to a degree, including histiocytes (see Chapter 13). Paraffin section, AEC with hematoxylin counterstain (× 200).

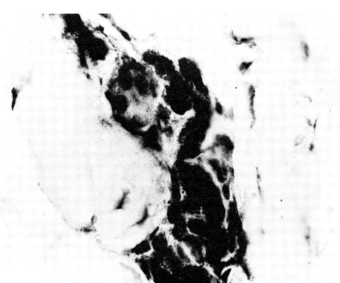

Figure 14–17. Anaplastic cells within muscle biopsy. Frozen section revealed no staining for keratins or CEA and weak reactivity for vimentin. S100 was strongly positive, and intense staining for melanoma-associated antigen was observed. Diagnosis: malignant melanoma. Frozen section, AEC with hematoxylin counterstain (× 500).

Figure 14–18. "Positive control" for common leukocyte antigen (CLA); section of normal tonsil processed in a manner identical to the test section shows intense positive staining (black) of leukocytes in and around follicles. Paraffin section, AEC with hematoxylin counterstain (× 125).

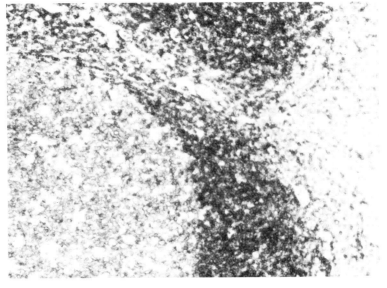

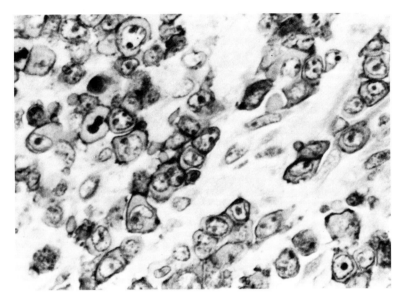

Figure 14–19. Anaplastic tumor showing positive cell surface membrane staining (black rim) with antibody to common leukocyte antigen. Positivity denotes derivation from leukocytes (lymphocytes, histiocytes, or granulocytes). In this instance the diagnosis was immunoblastic sarcoma of B cell type, confirmed by reactivity with LN1 and LN2 antibodies, and a "monoclonal" staining pattern for immunoglobulin. Paraffin section, AEC with hematoxylin counterstain ($\times$ 500).

ies are particularly valuable for certain of the B cell lymphomas (Figs. 14–21 to 14–24). True histiocytic tumors also tend to be positive for one or more of lysozyme, alpha$_1$-antitrypsin and alpha$_1$-antichymotrypsin; true lymphomas do not contain these antigens.

Desmin, Actin, Myosin. Desmin is a reliable marker of muscle cell tumors, but only in frozen sections,* whereas myoglobin typically is present in rhabdomyosarcomas and is frequently demonstrable in paraffin sections. Although some controversy exists, Zenker's

---
*A polyclonal antidesmin antiserum has been claimed to be effective in paraffin sections (Miles; see Fig. 13–11).

and B5 fixatives have been claimed to be superior to formalin for this purpose (Table 14–5). Staining for myoglobin is not seen in carcinomas or in sarcomas other than rhabdomyosarcomas; however, the proportion of positive cells may be small, and they may be distributed unevenly in the section (Figs. 14–25 and 14–26). Typically, the larger cells with more extensive cytoplasm are positive.

Staining for actin and myosin is less helpful, since both are quite widely distributed in normal and neoplastic tissues. Actin is demonstrable in paraffin sections and has been used to mark smooth muscle cells, pericytes, and myoepithelial cells and the corresponding neoplasms (Table 14–5).

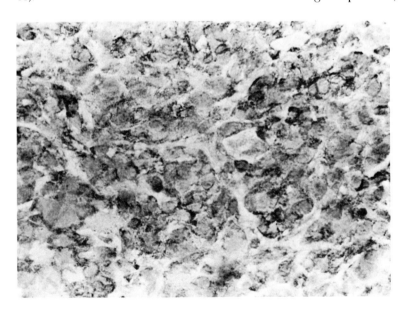

Figure 14–20. Anaplastic tumor showing irregular surface membrane staining for OKT10. OKT6 and OKT11 also gave positive reactions as did an anti-Ia antibody (Fig. 6–5). The eventual diagnosis was immunoblastic sarcoma of T cell type. Frozen section, AEC with hematoxylin counterstain ($\times$ 320).

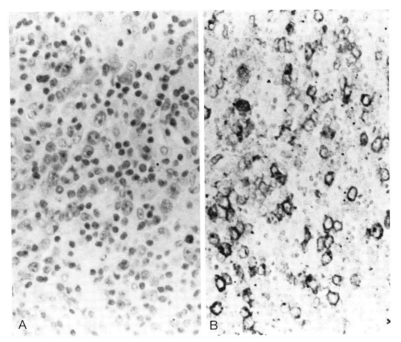

Figure 14–21. Large cell tumor with scattered lymphocytes (**A,** H&E section), diagnosis uncertain. Intense reactivity (**B,** black donuts) with LN1 reveals this as a follicular center cell tumor (large noncleaved type—see Chapter 4). Paraffin section, AEC with hematoxylin counterstain (× 200).

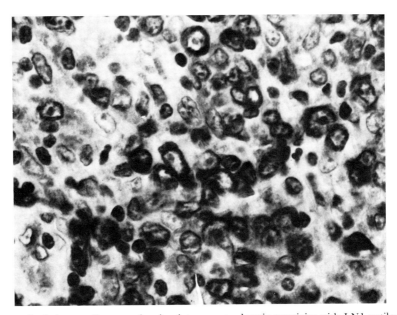

Figure 14–22. Anaplastic large cell tumor showing intense cytoplasmic reactivity with LN1 antibody (Chapter 4). Paraffin section, AEC with hematoxylin counterstain (× 500). Diagnosis: large noncleaved follicular center cell lymphoma.

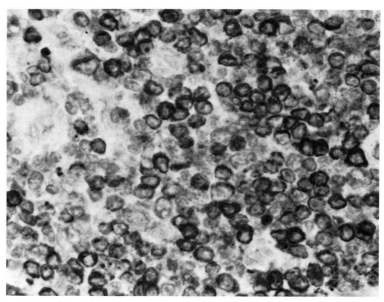

Figure 14–23. Small round cell tumor showing positive nuclear membrane and cytoplasmic staining with LN2 antibody (Chapter 4). Paraffin section, AEC with hematoxylin counterstain (× 500). Diagnosis: small noncleaved follicular center cell lymphoma (non-Burkitt).

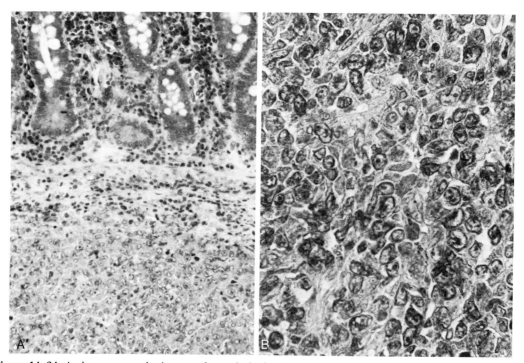

Figure 14–24. *A,* shows an anaplastic tumor beneath the lamina propria. Immunostaining for alpha chain reveals the normal IgA-containing plasma cells (black) in the gut wall (top); the tumor cells (bottom) do not stain (× 125). At a higher magnification (× 500), *B* shows positive staining for mu chain (IgM) within the cytoplasm of these tumor cells. This was a large cleaved follicular center cell lymphoma, marking monoclonally for IgM-lambda by surface marker studies. Paraffin sections, DAB with hematoxylin counterstain.

Table 14–5. Selected Bibliography: Actin, Myosin, Myoglobin

Mukai K et al 1979	Myoglobin in normal and neoplastic skeletal muscle
Corson & Pinkus 1981	Myoglobin in paraffin sections; positive in 13/17 rhabdomyosarcomas (including 5/7 alveolar, 5/5 embryonal, 3/5 pleomorphic); Zenker's fixative superior to formalin; other sarcomas negative
Brooks 1982	Myoglobin found exclusively in striated muscle: 80% of rhabdomyosarcomas positive; all other sarcomas and carcinomas negative; percentage of positive cells often small and patchily distributed
Mukai K et al 1980b	10/25 mixed Müllerian tumors showed evidence of skeletal muscle differentiation as detected by positivity with myoglobin antibody
Kindblom et al 1982	Myoglobin positive in cardiac and skeletal muscle and rhabdomyosarcomas; best fixatives: formalin and Bouin's; fixation time should be short
Storch 1981	Actin and myosin in a wide spectrum of cell types in frozen sections (including hepatocytes and skeletal muscle)
Mukai K et al 1981	Actin in smooth and striated muscle, in pericytes and myoepithelial cells
Osung et al 1980	Used an anti–smooth muscle antibody (antiactin) on frozen sections
Caselitz et al 1980	Actin in paraffin sections of parotid glands
Bussolati et al 1980a	Actin in fixed paraffin sections
Drenckhahn et al 1980	Myosin in brush borders
Bussolati et al 1980b	Actin-positive myoepithelial cells and their distribution in breast cancer; cells differentiate ductal vs lobular, but do not help in detecting invasion
Siegal et al 1983	Myoglobin in a rhabdomyosarcoma of the uterus
Jong et al 1984	20/23 rhabdomyosarcomas positive for myosin, 11/23 positive for myoglobin (paraffin sections)

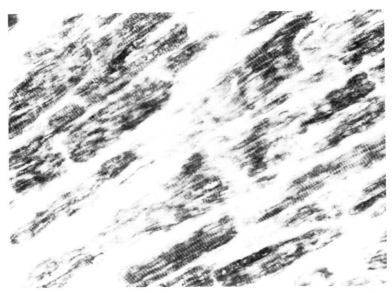

Figure 14–25. Striated muscle showing pattern of reactivity with antibody to myoglobin. This section serves as a positive control when investigating the presence of myoglobin in anaplastic tumors. Paraffin section, AEC with hematoxylin counterstain (× 200).

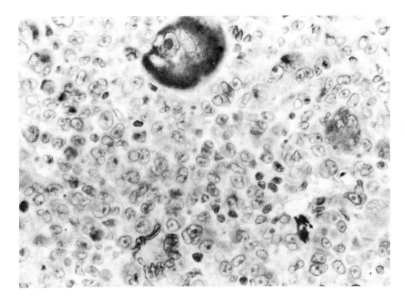

Figure 14–26. Anaplastic large cell tumor with occasional giant cells giving intense reactivity with antibody to myoglobin. Diagnosis: rhabdomyosarcoma. Paraffin section, DAB with hematoxylin counterstain (× 320).

Factor VIII Antigen. Factor VIII antigen is present in many normal endothelial cells, particularly within capillaries and venules (Fig. 14–27). It is demonstrable in paraffin sections (staining is enhanced by trypsinization) but is best evaluated in frozen sections. Staining for factor VIII is of value when considering a diagnosis of Kaposi's sarcoma or other angiomatoid tumor; a positive stain clearly displays the extent of neoplastic (and normal) endothelial cell proliferation within the sections (Fig. 14–28). Positive endothelial cells are thereby clearly distinguished from fibroblasts and other morphologically similar stromal elements. In Kaposi's sarcoma the better-formed vascular elements usually show strong factor VIII reactivity (Fig. 14–29), whereas the poorly defined slitlike channels may or may not show detectable staining (Table 14–6).

Benign vascular proliferations typically are strongly positive (eg, hemangiomas, angiokeratoma) or show patchy reactivity (eg, pyogenic granuloma, lymphangioma—Burgdorf et al, 1981a). Lymphangioma typically shows much less reactivity than hemangioma.

Hemangioblastomas are the subject of some debate as to whether or not the stromal cells are of endothelial origin (Table 14–6).

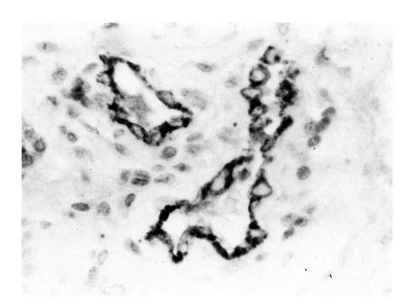

Figure 14–27. Factor VIII antigen within endothelial cells. Paraffin section, DAB with hematoxylin counterstain (× 500).

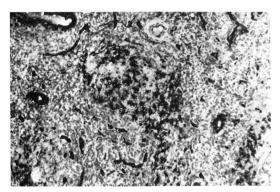

Figure 14–28. Lymph node focally invaded by Kaposi's sarcoma. The irregular sarcoma cells show positive cytoplasmic reactivity (red-black) for factor VIII antigen. Normal vessel endothelium also is positive. Paraffin section, AEC with hematoxylin counterstain (× 125). See color plate II–8.

A small number of tumors in the vimentin-positive group do not give characteristic patterns of reactivity with commonly available antibodies. Most of these tumors are rare; they include fibrosarcomas, chondrosarcomas, osteosarcomas, and Ewing's sarcoma.

Collagens, Laminin. There has been a considerable amount of work pertaining to the collagens, reticulin, and laminin (Table 14–7). Unfortunately, this has little bearing upon the recognition of mesenchymal neoplasms. There may be one possible application with reference to the distinction of in situ or intraductal carcinoma from invasive carcinoma: the basement membrane, revealed by staining for collagen IV and laminin, is de-

monstrably intact in the former but interrupted in the latter (Table 14–7).

GFAP. Staining for glial fibrillary acid protein (GFAP) has its main application in the evaluation of anaplastic intracerebral tumors; the staining facilitates the distinction of certain primary brain tumors from metastatic deposits of extracranial origin. Most astrocytomas and ependymomas contain GFAP; metastatic carcinomas or lymphomas do not. The patterns of reactivity of GFAP in tumors of the nervous system are considered more fully in Chapter 16.

Keratin- and Vimentin-Negative Group

Several diverse and somewhat rare tumor types typically show absence of reactivity for keratins and vimentin. A number of these show reactivity with antibody to neurofilament, the neuronal intermediate filament that is equivalent to keratin or vimentin. The true neuronal tumors fall into this group, including neuroblastomas, ganglioneuromas, and pheochromocytomas. Neuron-specific enolase serves as a useful confirmatory stain for these unusual tumors. Some of the neuroendocrine tumors also have been reported to show positivity for neurofilament (eg, neuroendocrine or Merkel cell carcinoma of the skin and oat cell carcinoma), although keratin has also been described in some of these tumors. Other than this area of uncertainty, neurofilament antigen has not been detected in nonneuronal tumors.

Some germ cell tumors lack all known

Figure 14–29. Kaposi's sarcoma in bladder wall; intense positivity within elongated epithelial cells treated with antibody to factor VIII antigen. Paraffin section, AEC; counterstain has been omitted to display the pattern more effectively in a black and white medium (× 200).

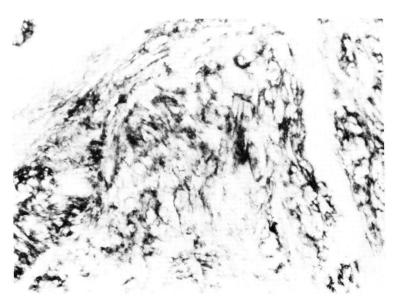

Table 14–6. Selected Bibliography: Factor VIII Antigen, Vascular Tumors

Mukai K et al 1980a Burgdorf et al 1981a	Hyperplastic and neoplastic vascular lesions; hemangioma-, angiokera-toma-positive; lymphangioma, pyogenic granuloma, patchy staining
Guarda et al 1981, 1982	23/28 angiosarcomas positive for factor VIII antigen
Jurco et al 1982	16/21 hemangioblastomas (cerebellum and spinal cord) showed staining of stromal cells for factor VIII antigen; in 13/21 GFAP was present in astrocytes centrally within the tumor
Nadji et al 1981	Histologic variants of Kaposi's all show factor VIII staining
McComb et al 1982a	Trypsinization improved staining of factor VIII antigen in paraffin sections
McComb et al 1982b	Factor VIII antigen and GFAP in hemangioblastomas
Sehested & Hou-Jensen 1981	Factor VIII antigen in endothelial cells, megakaryocytes and platelets
Böhling et al 1983	Factor VIII antigen and *Ulex europaeus* agglutinin (a lectin) both act as endothelial markers, but *Ulex* is more sensitive
Wilson 1984	Problems encountered in staining for factor VIII antigen in a small laboratory
Akhtar et al 1984	Kaposi's sarcoma in transplant recipients
Boxer 1984	11 atrial myxomas: pattern of selective positivity for factor VIII antigen and for actin suggests origin from primitive mesenchyme
Bell & Flotte 1982	Some adenomatoid tumors positive for factor VIII antigen (suggested endothelial origin); otherwise nonreactive (suggested mesothelial origin)

Table 14–7. Selected Bibliography: Collagen, Reticulin, Fibronectin, Laminin, and Others

Unsworth et al 1982	Antisera to reticulin, collagen III, and fibronectin showed distinct patterns serologically, but in tissue sections all gave similar pattern, suggesting tissue "reticulin" contains all three components
Burns et al 1980	Emphasized need for digestion (pepsin—4 mg/ml in 0.1 NHCl for 2 hrs at 37° C) in order to demonstrate fibronectin in formalin paraffin sections
Campbell JA et al 1980	Ligandin in paraffin sections; distribution in normal tissues and tumors
Stenman et al 1980	Fibronectin in developing fibrous plaques of atheroma (fibronectin is released during platelet aggregation)
Hedman 1980	Fibronectin in rough ER of embryonic fibroblasts; an EM study using protein A peroxidase
Grimaud et al 1980	Antisera vs types I, III, and IV collagens used in immunohistologic studies to explore tissue localization at light and electron microscopy
Oberley et al 1979	Fibronectin in the glomerulus, especially in relation to epithelial cell foot processes
Hølund et al 1982	Fibronectin in granulation tissue
SundarRaj et al 1982	Monoclonal antibodies to type III collagen
Dixon et al 1980	Fibronectin in renal biopsies (paraffin sections); glomerular fibronectin increased in most types of glomerular disease but reduced in diabetic nodules and hyalinized glomeruli
Scott et al 1981a	Fibronectin in arthritis
Furcht et al 1980	Affinity of purified antisera to fibronectin and collagen; both react with cellular collagen fibrils; fibronectin antibody shows axial periodicity
Scott et al 1981b	Fibronectin distribution in rectal mucosa
Wright & Leblond 1981	Antisera against procollagen I applied to frozen sections to analyze bone growth
Siegal et al 1981	Type IV collagen and laminin in study of fragmentation of basement membrane by invasive carcinoma (of breast)
Kallioinen et al 1984	Type IV collagen and laminin in basal cell carcinomas (intact in some) or squamous carcinoma (often fragmented)

intermediate filaments, possibly a parallel of the early embryonic cells that also are filament-free. Yolk cell carcinomas typically fall into this category, as do some seminomas or dysgerminomas. It should be noted, however, that embryonal carcinomas typically are keratin-positive, and faint reactivity for low molecular weight keratins may be seen in seminomas. Occasional yolk sac tumors and dysgerminomas have been described as having a few vimentin-positive tumor cells (Miettinen et al. 1983e). Confirmatory stains are discussed in Chapter 9.

Significance of a Positive Reaction for Both Keratin and Vimentin

Finally, if an anaplastic tumor is stained and shows positivity for both keratin and vimentin, and possibly also for CEA, the most likely explanation is some form of technical or processing artifact, such as inadvertently permitting the section to dry, utilizing primary or linking reagents at inappropriate dilutions, or the presence of nonblocked endogenous peroxidase. Transfer of antibodies from one side to another may also occur during the wash procedure. Also, necrotic tumors sometimes show unpredictable reactivity with many antibodies for reasons that are not apparent (see Chapter 4). Artifact should be suspected if the pattern of staining is virtually indistinguishable for the three or four antibodies employed, or if the "no primary" control shows a similar pattern.

A few tumors may exist in which there is staining for both vimentin and keratin. Certain so-called mixed tumors of carcino-sarcomas fall into this category, as do mesotheliomas of biphasic type. Also, synovial sarcomas, which many believe are epithelial neoplasms and thus keratin-positive, have been reported to stain for vimentin; the same has been claimed for renal carcinoma. In

Table 14–8. Selected Bibliography: Immunohistologic Approach to Anaplastic Tumors*

Taylor 1978a, b, 1983a Taylor & Kledzik 1981 Taylor et al 1985	Review of methods and principles for use of immunohistology in differential diagnosis of malignant disease—tissue sections
Ghosh et al 1983a, b	Differential diagnosis of pleural and peritoneal effusions using panels of antibodies (CEA, Ca 1, MFGM, keratin, common leukocyte antigen)
Gatter et al 1984a, 1985	Paraffin sections, CEA, common leukocyte antigen, MFGM, keratin: 120 cases with "difficult" diagnosis; 29 of 43 lesions thought to be anaplastic carcinomas were shown to be lymphomas; overall error rate of morphology alone was approximately 50%
Nagle et al 1983b	Use of antikeratin antibodies in differential diagnosis of tumors
Gabbiani et al 1981	Use of antibodies to intermediate filaments in differential diagnosis of tumors
Debus et al 1984	Use of antikeratin antibodies for classification of carcinomas
Van Muijen et al 1984	Use of antikeratin antibodies in normal tissues and tumors (antibodies 77, 78, and 80)
Osborn & Weber 1982	Use of antibodies to intermediate filaments in normal tissues and tumors
Brooks 1982	Review; immunohistochemical analysis of soft tissue tumors
Gown & Vogel 1982	Intermediate filaments, normal tissue, some reference to tumors
Gown & Vogel 1984	Intermediate filaments, normal tissue, and tumors; squamous and non-squamous keratins
Azar et al 1982	56 cases of anaplastic tumor, some immunohistochemistry plus EM studies
Schlegel et al 1980a	Antikeratin antibody in "poorly differentiated" malignant neoplasms
Battifora 1984	Excellent review, emphasizing antikeratin antibodies AE1 and AE3
Feller & Parwaresch 1983	Method for cytospins, smears, etc., using alkaline phosphatase and peroxidase
Giorno 1983	Cytospins and imprints—avidin-biotin method
Epenetos et al 1982	Detection of carcinoma cells in pleural effusions
Herbert & Gallagher 1982	Alpha$_1$-antichymotrypsin detects reactive mesothelial cells, and distinguishes them from mesothelioma or carcinoma
Blobel et al 1985	Mesotheliomas, keratin in epithelial type, vimentin in fibrous type

*These manuscripts are all listed elsewhere in the text with reference to particular tumor types but are collected here for their focus upon classification of tumor types.

cases in which both keratin and vimentin are positive, the pattern of staining nonetheless is usually different, more or fewer of the cells staining with one or other of the antibodies, often with a different cellular distribution. Before concluding that double staining is present, it is important to be sure that only tumor cells are being evaluated, not stromal cells, which will be vimentin-positive in all tumors.

A partial listing of some of the more recent studies that employed immunohistologic techniques specifically for the purpose of analysis of poorly differentiated tumors is given in Table 14–8.

15

INFECTIOUS DISEASE

"The Microbe is so very small
You cannot make him out at all,
But many sanguine people hope
To see him through a microscope."

HILAIRE BELLOC, 1870–1953
Cautionary Verses

"An immune stain just paves the way
To a bright salubrious day,
When through the lens you softly peep,
There's herpes simplex, fast asleep."

ANON.

The application of immunohistologic techniques for the diagnosis of infectious disease is included not so much for its immediate practical value as for its future potential.

The recognition of infectious disease within tissue is currently based upon successful growth in culture, with rare exceptions for organisms (usually large parasites) that are recognizable microscopically, or in which the cytologic features strongly suggest a particular infectious agent (eg, cytomegalovirus [CMV] infections). In the latter condition, culture or serologic confirmation is still usually required. Faced with a tissue section or cell preparation showing the general features of acute or chronic infection, the pathologist has had few options. If culture was not performed at the time of biopsy (or surgical removal or dissection at autopsy), by the time the need for such studies is realized, it is usually too late; the tissue is all in formalin. We do not have the leisure to routinely perform culture (for what organism?) or to routinely hold tissue for culture if needed, nor would these measures be cost-effective. Thus, in the absence of cultures, the pathologist may resort to electron microscopy (rarely helpful and both expensive and time-consuming) or "special stains." Histochemical stains for microorganisms are few and of limited utility (silver stains, acid-fast stains, and the like). There has thus been consider-

able interest in attempts to develop immunohistological stains for infectious agents.

Theoretically, this approach is promising, because many microorganisms possess a variety of distinctive antigens to which antibodies can be made, offering the potential of specific recognition of organisms by their antigenic constituents.

In practical terms the extent to which these antigens survive fixation or processing is crucial to the success of this technique in routine sections, as is the concentration of antigen present in the infected state. Sufficient antigen must be present in the tissue to produce a reaction product visible by light microscopy; electron microscopic recognition of microorganisms of course is possible but not practical for "routine diagnosis." For immunohistochemical diagnosis of infectious disease to be considered valuable, the findings by this technique must show a favorable correlation with culture or virus isolation methods.

If this last condition is met, then the techniques will become widely used, since the immunocytochemical method offers significant advantages: general utility even in small laboratories, rapidity, cost effectiveness, and avoidance of the necessity for growing potentially hazardous organisms. If the method has a sensitivity significantly lower than culture, it still can be used for an initial "rapid

Table 15–1. Selected Bibliography: Immunohistologic Recognition of Infectious Agents

Review

Löhler 1981 | Paraffin sections—demonstration of measles, polio, influenza, varicella-zoster, CMV, herpes simplex, parainfluenza T, lymphocytic choriomeningitis, Moloney's, and Friend's virus antigens

Viruses

Herpes Simplex Virus

Burns JC 1980 | Review of virus detection methods; emphasized need with reference to growing availability of specific antiviral therapy

Merkel & Zimmer 1981 | Detection of herpesvirus antigen in paraffin sections

Merkel & Zimmer 1982 | Diagnosis of herpes encephalitis on touch preparations

Moseley et al 1981 | Comparison of methods for recognition of genital herpes; peroxidase detected high proportion, including some that were negative on first culture but were positive on subsequent cultures

Schmidt et al 1983 | 82% agreement with virus isolation and immunoperoxidase

Esiri 1982 | Distribution of herpes antigen in 29 autopsied cases of herpes simplex encephalitis

Graham BS & Snell 1983 | Respiratory tract herpes, cytology and histology

Vernon 1982 | Herpetic tracheobronchitis, bronchial brushings

Hansen et al 1979 | Subcellular localization of herpes antigen in rabbit cornea monolayers

Davydova et al 1980 | Immunoperoxidase has advantages of specificity and simplicity for diagnosis of chronic herpes infection

Measles (and Related Viruses)

Budka et al 1982 | Measles antigen in subacute sclerosing encephalitis

Tokunaga et al 1980 | Measles giant cell pneumonia; Warthin-Finkeldy giant cells also present in GI tract, lymph nodes and spleen

Basle et al 1981 }
Rebel & Basle 1981 } | Measles antigen (or similar) within osteoclasts in Paget's disease of bone

Mills et al 1980, 1981 | Paget's disease contains respiratory syncytial virus-like antigen

Cevenini et al 1983 | Respiratory syncytial virus; agreed with virus isolation results at 89% level

Cytomegalovirus

Abramowitz et al 1982 | CMV antigen in paraffin sections of lymph node—in lymphocytes

Myerson et al 1984 | Presence of "occult" CMV in many normal-appearing cells; wide variety of cell types infected, including endothelial cells

Varicella-Zoster

Horten et al 1981 | VZ antigen in multifocal leukoencephalopathy, within astrocytes and neurons; Hodgkin's disease and cancer patients

Human Papilloma Virus (HPV) (see also Chapters 12, Cervix, and 13, Skin)

Meisels et al 1981 | Paraffin sections—cervical condylomata, including those with atypia

Woodruff et al 1980 | Paraffin sections, cervical condylomata

Syrjänen & Pyrhönen 1982a, b | Condylomata, dysplasia and neoplasia; discussion of role of virus

Jenson et al 1982b | About 50% of common and plantar warts positive for HPV

Mounts et al 1982 | HPV antigen in some cases of juvenile and adult laryngeal papilloma

Lass et al 1983 | HPV in 24/41 conjunctival papillomas

Quick et al 1980 | HPV antigen only at the surface of laryngeal papilloma; in many patients there had been maternal genital condylomata in pregnancy

Lack et al 1980 | HPV common antigen in 26/35 laryngeal papillomas, 5 different serotypes of HPV in different verrucae and papillomas

Morin et al 1981 | HPV antigen in cervical condylomata

Lutzner et al 1982 | Oral warts and different serotypes of HPV

Jenson et al 1982a | HPV antigen in 18/29 verrucae, 2/5 papillomas, 3/5 condylomata and 0/28 keratoacanthomas; positive intranuclear staining

SV40

Tabuchi et al 1980 }
Sheffield et al 1980 } | SV40 virus in rhesus monkey and mitotic cells

Table 15–1. Selected Bibliography: Immunohistologic Recognition of Infectious Agents
Continued

Shope Fibroma	
Bohn 1980	Development of virus particles and cell ultrastructure
Polyoma	
Gerber et al 1980	Polyoma virus common antigen in paraffin sections, including leukoencephalopathy and transplant patients
Influenza (and Sendai)	
Kohama et al 1981	Detected on surface of infected cells
Rotavirus	
Graham DY & Estes 1979 Chasey 1980	} Good technique papers for detection of viral antigens; paraffin sections, PAP method
Baboon Endogenous (BaEV)	
Schumacher et al 1981	BaEV antigen found at tips of cellular processes in acute lymphoblastic leukemia with "hand mirror" morphology
Distemper	
Ducatelle et al 1980	Described detection of distemper virus antigen in paraffin-embedded canine tissue

Miscellaneous Infectious Agents

Mycobacterium leprae	
Gillis & Buchanan 1982	Monoclonal antibodies versus leprosy bacillus and other mycobacteria
Mshana et al 1983	Utilized antibody to *M. bovis*, which cross-reacts with leprosy bacillus; correlated with histologic findings
Group B Streptococcus	
Andres & MacPherson 1980	PAP method with commercial group specific streptococcal antisera—formalin paraffin sections and autopsy material
Legionella pneumophilia	
Boyd & McWilliams 1982	Staining of involved lungs
Popov et al 1982	Rabbit antibody; immunoferritin and immunoperoxidase methods
Mycoplasma	
Imada et al 1979	Detection of colonies on agar plate; theoretically applicable to tissue sections
Chasey & Woods 1984	*Mycoplasma* demonstrated in thin sections
Chlamydia	
Elliott et al 1981	Description of antibodies and techniques; this study however found negative results for *Chlamydia* in bowel disease
Crum et al 1984	Chlamydial antigens in cervical biopsies; histology alone could not predict positive cases; sensitive and rapid immunoperoxidase method
Toxoplasma	
Conley & Jenkins 1981	Successful use of rabbit antisera to toxoplasma (in mice)
Tabei 1982	*Toxoplasma gondii*, immunohistologic detection (letter)
Cat-Scratch Disease	
Wear et al 1983	Use of convalescent sera revealed small bacilli
Trichomonas	
Bennett et al 1980 O'Hara et al 1980	} Use of rabbit antibodies for demonstration of trichomonads in paraffin sections and cytologic preparations
Trichophyton rubrum	
Holden CA et al 1981	Both light and electron microscopy
Fasciola hepatica	
Demaree & Hillyer 1982	Localization of coat antigens (EM)
Leishmania	
Livni et al 1983	Demonstration of leishmanial forms in macrophages in paraffin sections; used antibodies to *L. donovani*, *L. tropica*, and *L. mexicana*

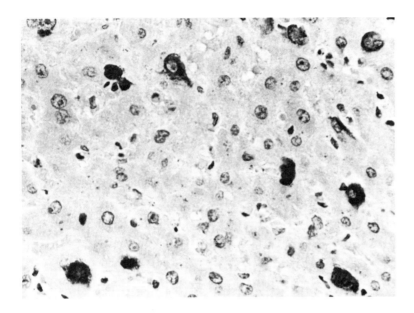

Figure 15–1. Liver: scattered cells show intense cytoplasmic reactivity (black) with antibody to HBsAg. Paraffin section, AEC with hematoxylin counterstain (× 320). HBcAg can be demonstrated by similar techniques and is primarily intranuclear in location.

diagnosis" or as a method of last resort if culture was not performed or was not technically satisfactory.

The work performed to date suggests that we are on the verge of fulfilling these various requirements for at least some organisms. Selected reports describing the successful immunohistologic demonstration of infectious agents under various conditions are given in Table 15–1. Particular emphasis is given to the immunohistologic demonstration of microorganisms in paraffin sections, since this is the pathologist's primary medium. The immunohistochemical identification of hepatitis B (Fig. 15–1), hepatitis A, and delta antigens, is described in some detail in Chapter 11 and clearly has an established role in the evaluation of needle biopsies of the liver. Similarly, extensive studies of human papilloma virus antigens (Fig. 15–2) have led to a diagnostic role in relation both to condylomatous and carcinomatous lesions of the uterine cervix (Chapter 12) and to some cutaneous and oral verrucae and papillomata (Chapter 13). Additional references to the demonstration of HPV antigens, particularly in laryngeal papillomata, are given in Table 15–1.

With herpes simplex the thrust, directed chiefly at the detection of herpesvirus antigen

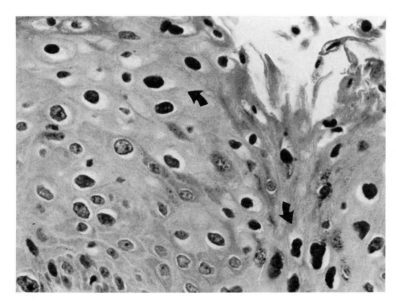

Figure 15–2. Skin papilloma (wart) treated with antibody to human papilloma virus (HPV) antigen. A positive reaction is seen within the nucleus of cells showing perinuclear vacuoles (koilocytes). Positive nuclei appear brown (dense black in the figure—arrows). Paraffin section, DAB with hematoxylin counterstain (× 320).

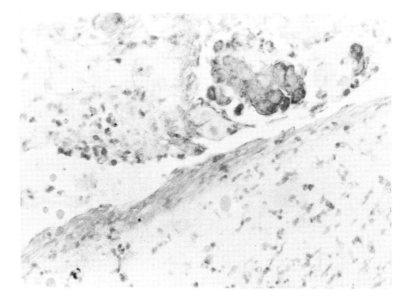

Figure 15–3. A cluster of cells (top right) at the base of an ulcerating lesion reveals granular cytoplasmic staining with antibody to Herpes simplex 2. Paraffin section, AEC with hematoxylin counterstain (× 200).

in cervical smear preparations (see also Chapter 12), has been a little different. The growing availability of useful therapy for herpesvirus enhances the need for a rapid and cost-effective test. Culture is considered to be accurate; indeed, it is the yardstick against which other methods are measured. However, to get a definitive answer takes a week or more. Rapid "immunoculture" techniques have shortened this time to 24 to 48 hours, with a correlation of approximately 90 percent with traditional virus isolation. In this approach the cervical scrape is cultured on a special monolayer for 24 to 48 hours, after which viral growth is detected by immunoperoxidase staining for herpesvirus antigen rather than waiting for formation of the characteristic "cytopathologic effects" (CPE) that occur only later. The short-term culture serves to "amplify" any viral antigen that is present to the level that it is easily detectable. There has been valid concern that direct staining of cervical (Pap) smears or of other herpetic lesions for herpesvirus antigen might be relatively insensitive, owing to the small amounts of antigen present. However, some investigators (eg, Schmidt et al, 1983) have claimed a correlation of 80 percent or

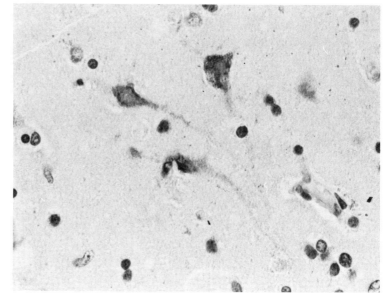

Figure 15–4. Herpes encephalitis showing a positive (black) cytoplasmic reaction for Herpesvirus antigen (type 1). Paraffin section, AEC with hematoxylin counterstain (× 320).

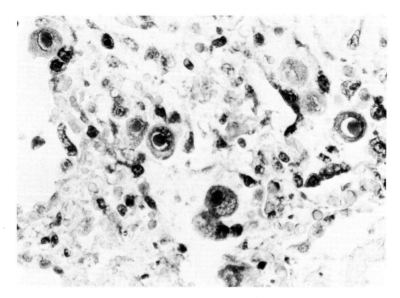

Figure 15–5. Neonatal pneumonitis treated with antibody to cytomegalovirus (CMV); large positively stained cells are clearly visible. Some contain characteristic inclusions; however, immunostaining has been described as giving positive results in the absence of recognizable inclusions. Paraffin section, AEC with hematoxylin counterstain (× 200).

more between direct immunoperoxidase (or direct immunofluorescence) methods and virus isolation. With improvement in antibody and more sensitive detection systems, this observation appears to be sufficient for this technique to find a place as the primary screening method. Indeed, the sensitivity problem may be exaggerated for many viral infections, since early infection is characterized not so much by a little virus in many cells, as by the presence of easily detectable virus in a very small proportion of cells. Diagnosis then becomes a function of sample size; positive results are obtainable in paraffin sections, but the sensitivity of this approach is not known (Figs. 15–3 and 15–4).

It is also apparent that for those viral infections associated with "characteristic inclusions or other cytologic features" the sensitivity of detection of disease by immunohistology far exceeds that of cytologic assessment alone. This is true for herpesvirus and *Chlamydia* in Pap smears, for HPV in verrucae and condylomata and for CMV in various tissue sites (Fig. 15–5; Myerson et al., 1984). To state the problem another way, the frequency of false negatives is much higher when relying upon cytologic features alone; additional immunocytologic stains selected upon the basis of clinical or cytologic suspicions serve to lower the frequency of false negatives, in some instances to a level that

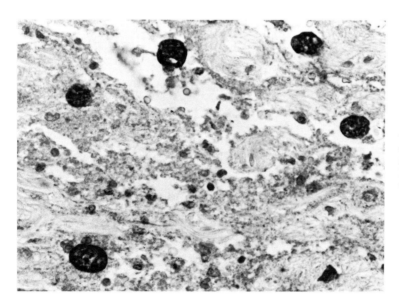

Figure 15–6. Severe colitis with ulceration; necrotic area showing intense reactivity of amebae with antibody to *Entamoeba histolytica*. Paraffin section, AEC with hematoxylin counterstain (× 200).

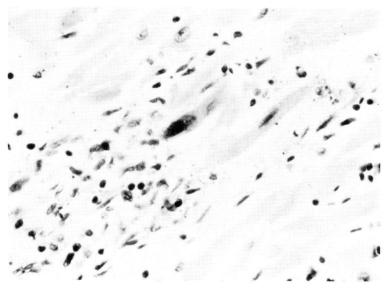

Figure 15–7. Myocarditis; section taken at autopsy shows inflammatory cells and cardiac muscle cells; one of the latter contains a cluster of black granules at one pole. This is the product of staining with antitoxoplasma antibody. Patient had acquired immunodeficiency. Paraffin section, DAB with hematoxylin counterstain (× 200).

Table 15–2. Infectious Agents for Which Antibodies Are Available for Use in Paraffin Sections

Baboon endogenous virus	Measles antigen
Buffalo pox	Moloney's virus
Chlamydia	Mouse mammary tumor
Cytomegalovirus	virus antigen
Distemper virus	*Mycobacteria*
Fasciola hepatica	*Mycoplasma*
Friend's virus	Parainfluenza
Group B streptococcus	Polio
Hepatitis B surface anti-	Polyoma virus
gen	Respiratory syncytial virus
Herpes simplex virus,	Rotavirus
1 & 2	Rubella
HTLV I	Shope's fibroma virus
HTLV III	SV40 virus
Human papilloma virus	*Toxoplasma*
Influenza	*Trichomonas*
Klebsiella	*Trichophyton*
Legionella	Varicella-zoster
Leishmania	
Lymphocytic choriomenin-	
gitis virus	

approaches the reliability of primary culture. Using immunocytochemical methods in the presence of proper controls, false positives are rare.

Table 15–1 lists some of the immunostains that may have practical diagnostic utility or may serve to illustrate approaches that are on the verge of becoming practicable (Figs. 15–6 and 15–7). For research purposes these as well as many other infectious agents may be studied by immunohistologic methods in cell preparations or tissue sections or by electron microscopy, and the list is growing daily (Table 15–2). The utilization of "in situ" tissue section hybridization using DNA or RNA probes for viral genetic material already is being widely used as an experimental technique and, with strong commercial interest, seems destined soon to become available as another form of specific staining for infectious agents.

16

DIAGNOSTIC IMMUNOSTAINING OF THE NERVOUS SYSTEM

Roy H. Rhodes, M.D., Ph.D.

"As long as our brain is a mystery, the universe, the reflection of the structure of the brain, will also be a mystery."

CAJAL, 1852–1934

"Brain. n. An apparatus with which we think that we think."

AMBROSE BIERCE, 1842–1914
The Devil's Dictionary

Progress in immunohistochemical staining of the nervous system has proceeded in step with studies of other tissues. The same basic principles apply and identical methods may be employed (Chapters 2 and 3).

There is an ever-increasing list of antigens that are relatively specific or even unique for neural cells. Many of the antibodies now available are monoclonals, and it is worth emphasizing that their exquisite sensitivity is understood only through empirical testing. The adverse effects of routine fixation and processing often preclude use of the monoclonals except on cryostat sections. In addition, very broad cellular immunoreactivity can be found with some monoclonals. Polyclonal antisera with monospecificity in immunohistochemical staining can label an epitope shared with other types of proteins when studied by immunochemical methods, and this fact can limit the means of confirming a set of data (Dahl et al, 1984). The material discussed here involves routine formalin fixation for the most part. The immunoperoxidase methods can thus be used on current or on archival material. In some instances, immunohistochemical studies allow refinements in the classification of lesions;

whereas in other cases etiologic data that can lead to rapid and specific therapy are provided.

ANTIGENS AND ANTISERA IN SURGICAL PATHOLOGY OF THE NERVOUS SYSTEM

Glial Fibrillary Acidic Protein (GFAP)

GFAP is a stable protein that is found in soluble and polymerized form in glial cells. In polymerized form it appears as the major glial cytoskeletal element in intermediate filaments. GFAP has been associated principally with astrocytes, but it also is found in ependymal cells and in folliculostellate cells of the anterior pituitary, and it has been identified in the peripheral nervous system (Table 16–1).

The demonstration of GFAP in Schwann cells of peripheral nerves by immunostaining has, however, been difficult to confirm by peptide mapping or by other immunochemical techniques. The source of the difficulty—fact or artifact–is an important ques-

Table 16–1. Selected Bibliography: Glial Fibrillary Acidic Protein (GFAP)

Eng 1980 Gheuens et al 1980 Roessmann et al 1980 Borit & McIntosh 1981 Shaw G et al 1981	GFAP in soluble and polymerized form in astrocytes and epen- dymal cells
Höfler et al 1984	GFAP in agranular folliculostellate cells of human anterior pitui- tary gland
Davison & Jones 1981 Jessen & Mirsky 1980 Dahl et al 1982 Fields & Raine 1982 Jessen et al 1984	GFAP present in peripheral nervous system as determined im- munohistochemically and electrophoretically but not by some other immunochemical methods based on central astrocytic GFAP; peripheral (Schwann cell and enteric astrocyte) GFA polypeptides differ slightly from central ones
Amaducci et al 1981 Dahl et al 1981a	Reactive astrocytes contain abundant GFAP
Deck et al 1978 Duffy et al 1978, 1980 Eng & Rubinstein 1978 van der Meulen et al 1978 De Armond et al 1980 Gambetti et al 1980 Pasquier et al 1980, 1981 Velasco et al 1980 Laverson et al 1981 Tascos et al 1982 Marsden et al 1983 Roessmann et al 1983a Bonnin & Rubinstein 1984	Most pediatric and adult astrocytomas are GFAP positive, but mixed tumors and others (eg, oligodendrogliomas) often have GFAP; GFAP negativity important in ruling out nonglial tu- mors, but the most malignant glial tumor (glioblastoma) often has little or no GFAP
Trojanowski et al 1984	

tion, because immunoperoxidase staining for GFAP may not always distinguish primary central nervous system glial tumors from central or peripheral neurilemmomas (schwannomas) if occasional examples of any of these tumors can be positive for GFAP. GFA polypeptides appear to be a heterogeneous group with a common molecular weight and with some shared antigenic determinants. Monoclonal antibodies that can define shared or absent determinants in testing astrocytic or peripheral GFAP (Jessen et al, 1984) can yield negative results on an unknown tumor that may be positively immunostained by other monoclonal or polyclonal antibodies to the group of GFA polypeptides.

GFAP or GFAP-like protein has been identified in a benign neurilemmoma (Tascos et al, 1982), in a recurrent central neurilemmoma (Bruner et al, 1984), and in a malignant, widely metastatic spinal nerve–root neurilemmoma by immunostaining (Fig. 16–1). GFAP or GFAP-like immunostaining also has been reported in pleomorphic adenomas of the salivary glands (Nakazato et al, 1982b). GFAP immunostaining is to be expected in normal astrocytes and in reactive astrocytes, as shown in Figure 16–2. GFAP also may be immunostained in phagocytic cells that have taken up this protein from the extracellular compartment (Deck and Rubinstein, 1981). These factors need to be considered when immunostaining for the presence of GFAP for diagnostic purposes.

Nonspecific binding of immunoglobulins in normal serum control slides may be the cause of the slight staining of enlarged (but not of normal) astrocytes in the absence of a primary specific antiserum. This type of nonspecific staining may be decreased by preincubation in normal serum (Paasivuo and Saksela, 1983; see also Chapter 3) or by cleaving the sialic acid binding sites for immunoglobulins with sodium metaperiodate and sodium borohydride (Langley et al, 1980). Preliminary work shows that reactive and neoplastic astrocytes, oligodendrocytes, and macrophages have IgG Fc receptors (Ma et al, 1981; Tsai et al, 1982). This circumstance does not appear to present a practical problem in diagnostic immunostaining in most cases, but covering such sites with a normal serum preincubation step may be prudent. Coverslips can be removed from routinely stained sections, which can be destained with alcohol and then restained for the presence of GFAP (Rhodes, 1982). The major diagnostic use of immunostaining for GFAP has been in neurooncology (Table 16–1).

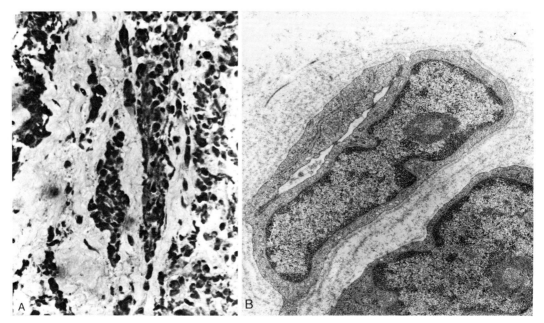

Figure 16–1. *A*, Glial fibrillary acidic protein (GFAP) is immunostained by the indirect immunoperoxidase method, using a 1:200 dilution of the primary antiserum, in a malignant neurilemmoma that arises from a spinal nerve root. The cellular nuclei are darkly counterstained with hematoxylin. The immunoreactive cytoplasmic GFAP is seen by the cytoplasmic reaction product of moderate density. The collagenous bands between the immunostained cells have some slight nonspecific staining (× 400). *B*, Electron microscopy of the malignant neurilemmoma shows individual tumor cells surrounded by redundant basement membrane material. The young adult patient died with widely metastatic disease (× 8800).

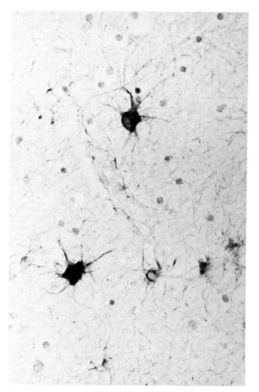

Figure 16–2. GFAP immunoreactivity using the PAP method shows reactive astrocytes in the cerebrum. There is a light hematoxylin counterstain (× 400).

Vimentin

Vimentin is an intermediate filament protein found in mesenchymal cells (see Chapters 13 and 14), melanocytes, astrocytes, ependymal cells, Schwann cells, and some developing neurons (Table 16–2). In the brain it is found in lesser amounts as development proceeds, with a concomitant increase in GFAP in the astrocytes. Reactive and neoplastic astrocytes in the brain and Schwann cells in transected nerves have an increase in vimentin. The astrocytes and Schwann cells may have mixtures of tightly packed, GFAP- and vimentin-containing intermediate filaments. It is possible that both GFAP and vimentin are structural proteins of the same individual filaments.

Mesenchymal tumors or meningiomas that contain vimentin are likely to contain an abundance of collagen that is easily demonstrated by a variety of routine stains (Gabiani et al, 1981; Yung et al, 1984). However, glial tumors rarely contain much collagen as part of their primary structure (Mathews and Moossy, 1974; Friede, 1978; Soeur et al, 1979; Iglesias et al, 1984; Kepes et al, 1984). Thus, in the absence of any but perivascular collagen, a tumor in the brain with vimentin

Table 16–2. Selected Bibliography: Vimentin in the Nervous System

Osborn et al 1981 Shaw G et al 1981 Schnitzer et al 1981 Autilio-Gambetti et al 1982	Vimentin in astrocytes, ependymal cells, and Schwann cells
Bignami et al 1982 Jacobs et al 1982	Vimentin in developing astrocytes and developing neurons
Dahl 1981 Dahl et al 1981b Schnitzer et al 1981 Bignami et al 1982 Pixley & de Vellis 1984	Vimentin in astrocytes decreases, whereas GFAP increases during development
Dahl et al 1981a Autilio-Gambetti et al 1982 Federoff et al 1983 Pixley & de Vellis 1984	Some reactive astrocytes and reactive Schwann cells have increased vimentin
Sharp et al 1982 Wang E et al 1984	Some intermediate filaments may contain both GFAP and vimentin
Roessmann et al 1983b Borit & Yung 1983	Some GFAP-deficient astrocytomas and ependymomas contain vimentin

immunoreactivity is likely to be an astrocytoma or ependymoma (Borit and Yung, 1983; Roessmann et al, 1983b).

Some astrocytomas have been shown to be deficient in GFAP but still to express vimentin. This work is preliminary, yet it would be an important finding if some glial tumors are vimentin-positive when GFAP is entirely lacking, since this might lead to difficulties in differentiation from other tumors. Primary central nervous system rhabdomyosarcomas are exceedingly rare, but they may contain immunoreactive vimentin (Hinton and Halliday, 1984) as well as myoglobin (Taratuto et al, 1985), and amelanotic melanomas typically show immunostaining for vimentin and also for S100 protein (vide infra). In most tumors it may also be helpful to demonstrate a lack of immunostaining for cytokeratins to rule out epithelial carcinomas (Gabbiani and Kocher, 1983; Huszar et al, 1983; Ramaekers et al, 1983).

S100 Protein

The acidic protein known as S100 has a wide distribution that includes various types of stromal cells (Chapter 13). Immunostaining for S100 protein is found in glial cells in the central and enteric nervous systems, in Schwann cells, in satellite cells in the autonomic ganglia and adrenal medulla, in sustentacular cells in the carotid body, in interstitial cells in the pineal body, in

folliculostellate cells in the anterior pituitary, in certain lymphoid tissue cells and in various myoepithelial and ductal epithelium cells (Table 13–1). Adipose tissue also contains immunoreactive S100 protein, as does human cartilage. Not all of the immunoreactive sites have a relationship to the neural crest (Nakajima et al, 1982a; Stefansson et al, 1982b; Kahn et al, 1983). The last examples seem to be exceptions to the supposed specificity of S100 protein as an antigen of the neuroectoderm.

S100 protein has been detected in brain tumors, including astrocytomas, oligodendrogliomas, ependymomas, choroid plexus papillomas, ganglioneuroblastomas, ganglioneuromas, gangliogliomas, meningiomas, hemangioblastomas, meningeal melanomas, craniopharyngiomas, chordomas, and medulloepitheliomas. Peripheral neuroblastomas, melanomas, Schwann cell tumors (including neurilemmomas, neurofibromas, and granular cell tumors), non-neural pleomorphic adenomas of the salivary glands, mixed sweat gland tumors, chondrosarcomas, breast tumors, eosinophilic granulomas, and other tumors have also been reported to immunostain for S100 protein. Furthermore, immunolocalization of S100 protein can be an aid in identifying amelanotic melanomas or demonstrating the Schwann cell component of some malignant nerve sheath tumors (Table 16–3). Amelanotic melanomas contain both alpha and beta subunits of S100 protein, whereas neurilemmomas contain only beta subunits (Isobe et al, 1984; Takahashi et al,

Table 16–3. Selected Bibliography: S100 Protein in the Nervous System

Haglid et al 1973 Dohan et al 1977 Nakajima et al 1982a Tabuchi et al 1982 Auer & Becker 1983 Ishiguro et al 1983a, b Kahn et al 1983 Nakamura et al 1983b Shimada et al 1985	S100 protein in glial, neuronal and meningeal tumors and in craniopharyngiomas
Nakamura et al 1983a	S100 protein in chordomas
Nakajima et al 1982b Kahn et al 1983 Cochran et al 1984	S100 protein in amelanotic melanomas
Nakajima et al 1982a Nakazato et al 1982a Stefansson & Wollmann 1982 Stefansson et al 1982 Kahn et al 1983 Mukai M 1983 Weiss SW et al 1983	S100 protein in neurilemmomas, neurofibromas and granular cell tumors
Nakajima et al 1982a Weiss SW et al 1983 Daimaru et al 1984 Herrera & Pinto de Moraes 1984	S100 protein in malignant nerve sheath tumors

1984). This fact would present a particular difficulty in immunostaining with a single monoclonal antibody when only one subunit or the other might be recognized. The practical use of immunostaining for S100 protein in surgical pathology of the nervous system may be limited to basically peripheral problems. This antigen may aid in the distinction between undifferentiated neuroblastomas with unequivocally positive S100 protein immunostaining and a favorable prognosis and a subgroup with negative or weak staining and a very poor prognosis (Shimada et al, 1985).

Myelin

The major problem encountered with myelin in pathology is its decrease or absence. Myelin basic protein (MBP) can be shown by immunostaining to decrease in demyelinating diseases. Multiple sclerosis plaques first show an initial increase in MBP immunostaining and then a profound deficit (Table 16–4). In addition, immunohistochemical studies reveal a deficiency in myelin-associated glycoprotein (MAG) far past the sharp border of the classic plaques of multiple sclerosis. This loss of immunoreactive MAG, however, is not specific for multiple sclerosis. The plaques themselves contain T cells that are heterogeneous with respect to T cell subsets from plaque to plaque in a given brain (Booss et al, 1983). In the acutely demyelinated lesions of progressive multifocal leukoencephalopathy (PML), both MBP and MAG are decreased (Itoyama et al, 1982).

Demyelination in peripheral nerve sections generally can be evaluated by routine and special stains, although teased nerve preparations are preferable. Immunostaining for MBP can show residual myelin in nerves involved by a widely destructive process as

Table 16–4. Selected Bibliography: Myelin

Whitaker 1978 Itoyama et al 1980a, b Prineas et al 1984	MBP and MAG levels and locations in multiple sclerosis
Abrams et al 1982 Melmed et al 1983 Steck et al 1983a, b Meier et al 1984	Association of idiopathic polyneuritis with a circulating monoclonal autoantibody (IgM kappa) against myelin or MAG

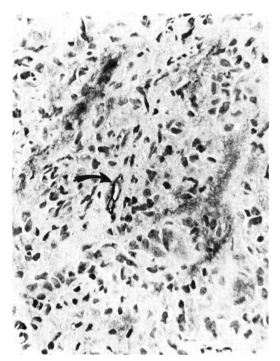

Figure 16–3. Myelin basic protein (MBP) is immuno-stained by an indirect immunoperoxidase method (1:50) in the malignant neurilemmoma described in Figure 16–1. There is a residual myelinated axon (arrow) surrounded by tumor cells. Note the diffuse granular reaction product that immunolocalizes MBP within tumor cells (× 400). (Immunostaining was kindly done by Dr. John N. Whitaker.)

an indication that one is indeed dealing with the residuum of a nerve (Fig. 16–3). Interestingly, it has been possible to demonstrate the presence of a monoclonal autoantibody, usually an IgM kappa, directed against MAG in the serum of some patients with a demyelinating neuropathy. In at least some of these patients, the demyelination may be secondary to a primary axonal degeneration, making the anti-MAG antibody of uncertain significance except as an aid in general classification (Mendell et al, 1985). Many patients with multiple sclerosis have in their serum an IgM autoantibody that binds to the surface of normal oligodendrocytes (Pedersen et al, 1983). Immunocytochemical studies show that such human monoclonal autoantibodies are not always neural specific. In a report of three patients with demyelinating neuropathy, an autoantibody demonstrated cross reactivity between MAG and a cell surface site of a subset of T lymphocytes, with a marked decrease in that subset of circulating T cells (Murray and Steck, 1984). MAG is probably only one of several neural glycoconjugates that shares antigenicity with the surface of T cells (Dobersen et al, 1985; Motoi et al, 1985; Sato S et al, 1985). There is a report of two patients with chronic polyneuropathy whose sera contained IgM fractions that were used to immunostain central and peripheral myelin with an apparent specificity for MBP (Panitch, 1982). These are instructive examples of clinical-immunohistochemical correlations that may aid in defining the pathophysiology of an obscure spectrum of conditions.

Other myelin-associated antigens that have been studied by immunoperoxidase staining in idiopathic polyneuritides include P0 glycoprotein and P1 and P2 basic proteins, which, along with MAG, appear to change in early lesions as a result of inflammation directed primarily at myelin (Schober et al, 1981). Myelin as the target may mean that there is a primary autoimmunity to myelin or a natural cross reactivity with it. Viral epitopes share amino acid sequences with MBP and P2, which may lead to a specific sensitization of lymphocytes to central and peripheral myelin (Jahnke et al, 1985). It has been suggested that demyelinating diseases such as the Guillain-Barré syndrome may follow a primary immune-complex vasculitis in which myelin is secondarily damaged, eliciting an inflammatory response (Reik, 1979). A vasculitis of this type additionally may open myelin to immunologic surveillance during which cross reactivity becomes a factor.

Enolase

Isoenzymes of the glycolytic–pathway enzyme enolase have differential body-wide distributions. Two enolases of interest here have been termed nonneuronal enolase (NNE) and 14-3-2 protein, and neuron-specific enolase (NSE), by most investigators (Marangos et al, 1979). NNE can be found by immunostaining in astrocytes, ependymal cells, arachnoidal cap cells, Schwann cells, and vascular endothelial cells. Astrocytomas, ependymomas, oligodendrogliomas, meningiomas, and neurilemmomas are immunostained varying amounts for NNE (Table 16–5).

NSE is found in normal neurons, and it has been reported in neuroblastomas, medulloblastomas, retinoblastomas, glioblastomas, astrocytomas, oligodendrogliomas, ependymomas, pineocytomas, choroid plexus

Table 16–5. Selected Bibliography: Enolase

Hullin et al 1980 Kato et al 1982	Enolase isoenzymes distributed differentially in various tissues
Langley & Ghandour 1981 Royds et al 1982	Location of NNE in normal tissue and in neural tumors by immunostaining
Vinores et al 1984	NSE in brain tumors, neurilemmomas, carcinomas, chordomas.
Dhillon et al 1982b Warner et al 1984	NSE in melanomas
Wick et al 1983 Sheppard et al 1984 Asa et al 1984	NSE in neuroendocrine tumors
Dhillon et al 1982b Ishiguro et al 1983b Triche & Askin 1983	NSE in peripheral neuroblastomas
Kyritsis et al 1984 Terenghi et al 1984	NSE in retinoblastomas
Asa et al 1984	NSE in pituitary tumors, carcinomas, lymphoma

papillomas, pituitary adenomas, meningiomas, neurilemmomas, melanomas, neuroendocrine tumors, some carcinomas, fibroadenomas, chordomas, and lymphomas. Most bronchial carcinomas of small cell type and some of glandular and squamous cell type may be immunostained for NSE (Table 16–5; see also Chapter 9). Although most melanomas contain immunoreactive NSE, a few that appear "negative" could contain an alternative or antigenically altered form of enolase. It is also worth remembering that tumors may produce enzymes not normally present in their progenitor cell lines, and therefore NSE immunoreactivity must be assessed with care in the study of neoplasia. Thus, NSE immunoreactivity may be of value in lesions outside the central nervous system, but its reported presence in tumors that include melanoma, neurilemmoma, carcinoma, and lymphoma must always be considered prior to accepting a positive stain as evidence of neuronal differentiation. The immunostaining of ganglion cells by NSE can be part

of the evaluation of rectal mucosal biopsies for Hirschsprung's disease (Hall and Lampert, 1984).

Neurofilaments

Neurofilaments comprise an immunologically distinct class of intermediate filaments that are cell type–specific, at least in normal cells, when their protein constituents are demonstrated by immunostaining. One exception to this specificity has been reported in a pulmonary squamous cell tumor. In attempting to evaluate tumors for the presence of neurofilaments, the pathologist should beware of false-negative results that may be attributable to the adverse effects of fixation or to the extremely narrow range of specificity possessed by some monoclonal antibodies that fail to recognize slightly aberrant molecules. There could be false-positive results from cross reactivity or from the synthesis by neoplastic cells of products not nor-

Table 16–6. Selected Bibliography: Neurofilaments

Lazarides 1981 Shaw G et al 1981 Yen & Fields 1981 Osborn & Weber 1982 Dahl 1983 Fuchs & Hanukoglu 1983	Immunoreactive neurofilament triplet protein marker of neurons in normal cells
Lehto et al 1983, 1984	Polyclonal antiserum to neurofilament proteins positive in pulmonary small cell tumors
van Muijen et al 1984	Monoclonal antibodies to neurofilament proteins positive in a poorly differentiated pulmonary squamous cell tumor, but negative in small cell tumors
Trojanowski et al 1982	Olfactory neuroblastoma positive with monoclonal antibody to 70-kd neurofilament subunit but negative for other neurofilament subunits with other monoclonals
Roessmann et al 1983a	Neurofilaments immunostained in some neuroblastomas, medulloblastomas, ganglioma, pineoblastoma; Homer-Wright rosettes negative; some tumors negative by silver-impregnation for neurofilaments are positive by immunostaining

mally found in their cells of origin. The only normal neurons reported to be nonreactive for neurofilament protein are the interneurons of the cerebellar internal granule cell layer (Table 16–6).

Neurofilaments contain three cross-reacting polypeptides (70, 150, and 200 kd subunits). The extent of the cross reactivity of the antibodies against these different polypeptides depends in part on the method of isolating them as antigens. The 150kd polypeptide may be selectively distributed, or at least antibodies may not show immunologic reactivity to it in all neurofilaments. Since some tumors (eg, neuroblastoma) contain only one of the triplet proteins, it is important that a reagent for use on tissue sections should contain immunoglobulins reactive against the entire major set of neurofilament antigens.

A helpful classic adjunct to the identification of neurons is silver impregnation. Bodian's silver method appears to impregnate neurofilaments themselves (Gambetti et al, 1981; Phillips et al, 1983), although like any silver method, it also can impregnate other tissue components nonspecifically. Overall, relative specificity of this method can be valuable, but in brain tumors that contain neoplastic neurons, Bodian's method may be negative when the much more sensitive and specific immunostaining method for neurofilament proteins is positive. Both the Bodian method and neurofilament immunostaining may be positive in neuronal cell bodies, but the highest positivity is typically in axons. Swollen and irregular axons are to be ex-

pected in neuronal neoplasms (Russell and Rubinstein, 1977), yet some swollen and varicose axons are seen in apparently normal brains with silver impregnation (Brodal, 1982). Such dystrophic axons are certainly to be expected in damaged but non-neoplastic brain tissue, including brain regions into which tumor cells have infiltrated. Axonal swellings in infarcts, contusions, or other lesions may be very large (neuronal spheroids, axonal retraction balls, or neuraxonal dystrophy), and a positive immunostain for neurofilaments in abnormal axons must be interpreted with the usual caution related to the general histologic findings in the tissue.

Other Neural Cell Markers

An isoenzyme of carbonic anhydrase is an oligodendrocyte-specific marker (as well as a red blood cell marker) of potential utility in identifying oligodendrogliomas or in differentiating residual oligodendrocytes from chronic inflammatory cells in demyelinating lesions. It has not yet been used for such purposes, although its absence in astrocytomas has been reported. Antiserum raised against galactocerebroside specifically labels oligodendrocytes and Schwann cells, and this antigen is expressed in these cells before myelin formation begins. Neither galactocerebroside, MBP nor MAG, has been positively identified in oligodendrogliomas, but MBP may be found in neurilemmomas (Figure 16–3). Cathepsin D is an endopeptidase that can be localized in oligodendrocytes by immu-

Table 16–7. Selected Bibliography: Miscellaneous Neural Cell Markers

Ghandour et al 1979, 1980a, b Langley et al 1980 Kumpulainen et al 1983	Carbonic anhydrase isoenzyme in normal oligodendrocytes
Kumpulainen & Nyström 1981	Carbonic anhydrase positive in paraffin-embedded autopsy brain, but specificity for oligodendrocytes not clear; astrocytomas negative
Ranscht et al 1982	Galactocerebroside positive in oligodendrocytes and Schwann cells
Whitaker et al 1981	Cathepsin D in oligodendrocytes and some astrocytes and neurons
Parham et al 1985	Cathepsin D positivity best in neoplastic ganglion cells and in macrophages; also in Ewing's sarcoma and rhabdomyosarcoma
Norenberg & Martinez-Hernandez 1979	Glutamine synthetase in brain is specific for astrocytes
Pilkington & Lantos 1982	Glutamine synthetase positive for astrocytomas
Schachner 1979 Franko et al 1981 Miller CA & Benzer 1983 Venter et al 1984	Monoclonal antibodies labeling antigens often of uncertain functional significance, could be of diagnostic aid with careful evaluation
Kemshead & Coakham 1983	Monoclonal antibodies set up in batteries to evaluate potential for diagnostic use on frozen sections
Sikora 1984	Monoclonal antibodies given IV may localize tumor; potentially useful in therapy, but for diagnosis by immunostaining as well

noperoxidase staining, but it also may be seen in other glial cells, in neurons and in macrophages. It can be immunostained in neoplastic neurons. Glutamine synthetase is a specific marker in the brain for astrocytes with an immunohistochemical distribution in astrocytomas similar to that of GFAP (Table 16–7).

Monoclonal antibodies are of great potential benefit in diagnostic neuropathology. Most work to date has been of research interest; it does not have immediate diagnostic application, although some monoclonal antibodies to replace polyclonal antisera currently being marketed have proven useful. Many monoclonal antibodies developed against neural tissue have interesting specificities, but often there are significant cross reactions, and the molecular nature and functional properties of many of the involved antigens are unknown. Monoclonal antibodies raised against brain tumors may be of diagnostic and even of therapeutic value, but, generally, only fresh-frozen tissue is useful with these reagents.

Serum Proteins

Immunostaining for albumin, fibrin, globulins, and complement factors has demonstrated them in a variety of lesions in the brain and in peripheral nerves (Table 16–8). This approach brings hope of a better understanding of the pathophysiology of these lesions and, possibly, the beginning of a new classification and the standardization of testing for some enigmatic neural problems. An important note of caution is that abnormal cellular and extracellular brain proteins or the inflammatory process itself may simply trap or bind serum proteins that are not primarily involved in the pathogenesis of the particular lesions (Stiller and Katenkamp,

1975; Powers et al, 1981; Allsop et al, 1983; Wisniewski et al, 1983c).

Inflammatory Cells/Microglia

The cell that classically responds to injury in the brain has been called the microglial cell (as opposed to macroglia, ie, astrocytes and oligodendrocytes). It is said to be a reticuloendothelial cell that migrates into the brain in the perinatal period and remains as the "resting" microglial cell (del Rio-Hortega, 1932). No direct evidence for such a cell has been offered. At least some macrophages in the developing brain are exogenous monocytes (Murabe and Sano, 1983; Miyake et al, 1984). Some of the phagocytes active in the developing central nervous system may be glioblasts and astrocytes (Rhodes, 1982), and both astrocytes and oligodendrocytes can have at least limited phagocytic function in the mature brain (Shuangshoti et al, 1979; Trachtenberg, 1983; Triarhou et al, 1985). Endogenous brain cells may form a small part of the response to larger or more destructive lesions (Table 16–9). These cells may correspond to the "resting" microglial cell, the nature of which may actually be that of a reserve neuroglial cell that responds to injury, not by becoming a foamy macrophage but possibly by forming fibrous astrocytes (Fujita et al, 1981).

Resting microglia do not have the usual monocytic or lymphoid membrane markers (Table 16–9). On the other hand, silver carbonate impregnation, supposedly specific for microglia, is found on a variety of reactive inflammatory cells and on non-Hodgkin lymphomas both in the central nervous system and outside it, and it is clearly not specific (Oehmichen and Huber, 1976; Houthoff et al, 1978; Esiri and Booss, 1984). This method of microglial silver impregnation also dem-

Table 16–8. Selected Bibliography: Serum Proteins in the Nervous System

Stiller & Katenkamp 1975 Esiri et al 1976 Mussini et al 1977 Powers et al 1981 Tabuchi et al 1981 Eikelenboom & Stam 1982 Shirahama et al 1982 Kalyan-Raman & Kalyan-Raman 1984 Scheithauer et al 1984	Serum proteins in nervous tissue in a variety of lesions but not in normal brain
Nardelli E et al 1981 Steck et al 1983a, b	Immunoglobulin in peripheral nerves in idiopathic polyneuritis.

Table 16–9. Selected Bibliography: Inflammatory Cells, Ia Antigen in
the Nervous System

Oehmichen & Huber 1976 Oehmichen & Torvik 1976 Tsuchihashi et al 1981	Small endogenous cells in the nervous system that are without Fc receptors or monocytic markers participate to some degree in phagocytosis
Esiri et al 1976 Fujita et al 1978, 1981 Oehmichen et al 1979 Wood GW et al 1979 Tsuchihashi et al 1981 Valentino & Jones 1981 Ling et al 1982 von Hanwehr et al 1984	Most immunohistochemical markers for monocytes and lymphocytes are absent from normal nervous system parenchyma
Valentino & Jones 1981 Murabe & Sano 1983	Monocytes invade brain in fetal development Monocytes disappear from brain after neonatal period
Miyake et al 1984 Natali et al 1981c Hauser et al 1983 Hirsch et al 1983 Fontana et al 1984 Kim et al 1984 Wong GHW et al 1984 Traugott et al 1985	Ia antigens are difficult to detect in normal brain, but reactive astrocytes have Ia antigens
Traugott et al 1985	Ia antigens found on cerebral vascular endothelial cells in multiple sclerosis
Garson et al 1982 Schuller-Petrovic et al 1983 Kim et al 1984 Dobersen et al 1985 Suzumura & Silberberg 1985	Some markers for T cell subsets cross-react with neural cells
Tsutsumi 1984 Motoi et al 1985	Leu 7 labels T cells and various neural tumors
Mathew et al 1983	Monoclonal antibody against monocytes labels "resting" microglial cells; nature of antigen unspecified
Fontana 1982 Fontana et al 1983, 1984	Stimulated astrocytes secrete interleukin 1
Budka et al 1984	Monoclonal antibodies against monocyte and lymphoid markers label normal glial cells and glial tumors; nature of antigens unspecified
Esiri & Booss 1984	alpha₁-Antichymotrypsin, alpha₁-antitrypsin and lysozyme positive in macrophages and reactive astrocytes in brain lesions
Justice et al 1985	alpha₁-Antichymotrypsin immunoreactivity in normal human neurons, astrocytes, oligodendrocytes, ependymal cells, and choroid plexus epithelium; blocked by purified alpha₁-antichymotrypsin
Rhodes & Tőkés (unpublished)	alpha₁-Antichymotrypsin but not alpha₁-antitrypsin in astrocytes, and immunoreactivity increases with acute phase of lesion; acute-phase reactant crossing blood-brain barrier and blood-cerebrospinal fluid barrier, or de novo synthesis in situ?
Shuangshoti et al 1979 Rhodes 1982, 1984 Tsai et al 1982 Choi et al 1983 Paasivuo & Saksela 1983 Raff et al 1983, 1984 Van Alstyne et al 1983 Fontana et al 1983, 1984 Choi & Kim 1984 Merrill et al 1984 Stefansson et al 1984 Temple & Raff 1985	Multipotential features of glial cells suggest roles in multiple functions in nervous system; aside from neurons and endothelial cells, only glial cells are available to limit and control immune reactions and general homeostasis
Stam et al 1980 Tabuchi et al 1981 Eikelenboom & Stam 1982 Wisniewski & Kozlowski 1982 Oehmichen 1983 Wisniewski et al 1983b, c	Immunoreactive markers for serum proteins and leukocytes in nervous system after lesions break down blood-brain barrier

onstrates glioblasts in early human development (Fujita and Kitamura, 1976) and reacts with monocytic macrophages identified by immunostaining in the neonatal rodent brain, showing a lack of specificity for the classically defined microglial cell (Miyake et al, 1984).

Blood-borne monocytes can be tagged in various ways, and these cells can be followed into injured brain parenchyma in which they become the foamy macrophages or "gitter cells" that correspond to the "activated" microglial cell. The monocytic macrophages that appear in the developing brain and then disappear by maturity, at least as detected by specific marker studies, do not appear to remain resting microglia; rather, they disappear from the brain immediately following the neonatal period. The abundant resting microglia in the adult brain appear to be derivatives of glioblasts when their origin is traced developmentally (Rhodes, 1982), including tracing by ultrastructural radioautography (Kitamura et al, 1984).

Whatever the true nature of resting microglial cells, recent evidence strongly supports the concept that the bone marrow–derived, blood-borne monocyte is the typical foamy macrophage (activated microglial cell) seen in widely destructive and rapidly evolving brain lesions (Oehmichen, 1983). One proposed role for exogenous macrophages in the injured brain is to influence the migration of newly developing vascular endothelial cells (Beck et al, 1983). If such an activity occurs during fetal neurogenesis, this timing could be part of the reason for the presence of exogenous macrophages in the developing brain, but not in the mature normal brain.

Immune response-associated (Ia) antigens may be part of an accessory system that was first described as lymphoid-tissue specific, but Ia antigens have been immunostained on normal and activated glial cells and cerebral vascular endothelial cells. As described elsewhere (Chapter 13), Ia antigens are also found on melanocytes in sections and on cultured melanoma cells (Winchester et al, 1978). They are not present in human fetal brain (Hofman et al, 1984b). Several markers for subsets of T cells show cross reactivity with human oligodendrocytes, ependymal cells, Schwann cells, myelin, cerebellar neurons, and several neural tumors. Interleukin 1, a factor in immune stimulation generally associated with macrophages, reportedly is secreted by stimulated astrocytes. Several antigenic markers prepared against lymphoid cells or monocytic macrophages may be found on normal, reactive, or neoplastic glial cells or on neurons. Antigenic determinants such as these may be essential for cells that have a phagocytic function, and as new immunoregulation determinants are described, they need to be evaluated carefully for cellular specificity. Some of these reports utilize antibodies not readily available or not well characterized, so that specific relationships of leukocytic and glial antigenic determinants are presently tentative. The function of Ia determinants on glial cells and cerebral endothelial cells apparently is to make the inside of the brain accessible to immunologic surveillance on a limited and controlled basis, by which lymphocytes, endothelial cells, and astrocytes communicate by mutual interactions when antigen presentation is required (Fontana and Fierz, 1985; Traugott et al, 1985; Wong GHW et al, 1985).

Given the multipotential features of glial cells, it is not too surprising that they share mesodermal macrophage antigens. However, such well-characterized immunohistochemical markers for leukocytes as muramidase or immunoglobulin light chains should be expected in the brain only in connection with a significant lesion such as an infarct, infection, contusion, tumor, or degenerative process in which there may be a breakdown in the blood-brain barrier. Caution should be observed in the investigation of brain tissue from patients with seizures, since these alone can cause a breach of the blood-brain barrier (Lee and Olszewski, 1961; Westergaard et al, 1978).

Infectious Agents

Viruses

The brain has a stereotyped response to conventional viruses that includes focal or generalized edema, perivascular and leptomeningeal chronic inflammatory cellular infiltrate, cellular degeneration or tissue necrosis, and sometimes gliomesenchymal cell nodules. These same findings can be seen in rickettsial and protozoal encephalitis (Dudley, 1982). Similar changes also can be seen in some noninfectious inflammatory conditions, but intranuclear and cytoplasmic inclusions are typical findings of viral encephalitides (Lindenberg and Haymaker, 1982). A specific diagnosis made on the basis of serum and cerebrospinal-fluid antibody changes may be inaccurate (Olson et al, 1967; Johnson et al, 1968). Brain biopsy for tissue culture or for immunostaining of specific viral antigens is the usual method of assuring an accurate diagnosis (Olson et al, 1967; Johnson RT et al, 1968; Whitley et al, 1981). The limit to the number of viruses that can be sought is related to the amount of tissue available, the amount of viral antigen present, the number of specific antisera at hand, and the degree of survival of viral antigens after tissue processing (Table 16–10).

Herpes simplex virus antigen can readily be demonstrated by immunoperoxidase methods. Although not as rapid as the direct immunofluorescence technique, the immunoperoxidase method offers the advantage of enhanced sensitivity and yields a permanent slide in which the morphology of the lesion can be observed (Fig. 16–4). A combination of cell culture and immunoperoxidase methods provides for sensitive and rapid identification of virus (Meyer and Amortegui, 1984). Archival studies are possible on fixed tissues, but retrospective studies even on fresh tissue are limited in herpes simplex encephalitis because viral antigen disappears from the brain about three weeks

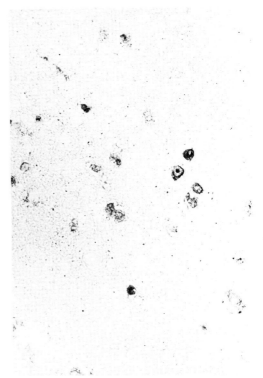

Figure 16–4. Herpes simplex virus type 1 is immunostained with the PAP method (1:100) without using proteolytic preincubation. Its glycoprotein antigen is localized in an intranuclear inclusion and in the cytoplasm of several neurons in the cingulate gyrus (× 400).

Table 16–10. Selected Bibliography: Infections in the Nervous System

Kumanishi & Hirano 1978 Kumanishi & In 1979 Gerber et al 1980 Budka & Popow-Kraupp 1981 Sethi & Lipton 1981 Esiri et al 1982 Löhler 1982	Antigens of many different viruses immunoreactive in the infected nervous system
Benjamin & Ray 1975 Budka & Popow-Kraupp 1981 Merkel & Zimmer 1981 Esiri 1982 Mann et al 1983	Herpes simplex virus immunoreactivity in nervous system infection (refer also to text)
Moskowitz et al 1984a, b	Cytomegalovirus immunoreactivity in the AIDS syndrome central nervous system
Budka et al 1982 Esiri et al 1982 Wisniewski et al 1983a	Measles virus antigen immunoreactivity in brain in subacute sclerosing panencephalitis
Gerber et al 1980 Budka & Shah 1982 Itoyama et al 1982	Papovavirus antigen immunoreactivity in the brain in PML
Ruppenthal 1980 Horten et al 1981 Gullotta & Dickopf 1982 Blue & Rosenblum 1983 Morgello et al 1984	Herpes virus immunoreactivity in the brain in a progressive multifocal encephalitis (as opposed to leukoencephalopathy of PML in white matter only)
Johnson KP et al 1980 Budka & Popow-Kraupp 1981	Rabies virus immunoreactivity in the brain
Moskowitz et al 1984a Martinez AJ 1982	*Toxoplasma* immunostaining is the method of choice for tissue diagnosis Ameba-immunostaining in the brain

after the onset of clinical disease (Olson et al, 1967; Esiri, 1982).

An emerging problem is herpes simplex virus type 2 encephalitis, rather than the expected type 1 encephalitis, in the adult. Changing social practices may be a factor in the increase in herpes simplex type 2 in facial lesions (Gunby, 1981). We have seen one tissue culture–confirmed case of herpes simplex type 2 encephalitis in a young adult male. A similar case was seen in an elderly man, in which herpes simplex was identified in tissue culture and immunostaining for herpes simplex types 1 and 2 showed only type 2 immunoreactivity. Both cases were relatively mild with significant recovery of neurological function. Neither patient had evidence of immunosuppression. Even more mild was a temporal lobe lesion that improved sufficiently for the otherwise healthy adult male to return to work. His small needle biopsy showed some amphiphilic intranuclear inclusions. Immunostaining showed herpes simplex virus type 2 antigen in the cytoplasm of many of the cells. A fourth case was seen in a homosexual male with the acquired immunodeficiency syndrome (AIDS) as a progressive multifocal encephalitis (on serial CT scans) with necrotic, cavitated foci. Spongiform areas between relatively normal tissue and regions of necrosis contained some cells with eosinophilic intranuclear inclusions. These cells stained for herpes simplex virus type 2 (Fig. 16–5) but not for type 1, papovavirus (polyomavirus common internal antigen), or cytomegalovirus. This condition might be considered as being a herpetic progressive multifocal encephalitis as opposed to the classical PML of papovavirus (vide infra). In nine cases of herpes simplex type 2 encephalitis and one case of myelitis reported past infancy and also in cases cited here, a favorable outcome tended to be seen in the absence of immunosuppression (Sutton et al, 1974; Linnemann et al, 1976; Manz et al, 1979; Nahmias et al, 1982; Oommen et al, 1982; Britton et al, 1985; Dix et al, 1985).

Cross reactions between antisera to herpes simplex types 1 and 2 are generally expected (Benjamin and Ray, 1975), but results with hyperimmune antisera to types 1 and 2 have demonstrated that this cross reaction can be minimal (Rhodes et al, 1984; Dix et al, 1985; Figure 16–5). Herpes simplex antigens may be masked in tissue sections, presumably by overfixation with formalin. This circum-

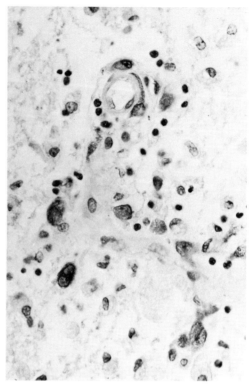

Figure 16–5. Herpes simplex virus type 2 (HSV 2) is immunostained by the avidin-biotin-peroxidase method (1:500) at the edge of a necrotic lesion in the brain of a homosexual male with the acquired immunodeficiency syndrome. Some enlarged cells are immunostained around a small blood vessel in the upper part of the field. Other positive cells are scattered among the necrotic tissue debris. Macrophages are negative. There is a hematoxylin counterstain. Immunostaining (1:100) was reduced or abolished when antiserum to HSV 2 diluted 1:25 was incubated overnight at 4°C in a culture tube containing cells infected with valid HSV 2 prior to immunostaining for HSV 2. Incubation of antiserum to HSV 2 in the presence of HSV 1 infected cells had no effect on subsequent immunostaining for HSV 2 (× 400).

stance is overcome by preincubation of deparaffinized sections in a proteolytic enzyme solution such as 0.1% trypsin for 20 minutes at room temperature (see Chapters 2 and 3).

Cytomegalovirus encephalitis generally presents a typical picture with large cells containing intranuclear and cytoplasmic inclusions. Immunostaining can be performed to confirm the diagnosis (Fig. 16–6). Involvement of cytomegalovirus in the brain and spinal cord has been reported in AIDS. Cytomegalovirus has been identified in focal areas of demyelination (Moskowitz et al, 1984b), and it can be immunostained in such areas in capillary endothelial cells (Fig. 16–

7), but an etiological role has not been demonstrated in AIDS encephalomyelitis. Cytomegalovirus may be mostly a secondary infection in AIDS brains superimposed on a retroviral infection (Britton et al, 1985; Shaw GM et al, 1985).

Subacute sclerosing panencephalitis, caused by a variant of measles virus, results in viral antigen in neurons (Fig. 16–8), in some oligodendrocytes, and in vascular wall cells as seen by immunostaining methods. A higher antigenic load detectable by immunostaining may correlate with a shortened prognosis.

PML is a subacute demyelinating disorder caused by a papovavirus infection and it is often associated with disorders of the reticuloendothelial system. Foamy macrophages abound and reactive astrocytes may be very large with bizarre nuclei. Enlarged nuclei of oligodendrocytes in and near the lesions have dense staining of basophilic or acidophilic viral inclusions. JC, SV40, and BK papova-

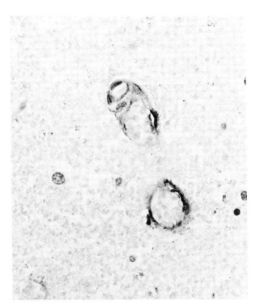

Figure 16–7. Cytomegalovirus cytoplasmic antigen is immunostained in endothelial cells in a spongiform region of axonal loss and demyelination in the dorsal columns of the spinal cord of a patient with the acquired immunodeficiency syndrome. There is a hematoxylin counterstain (× 400).

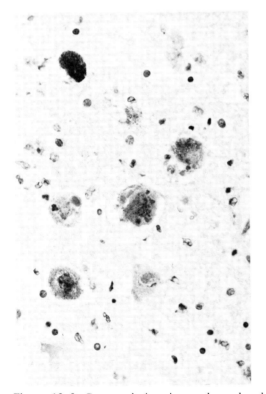

Figure 16–6. Cytomegalovirus in a subependymal lesion is immunostained by the avidin-biotin-peroxidase method (1:500). An antigen confined to the cytoplasm is localized in greatly enlarged glial cells. With this antiserum, large intranuclear inclusions are negative, and they show only the hematoxylin counterstain (× 400).

viruses have been isolated in this disease, and viral particles have been shown by electron microscopy in glial cells (Lindenberg and Haymaker, 1982). Antiserum to papovavirus demonstrates immunoreactivity in the enlarged oligodendrocyte nuclei in PML (Fig. 16–9). Immunoreactivity for viral antigens in the large abnormal astrocytes also has been reported. Glial cell tumors, meningiomas, and various other primary and metastatic brain tumors contain SV40 sequences when studied by DNA hybridization methods. Whether this finding is fortuitous or is of etiological significance is unknown (Ibelgaufts and Jones, 1982; Rachlin et al, 1984). The ability of SV40 virus to transform human neural cells has been demonstrated in tissue culture (Daya-Grosjean et al, 1984), and tissue or viruses from human cases of PML produce neuroepithelial tumors when inoculated into animals (Brun and Jonsson, 1984; Nagashima et al, 1984).

Encephalitis produced by several types of herpesvirus, including varicella-zoster, herpes simplex types 1 and 2 (see Figure 16–5), and cytomegalovirus may on rare occasion produce a PML-like clinical picture with cerebral demyelination. The CT scan, in addition to low density of white matter, may show hemorrhage or a mass effect. Other differ-

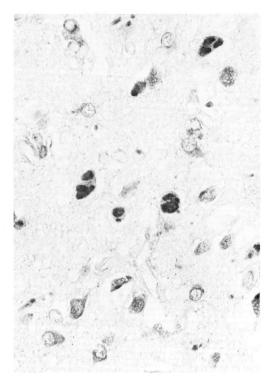

Figure 16–8. The altered measles virus that causes subacute sclerosing panecephalitis (SSPE) has been localized in intranuclear and cytoplasmic inclusions of cerebral neurons by use of an indirect immunoperoxidase method that employs a human antiserum to measles virus (provided by Dr. Carol A. Miller). Application of the primary antiserum (1:100) was followed by peroxidase-conjugated goat antihuman immunoglobulin. The secondary antiserum was initially absorbed by being placed overnight at 4°C on a section of the brain from the block of tissue being tested to decrease nonspecific staining (× 400).

ences from the classical PML caused by papovaviruses include more prominent necrosis, gray matter involvement, leptomeningitis, and vasculitis. Because of the possibility of more effective treatment, it is important that immunohistochemical techniques be employed to reach the correct diagnosis on brain biopsy.

Histologic confirmation of rabies infection can be achieved by immunoperoxidase methods. Immunostaining for rabies is reportedly enhanced by preincubation with a proteolytic enzyme.

The slow-virus agent of Creutzfeldt-Jakob disease has not been definitely identified, but it very likely is the prion demonstrated as an amyloid-type protein in scrapie. Prions have been immunostained in amyloid plaques in animal brains inoculated with scrapie or with human Creutzfeldt-Jakob brain tissue (Bendheim et al, 1984). This agent has been identified in splenic (Merz et al, 1983) and cerebral fractions from patients with Creutzfeldt-Jakob disease (Bockman et al, 1985).

Protozoa

It is possible to make a tissue diagnosis of a protozoal encephalitis when the appropriate antiserum can be obtained. *Toxoplasma gondii* is difficult to find, and when found, it is difficult to distinguish from some other protozoa in routine sections (Frenkel, 1971). Electron microscopy is a valuable diagnostic aid (Rhodes et al, 1977), but immunostaining for suspected toxoplasma encephalitis is eas-

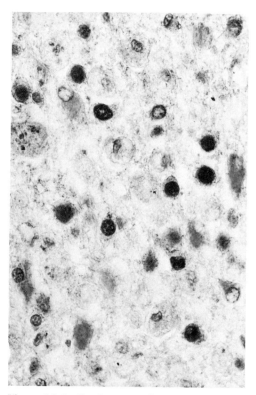

Figure 16–9. Classic progressive multifocal leukoencephalopathy (PML) oligodendrocytes have enlarged nuclei that are heavily immunostained by the avidin-biotin-peroxidase method (1:1000) for the polyomavirus common internal antigen. These cellular nuclei are enlarged compared with nuclei of normal oligodendrocytes, or even compared with the enlarged nuclei of the reactive astrocytes in the photomicrograph. There is a hematoxylin counterstain (× 400). (The primary antiserum was kindly provided by Dr. Duard L. Walker.)

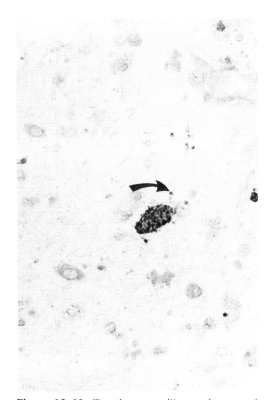

Figure 16–10. *Toxoplasma gondii* organisms are immunostained in a parasitic cyst and as free-tissue tachyzoites (arrow) by the avidin-biotin-peroxidase method (1:500). The tissue is from a cerebral biopsy that was performed for the diagnosis of multiple lucent lesions found on a CT scan in a patient with the acquired immunodeficiency syndrome (× 400).

ier and faster (Fig. 16–10), and it appears to be the method of choice. *Acanthamoeba castellanii* has been immunostained in the brain and some cross reactivity with several other *Acanthamoeba* species has been shown. Immunoperoxidase staining for *Entamoeba histolytica* has been attempted in brain tissue, but the diagnosis had to rely on other factors (Becker GL et al, 1980).

PITUITARY TUMORS AND RELATED LESIONS

Problems in fixation and the ultrastructural pleomorphism of secretory granules have made the distinction of subtypes among pituitary adenomas a cytochemical rather than a morphologic study (Schechter, 1973; Adelman, 1980; Esiri et al, 1983). Immunoperoxidase staining has been readily applicable to the demonstration of hormonal peptides in

the anterior pituitary, and it is now the method of choice for analysis (see also Chapter 8). Immunostaining for pituitary hormones may be successfully performed on current and archival material, and immunostaining of previously stained sections is possible (Table 16–11).

Cytokeratins have been localized by immunostaining in the pars intermedia and in the endocrine cells of the anterior pituitary (Asa et al, 1981; Höfler et al, 1984). Cytokeratins are also found in craniopharyngiomas (Asa et al, 1981). In pituitary adenomas the pattern of cytokeratin immunostaining differs between cells containing different hormones (Höfler et al, 1984). Also relevant is the finding of immunoreactive cytokeratin in chordomas (Adelman et al, 1983; Miettinen et al, 1983b), since these may present in the vicinity of the sella turcica. Rare mixed tumors and hamartomatous lesions associated with the pituitary and hypothalamus can now be classified more accurately by immunostaining for antigens related to these structures. It should also be noted that extrasellar tumors can produce hypothalamic and pituitary hormones, and these can be identified by immunostaining methods (Table 16–11).

Immunostaining for growth hormone (GH), prolactin (PRL), gonadotropins, adrenocorticotropic hormone, or thyroid-stimulating hormone appears to be more reliable in characterizing a pituitary adenoma than light or electron microscopy (for an immunohistologic classification of pituitary adenomas, see Chapter 8). However, not all pituitary adenomas contain detectable immunoreactive hormone (the so-called undifferentiated cell adenomas described in Chapter 8). It is not unusual for a pituitary adenoma to contain two immunoreactive hormones (one of them usually PRL) or even three or more hormones on occasion. Para-adenomatous cells of the normal pituitary surrounding an adenoma may be cytochemically reactive and display abundant immunostained PRL, GH, or both, depending upon the state of cytochemical transformation of the cells at the time of biopsy (Landolt and Minder, 1984).

Martinez AJ et al (1980) found that although clinical features, serum hormonal levels, ultrastructural features, and immunoperoxidase staining generally correlated well, several problems may be encountered that may preclude a definite diagnosis: (1) small size of biopsy, (2) uncertainty about total

Table 16–11. Selected Bibliography: Pituitary Region

Osamura et al 1978 Baskin et al 1979 Beauvillain & Tramu 1980	Peptide hormones immunoreactive in the pituitary and hypothalamus
Halmi 1978	Pituitary hormone immunoreactivity in previously stained sections
Asa et al 1980 Rhodes et al 1982 Burchiel et al 1983 Fischer et al 1983 Scheithauer et al 1983 Price et al 1984 Serebrin & Robertson 1984	Hormonal and neuropeptide immunoreactivity in rare intrasellar and hypothalamic lesions not classified as pituitary adenomas; most are ganglioneuromas or gangliocytomas
Alumets et al 1983 Berger et al 1984b	Immunoreactivity of pituitary and hypothalamic hormones in extrasellar tumors
Landot 1979 Martinez AJ et al 1980 Cravioto et al 1981 Horvath et al 1981 Martinez D & Barthe 1982 Esiri et al 1983 McComb DJ et al 1984 Wowra & Peiffer 1984	Immunoreactivity of pituitary hormones in pituitary adenomas

removal of tumor or quality of the sample, (3) operative artifact, (4) inclusion of an altered but non-neoplastic pituitary gland, (5) difficulty in distinguishing hyperplasia from adenoma, (6) mixture of a few cells immunoreactive for other than the predominant hormone, and (7) paradoxical serum hormonal level abnormalities, especially prolactinemia in patients with an undifferentiated cell adenoma and no endocrinologic symptoms.

TUMORS OF THE NERVOUS SYSTEM

The World Health Organization classification of brain tumors (Zülch, 1980) with some modifications taken mainly from Russell and Rubinstein (1977) is followed in this discussion.

Neuroepithelial Tumors

Astrocytoma

This group of tumors includes relatively benign optic nerve gliomas and cystic cerebellar astrocytomas of childhood (both better referred to as juvenile pilocytic astrocytomas), adult pilocytic astrocytomas, protoplasmic and fibrillary astrocytomas that generally occur in a mixture, gemistocytic astrocytomas formed of swollen-bodied astro-

cytes and anaplastic astrocytomas. This list is given with an increasing tendency toward malignant biologic behavior. Uncertainties in prognosis also increase down this list, making the traditional grading system of little if any practical value except to state that a particular tumor should be treated more aggressively if its "grade" is high. Gemistocytic and anaplastic astrocytomas can be grouped with glioblastoma multiforme in general prognosis and clinical approach. True gemistocytic astrocytomas are too rare to venture a predictive opinion (Russell and Rubinstein, 1977). Most of these, as seen on biopsy material, are probably revealing only one cytologic component of a more complex malignant glioma (Pasquier et al, 1981; Davis and Erlich, 1983). The prognosis for an anaplastic astrocytoma (neoplastic astrocytes with hypercellularity and pleomorphism and perhaps some mitoses) is better than for a glioblastoma on average. The principal differentiating feature between these two tumors is the presence of necrosis in the latter. However, tumor sampling is always a problem. The necrosis may not be sampled in some of these patients because the necrotic foci tend to be deep in the white matter and because, in practice, biopsies are often taken superficially to avoid excessive surgical hemorrhage. Stereotaxic biopsies help to overcome this difficulty, but their usefulness is limited by the small size of the tissue sample.

How can immunohistochemistry be of help

(Table 16–12)? GFAP immunostaining can help to differentiate the following:

1. Glial tumors from meningiomas, sarcomas or tumors metastatic to the brain

2. Heterotopic leptomeningeal astrocytomas, mixed gliomas and glioblastomas from meningiomas

3. Unusual malignant meningeal mesenchymal tumors from glial tumors

4. Pleomorphic xanthoastrocytomas from fibrous xanthomas

In addition, the astrocytic nature of some pineal neoplasms has been confirmed by immunostaining, and the origin of leptomeningeal and bone marrow metastases from cerebral glioblastomas has been indicated by immunostaining of lumbar puncture and biopsy material for GFAP. In general, immunoperoxidase staining has provided a firmer basis for classification of these tumors (Table 16–1). The immunoperoxidase method has shown that GFAP is an excellent marker for astrocytomas (Fig. 16–11); the more malignant or undifferentiated the tumor, the fewer of its cells contain immunoreactive GFAP.

Preliminary work suggests that vimentin may predominate over GFAP in some neoplastic astrocytes (Table 16–2). Given careful consideration, the presence of vimentin in poorly differentiated tumor cells may suggest a glial cell origin if collagen is not present. However, in evaluating the immunostaining results, reactive astrocytes within a tumor either metastatic to the brain or locally invasive from a primary mesenchymal leptomeningeal tumor must be ruled out (Stone et al, 1979; De Armond et al, 1980). A connective tissue response to leptomeningeal invasion of an astrocytoma also must be considered (De Armond et al, 1980; Taratuto et al, 1984). A *light* hematoxylin counterstain is advisable on at least one slide; this measure is often critical to the histopathologic analysis.

The correspondence of the localization of glutamine synthetase and GFAP, including the decrease in immunoreactivity of both as the degree of differentiation of glial tumors decreases, could prove to have practical value (Pilkington and Lantos, 1982), but data are insufficient to warrant a general recommendation at this time.

Astroblastoma

Astroblastomas have a monotonous pattern of perivascular structuring of neoplastic as-troblastic cells with cellular foot processes that are thicker than in ependymomas. These rare tumors have few stained glial fibrils with Mallory's phosphotungstic acid-hematoxylin (PTAH) stain, but their astrocytic nature has been confirmed with immunostaining for GFAP (Table 16–12). Most of the GFAP is in the cellular processes near their contacts with vascular walls (Fig. 16–12). The appearance of GFAP in this specific location may be related to the induction of GFAP by adjacent connective tissue components (Herpers et al, 1984). The discrepancy between PTAH staining and immunostaining may be due to a relatively soluble and abundant fraction of GFAP that is immunostained but cannot be identified by PTAH staining because it is not contained in intermediate filaments (De Armond et al, 1980).

Subependymal Giant Cell Astrocytoma

These peculiar lesions are found most often in patients with tuberous sclerosis. In some instances a proportion of the cells stain for GFAP, whereas in other cases all of the cells are nonreactive for GFAP. NSE also has been immunostained in the cells of these lesions, but as already discussed, this fact does not necessarily indicate a neuronal origin. The occurrence of immunostained neurofilament protein in some of these tumors arguably makes them bidirectional or mixed tumors versus astrocytomas with an aberrant and restricted neuronal expression (Bonnin et al, 1984).

Oligodendroglioma

Although various antigens such as galactocerebroside and carbonic anhydrase have been described in oligodendrocytes, their role in the recognition of oligodendrogliomas is not yet clear (Table 16–7). Leu 7 is present in oligodendrogliomas, although other brain tumors may also be immunoreactive to Leu 7 to a lesser extent. MBP and MAG immunoreactivities are reported as absent in oligodendrogliomas, while positive immunostaining for GFAP has been interpreted either as demonstrating an inclusion of reactive astrocytes, an intermixing of some neoplastic astrocytes, or the synthesis of GFAP by neoplastic oligodendrocytes that have a dual glial phenotype. None of these suggestions are mutually exclusive and all may occur.

Table 16–12. Selected Bibliography: Immunohistochemistry of Tumors of the Nervous System

Duffy et al 1978, 1980 Pasquier et al 1980 Taratuto et al 1984	GFAP immunoreactivity differentiates glial and nonglial tumors in brain
Horoupian et al 1979 Kepes et al 1979b Kalyan-Raman et al 1981	GFAP immunoreactivity differentiates heterotopic or superficial astrocytomas from meningiomas or meningeal mesenchymal tumors
Shuangshoti et al 1984	GFAP immonoreactivity differentiates mixed gliomas from meningiomas
Kalyan-Raman et al 1983	GFAP immunoreactivity differentiates glioblastomas from meningiomas
Herrick & Rubinstein 1979 De Armond et al 1980 Velasco et al 1980 Papasozomenos & Shapiro 1981	GFAP immunoreactivity confirms glial differentiation in some pineal neoplasms
Yung et al 1983 Wechsler et al 1984	GFAP immonoreactivity identifies systemic metastases of glioblastoma
Bonnin & Rubinstein 1984	GFAP immunoreactivity confirms glial differentiation in astroblastomas and in some subependymal giant cell astrocytomas
Stefansson & Wollman 1980, 1981 Velasco et al 1980 Tascos et al 1982 Bonnin et al 1984	GFAP, NSE, and neurofilament protein in subependymal giant cell astrocytomas
Motoi et al 1985	Leu 7 in oligodendrogliomas and other brain tumors
Meneses et al 1982	MBP and MAG not in oligodendrogliomas
van der Meulen et al 1978 De Armond et al 1980 Velasco et al 1980 Meneses et al 1982 Herpers & Budka 1984	GFAP immunoreactivity in oliogodendrogliomas
van der Meulen et al 1978 De Armond et al 1980 Velasco et al 1980 Tascos et al 1982 Roessmann et al 1983a	GFAP immunoreactivity in mixed gliomas, including gangliogliomas, and in ependymomas
Rubinstein & Brucher 1981	GFAP immunoreactivity in choroid plexus papillomas
Møller et al 1978 Lowenthal et al 1982 Papasozomenos 1983	S100 protein and GFAP in normal pineal astrocytes
Herrick & Rubinstein 1979 Borit & Yung 1983 Roessmann et al 1983a	Pineal tumors may have GFAP, vimentin, or neurofilament protein immunoreactivity
Roessmann et al 1983a Carlei et al 1984 Choi & Anderson 1985	Neurofilament protein, NSE, GFAP, and S100 protein immunoreactivity in neuroblastomas and ganglioneuromas
Trojanowski et al 1984	Neurofilament protein immunoreactivity in paragangliomas, pheochromocytomas, and teratomas
Hassoun et al 1984 Lloyd RV et al 1984 Tsutsumi 1984	Neuropeptide, NSE, and Leu 7 immunoreactivity in pheochromocytomas
De Armond et al 1980 Duffy et al 1980 Velasco et al 1980 Pasquier et al 1981 Tascos et al 1982	GFAP immunoreactivity in glioblastomas usually less than in astrocytomas; amount immunostained decreases as degree of malignancy increases

Table 16–12. Selected Bibliography: Immunohistochemistry of Tumors of
the Nervous System *Continued*

Kepes et al 1982	GFAP immunoreactivity in "adenoid" regions of gliosarcomas
De Armond et al 1980 Velasco et al 1980 Mannoji et al 1981 Palmer et al 1981 Coffin et al 1983 Roessmann et al 1983a	GFAP immunoreactivity in some medulloblastomas; in reactive astrocytes, small morphologically undifferentiated neoplastic astrocytes and swollen-bodied neoplastic astrocytes
Dickson et al 1983 Smith & Davidson 1984 Chowdhury et al 1985	Myoglobin immunoreactivity in medulloblastomas and medul-lomyoblastoma
Biggs & Powers 1984	Actin immunoreactivity in medulloblastoma
Mogollon et al 1984	MBP immunoreactivity in nerve sheath tumors
Tascos et al 1982 Bruner et al 1984	GFAP immunoreactivity in nerve sheath tumors
Brooks et al 1985	Myoglobin immunoreactivity in "Triton" tumor variant of neuri-lemmoma
Miettinen et al 1984	Vimentin immunoreactivity in granular cell tumors
Mukai M 1983	PO, P2 and S100 antigen immunoreactivity in granular cell tumors
Schwechheimer et al 1984 Yung et al 1984	Vimentin and desmoplakins in meningiomas; cytokeratin "positivity" depends on antiserum used; no GFAP immunoreactivity
Kepes et al 1979a Deck and Rubinstein 1981 McComb RD et al 1982b Tanimura et al 1984	GFAP immunoreactivity in capillary hemangioblastomas
Jurco et al 1982	Factor VIII–related antigen immunoreactivity positive in hemangioblastoma stromal cells
McComb RD et al 1982b Böhling et al 1983 Epstein JI et al 1984 Tanimura et al 1984	Factor VIII–related antigen immunoreactivity negative in hemangioblastoma stromal cells
Böhling et al 1983 Llena & Hirano 1983	Factor VIII–related antigen immunoreactivity positive in tumor cells away from vessels in hemangioendotheliomas
Houthoff et al 1978 Taylor et al 1978c Slager et al 1982 Graham et al 1983 Allegranza et al 1984	Immunoglobulin light chains in primary lymphomas of nervous system
Kurman & Scardino 1981 Ahmed et al 1983 Said 1983 Naganuma et al 1984 Bjornsson et al 1985	Immunostaining in intracranial germinomas
Trojanowski & Hickey 1984 Bjornsson et al 1985 Nakamura et al 1985	Immunostaining in intracranial teratomas
Nakakuma et al 1983 Said 1983 Packer et al 1984b	Immunostaining in intracranial embryonal-cell carcinomas
Sheibani et al 1979 Naganuma et al 1984	Immunostaining in intracranial choriocarcinomas
Shirai et al 1976 Stachura & Mendelow 1980 Naganuma et al 1984 Bjornsson et al 1985	Immunostaining in intracranial endodermal-sinus tumors

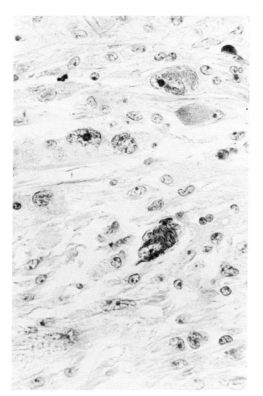

Figure 16–11. GFAP immunostained by the PAP method (1:100) is found in various amounts in only a few of the pleomorphic tumor cells in this astrocytoma. There is a hematoxylin counterstain (× 400).

Oligodendrogliomas may contain a significant number of neoplastic astrocytes before being regarded as a mixed glioma, and GFAP immunoreactivity has been reported in the cytoplasm of cells that morphologically are typical neoplastic oligodendrocytes. Oligodendrocytes and astrocytes appear to share some features in normal development, such as the synthesis of GFAP (Rhodes, 1982; Choi et al, 1983; Ogawa et al, 1985). The progenitor cell of the oligodendrocyte and of the astrocyte may, in fact, be one and the same (Rhodes, 1982, 1984; Temple and Raff, 1985), a situation of particular interest and significance in neurooncology.

Mixed Gliomas

When unqualified, the term *mixed glioma* includes tumors with various admixtures of neoplastic astrocytoma and oligodendroglioma cells, either intimately intermingled or in discrete foci. As would be expected, the neoplastic astrocytes are immunostained for

GFAP, whereas the oligodendrocytes are not. The regions that have a mixture of neoplastic cells show immunostained cells or their processes containing GFAP adjacent to negative oligodendrocytes. In other regions immunostaining confirms the separate areas of each cellular type. As mentioned, the actual cellular type to which some of the GFAP–positive cellular processes belong cannot always be ascertained, and typical neoplastic oligodendrocytes may have GFAP in their cytoplasm. Some mixed gliomas consist of astrocytic and ependymal cells with GFAP immunostaining in typical astrocytic cells and in elongated tanycytes that may represent an "astrocytic" form of ependymal cells.

Astrocytic cells in gangliogliomas contain GFAP. Immunostaining for neurofilament triplet protein will demonstrate cytochemically differentiated neoplastic neurons, both of small immature forms and of enlarged ganglion cell types.

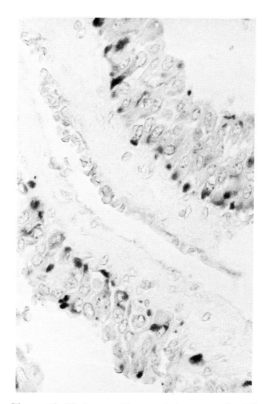

Figure 16–12. An astroblastoma is immunostained for GFAP by the PAP method (1:100). Most of the immunoreactivity is in the stout cellular processes where they contact the connective tissue adventitia of a blood vessel wall (located across the center of the field). There is a hematoxylin counterstain (× 400).

Ependymoma

Ependymomas may be positive or negative for GFAP, and they may or may not contain demonstrable vimentin.

Choroid Plexus Papilloma

Some of these tumors can be immuno-stained for GFAP in focal areas. This circumstance has been interpreted as focal glial differentiation.

Pineal Cell Tumors

Pineoblastomas are small cell tumors that are similar to medulloblastomas, but transitions to more mature pineocytomas can be seen. Pineocytomas have a lobular architecture and a tendency for some astrocytic and ganglion cell differentiation. About a third of pineal parenchymal tumors (excluding germ cell tumors) are partially differentiated. These tend to occur past childhood, are relatively radioresistant, and also are relatively benign (Herrick and Rubinstein, 1979). Tissue diagnosis including immunostaining for GFAP, vimentin, and neurofilaments may aid in the assessment of these tumors. Occasionally, a pineal tumor is fully differentiated as an astrocytoma and may then be expected to stain for GFAP. Astrocytes in the normal pineal body contain immunoreactive GFAP and S100 protein.

Neuronal Tumors

Neuroblastomas usually occur as abdominal tumors of childhood and consist largely or entirely of undifferentiated small cells (Donohue et al, 1974). Cerebral and peripheral nerve forms outside of the sympathetic nervous system are rare. Most cerebral neuroblastomas have some differentiated ganglion cells, and they can then be termed differentiating neuroblastomas or ganglioneuroblastomas.

Glial differentiation in some central and peripheral neuroblastomas is revealed by immunostaining for GFAP, whereas the expected neuronal differentiation is confirmed by the presence of immunoreactive neurofilament protein. The less the morphologic differentiation toward ganglion cells, the more likely a neuroblastoma is to express GFAP. This likelihood may indicate a pluripotential nature of the cells in primitive neuroblastomas (Carlei et al. 1984).

Ganglioneuromas are predominantly formed of mature, but sometimes bizarre, neoplastic neurons and they contain some small cells that are thought to be neuroblasts. Their glial component is of an innocuous spindle cell type that is not neoplastic. They often have a prominent vascular connective-tissue component. When the glial component is neoplastic, the tumors are termed ganglio-gliomas, and their behavior is sometimes closer to that of an astrocytoma. Rarely is malignant behavior seen in brain tumors in which morphologically differentiated neuronal cells predominate. A recent report of a cerebral ganglioglioma records GFAP-positive neoplastic astrocytes and also typical Schwann cells by ultrastructural criteria (see also Figure 16–1B). This tumor displays the major elements to be expected in a neuroectodermal neoplasm that might represent, not the neural tube or crest, but the neural plate (Gambarelli et al, 1982).

Immunohistochemistry has helped to clarify the classification of peripheral neuronal tumors by demonstrating neurofilament proteins in poorly differentiated and well-differentiated ganglion cell tumors that include paragangliomas, pheochromocytomas, and focal areas in teratomas. The cytogenesis of small cell pulmonary tumors is not certain, but they contain neurofilament triplet protein as studied immunohistochemically (Table 16–6; see also Chapter 11). Polyclonal antisera are more likely to immunostain these tumors than monoclonal antibodies, which might recognize antigenic determinants that only exist in non-neoplastic cells or that have been lost in tissue-processing (van Muijen et al, 1984). Immunostaining for substance P may also be helpful in assessing neuronal differentiation in a tumor (Tarkkanen et al, 1983). Immunoreactivity for NSE in neoplastic neurons is not helpful because of the widespread occurrence of NSE in neoplastic cells of many types, as indicated elsewhere (see also Chapter 7).

Pheochromocytomas

Immunocytochemical staining has demonstrated several neuropeptides in pheochromocytomas, but the results are not helpful in terms of prognostic implications, and they do not constitute specific immunohistochemical markers. NSE is not found in tumors of the adrenal cortex, whereas benign and malignant pheochromocytomas do have NSE immunoreactivity that may aid in distinguishing the origin of the adrenal mass in unusually difficult cases. Leu 7 immunoreactivity on pheochromocytoma cells is also helpful since this finding generally is demonstrable in routinely processed tissue (see also Chapter 7). Some investigators regard this occurrence as further evidence of shared epitopes between neural tumors and T cells.

Poorly Differentiated and Embryonal Tumors

Glioblastoma Multiforme. Glioblastoma multiforme may be considered a high-grade astrocytoma, but because of inconsistent use of the grades relating to it, the tumor is better considered as a separate entity (Davis, 1977). As mentioned, its high degree of malignancy is reflected by the decreased number of cells with positive immunostaining for GFAP compared with less aggressive astrocytomas. Glioblastomas may have cells that can be immunostained for both vimentin and GFAP and also for vimentin alone when GFAP is absent. The gliosarcoma variant of

glioblastoma, in which there is a perivascular fibrosarcoma coexisting with a glioblastoma, displays only vimentin and no GFAP immunostaining in its strictly sarcomatous regions. Some gliosarcomas have regions resembling a metastatic adenocarcinoma with "adenoid" formations but the duct- or glandlike cells contain immunoreactive GFAP rather than cytokeratins. Giant cell glioblastomas, previously known as monstrocellular sarcomas, have GFAP-positive cells of various sizes as seen in Figure 16–13.

Medulloblastoma and Other Small Cell Tumors. Some of the small cells in these tumors may be cytochemically differentiated as demonstrated by immunoreactive neurofilament protein. Some medulloblastomas and neuroblastomas also contain neoplastic and/or reactive astrocytes identified by immunostaining for GFAP, and careful interpretation is necessary. Still other cases have cells with both immunoreactive GFAP and neurofilament protein in the neoplastic cells. Immunoreactive GFAP and also myoglobin in striated muscle cells that form part of some medulloblastomas have been reported in the

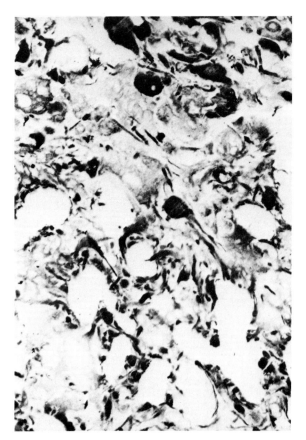

Figure 16–13. A giant cell glioblastoma viewed at medium power has both large and small cells immunostained for GFAP by an indirect immunoperoxidase method (1:100). The sharply circumscribed negative regions contain blood vessels (× 160).

same tumor, including the medullomyoblastoma variant. One reported medulloblastoma had only immunoreactive actin in tumor cells with many microfilaments but with ultrastructural criteria otherwise consistent with neuronal differentiation.

Most medulloblastomas are small cell tumors in which little if any differentiation is found except perhaps by immunostaining of products within the cytoplasm of small, morphologically undifferentiated cells. Cytochemical differentiation has not yet been related to prognosis. There is an obvious morphologic relationship between small cell tumors termed neuroblastoma, medulloblastoma, pineoblastoma, and retinoblastoma (Davis and Erlich, 1983). Tumors with neuronal antigenic differentiation may be called neuroblastomas; those with mostly GFAP-positive cells, small cell gliomas (or astrocytomas); those with both neuronal and glial immunoreactive antigens, glioneuroblastomas or mixed glial-neuroblastic tumors; and those with undifferentiated small cells, primitive neuroectodermal tumors, or PNET (Roessmann et al, 1983a). The practical problems with these designations are that immunostaining is a requirement for consistency, and terms such as *medulloblastoma* (as opposed to the alternative designation *cerebellar neuroblastoma*) are embedded in the literature and in the clinical approach to the patient.

A more streamlined approach to terminology revolving around the term PNET has been suggested, with the addition of applicable qualifying terms such as *undifferentiated, with glial differentiation* (Fig. 16–14), etc (Rorke, 1983). This approach may be preferable to the present nomenclature, because it orders current thinking on classification quite nicely, but in practice it may hold similar problems in attempting to change existing terminology. The prognosis for all of these tumors is not necessarily the same, although treatment is similar. PNET with neuronal differentiation in the retroperitoneum may carry a relatively favorable prognosis compared with PNET-undifferentiated (Beckwith and Martin, 1968), whereas the opposite may be true of PNET in the posterior fossa (Packer et al, 1984a). Terminology for this group will probably follow clinical advances in prognostication, and such advances may in part rely in the future on immunostaining results.

Medulloepithelioma. Medulloepitheliomas are perhaps the most primitive tumors of the

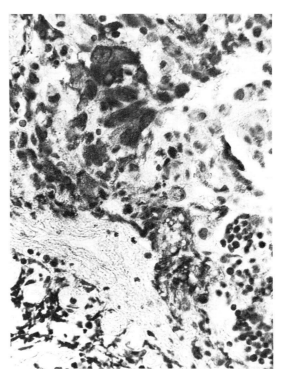

Figure 16–14. A primitive neuroectodermal tumor (PNET) with glial differentiation is seen with immunostaining for GFAP in large cells by an indirect immunoperoxidase method (1:100). The small tumor cells with darkly counterstained nuclei are negative for GFAP. A few strictly perivascular foci of enlarged cells such as the one shown here had astrocytic differentiation based on GFAP immunostaining. Their appearance with other stains did not convincingly reveal their identity. This is a particularly unusual tumor in that it occurred in the cerebrum of an adult (× 400).

neuroepithelium and may be central or peripheral. Diverse maturation of glial or neuronal cells and even of mesodermal elements has been described. Auer and Becker (1983) argue that all of these elements may be classified as neuroectodermal derivatives, since the mesodermal elements, including striated muscle, could be neural-crest products. These researchers report immunoreactivity for GFAP and for S100 protein in their case. This finding may be one further example of a neoplasm of neural plate derivation.

Nerve Sheath Tumors

Neurilemmomas are Schwann cell tumors. Neurofibromas can be considered as neoplasms or as hamartomas of peripheral nerves (Russell and Rubinstein, 1977). Neurofibromas contain Schwann cells, fibroblasts, and blood vessels, the normal tissue components of nerves aside from neuronal processes. Typical lesions in this group present no difficulties. When a spindle cell tumor arising from a peripheral nerve contains more than a rare mitotic figure, has pleomorphism and hypercellularity, and has invaded a significant part of a previously operated field, it can be called a malignant nerve sheath tumor, whatever its derivation (Trojanowski et al, 1980).

MBP may be found as a granular reaction product in benign and malignant nerve sheath tumors (see Fig. 16–3). Neoplastic Schwann cells typically are reactive for S100 protein and rarely for GFAP (see Fig. 16–1). There is cellular immunoreactivity for myoglobin in the "Triton" tumor variant of neurilemmoma. Granular cell tumors, which are probably of Schwann cell origin, contain immunoreactive vimentin, S100 protein, PO glycoprotein, and P2 basic protein.

Meningiomas

Meningiomas typically are formed of arachnoidal cap cells of a fibroblastic, syncytial, or transitional (combined) histologic appearance. Antibodies that may be specific for arachnoidal cap cell antigens have been partially characterized (Kepes, 1982). The arachnoidal cap cells in meningiomas may contain S100 protein, vimentin, cytokeratin, and desmoplakins. They do not react for GFAP. Meningeal melanomas may be immunoreactive for S100 protein and vimentin, and they should be distinguished from meningiomas (the typical reactions of melanomas are given in Chapter 13.)

Tumors of Vascular or Putative Vascular Origin

Immunostaining for brain tumors suspected to be of vascular origin involves mainly the investigation of the histogenesis of capillary hemangioblastomas. The morphologically closely related subgroup of angioblastic meningioma traditionally includes angioblastic meningiomas themselves, which are benign tumors arising in the supratentorial meninges, and hemangiopericytomas, which are a completely different type of tumor that may be rapidly recurrent and may have a real potential for distant metastasis. Immunoreactive laminin is restricted to the basement membrane of the vascular walls of hemangioblastomas and of hemangiopericytomas, and laminin immunostaining is not found between the tumor cells, even when silver-impregnated components of a basement membrane can be identified (Böhling et al, 1983).

Capillary hemangioblastomas are histologically closely related to or identical with angioblastic meningiomas. They are benign, usually single, parenchymal tumors in the posterior fossa. They can produce erythropoietin, and they may form part of the von Hippel-Lindau syndrome. More rarely, they are found in the cerebrum, peripheral nerves, or a spinal cord site. There are two basic tissue components in hemangioblastomas and in angioblastic meningiomas. These components are lipid-laden foamy "stromal cells" and large-bore, thin-walled blood vessels. Some of the stromal cells can be immunostained for GFAP, which has been interpreted either as an inclusion of reactive lipidized astrocytes, phagocytosis of extracellular GFAP by stromal cells, or a partial population of lipidized neoplastic astrocytes. The vascular endothelial cells of hemangioblastomas, as in other tumors, stain positively for factor VIII–related antigen, which may be contained mostly in endothelial cell–specific Weibel-Palade bodies. Jurco et al (1982) have shown that stromal cells in these tumors may contain immunoreactive factor VIII–related antigen and thus may also be of vascular endothelial origin (Fig. 16–15). The immunoreactivity of the stromal cells to factor VIII–related antigen may depend upon their degree of maturity, and this possibility may account for negative findings for immunoreactive factor VIII–related antigen in stromal cells even after preincubation with trypsin. It is worthwhile emphasizing that factor VIII–related protein is best demonstrated in frozen sections. If paraffin sections are employed, then trypsin digestion is considered essential to avoid a false negative. Also, the purity and specificity of antisera for factor VIII–related antigen have been questioned (Wilson AJ, 1984).

Another vascular tumor that rarely is found in the brain parenchyma is the hemangioendothelioma. A possible relationship of this tumor to hemangioblastomas and angioblastic meningiomas is suggested by positive immunostaining for factor VIII–related antigen.

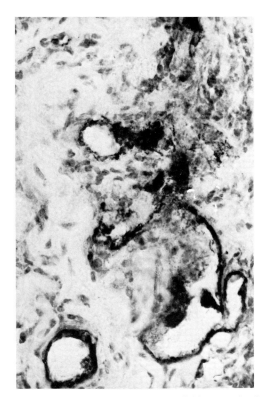

Figure 16–15. A capillary hemangioblastoma in the spinal cord is immunostained by a polyclonal antiserum to factor VIII–related protein with the PAP method (1:500) after preincubation with trypsin. There is very light hematoxylin counterstain. The vascular endothelial cells are heavily immunostained, and, in addition, there is granular immunostaining in many of the foamy stromal cells in the upper right (× 400).

Primary Lymphomas

Primary lymphomas of the central nervous system have been termed microgliomas or reticulum cell sarcomas (Russell and Rubinstein, 1977), although currently they are recognized as lymphomas generally of B cell type (Bonnin and Rubinstein, 1984). A primary T cell lymphoma of the leptomeninges has been recorded (Marsh et al, 1983). The B cell tumors can be immunostained in most cases for the presence of cytoplasmic immunoglobulins (see Chapters 4 and 5), but sometimes they are not diagnosed until autopsy, and postmortem autolysis may hinder positive immunostaining. These lymphomas are generally monoclonal but staining for both kappa and lambda light chains has been reported. In some cases, this may represent a processing artifact, but in other cases, a "polyclonal" lymphoma appears to be present (see Chapters 4 and 5). The incidence of

these tumors is increased in immunosuppressed patients, including those receiving a renal transplant and patients with AIDS. Graham DI et al (1983) believe the presence of more than one immunoglobulin in some cases of immunosuppression-related brain lymphomas may indicate that these are reactive processes rather than tumors. In this circumstance they may be akin to angioimmunoblastic lymphadenopathy which, although polyclonal in many cases, very often progresses rapidly to death (see Chapter 4).

Germ Cell Tumors

Germinomas, teratomas, embryonal cell carcinomas, choriocarcinomas, and endodermal sinus tumors are found in the midline as pineal region and diencephalon-related masses. The large cells in germinomas are radiosensitive neoplastic germ cells. The small-cell component in germinomas appears to be inflammatory. This component includes cells that can be immunostained by B lymphocyte markers and cells that form E-rosettes to mark them as T lymphocytes (Neuwelt and Smith, 1979). Pineal germinomas may secrete human chorionic gonadotropin that can be demonstrated by immunostaining.

The immunohistochemical reactions of intracranial germ cell tumors correspond to those of germ cell tumors and teratomas elsewhere (see Chapter 9). Teratomas show the greatest variation according to the various components present: the neural components may contain immunoreactive GFAP, MBP, NSE, S100 protein, or neurofilament triplet protein.

DEGENERATIVE CENTRAL NERVOUS SYSTEM DISEASES

Altered Neuronal Fibrous Proteins and Cerebral Amyloid

Occasional neurofibrillary tangles and senile (neuritic) plaques can be found in aged brains (Tomlinson, 1979; Kurucz et al, 1981). An abundance of plaques and tangles together is the classic hallmark of Alzheimer's disease, and these lesions are found together most prominently in the hippocampus (Tomlinson, 1979; Terry and Katzman, 1983).

Silver-impregnated neurofibrillary tangles and bundles of filaments in the neurites of the plaque coronas are formed of paired helical filaments containing antigens which are shared by other neuronal fibrous proteins, with the particular protein implicated being dependent upon the method of study (Table 16–13). Paired helical filaments are formed at least partially from peptides identified in normal human brain. These peptides may be derived from a combination of normal proteins thus far incompletely characterized, from microtubules and neurofilaments,

and from newly formed abnormal cellular products. The chemical heterogeneity of paired helical filaments must be reconciled with their uniform morphology, which is found by ultrastructural studies in Alzheimer's disease and in aged Down's syndrome brains. Some Alzheimer-type paired helical filaments also are seen in Pick bodies, in Pick's disease (Rasool and Selkoe, 1985), and in cultured human fetal neurons altered by excitotoxic amino acids (De Boni and Crapper McLachlin, 1985). These observations indicate that several mechanisms of

Table 16–13. Selected Bibliography: Degenerative Diseases of the Nervous System

Grundke-Iqbal et al 1979, 1984, 1985 Powers et al 1981 Yen et al 1981, 1983a Anderton et al 1982 Elovaara et al 1983 Gambetti et al 1983a, b Wisniewski et al 1983c Bignami et al 1984 Rasool et al 1984 Wang GP et al 1984b Rasool & Selkoe 1985	Alzheimer's paired helical filaments: immunoreactivity heterogeneous for various neuronal fibrous proteins and for uncharacterized antigens
Wisniewski et al 1984 Wischik et al 1985	Paired helical filaments in Alzheimer's disease have uniform ultrastructure
Gambetti et al 1983b Yen et al 1983b	Cross-reaction between straight filaments in progressive supranuclear palsy, normal neuronal fibrous protein fractions (microtubules & neurofilaments), and Alzheimer's neurofibrillary tangles
Probst et al 1983 Munoz-Garcia & Ludwin 1984 Rasool & Selkoe 1985	Cross-reactions of Pick bodies with Alzheimer's neurofibrillary tangles or normal microtubules and neurofilaments; varies between studies
Borthwick et al 1985a, b	Marked reduction of tubulin in affected areas of Alzheimer brain tissue; some reduction of other partially characterized proteins
Stiller and Katenkamp 1975 Powers et al 1981 Shirahama et al 1982 Wisniewski and Kozlowski 1982 Allsop et al 1983 Elovaara et al 1983 Torack and Gebel 1983 Wisniewski et al 1983c Goust et al 1984	Immunostaining in Alzheimer's disease complicated by possible artifacts or breach of blood-brain barrier by serum proteins
Terry et al 1964 Wisniewski et al 1970 Powers et al 1981	Development of senile plaque: ultrastructure and serum protein component immunoreactivity
Morrison et al 1985 Roberts et al 1985	Somatostatin immunoreactivity corresponds closely to neurons with tangles and to neurites in senile plaques
Beal et al 1985	Somatostatin immunoreactivity in Alzheimer frontal and temporal cortex decreases linearly with somatostatin receptor decrease, indicating a system degeneration.
Eikelenboom and Stam 1984	Immunoreactivity and histochemistry of senile plaques in younger Alzheimer brains; possible residuum of chronic inflammatory response
Goust et al 1984	Immunoglobulin not bound to tissue components in aged Alzheimer brains; disappearance of dead neurons/antigen?

neuronal damage result in very similar alterations of the neuronal cytoskeleton. As a further example of these changes, straight filaments 15 nm in diameter characterize the neurofibrillary tangles in progressive supranuclear palsy, and some similar straight filaments also are found in Alzheimer's neurofibrillary tangles and in Pick bodies; these abnormal straight filaments share antigenic determinants with paired helical filaments, microtubules, and neurofilaments.

The loss of neurons or the presence of tangles in Alzheimer's disease is correlated with a marked reduction in tubulin and a smaller loss of other proteins. Thus, tubulin loss results from neuronal death or possibly from a conversion into paired helical filaments in neurofibrillary tangles. Experimentally, an induced decrease in neuronal microtubules causes a collapse and rearrangement of the neurofilaments to which they were formerly attached. The neurofilaments subsequently form perinuclear tangles (Sato Y et al, 1985). If, in disease, a proteolytic enzyme were to partially degrade microtubules and other neuronal fibrous proteins in a posttranslational process, these altered fibrous polypeptide subunits might reaggregate into the uniform spheroidal structures that form paired helical filaments (Wischick et al, 1985).

The chemical heterogeneity of paired helical filaments is complicated by the likelihood that abnormal protein bundles trap or bind serum proteins, or even elicit an inflammatory response upon becoming extracellular when a neuron is damaged. These factors have greatly complicated the interpretation of studies of the histochemistry and immunohistochemistry of plaques and tangles.

Senile plaques begin with swelling and irregularities in cortical neurites, and soon amyloid appears as the core of each plaque. Reactive astrocytes and some reactive mononuclear cells appear in the plaque, and as the core matures, becoming more compact, immunoreactive IgG and light chains increase in the neuritic corona and in the core. Changes in vascular permeability may be responsible for the presence of immunoglobulins and other serum proteins in senile plaques. The major core protein of the senile plaque in Alzheimer's disease reportedly has an amino acid composition different from that of any other known amyloid (Allsop et al, 1983; Glenner and Wong, 1984; see Chapter 5). Cerebral amyloid is rarely found in cases of systemic amyloidosis (Haber-

land, 1964; Wright and Calkins, 1974), and it may include endogenous brain proteins such as neurofilaments (Powers et al, 1981), paired helical filaments (Iqbal et al, 1984), substance P, and cholecytokinin that become exteriorized as degenerating neurons die and release them (Candy et al, 1981; Perry et al, 1981).

Neurons that form intrinsic neocortical association pathways have global cerebral cortical afferents, show a functional deficit in Alzheimer's disease (Foster et al, 1984), have increased plaques and tangles, and contain immunoreactive somatostatin. As plaques increase, somatostatin decreases (Perry and Perry, 1982). There may be a primary lesion to this intrinsic system or these association neurons may be especially susceptible to environmental factors. Senile plaques in younger Alzheimer brains contain macrophages, acid hydrolases, and immunoreactive complement factors as indicators of a chronic inflammatory response (Eikelenboom and Stam, 1984), and the neurites of the plaque coronas generally contain some immunoreactive somatostatin.

The type of rapid and extensive cellular inflammatory response in the brain that removes most degraded native proteins is seen only after rapidly evolving or widely destructive lesions (Brierley and Brown, 1982; Schröder, 1983; Sadun and Schaechter, 1985). The cell-by-cell degeneration and death in cerebral degenerative diseases may be sampled but is responded to in a limited way by the immune system, so that the normally low level of indigenous cerebral phagocytic function may allow the initial extracellular accumulation of insoluble waste proteins as a nidus for senile plaque formation.

Neurotransmitter-Related Changes

Changes in the amounts of choline acetyltransferase and acetylcholinesterase have been found in Alzheimer's disease. These changes may be secondary to neuronal degeneration, but diminution in these enzymes in the cerebrum can be shown by immunostaining methods and appear to be correlated with an increase in the number of senile plaques and with the presence of dementia (Bowen et al, 1976; Perry et al, 1978; Perry and Perry, 1982; Atack et al, 1983; Pearson RCA et al, 1983).

Tyrosine hydroxylase immunoreactivity is

greatly diminished in the substantia nigra in Parkinson's disease secondary to neuronal loss (Pearson J, 1983).

Substance P, an undecapeptide thought to be associated with the synaptic transmission of pain-related information, has markedly decreased immunoreactivity in the substantia gelatinosa of the spinal cord in patients with familial dysautonomia. These patients have normal immunoreactivity for substance P in brain regions tested. The selective loss in the spinal cord of substance P–containing axons in the region of primary sensory neuronal terminals may be related to clinical deficits. The primary lesion may be a loss of dorsal-root axons with a secondary intramedullary axonal loss (Pearson J, 1983). Axons containing substance P also are greatly diminished in the basal ganglia and midbrain in Huntington's disease (Marshall et al, 1983; Pearson J, 1983; Grafe et al, 1985) and in at least some cases of Parkinson's disease (Tenovuo et al, 1984; Grafe et al, 1985).

Paraneoplastic Degeneration

This type of paraneoplastic syndrome is thought to result either from the production of a tumor product or from the occurrence of an ineffective immune response to tumor or tissue products that show cross reactivity with neurons. Purkinje cell, and sometimes granule cell, loss can be demonstrated in patients dying with a variety of carcinomas. Circulating antibodies to cerebellar Purkinje cells have been demonstrated by immunostaining methods in patients with ovarian carcinoma both with and without paraneoplastic cerebellar degeneration (Greenlee and Brashear, 1983). Antibodies to dorsal root ganglia have been described in lung cancer patients with immunostaining, principally of neuronal nuclei, by these autoantibodies (Graus et al, 1985).

Gangliosidoses

Gangliosidoses are genetically transmitted storage diseases for which specific enzyme deficits are well characterized (Lake, 1984). Immunostaining with a specific antiserum raised in rabbits against the abnormal storage material in G_{M2} gangliosidosis shows a granular reaction product in cortical neurons. Electron microscopic immunoperoxidase staining shows labeling of the surface of the membranous cytoplasmic bodies that contain the abnormal stored ganglioside (Schwerer et al, 1982). Employing cholera-toxin affinity for G_{M1} ganglioside and immunostaining of the cholera toxin (Ganser et al, 1983) or using nonimmunologic staining for G_{M1}, with a modification of the avidin-biotin-peroxidase method, may allow identification of this stored material in samples obtained by biopsy (Asou et al, 1983).

APPENDICES

"'It's a poor memory that only works backwards,' the Queen remarked."

Lewis Carroll (1832–1898)
Through the Looking Glass

Appendix 1

Staining Protocols and Practical Procedures

Three model protocols are given for guidance. Each serves only as a central theme; other investigators may utilize variations, sometimes quite extensive, with equal success. Undoubtedly, many of you will experiment and develop further changes to meet your particular needs.

As already noted, if using a "kit", it is advisable to utilize the protocol strictly as given by the manufacturer, even if it differs from your general practice.

Three basic models are given here; for other methods see Chapter 2.

Table A1–1: ABC method (for either antisera or mouse monoclonal antibodies in paraffin sections):
The appropriate linking reagent must be used (eg, biotinylated horse antimouse Ig with mouse monoclonal antibodies).

Table A1–2: PAP method (for either antisera or mouse monoclonal antibodies in paraffin sections):
For monoclonal (mouse) antibodies, mouse PAP must be used.
For rabbit antisera use rabbit PAP.
For goat antisera use goat PAP.
For human antibodies see Chapters 2 and 3.

Table A1–3: Indirect Conjugate Procedure

These are a few practical points that are worth reiteration:

1. Using a diamond pencil to etch a circle on the slide around the section helps retain reagents over the section and prevents drying. This is particularly important with cell smears or cytocentrifuge preparations, in order to demarcate the area of the slide for application of antibodies.

2. All stains should be carried out in a humidity chamber to prevent drying; this is particularly important if overnight incubation is performed or if accelerated staining at 37°C is attempted. Humidity chambers can be purchased. Simple homemade versions consist of glass or plastic trays with lids, containing flat racks or rods upon which the slides rest. To remain humid, a humidity chamber must contain plenty of water, not just the reagents on the slides!

3. Trypsinization may be necessary for some antigens in formalin sections (see text), but trypsinization can turn sections into soup. Use at lowest possible concentration (0.01% upwards) for least possible time (5–30 minutes) at 37°C.

4. Mercury pigment (in B5-fixed sections) may readily be removed by placing dewaxed sections in iodine solution (0.5% in 70% alcohol) for 5 min, followed by 2.5% sodium thiosulphate for 1 minute. This removal may be performed prior to immunostaining or immediately prior to development of the chromogen.

5. If sections detach during staining, it may be that washing, etc, has been too violent. Gently drain reagents; gently add wash solutions, or wash in a Coplin jar. Gelatin- or albumin-treated slides may be used to promote adhesion, and overnight drying prior to staining also helps. If all else fails, simply glue the sections on by pretreating slides with dilute (10% aqueous) Elmer's glue or Tissue Tack (Polysciences, Warrington, Pennsylvania).

6. Phosphate-buffered saline (PBS) or modified PBS (stock solution—NcCl 180 gm, NaH_2PO_4 33 gm; $K_2 HPO_4$ 188 gm in 1 L of distilled water [add K_2HPO_4 first, heat if necessary with stirring]; working solution—dilute 40 ml stock to 1 L in distilled water) may be substituted for Tris-saline.

7. For snap-freezing and storing tissues, take care to use safety flasks for liquid nitrogen or isopentane; ordinary vacuum flasks are apt to explode. Neslab Instruments (of Portsmouth, New Hampshire) produces several freezing apparatuses that simplify and standardize the process. Long-term storage should be in air-tight containers (aluminum foil in Ziploc plastic bags or in small plastic containers such as those used for film storage) to prevent dehydration. Storage temper-

Table A1–1. Direct and Indirect Avidin-Biotin Conjugate (ABC) Peroxidase
Techniques

Frozen Sections	**Paraffin Sections**
1. Cut, air dry overnight, fix 5 min in reagent-grade acetone, dry[1]	1. Cut 5 μm paraffin sections, rehydrate with xylol-absolute ethanol

2. Block endogenous peroxidase with 80% methanol containing 0.6% H_2O_2, 15 min (optional—see Chapter 3)
3. Add nonimmune serum from the species from which the secondary antibody was obtained or 10% egg albumin in Tris buffer, 10 min (optional);[2] drain, do not wash

Direct	**Indirect**
4a. Add biotin-labelled primary antibody against the specific antigen, 30 min	4a. Add unlabelled primary antibody,[3] 30 min
4b. Wash in Tris-saline, 5 min	4b. Wash in Tris-saline, 5 min
	4c. Add biotinylated secondary antibody, 30 min
	4d. Wash in Tris-saline, 5 min

5a. Add ABC reagent, complexes of avidin with biotinylated horseradish peroxidase,[4] 10–60 min
5b. Wash in Tris-saline, 5 min
6. Add diaminobenzidine (0.6 mg/ml)[5] plus 0.03% H_2O, 5 min
7. Add Mayer's hematoxylin, 1–3 min
8. Dehydrate, clear, and mount in Permount

[1]Cut frozen sections to 5 μm or less; overnight drying promotes adhesion to slide, or use gelatin-coated slide. Some advocate desiccation by freeze-drying. Fix in acetone (10 seconds to 10 minutes; 5 minutes suffices for most antigens), and dry thoroughly prior to adding buffer or primary antibody.

[2]This is an optional step designed to reduce nonspecific attachment of primary or secondary antibodies to the section by Fc-binding or other mechanism. The rationale is that the normal serum (or albumin) occupies these nonspecific binding sites to the exclusion of the specific antibodies added subsequently. This "blocking" reagent clearly must not be detected by any of the specific antibodies that follow; the best choice is to use nonimmune serum from the same species as the linking or secondary antibody.

[3]All antibodies at optimal dilution (see Chapter 2).

[4]The final concentration of avidin and biotinylated peroxidase should be 20 μg/ml and 5 μg/ml, respectively; the complexes should be prepared 30 minutes before use. In the simple biotin-avidin technique, avidin-peroxidase conjugate is used directly at this point.

[5]Other chromogens may be used (Chapter 3); remember that Mayer's hematoxylin, a progressive stain that does not require alcoholic differentiation, must be used with the alcohol-soluble chromogens (eg, amino-ethyl carbazole). Diaminobenzidine is not alcohol-soluble, and Harris's hematoxylin may be used. Likewise, alcoholic dehydration and Permount must be avoided with AEC (Chapter 3).

ature should be −70°C or lower; for best long-term storage, use a liquid nitrogen refrigerator. Storage in the cryostat is acceptable for only a few days.

8. Although diaminobenzidine, amino-ethyl carbazole, etc, are not light-sensitive to the same degree as fluorescent dyes, slides will tend to fade if exposed to light. For prolonged storage of stained slides, use a cool place in closed boxes; diaminobenzidine and amino-ethyl carbazole will remain bright under these conditions for years.

For other practical points, the reader is referred back to Chapters 2 and 3 or to the text *Diagnostic Histopathology* by Jules Elias (1982).

Table A1–2. Peroxidase-Antiperoxidase (PAP) Method for Paraffin or Frozen Sections

Frozen Sections	Paraffin Sections
1. Cut, air dry overnight, fix 5 min in reagent-grade acetone, dry[1]	1. Cut 5 μm paraffin sections, rehydrate with xylol-absolute ethanol

2. Block endogenous peroxidase with 80% methanol containing 0.6% H_2O_2, 15 min (optional—see Chapter 3)
3. Add nonimmune serum from the species from which the secondary antibody was obtained or 10% egg albumin in Tris buffer, 10 min (optional);[2] drain, do not wash
4a. Add unlabelled primary antibody,[3] 30 min
4b. Wash in Tris-saline, 5 min
5a. Add linking antibody, 30 min
5b. Wash in Tris-saline, 5 min
6a. Add PAP reagent[4]
6b. Wash in Tris-saline, 5 min
7. Add diaminobenzidine (0.6 mg/ml)[5] plus 0.03% H_2O_2, 5 min
8. Add Mayer's hematoxylin, 1–3 min
9. Dehydrate, clear, and mount in Permount

[1]Cut frozen sections to 5 μm or less; overnight drying promotes ahesion to slide, or use gelatin-coated slide. Some advocate desiccation by freeze-drying. Fix in acetone (10 seconds to 10 minutes; 5 minutes suffices for most antigens), and dry thoroughly prior to adding buffer or primary antibody.

[2]This is an optional step designed to reduce nonspecific attachment of primary or secondary antibodies to the section by Fc-binding or other mechanism. The rationale is that the normal serum (or albumin) occupies these nonspecific binding sites to the exclusion of the specific antibodies added subsequently. This "blocking" reagent clearly must not be detected by any of the specific antibodies that follow; the best choice is to use nonimmune serum from the same species as the linking or secondary antibody.

[3]All antibodies at optimal dilution (see Chapter 2).

[4]PAP at optimal dilution; note that species of origin of PAP and primary antibody must be such that linking antibody binds with both— ie, from the same or cross-reacting species (see Chapters 2 and 3).

[5]Other chromogens may be used (Chapter 3); remember that Mayer's hematoxylin, a progressive stain that does not require alcoholic differentiation, must be used with the alcohol-soluble chromogens (eg, amino-ethyl carbazole). Diaminobenzidine is not alcohol-soluble, and Harris's hematoxylin may be used. Likewise, alcoholic dehydration and Permount must be avoided with AEC (Chapter 3).

Table A1–3. Indirect Conjugate Procedure

Frozen Sections	Paraffin Sections
1. Cut, air dry overnight, fix 5 min in reagent-grade acetone, dry[1]	1. Cut 5 μm paraffin sections, rehydrate with xylol-absolute ethanol

2. Block endogenous peroxidase with 80% methanol containing 0.6% H_2O_2, 15 min (optional—see Chapter 3)
3. Add nonimmune serum from the species from which the secondary antibody was obtained or 10% egg albumin in Tris buffer, 10 min (optional);[2] drain, do not wash
4a. Add unlabelled primary antibody against the specific antigen, 30 min[3]
4b. Wash in Tris-saline, 5 min
5a. Add peroxidase-conjugated antibody with specificity against the primary antibody[4]
5b. Wash in Tris-saline, 5 min
6. Add diaminobenzidine (0.6 mg/ml)[5] plus 0.03% H_2O_2, 5 min
7. Add Mayer's hematoxylin, 1–3 min
8. Dehydrate, clear, and mount in Permount

[1]Cut frozen sections to 5 μm or less; overnight drying promotes adhesion to slide, or use gelatin-coated slide. Some advocate desiccation by freeze drying. Fix in acetone (10 seconds to 10 minutes; 5 minutes suffices for most antigens), and dry thoroughly prior to adding buffer or primary antibody.

[2]This is an optional step designed to reduce nonspecific attachment of primary or secondary antibodies to the section by Fc-binding or other mechanism. The rationale is that the normal serum (or albumin) occupies these nonspecific binding sites to the exclusion of the specific antibodies added subsequently. This "blocking" reagent clearly must not be detected by any of the specific antibodies that follow; the best choice is to use nonimmune serum from the same species as the linking or secondary antibody.

[3]All antibodies at optimal dilution (see Chapter 2).

[4]For peroxidase-conjugated antibody one may substitute alkaline phosphatase or glucose oxidase–labelled reagents for single stains or as second-phase reagents in double stains.

[5]Other chromogens may be used (Chapter 3); remember that Mayer's hematoxylin, a progressive stain that does not require alcoholic differentiation, must be used with the alcohol-soluble chromogens (eg, amino-ethyl carbazole). Diaminobenzidine is not alcohol-soluble, and Harris's hematoxylin may be used. Likewise, alcoholic dehydration and Permount must be avoided with AEC.

Appendix 2

Commercial Sources for Antibodies

A number of companies, small and large, now market reagents for immunohistologic staining. Primary antibodies, labelling reagents, and chromogens may be purchased separately or combined together in "kit" form.

Kits offer some advantages to the occasional user, since they contain essentially all of the necessary reagents for the performance of the stain, with the exception of such common laboratory items as glass slides, mounting media, solvents, buffers, and the like. Generally, these kits include detailed staining instructions, which should be followed to achieve successful staining. The temptation to introduce one's own embellishments should be resisted, because the kits usually contain matched pretitered reagents, and interference with the protocol is more likely to hinder staining than to enhance it.

The following table lists the principal manufacturers selling reagents designed for immunohistology in the United States; many of these companies also market them in Europe or the Far East. Many other vendors of antibodies exist, and these antibodies may of course be adapted for use in immunohistology by combining with a suitable labelling system. In this instance it should be stressed that the burden of proof of specificity of these antibodies, both for primary and for any secondary antibodies, is on the user. The ultimate proof of specificity of an antibody for use in immunohistologic procedures is, as described in Chapter 2, largely empirical, but must involve an immunohistologic demonstration of specificity.

Shelf life of these reagents is listed as six months to one year or more. In our experience, when they are maintained at 4° C and are dispensed from dropper bottles rather than by pipettes, it is possible to achieve an even longer useful life.

For details of the exact types of kits available, consult the individual manufacturer; no attempt is made to give other than a general guide here since availability of reagents changes regularly, with many new antibodies appearing every few months.

One word of warning: combining reagents from different manufacturers should only be attempted if details of the species and subclass of immunoglobulin are given so that appropriate choices can be made; eg, the blind admixture of surplus Ortho anti-insulin with Dako PAP systems may fail if the Ortho reagent is guinea pig antibody, whereas the Dako PAP system is designed for rabbit antiserum.

Table A2–1. Commercial Availability of Immunostaining Kits and Reagents

Abbott Laboratories Chicago, Illinois	Kit with monoclonal antibody for estrogen receptor
Becton Dickinson Mountain View, California	B and T cell kits; range of monoclonal antibodies; Leu series
Bethesda Research Laboratories Gaithersberg, Maryland	Antibody to TDT, among others
Biogenex Dublin, California	Approximately 40 immunohistology kits, plus individual antibodies
Biomeda Foster City, California	Approximately 20 immunohistology kits
Cappel Malvern, Pennsylvania	Range of antibodies and conjugates
Coulter Hialeah, Florida	Range of monoclonal antibodies to leukocytes
Dako Santa Barbara, California	Approximately 40 immunohistology kits, individual antibodies, conjugates, and PAP
Diagnostic Technology Inc Hauppauge, New York	Limited range of monoclonals, mostly versus immunoglobulins
Geometric Data Systems Wayne, Pennsylvania	Immunogold system
Hybritech San Diego, California	Range of monoclonal antibodies to CEA, prostatic acid phosphatase, and specific antigen, T and B cells, etc
Immunonuclear Corp Stillwater, Minnesota	Approximately 40 kits and antibodies, PAP, and ABC
Labsystems Chicago, Illinois	Monoclonal antibodies to intermediate filaments
Lipshaw · Detroit, Michigan	Antibodies, approximately 50 kits, PAP, and avidin-biotin reagents
Meloy Springfield, Virginia	Range of antibodies and reagents
Miles Naperville, Illinois	Approximately 50 immunohistology kits plus broad range of antibodies, conjugates, PAP reagents, peroxidase, alkaline phosphatase, and biotin-conjugated antibodies
Nordic El Toro, California	Extensive range of antibodies and conjugates

Ortho
  Carpinteria, California,
    Raritan, New Jersey
	Broadest range of kits and antibodies including hormones, immunoglobulins, CEA, etc; URO and MEL series of monoclonal antibodies plus monoclonal antibodies to T and B cells; incubation chamber; PAP and ABC reagents

Polysciences Warrington, Pennsylvania	Range of antibodies, conjugates, PAP reagent, clearing agents, and mounting media
Sigma St. Louis, Missouri	Basic stains and reagents
Supertechs Bethesda, Maryland	Anti-TDT antibody
Tago Inc Burlingame, California	Good quality conjugates, peroxidase, alkaline phosphatase, glucose oxidase
Techniclone Anaheim, California	LN series of antibodies, reactive with lymphocytes in paraffin sections
Vector Burlingame, California	ABC kits and biotinylated reagents; normal sera

Also of value is Linscott's *Directory of Immunologic and Biologic Reagents* (40 Glen Drive, Mill Valley, CA 94941). This lists many sources, including private investigators, for many antibodies, including the rare and exotic.

Appendix 3

Monoclonal Antibodies Versus Leukocyte Membrane Antigens

The following three tables are modified from those given for the T cell, B cell, and monocyte–granulocyte antibody protocols (designated T2, B2, and M2, respectively) at the First International Workshop on Human Leucocyte Differentiation Antigens. The tables are given in full in *Leucocyte Typing* (A. Bernard et al, eds. New York, Springer-Verlag, 1984), together with many original articles, details of the patterns of cross reactivity of the various antibodies, and the nature of the antigens recognized.*

*Since this book went to press, the Proceedings of the Second International Workshop (1984) have also been published: Reinherz et al. Leucocyte Typing II, vols 1–3. New York, Springer-Verlag, 1985.

Table A3–1. Anti–T Cell Antibodies: Reagents with Reactivity Mainly for T Cells*

Antibody	First Author	Reference
T29/33	Omary BM	(1980) J Exp Med 152:842
A3D8	Telen MJ	(1983) J Clin Invest 71:1878
NA1/34	McMichael AJ	(1979) Eur J Immunol 9:205
	McKie RM	(1982) Clin Exp Dermatol 7:43
26.2	Deng CT	
UCHT1	Beverley PCL	(1981) Eur J Immunol 11:329
	Linch DC	(1982) Prenatal Diagn 2:211
UCHT2	Beverley PCL	(1981) In: Peeters H, ed. Protides of the Biological Fluids, vol 29, p 653
BL6	Yonish-Rouach E	(1982) In: Serrou B, Rosenfeld C, Daniels J, eds. Current Concepts in Human Immunology and Cancer Immunotherapy, Amsterdam, Elsevier/North Holland
F15.42.1	McKenzie JL	(1981) J Immunol 126:843
	McKenzie JL	(1981) Brain Res 230:307
MBG6	Bastin JM	(1981) Clin Exp Immunol 46:597
SC1	Fox RI	(1982) J Immunol 129:401
	Fox RI	(1982) J Immunol 128:351
D47	Boumsell L	(1984) In: Bernard A et al, eds. Leucocyte Typing. New York, Springer-Verlag
H207	Bai Yan	(1984) In: Bernard A et al, eds. Leucocyte Typing. New York, Springer-Verlag
T3(2AD2)	Reinherz EL	(1980) Eur J Immunol 10:758
	Reinherz EL	(1982) Cell 30:735
9.6	Kamoun MM	(1981) J Exp Med 153:207
	Martin PJ	(1981) J Immunol 127:1920
10.2	Martin PJ	(1980) Immunogenetics 11:429
	Martin PJ	(1981) J Immunol 128:1920
A50	Boumsell L	(1980) J Exp Med 152:229
M241	Knowles RW	(1982) Eur J Immunol 12:676
38.1	Hansen JA	(1982) Prog Cancer Res Ther 21:75
T411	Rieber P	(1981) Hybridoma 1:59
T101	Royston I	(1980) J Immunol 125:725
	Dillman RO	(1982) Blood 59:1036
3.40	Naito K	(1984) In: Bernard A et al, eds. Leucocyte Typing. New York, Springer-Verlag
67B7	Billing R	(1984) In: Bernard A et al, eds. Leucocyte Typing. New York, Springer-Verlag
T6(19Thy1A8)	Reinherz EL	(1980) Proc Natl Acad Sci USA 77:1588
	Umiel T	(1982) J Immunol 129:1054
35.1	Martin PJ	(1982) Hum Immunol 5:160
D66	Bernard A	(1982) J Exp Med 155:1317

Table A3–1. Anti–T Cell Antibodies: Reagents with Reactivity Mainly for T Cells* *Continued*

Antibody	First Author	Reference
T11(3Pt2H9)	Meuer SC	(1982) Proc Natl Acad Sci USA 79:4395
	Meuer SC	(1982) Science 218:471
12.1	Kamoun MM	(1981) J Immunol 127:987
	Martin PJ	(1982) Immunogenetics 15:385
DU.SKW.3.1	Haynes BF	(1982) Science 215:298
	Dowell	(1983) Hum Immunol 7:95
AMG4	Gordon	(1984) In: Bernard A et al, eds. Leucocyte Typing. New York, Springer-Verlag
T1(24T6G12)	Reinherz EL	(1979) J Immunol 123:1312
	Reinherz EL	(1982) Cell 30:735
Cris1	Vilella R	(1982) Immunologia 1:58
FMC31	Beckman IG	(1984) In: Bernard A et al, eds. Leucocyte Typing. New York, Springer-Verlag
Tü33	Ziegler W	(1984) In: Bernard A et al, eds. Leucocyte Typing. New York, Springer-Verlag
3a1	Haynes BF	(1979) Proc Natl Acad Sci USA 76:5829
	Haynes BF	(1981) N Engl J Med 304:1319
4a	Mosishima Y	(1982) J Immunol 129:1091
H65	Bai Yan	(1984) In: Bernard A et al, eds. Leucocyte Typing. New York, Springer-Verlag
Q151.196	Crepaldi T	(1982) Tissue Antigens 20:282
89b1	Szer IS	(1982) Abstracts, 15th International Leucocyte Culture Conference, Chichester, Eng., Wiley
9.3	Hansen JA	(1980) Immunogenetics 10:247
	Lum LG	(1982) Cell Immunol 72:122
Leu 3a	Evans RL	(1981) Proc Natl Acad USA 78:544
	Gatenborg PA	(1982) J Immunol 129:1997
UCHT4	Beverley PCL	(1982) Proc R Soc (Ed) 818:221
T1020	Rieber P	(1984) In: Bernard A et al, eds. Leucocyte Typing. New York, Springer-Verlag
TAC	Uchiyama T	(1981) J Immunol 126:1393
	Leonard W	(1982) Nature 300:267
B614	Lansdorp PM	(1984) In: Bernard A et al, eds. Leucocyte Typing. New York, Springer-Verlag
B9.11.10	Malissen B	(1982) Eur J Immunol 12:739
91D6	Szer IS	(1982) Abstracts, American Federation for Clinical Research, Fed Proc, Sept 1982
B9.1.1	Malissen B	(1982) Eur J Immunol 12:739
T4(12T4D11)	Reinherz EL	(1979) Proc Natl Acad Sci USA 76:4061
	Meuer SC	(1982) Proc Natl Acad Sci USA 79:4395
T811	Rieber P	(1981) Hybridoma 1:59
	Lohmeyer J	(1981) Eur J Immunol 11:997
E10	Boumsell L	(1984) In: Bernard A et al, eds. Leucocyte Typing. New York, Springer-Verlag
T8(21Thy)	Reinherz EL	(1980) J Immunol 124:1301
	Reinherz EL	(1981) Nature 294:168
51.1	Hansen JA	(1984) In: Bernard A et al, eds. Leucocyte Typing. New York, Springer-Verlag
Leu 2a	Evans RL	(1981) Proc Natl Acad Sci USA 78:544
	Gatenborg PA	(1982) J Immunol 129:1997
HH9	Naoe T	(1984) In: Bernard A et al, eds. Leucocyte Typing. New York, Springer-Verlag
B9.8.6	Malissen B	(1982) Eur J Immunol 12:739
ATL27	Ueda R	(1984) In: Bernard A et al, eds. Leucocyte Typing. New York, Springer-Verlag
B9.2.4	Malissen B	(1982) Eur J Immunol 12:739
Tü14	Ziegler W	(1984) In: Bernard A et al, eds. Leucocyte Typing. New York, Springer-Verlag
2D2	Clement L	(1984) In: Bernard A et al, eds. Leucocyte Typing. New York, Springer-Verlag
AA1	Chiorazzi N	(1984) In: Bernard A et al, eds. Leucocyte Typing. New York, Springer-Verlag
B9.7.6	Malissen B	(1982) Eur J Immunol 12:739
CL1-3	Morishima Y	(1982) J Immunol 129:1091
C10	Galton J	(1984) In: Bernard A et al, eds. Leucocyte Typing. New York, Springer-Verlag

Table A3–1. Anti–T Cell Antibodies: Reagents with Reactivity Mainly for T Cells* *Continued*

Antibody	First Author	Reference
AA2	Chiorazzi N	(1984) In: Bernard A et al, eds. Leucocyte Typing. New York, Springer-Verlag
B9.3.1	Malissen B	(1982) Eur J Immunol 12:739
E6.2	Lansdorp PM	(1984) In: Bernard A et al, eds. Leucocyte Typing. New York, Springer-Verlag
B9.4.1	Malissen B	Eur J Immunol 12:739
T29/33	Omary BM	(1980) J Exp Med 152:842
M236	Knowles RW	(1984) In: Bernard A et al, eds. Leucocyte Typing. New York, Springer-Verlag
B721	Frisman	(1984) In: Bernard A et al, eds. Leucocyte Typing. New York, Springer-Verlag
A3D8	Telen MJ	(1983) J Clin Invest 71:1878
M1D4	Guarnotta G	(1984) In: Bernard A et al, eds. Leucocyte Typing. New York, Springer-Verlag

*Some non–T cell reagents were included as controls; tests were run against a variety of leukocyte populations for the purposes of comparison.

Table A3–2. Anti–B Cell Antibodies: Reagents with Reactivity Mainly for B Cells

Antibody	First Author	Reference
T29/33	Omary BM	(1980) J Exp Med 152:842
A3D8	Telen MJ	(1983) J Clin Invest 71:1878
58G12	Billing R	(1984) In: Bernard A et al, eds. Leucocyte Typing. New York, Springer-Verlag
L22	Royston I	(1984) In: Bernard A et al, eds. Leucocyte Typing. New York, Springer-Verlag
35.1	Deng CT	(1984) In: Bernard A et al, eds. Leucocyte Typing. New York, Springer-Verlag
F8.11.13	Dalchau R	(1981) J Exp Med 153:753
FMC1	Brooks DA	(1980) Clin Exp Immunol 39:477
	Seymour GJ	(1982) J Periodont Res 17:247
FMC8	Brooks DA	(1982) Pathology 14:5
DU-ALL-1	Jones NH	(1982) Leukem Res 6:449
BA2	Kersey JH	(1981) J Exp Med 153:726
	Platt JL	(1983) J Exp Med 157:155
B532	Frisman DM	(1984) In: Bernard A et al, eds. Leucocyte Typing. New York, Springer-Verlag
VIL-A1	Knapp W	(1982) Leuk Res 6:137
	Knapp W	(1983) Ann NY Acad Sci
BA3	LeBien TW	(1982) J Immunol 129:2287
	Platt JL	(1983) J Exp Med 157:155
24.1	Braun M	(1982) Blood 61:718
NL-1	Ueda R	(1982) Proc Natl Acad Sci USA 79:4386
SJ9A4	Komada Y	(1983) Blood 7:487
GB13	Funderud S	(1983) Scand J Immunol 17:161
TC3/61	Maeda H	(1984) In: Bernard A et al, eds. Leucocyte Typing. New York, Springer-Verlag
BB.1	Yokochi T	(1982) J Immunol 129:923
3HBB14	Hartmann KU	(1984) In: Bernard A et al, eds. Leucocyte Typing. New York, Springer-Verlag
3HBB2	Hartmann KU	(1984) In: Bernard A et al, eds. Leucocyte Typing. New York, Springer-Verlag
Tü1	Ziegler W	(1984) In: Bernard A et al, eds. Leucocyte Typing. New York, Springer-Verlag
B1(8)	Stashenko P	(1980) J Immunol 125:1678
J5	Ritz J	(1980) Nature 283:583
Y29/55	Forster HK	(1981) The Immune System 2:425
	Forster HK	(1982) Cancer Res 42:1927
B2(9)	Nadler L	(1981) J Immunol 126:1941
I2	Nadler L	(1981) Hum Immunol 1:77

Table A3–3. Anti-Monocyte/Granulocyte Antibodies: Reagents with Reactivity Mainly for Cells of the Monocyte/Granulocyte Series

Antibody	First Author	Reference
T29/33	Omary BM	(1980) J Exp Med 152:842
A3D8	Telen MJ	(1983) J Clin Invest 71:1879
TG1	Beverley PCL	(1980) Nature 387:332
	Linch DC	(1982) Prenatal Diagnosis 2:211
M67	Rieber P	(1984) In: Bernard A et al, eds. Leucocyte Typing. New York, Springer-Verlag
V IM-D2	Majdic O	(1982) Wien Klin Wochenschr 94:387
MCS.1	Tatsumi E	(1981) Proc Am Assoc Cancer Res 22:181
VI M-D5	Majdic O	(1981) Blood 58:1127
	Knapp W	(1985) Ann NY Acad Sci, in press
MCS.2	Tatsumi E	(1981) Proc Am Assoc Cancer Res 22:181
M522	Lohmeyer	(1981) Eur J Immunol 11:997
FMC17	Brooks DA	(1981) Clin Exp Pharmacol Physiol 8:415
	Brooks DA	(1985) Pathology, in press
20.2	Kamoun MM	(1984) In: Bernard A et al, eds. Leucocyte Typing. New York, Springer-Verlag
FMC13	Zola H	(1981) Br J Haematol 48:481
IG10	Bernstein ID	(1982) J Immunol 128:876
	Andrews RG	(1982) In: Mitchell MS, Oettgen HF, eds. Hybridomas in Cancer Diagnosis and Treatment, vol 21, p 147. New York, Raven Press
FMC12	Zola H	(1981) Br J Haematol 48:481
5F1	Bernstein ID	(1982) J Immunol 128:876
	Andrews RG	(1982) In: Mitchell MS, Oettgen HF, eds. Hybridomas in Cancer Diagnosis and Treatment, vol 21, p 147. New York, Raven Press
FMC11	Zola H	(1981) Br J Haematol 48:481
B2.12	Tetteroo PAT	(1984) In: Bernard A et al, eds. Leucocyte Typing. New York, Springer-Verlag
FMC10	Zola H	(1981) Br J Haematol 48:481
B13.9	Tetteroo PAT	(1984) In: Bernard A et al, eds. Leucocyte Typing. New York, Springer-Verlag
G2	Martin LS	(1984) In: Bernard A et al, eds. Leucocyte Typing. New York, Springer-Verlag
B4.3	Tetteroo PAT	(1984) In: Bernard A et al, eds. Leucocyte Typing. New York, Springer-Verlag
TG8	Maeda H	(1984) In: Bernard A et al, eds. Leucocyte Typing. New York, Springer-Verlag
D5	Lansdorp PM	(1984) In: Bernard A et al, eds. Leucocyte Typing. New York, Springer-Verlag
TM18	Maeda H	(1984) In: Bernard A et al, eds. Leucocyte Typing. New York, Springer-Verlag
82H7	Mannoni P	(1984) In: Bernard A et al, eds. Leucocyte Typing. New York, Springer-Verlag
G.1120	Rieber P	(1984) In: Bernard A et al, eds. Leucocyte Typing. New York, Springer-Verlag
20.3	Kamoun MM	(1984) In: Bernard A et al, eds. Leucocyte Typing. New York, Springer-Verlag
M0-1	Todd RF	(1981) J Immunol 126:1435
	Todd RF	(1982) Hybridoma 1:329
75B10	Billing R	(1984) In: Bernard A et al, eds. Leucocyte Typing. New York, Springer-Verlag
DU-HL60-1	McKolanis JR	(1984) In: Bernard A et al, eds. Leucocyte Typing. New York, Springer-Verlag
80H3	Mannoni P	(1982) Hum Immunol 5:309
3C4	Kayser	(1984) In: Bernard A et al, eds. Leucocyte Typing. New York, Springer-Verlag
M0-2	Todd RF	(1981) J Immunol 126:1435
	Todd RF	(1982) Hybridoma 1:329
DU-HL60-3	McKolanis JR	(1984) In: Bernard A et al, eds. Leucocyte Typing. New York, Springer-Verlag

Table A3–3. Anti-Monocyte/Granulocyte Antibodies: Reagents with Reactivity Mainly for Cells of the Monocyte/Granulocyte Series *Continued*

Antibody	First Author	Reference
Tü3	Ziegler W	(1984) In: Bernard A et al, eds. Leucocyte Typing. New York, Springer-Verlag
DU-HL60-4	McKolanis Jr	(1984) In: Bernard A et al, eds. Leucocyte Typing. New York, Springer-Verlag
M0P9	Dimitriu-Bona A	(1981) Fed Proc 40:988
	Dimitriu-Bona A	(1983) J Immunol 130:145
MY4(322)	Griffin JD	(1981) J Clin Invest 68:932
	Griffin JD	(1983) Blood 61:408
Tü5	Ziegler W	(1984) In: Bernard A, et al, eds. Leucocyte Typing. New York, Springer-Verlag
MCCH36.71	Sullivan A	(1984) In: Bernard A, et al, eds. Leucocyte Typing. New York, Springer-Verlag
M0P15	Dimitriu-Bona A	(1981) Fed Proc 40:988
	Dimitriu-Bona A	(1983) J Immunol 130:145
MY7(366)	Griffin JD	(1981) J Clin Invest 68:932
	Griffin JD	(1983) Blood 61:408
Tü9	Ziegler W	(1984) In: Bernard A, et al, eds. Leucocyte Typing. New York, Springer-Verlag
M0S-1	Dimitriu-Bona A	(1981) Fed Proc 40:988
	Dimitriu-Bona A	(1983) J Immunol 130:145
MY8(374)	Griffin JD	(1981) J Clin Invest 68:932
	Griffin JD	(1983) Blood 61:408
M0S-39	Dimitriu-Bona A	(1983) J Immunol 130:145
Tü2	Ziegler W	(1984) In: Bernard A, et al, eds. Leucocyte Typing. New York, Springer-Verlag
A3D8	Telen MJ	(1983) J Clin Invest 71:1878

Appendix 4. Tabulated Patterns of Immunohistochemical Staining

During many lectures on this topic, it has become apparent that audiences commonly express a liking for tables that purport to summarize the typical immunohistochemical reaction to different tumors. Such tables admittedly are of value in a teaching forum, providing a basis for discussion and comparison. However, it must be emphasized that findings condensed into tabular form can only provide an indication of the most commonly encountered patterns. Variability stems from several factors: the antibodies employed differ, the tumors differ, and the investigators differ.

For these reasons I have elected not to include such tables in the text, in which more detailed discussion of the variable staining patterns of different tumors has been attempted. The tables included in this appendix may prove useful for teaching and reference; they should be interpreted in conjunction with the appropriate text.

Abbreviations

AACT	alpha$_1$-antichymotrypsin
AAT	alpha$_1$-antitrypsin
AFP	alpha fetoprotein
CEA	carcinoembryonic antigen
CLA	common leukocyte antigen
EMA	epithelial membrane antigen (see mammary EMA or milk–fat globule membrane)
GFA	glial fibrillary acidic protein
HbA/F	hemoglobin A or F (adult or fetal)
HBsAg	hepatitis B surface antigen
hCG	human chorionic gonadotrophin
Ker	keratin
K/L	kappa/lambda
LN2	an anti–B cell/monocyte monoclonal antibody
MBP	myelin basic protein
Mx	muramidase (lysozyme)
neurofil	neurofilament (intermediate filament)
NSE	neuron-specific enolase
PSAP	prostate-specific acid phosphatase
PSEA	prostate-specific epithelial antigen
S100	S100 protein
Vim	vimentin
818	myeloid antigen (Techniclone)

Table A4–1. Bone Marrow Tumors

	Granulocytic	Monocytic Histiocytic	Erythroid	Lymphoid	Megs	Secondary
AAT/AACT	+	+	−	−	−	−
Mx	+ +	+	−	−	−	(∓)[1]
Cathepsin G	+	−	−	−	−	−
Myeloid (818)	+ +	−	−	−	−	−
Hb A/F	−	−	+	−	−	−
CLA	+	+	−	+	−	−
LN2	−	+	−	+	−	−
Ker (pan)	−	−	−	−	−	±[2]

[1]Rare carcinomas have the potential for muramidase production (e.g., lacrimal gland, sometimes stomach).
[2]Carcinoma

Table A4–2. Germ Cell Tumors

	Pure Seminoma	Seminoma (with giant cells)	Embryonal Carcinoma	Chorio-carcinoma	Yolk-Sac Tumor	Teratoma
hCG	±	+	±	+	−	±
Ker (pan)	−	−	+	+	±	+[1]
Vimentin	+	+	−	−	±	+[1]
AFP	−	−	±	−	+	±
CEA	−	−	−	−	−	+
Ferritin	+	+	±	−	±	−
AAT	−	−	−	−	+	−

[1]Keratin in epithelial elements, vimentin in mesenchymal elements.

375

Table A4–3. Thyroid Tumors

	Follicular Epithelium	Papillary/ Follicular Carcinoma	C Cell Hyperplasia	Medullary Carcinoma
Thyroglobulin (or T3/T4)	+	+	−	−
Calcitonin	−	−	+	+
CEA	−	±	±	±

Table A4–4. Gastrointestinal Tumors

	Carcinoma	Carcinoid	Lymphoma
Ker (Pan)	+	±	−
CEA	+	−	−
NSE*	−	+	−
CLA	−	−	+
LN2	−	−	+

*Leu 7 also marks neuroendocrine cells.

Table A4–5. Tumors of the Pancreas

	Adeno-carcinoma	Islet Cell Tumors
CEA	+	−
NSE	−	+
Specific hormones	−	+
Ker (high MW)	+	−

Table A4–6. Tumors of the Liver

	Hepatoma	Secondary Carcinoma	Cholangio-carcinoma
HBsAg	±	−	−
AFP	+ +	−	−
AAT	+ +	−	−
Ker (high MW)	−	±	±
CEA	−(+)	±	+

(+) equals rare.

Table A4–7. Lung Tumors

	Primary Squamous Carcinoma	Primary Adenocarcinoma	Oat Cell	Secondary Carcinoma	Mesothelium
Ker (high MW)	+	−(+)	−	±	+
Ker (low MW)	−(+)[1]	+	±	±	+
CEA	−(+)	±	−	±	−[2]
EMA	−	+	−	±	−
Bombesin	−	−	±	−	−
NSE	−	−	±	−	−
Lung carcinoma–specific	(+)[3]	(+)[3]	(+)[3]	−	−
OC125(F)[4]	−	−	−	−	+

[1](+) equals weak positivity or rare positive cells.
[2]Some studies have reported weak reactivity.
[3]Monoclonals with claimed specificity for each of squamous, adeno- and small cell carcinoma types have been reported.
[4]Frozen sections only.

Table A4–8. Tumors of the Prostate

	Prostatic Cancer	Other Cancer (eg, of colon)
PSAP	+	−
PSEA	+	−
Ker (high MW)	−	±
CEA	−(+)	+

Table A4–9. Central Nervous System Tumors

	Astrocytomas	Ependymomas	Oligodendroglioma	Neuroblastoma	Medulloblastoma	Meningioma	Secondary Tumors
GFA	+	+	+	−	±	−	−
NSE	±	−	±	+	+	−	−
S100	±	±	−	−	−	±	±[1]
Vim	−	−	−	−	−	+	±[1]
CLA	−	−	−	−	−	−	±[1]
Ker	−	−	−	−	−	−	±[1]

[1]Metastatic melanoma is S100-positive; lymphoma, CLA-positive; carcinomas, keratin-positive; lymphomas, vimentin-positive.

Table A4–10. Neural and Related Tumors

	Neurofibroma Schwannoma	Granular Cell Tumor	Ganglioneuroma	Neuroblastoma	Gliomas	Melanoma
S100	+	+	+	−	−	+
GFAP	−	−	−	−	+	−
NSE	−	−	+	+	−	−
MBP	+	−	+	−	−	−
Neurofil	−	−	+	+	−	−
Vimentin	+	+	−	−	±	+

Table A4–11. Sarcomas

	Spindle Epithelioid	Chondro-sarcoma	Osteo-sarcoma	Fibro-sarcoma	Angio-(Kaposi) sarcoma	MAL[1] Fibrous	Leio-Myo-sarcoma	Rhabdo-myosar-coma	Mela-noma	Lym-phoma
Ker	+	−	−	−	−	−	−	−	−	−
Vim	±	+	+	+	+	+	+	+	+	+
S100	−	+[2]	−	−	−	−	−	−	+ +	−
Actin/Myosin	−	−	−	±	−	±	+	+	−	−
Desmin	−	−	−	−	−	−	+	+	−	−
Myoglobin	−	−	−	−	−	−	−	+	−	−
Factor VIII	−	−	−	−	+	−	−	−	−	−
AACT	−	−	−	−	−	+	−	−	−	−
CLA	−	−	−	−	−	−	−	−	−	+

[1]MAL fibrous equals malignant fibrous histiocytoma.
[2]Note that chondromas and granular cell tumors also are S100 positive.

Table A4–12. Anaplastic Tumors

	Lym-phoma	Carci-noma	Other Sarcomas	Mela-noma
CLA	+	−	−	−
LN2	±	−	−	−
K/L	±	−	−	−
Ker (Pan)	−	+	−[1]	−
CEA	−	±	−	−
EMA	−	±	−[1]	−
S100	−	−	−	+
Vimentin	+	−	+	+

[1]Note that so-called spindle-cell and epithelioid sarcomas are keratin-positive (ie, epithelial).

BIBLIOGRAPHY

"As a rule disease can scarcely keep pace with the itch to scribble about it."

JOHN MAYOW (1640–1674)
De Rachitide

Abramowitz A, Livni N, Morag A, et al. An immuno-peroxidase study of cytomegalovirus mononucleosis. Arch Pathol Lab Med 106:115, 1982

Abrams GM, Latov N, Hays AP, et al. Immunocytochemical studies of human peripheral nerve with serum from patients with polyneuropathy and paraproteinemia. Neurology 32:821, 1982

Adams RL, Springall DR, Levene MM, et al. The immunocytochemical detection of herpes simplex virus in cervical smears—a valuable technique for routine use. J Pathol 143:241, 1984

Addis BJ, Isaacson P, Billings JA. Plasmacytoma of lymph nodes. Cancer 46:340, 1980

Adelman LS. The pathology of pituitary adenomas. In: Post KD, Jackson IMD, Reichlin S, eds. The Pituitary Adenoma. New York, Plenum, p 47, 1980

Adelman LS, Dahl D, Bignami A. Chordomas stain with keratin antiserum. J Neuropathol Exp Neurol 42:314, 1983

Afroudakis AP, Liew CT, Peters RL. An immunoperoxidase technic for the demonstration of the hepatitis B surface antigen in human livers. Am J Clin Pathol 65:533, 1976

Aguirre P, Scully RE, Wolfe HJ, et al. Endometrial carcinoma with argyrophil cells: a histochemical and immunohistochemical analysis. Hum Pathol 15:210, 1984

Ahmed SR, Shalet SM, Price DA, et al. Human chorionic gonadotrophin secreting pineal germinoma and precocious puberty. Arch Dis Child 58:743, 1983

Ahnen DJ, Nakane PK, Brown WR. Ultrastructural localization of carcinoembryonic antigen in normal intestine and colon cancer: abnormal distribution of CEA on the surfaces of colon cancer cells. Cancer 49:2077, 1982

Aho HJ, Patzke HP, Nevalainen TJ, et al. Immunohistochemical localization of trypsinogen and trypsin in acute and chronic pancreatitis. Digestion 27:21, 1983

Akhtar M, Bunuan H, Ali MA, et al. Kaposi's sarcoma in renal transplant recipients. Ultrastructural and immunoperoxidase study of four cases. Cancer 53:258, 1984

Al Adnani MS, Ali SM. Patterns of chronic liver disease in Kuwait with special reference to localisation of hepatitis B surface antigen. J Clin Pathol 37:549, 1984

Al Saate T, Laurent G, Caveriviere P, et al. Reactivity of Leu 1 and T101 monoclonal antibodies with B cell lymphomas (correlations with other immunological markers). Clin Exp Immunol 58:631, 1984

Alario A, Ortonne J-P, Schmitt D, et al. Lichen planus: study with anti-human T lymphocyte antigen (anti-HTLA) serum on frozen tissue sections. Br J Dermatol 98:601, 1978

Alberti VN, Neiman RS. Lymphoplasmacytic lymphoma. A clinicopathologic study of a previously unrecognized composite variant. Cancer 53:1103, 1984

Albores-Saavedra J, de Jesus Manrique J, Angeles-Angeles A, et al. Carcinoma in situ of the gallbladder. A clinicopathologic study of 18 cases. Am J Surg Pathol 8:323, 1984

Albores-Saavedra J, Nadji M, Morales AR, et al. Carcinoembryonic antigen in normal, preneoplastic and neoplastic gallbladder epithelium. Cancer 52:1069, 1983

Albrechtsen R, Wewer U, Wimberley PD. Immunohistochemical demonstration of a hitherto undescribed localization of hemoglobin A and F in endodermal cells of normal human yolk sac and endodermal sinus tumor. Am J Med 69:140, 1980

Ali M, Fayemi O, Nalebuff DJ. Localization of IgE in adenoids and tonsils: an immunoperoxidase study. Arch Otolaryngol 105:695, 1979

Allegranza A, Mariani C, Giardini R, et al. Primary malignant lymphomas of the central nervous system: a histological and immunohistological study of 12 cases. Histopathology 8:781, 1984

Allen DC, Biggart JD, Orchin JC, et al. An immunoperoxidase study of epithelial marker antigens in ulcerative colitis with dysplasia and carcinoma. J Clin Pathol 38:18, 1985

Allsop D, Landon M, Kidd M. The isolation and amino acid composition of senile plaque core protein. Brain Res 259:348, 1983

Alm P, Hultberg B, Olsson AM. Testicular tumour markers in tissue correlated to serum levels and clinical stage. Scand J Urol Nephrol 18:283, 1984

Almagro UA. Argyrophilic prostatic carcinoma. Case report with literature review on prostatic carcinoid and "carcinoid-like" prostatic carcinoma. Cancer 55:608, 1985

Alumets J, Sundler F, Falkmer S, et al. Neurohormonal peptides in endocrine tumors of the pancreas, stomach, and upper small intestine: I. An immunohistochemical study of 27 cases. Ultrastruct Pathol 5:55, 1983

Amaducci L, Forno KI, Eng LF. Glial fibrillary acidic protein in cryogenic lesions of the rat brain. Neurosci Lett 21:27, 1981

379

Ammirati PM, Wang C-Y, Evans RL, et al. Ia alloantigens on human T cells. Expression and synthesis by human autologous reactive T cells. In: Aiuti F, Wigzell H, eds. Thymus, Thymic Hormones and T Lymphocyte. p 59, 1980

Amouric M, Lechene de la Porte P, Figarella C. Immunocytochemical localization of pancreatic kallikrein in human acinar cells. Hoppe Seylers Z Physiol Chem 363:515, 1982

Andersen W, Kang YH, DeSombre ER. Endogenous peroxidase: specific marker enzyme for tissues displaying growth dependency on estrogen. J Cell Biol 64:668, 1975

Anderson KC, Bates MP, Slaughenhoupt BL, et al. Expression of human B cell–associated antigens on leukemias and lymphomas: a model of human B cell differentiation. Blood 63:1424, 1984

Anderton BH, Breinburg D, Downes MJ, et al. Monoclonal antibodies show that neurofibrillary tangles and neurofilaments share antigenic determinants. Nature 298:84, 1982

Andres T, MacPherson B. Identification of group B streptococci in tissue sections using the peroxidase-antiperoxidase method: a retrospective necropsy study. J Clin Pathol 33:1165, 1980

Ansari MA, Pintozzi RL, Choi YS, et al. Diagnosis of carcinoid-like metastatic prostatic carcinoma by an immunoperoxidase method. Am J Clin Pathol 76:94, 1981

Aozasa K, Inoue A. Malignant histiocytosis presenting as lethal midline granuloma: immunohistological study. J Pathol 138:241, 1982

Arends JW, Groniowski MM, de Koning Gans HJ, et al. Immunohistochemical study of the distribution of secretory component and IgA in the normal and diseased uterine mucosa. Int J Gynecol Pathol 2:171, 1983a

Arends JW, Verstynen C, Bosman FT, et al. Distribution of monoclonal antibody–defined monosialoganglioside in normal and cancerous human tissues: an immunoperoxidase study. Hybridoma 2:219, 1983b

Arends JW, Wiggers T, Verstijnen C, et al. Gastrointestinal cancer-associated antigen (GICA) immunoreactivity in colorectal carcinoma in relation to patient survival. Int J Cancer 34:193, 1984

Arnold W, Mitrenga D, von Mayersbach H. The preservation of substance and immunologic activity of intravenously injected human IgG in the mouse liver. (Comparative studies on various tissue preparation and fixation methods). Acta Histochem 49:161, 1974

Arnold WA, Kalden JR, von Mayersbach H. Influence of different histologic preparation methods on preservation of tissue antigens in the immunofluorescent antibody technique. Ann NY Acad Sci 254:27, 1975

Aroni K, Kittas C, Papadimitriou CS, et al. An immunocytochemical study of the distribution of lysozyme, alpha-1-antitrypsin and alpha-1-antichymotrypsin in the normal and pathological gall bladder. Virchows Arch [A] 403:281, 1984

Asa SL, Kovacs K, Bilbao JM, et al. Immunohistochemical localization of keratin in craniopharyngiomas and squamous cell nests of the human pituitary. Acta Neuropathol 54:257, 1981a

Asa SL, Kovacs K, Bilbao JM. The pars tuberalis of the human pituitary. A histologic, immunohistochemical, ultrastructural and immunoelectron microscopic analysis. Virchows Arch [A] 399:49, 1981b

Asa SL, Kovacs K, Killinger DW, et al. Pancreatic islet cell carcinoma producing gastrin, ACTH, alpha-endorphin, somatostatin and calcitonin. Am J Gastroenterol 74:30, 1980

Asa SL, Penz G, Kovacs K, et al. Prolactin cells in the human pituitary. A quantitative immunocytochemical analysis. Arch Pathol Lab Med 106:360, 1982

Asa SL, Ryan N, Kovacs K, et al. Immunohistochemical localization of neuron-specific enolase in the human hypophysis and pituitary adenomas. Arch Pathol Lab Med 108:40, 1984

Ashall F, Bramwell ME, Harris H. A new marker for human cancer cells. 1. The Ca antigen and the CA1 antibody. Lancet 2:1, 1982

Askew AR, Grant BJ, Vinik AI. G cells and gastrin release from human antral mucosa in vitro. Aust NZ J Surg 50:317, 1980

Asou H, Brunngraber Eg, Jeng I. Cellular localization of GM1-ganglioside with biotinylated choleragen and avidin peroxidase in primary cultured cells from rat brain. J Histochem Cytochem 31:1375, 1983

Astarita RW, Minckler D, Taylor CR, et al. Orbital and adnexal lymphomas: a multiparameter approach. Am J Clin Pathol 73:615, 1980

Atack JR, Perry EK, Bonham JR, et al. Molecular forms of acetylcholinesterase in senile dementia of Alzheimer type: selective loss of the intermediate (10S) form. Neurosci Lett 40:199, 1983

Atkinson BF, Ernst CS, Herlyn M, et al. Gastrointestinal cancer-associated antigen in immunoperoxidase assay. Cancer Res 42:4820, 1982

Au FC, Stein BS, Gennaro AR, et al. Tissue CEA in colorectal carcinoma. Dis Colon Rectum 27:16, 1984

Auer RN, Becker LE. Cerebral medulloepithelioma with bone, cartilage, and striated muscle: light microscopic and immunohistochemical study. J Neuropathol Exp Neurol 42:256, 1983

Aufdemonte TB, Humphrey DM. Immunoperoxidase characterization of a malignant plasma cell tumor involving the mandible. J Oral Maxillofac Surg 40:197, 1982

Autilio-Gambetti L, Sipple J, Sudilovsky O, et al. Intermediate filaments of Schwann cells. J Neurochem 38:774, 1982

Avagnina MA, Elsner B, López SS, et al. Demostración de antígeno carcinoembrionario en tumores benignos y malignos colónicos con el método de inmunoperoxidasa. Medicina 40:375, 1980

Avrameas S. Coupling of enzymes to proteins with glutaraldehyde. Use of the conjugates for the detection of antigens and antibodies. Immunochemistry 6:43, 1969

Avrameas S. Studies on antibody formation with enzyme markers. Ann NY Acad Sci 254:175, 1975

Avrameas S, Ternynck T, Guesdon JL. Coupling of enzymes to antibodies and antigens. Scand J Immunol 8:7, 1978

Azar HA, Espinoza CG, Richman AV, et al. "Undifferentiated" large cell malignancies: an ultrastructural and immunocytochemical study. Hum Pathol 13:323, 1982

Azar HA, Jaffe ES, Berard CW, et al. Diffuse large cell lymphomas (reticulum cell sarcomas, histiocytic lymphomas). Correlation of morphologic features with functional markers. Cancer 46:1428, 1980

Azer PC, Braunstein GD, Van de Velde RL, et al. Ectopic production of pregnancy-specific beta 1-glycoprotein by a nontrophoblastic tumor in vitro. J Clin Endocrinol Metab 50:234, 1980

Azumi N, Shibuya H, Ishikura M. Primary prostatic carcinoid tumor with intracytoplasmic prostatic acid phosphatase and prostate-specific antigen. Am J Surg Pathol 8:545, 1984

Bailey AJ, Sloane JP, Trickey BS, et al. An immunocytochemical study of alpha-lactalbumin in human breast tissue. J Pathol 137:13, 1982

Balázs L. [Intracellular immunoglobulins in lymphogranulomatosis (Hungarian; Engl. abstr).] Morphol Igazsagugyi Orv Sz 21:59, 1981

Balázs L, Kelenyi G. [Intracellular immunoglobulins in lymphogranulomatosis. (German; Engl. abstr.)] Folia Haematol 107:621, 1980

Banerjee D, Pettit S. Endogenous avidin-binding activity in human lymphoid tissue. J Clin Pathol 37:223, 1984

Banks PM. Diagnostic applications of an immunoperoxidase method in hematopathology. J Histochem Cytochem 27:1192, 1979

Banks PM, Long JC, Howard CA. Preparation of lymph node biopsy specimens. Hum Pathol 10:617, 1979

Banks-Schlegel SP, McDowell EM, Wilson TS, et al. Keratin proteins in human lung carcinomas. Combined use of morphology, keratin immunocytochemistry, and keratin immunoprecipitation. Am J Pathol 114:273, 1984

Bannatyne P, Russell P, Wills EJ. Argyrophilia and endometrial carcinoma. Int J Gynecol Pathol 2:235, 1983

Barr RJ, Sun NC, King DF. Immunoperoxidase staining of cytoplasmic immunoglobulins. A diagnostic aid in distinguishing cutaneous reactive lymphoid hyperplasia from malignant lymphoma. J Am Acad Dermatol 3:58, 1980

Barry JD, Koch TJ, Cohen C, et al. Correlation of immunohistochemical markers with patient prognosis in breast carcinoma: a quantitative study. Am J Clin Pathol 82:582, 1984

Bartl R, Frisch B, Burkhardt R, et al. Bone-marrow histology in myeloma—its importance in diagnosis, prognosis, classification and staging. Br J Haematol 51:361, 1982

Baskin DG, Erlandsen WL, Parsons JA. Immunochemistry with osmium-fixed tissue. I. Light microscopic localization of growth hormone and prolactin with the unlabeled antibody-enzyme method. J Histochem Cytochem 27:867, 1979

Baskin DG, Mar H, Gorray KC, et al. Electron microscopic immunoperoxidase staining of insulin using 4-chloro-1-naphthol after osmium fixation. J Histochem Cytochem 30:710, 1982

Basle M, Rebel A, Pouplard A, et al. [Viral origin of Paget's disease of bone. Contribution of electron microscopy and immunocytology to the aetiological diagnosis.] Nouv Presse Med 10:1193, 1981

Basten A, Miller JF, Loblay R, et al. T cell–dependent suppression of antibody production. I. Characteristics of suppressor T cells following tolerance induction. Eur J Immunol 8:360, 1978

Bates RJ, Chapman CM, Prout GR Jr, et al. Immunohistochemical identification of prostatic acid phosphatase: correlation of tumor grade with acid phosphatase distribution. J Urol 127:574, 1982

Battifora H. Recent progress in the immunohistochemistry of solid tumors. Sem Diag Pathol 1:251, 1984

Battifora H, Kopinski MI. Distinction of mesothelioma from adenocarcinoma. An immunohistochemical approach. Cancer 55:1679, 1985

Bauer TW, Mendelsohn G, Humphrey RL, et al. Angioimmunoblastic lymphadenopathy progressing to immunoblastic lymphoma with prominent gastric involvement. Cancer 50:2089, 1982

Beal MF, Mazurek MF, Tran VT, et al. Reduced numbers of somatostatin receptors in the cerebral cortex in Alzheimer's disease. Science 229:289, 1985

Beauvillain JC, Tramu G. Immunocytochemical demonstration of LH-RH, somatostatin, and ACTH-like peptide in osmium-postfixed, resin-embedded median eminence. J Histochem Cytochem 28:1014, 1980

Beck DW, Hart MN, Cancilla PA. The role of the macrophage in microvascular regeneration following brain injury. J Neuropathol Exp Neurol 42:601, 1983

Becker GJ, Hancock WW, Kraft N, et al. Monoclonal antibodies to human macrophage and leucocyte common antigens. Pathology 13:669, 1981

Becker GL Jr, Knep S, Lance KP, et al. Amebic abscess of the brain. Neurosurgery 6:192, 1980

Becker KL, Nash D, Silva OL, et al. Increased serum and urinary calcitonin levels in patients with pulmonary disease. Chest 79:211, 1981

Beckstead JH, Halverson PS, Ries CA, et al. Enzyme histochemistry and immunohistochemistry on biopsy specimens of pathologic human bone marrow. Blood 57:1088, 1981

Beckstead JH, Wood GS, Turner RR. Histiocytosis X cells and Langerhans cells: enzyme histochemical and immunologic similarities. Hum Pathol 15:826, 1984

Beckwith JB, Martin RF. Observations on the histopathology of neuroblastomas. J Pediatr Surg 3:106, 1968

Beilby JO, Horne CH, Milne GD, et al. Alpha-fetoprotein, alpha-1-antitrypsin, and transferrin in gonadal yolk-sac tumours. J Clin Pathol 32:455, 1979

Bejui-Thivolet F, Viac J, Thivolet J, et al. Intracellular keratins in normal and pathological bronchial mucosa. Immunocytochemical studies on biopsies and cell suspensions. Virchows Arch [A] 395:87, 1982

Bell DA, Flotte TJ. Factor VIII related antigen in adenomatoid tumors: implications for histogenesis. Cancer 50:932, 1982

Bellet D, Arrang JM, Contesso G, et al. Localization of the beta subunit of human chorionic gonadotrophin on various tumors. Eur J Cancer 16:433, 1980

Bellomi A, Gamoletti R. Malignant histiocytic tumour presenting as a primary uterine neoplasm: a cytochemical and electron microscopy study. J Pathol 134:233, 1981

Bender BL, Jaffe R. Immunoglobulin production in lymphomatoid granulomatosis and relation to other "benign" lymphoproliferative disorders. Am J Clin Pathol 73:41, 1980

Bendheim PE, Barry RA, DeArmond SJ, et al. Antibodies to a scrapie prion protein. Nature 310:418, 1984

Benjamin DR, Ray CG. Use of immunoperoxidase on brain tissue for the rapid diagnosis of herpes encephalitis. Am J Clin Pathol 64:472, 1975

Bennett BD, Bailey J, Gardner WA Jr. Immunocytochemical identification of trichomonads. Arch Pathol Lab Med 104:247, 1980

Bentz MS, Cohen C, Budgeon LR, et al. Evaluation of commercial immunoperoxidase kits in diagnosis of prostate carcinoma. Urology 23:75, 1984

Bentz MS, Cohen C, Demers LM, et al. Immunohistochemical acid phosphatase level and tumor grade in prostatic carcinoma. Arch Pathol Lab Med 106:476, 1982

Berger G, Berger F, Bejui F, et al. Bronchial carcinoid with fibrillary inclusions related to cytokeratins: an immunohistochemical and ultrastructural study with subsequent investigation of 12 foregut APUDomas. Histopathology 8:245, 1984a

Berger G, Trouillas J, Bloch B, et al. Multihormonal

carcinoid tumor of the pancreas: secreting growth hormone–releasing factor as a cause of acromegaly. Cancer 54:2097, 1984b

Bergholz M, Bartsch HH, Krueger GR, et al. Angioimmunoblastic lymphadenopathy and persistent virus infection: Discussion of immunohistological findings on two cases. (German; Engl Abstr). Klin Wochenschr 57:1317, 1979

Bergroth V, Reitamo S, Konttinen T, et al. Sensitivity and nonspecific staining of various immunoperoxidase techniques. Histochemistry 68:17, 1980

Bergroth V, Reitamo S, Konttinen YT, et al. Fixation-dependent cytoplasmic false-positive staining with an immunoperoxidase method. Histochemistry 73:509, 1982

Berkowitz RS, Alberti O Jr, Hunter NJ, et al. Localization of stage-specific embryonic antigens in hydatidiform mole, normal placenta, and gestational choriocarcinoma. Gynecol Oncol 20:71, 1985

Berman JW, Basch RS. Amplification of the biotin-avidin immunofluorescence technique. J Immunol Meth 36:335, 1980

Bernard A, Boumsell L, Dausett J, et al. Leucocyte typing. In: Proceedings of the First International Reference Workshop, New York, Springer-Verlag, 1984

Bernard D, Maurizis JC, Rusé F, et al. Presence of HLAD/DR antigens on the membrane of breast tumour cells. Clin Exp Immunol 56:215, 1984

Berry N, Jones DB, Smallwood J, et al. The prognostic value of the monoclonal antibodies HMFG1 and HMFG2 in breast cancer. Br J Cancer 51:179, 1985

Bhagavan BS, Dorfman HD, Murthy MS, et al. Intravascular bronchiolo-alveolar tumor (IVBAT): a low-grade sclerosing epithelioid angiosarcoma of the lung. Am J Surg Pathol 6:41, 1982

Bhan AK, DesMarais CL. Immunohistologic characterization of major histocompatibility antigens and inflammatory cellular infiltrate in human breast cancer. J Natl Cancer Inst 71:507, 1983

Bhan AK, Reinherz EL, Poppema S, et al. Location of T cell and major histocompatibility complex antigens in the human thymus. J Exp Med 152:771, 1980

Bhattacharya M, Chatterjee SK, Barlow JJ. Identification of a human cancer-associated antigen defined with monoclonal antibody. Cancer Res 44:4528, 1984

Biberfeld P, Ghetie V, Sjöquist J. Demonstration and assaying of IgG antibodies in tissues and on cells by labelled staphylococcal protein A. J Immunol Meth 6:249, 1975

Biberfeld P, Mellstedt H, Pettersson D. Immunocytochemical studies of human myeloma cells by light and electron microscopy. Isr J Med Sci 15:687, 1979

Bigbee JW, Kosek JC, Eng LF. Effects of primary antiserum dilution on staining of "antigen rich" tissues with the peroxidase-antiperoxidase technique. J Histochem Cytochem 25:443, 1977

Biggs PJ, Powers JM. Neuroblastic medulloblastoma with abundant cytoplasmic actin filaments. Arch Pathol Lab Med 108:326, 1984

Bignami A, Raju T, Dahl D. Localization of vimentin, the nonspecific intermediate filament protein, in embryonal glia and in early differentiating neurons. In vivo and in vitro immunofluorescence study of the rat embryo with vimentin and neurofilament antisera. Dev Biol 91:286, 1982

Bignami A, Selkoe DJ, Dahl D. Amyloid-like (congophilic) neurofibrillary tangles do not react with neurofilament antisera in Alzheimer's cerebral cortex. Acta Neuropathol (Berl) 64:243, 1984

Björklund V, Björklund B, Wittekind C, et al. Immunohistochemical localization of tissue polypeptide antigen (TPA) and carcino-embryonic antigen (CEA) in breast cancer. A comparative study. Acta Pathol Microbiol Immunol Scand [A] 90:471, 1982

Bjornsson J, Scheithauer BW, Okazaki H, et al. Intracranial germ cell tumors: pathobiological and immunohistochemical aspects of 70 cases. J Neuropathol Exp Neurol 44:32, 1985

Blobel G, Moll R, Franke W, et al. The intermediate filament cytoskeleton of malignant mesotheliomas and its diagnostic significance. Am J Pathol 121:235, 1985

Block M. Bone marrow examination. Aspiration of core biopsy, smear or section, hematoxylin-eosin or Romanowsky stain—which combination? Arch Pathol Lab Med 100:454, 1976

Blue MC, Rosenblum WI. Granulomatous angiitis of the brain with herpes zoster and varicella encephalitis. Arch Pathol Lab Med 107:126, 1983

Blum HE, Haase AT, Vyas GN. Molecular pathogenesis of hepatitis B virus infection: simultaneous detection of viral DNA and antigens in paraffin-embedded liver sections. Lancet 2:771, 1984

Böcker W, Dralle H, Dorn G. Thyroglobulin: an immunohistochemical marker in thyroid disease. In: Diagnostic Immunohistochemistry. DeLellis RA, ed. Masson Monographs in Diagnostic Pathology. Sternberg SS, series ed. New York, Masson 1981, p 37

Bockman JM, Kingsbury DT, McKinley MP, et al. Creutzfeldt-Jakob disease proteins in human brains. N Engl J Med 312:73, 1985

Boenisch T. Reference Guide to Immunoperoxidase Techniques: A Manual and Bibliography. Dako Corporation, 22 N Milpas, Santa Barbara, Calif, 1980

Bogomoletz WV, Bernard J, Capron F, et al. T-cell origin of Lennert's lymphoma. Immunohistochemical and immunologic study of one case. Arch Pathol Lab Med 107:586, 1983

Böhling T, Paetau A, Ekblom P, et al. Distribution of endothelial and basement membrane markers in angiogenic tumors of the nervous system. Acta Neuropathol (Berl) 62:67, 1983

Bohn W. Electron microscopic immunoperoxidase studies on the accumulation of virus antigen in cells infected with Shope fibroma virus. J Gen Virol 46:439, 1980

Bollum FJ. Antibody to terminal deoxynucleotidyl transferase. Proc Natl Acad Sci USA 72:4119, 1975

Bollum FJ, Hassur S, Chang LMS. The limited localization and conserved structure of terminal deoxynucleotidyl transferase. In: Knapp W, ed. Leukemia Markers. Academic Press, 1981, p 33

Bolton EM, Thompson JF, Wood RF, et al. Immunoperoxidase staining of fine-needle aspiration biopsies and needle core biopsies from renal allografts. Transplantation 36:728, 1983

Bonetti F, Chilosi M, Pisa R, et al. Epithelial membrane antigen expression in cholangiocarcinoma. A useful immunohistochemical tool for differential diagnosis with hepatocarcinoma. Virchows Arch [A] 401:307, 1983

Bonnin JM, Rubinstein LJ. Immunohistochemistry of central nervous system tumors. Its contributions to neurosurgical diagnosis. J Neurosurg 60:1121, 1984

Bonnin JM, Rubinstein LJ, Papasozomenos SC, et al. Subependymal giant cell astrocytoma. Significance and possible cytogenic implications of an immunohistochemical study. Acta Neuropathol (Berl) 62:185, 1984

Boorsma DM, Streefkerk JG. Periodate or glutaraldehyde for preparing peroxidase conjugates? J Immunol Meth 30:245, 1979

Booss J, Esiri MM, Tourtellotte WW, et al. Immunohistological analysis of T lymphocyte subsets in the central nervous system in chronic progressive multiple sclerosis. J Neurol Sci 62:219, 1983

Borges M. The cytochemical application of new potent inhibitors of alkaline phosphatases. J Histochem Cytochem 21:812, 1973

Borit A, McIntosh GC. Myelin basic protein and glial fibrillary acidic protein in human fetal brain. Neuropathol Appl Neurobiol 7:279, 1981

Borit A, Yung A. Glial fibrillary acidic protein (GFAP) and vimentin in brain tumors. J Neuropathol Exp Neurol 42:308, 1983

Boros L, Bhaskar AG, D'Souza JP. Monoclonal evolution of angioimmunoblastic lymphadenopathy. Am J Clin Pathol 75:856, 1981

Borowitz MJ, Croker BP, Metzgar RS. Immunohistochemical analysis of the distribution of lymphocyte subpopulations in Hodgkin's disease. Cancer Treat Rep 66:667, 1982

Borowitz MJ, Croker BP, Metzgar RS. Lymphoblastic lymphoma with the phenotype of common acute lymphoblastic leukemia. Am J Clin Pathol 79:387, 1983

Borowitz MJ, Tuck FL, Sindelar WF, et al. Monoclonal antibodies against human pancreatic adenocarcinoma: distribution of DU-PAN-2 antigen on glandular epithelia and adenocarcinomas. J Natl Cancer Inst 72:999, 1984

Borthwick NM, Gordon A, Yates CM. Reductions in soluble brain proteins in older subjects with Down's syndrome. J Neurol Sci 68:205, 1985a

Borthwick NM, Yates CM, Gordon A. Reduced proteins in temporal cortex in Alzheimer's disease: an electrophoretic study. J Neurochem 44:1436, 1985b

Bos JD, Sillevis Smitt JH, Krieg SR, et al. Acute disseminated histiocytosis-X: in situ immunophenotyping with monoclonal antibodies. J Cutan Pathol 11:59, 1984

Bosman FT, Cramer-Knijnenburg G, van Bergen Henegouw J. A simplified method for the rapid preparation of peroxidase-antiperoxidase (PAP) complexes. Histochemistry 67:243, 1980a

Bosman FT, Giard RW, Nieuwenhuijzen Kruseman AC, et al. Human chorionic gonadotrophin and alphafetoprotein in testicular germ cell tumours: a retrospective immunohistochemical study. Histopathology 4:673, 1980b

Bosman FT, Lindeman J, Kuiper G, et al. The influence of fixation on immunoperoxidase staining of plasma cells in paraffin sections of intestinal biopsy specimens. Histochemistry 53:57, 1977

Bosman FT, Louwerens JW. Neuroendocrine (APUD) cells in ovarian teratomas and testicular teratocarcinomas. Cell Biol Int Rep 5:464, 1981

Bosman FT, Nieuwenhuijzen Kruseman AC. Clinical applications of the enzyme labeled antibody method. Immunoperoxidase methods in diagnostic histopathology. J Histochem Cytochem 27:1140, 1979

Bostwick DG, Roth KA, Barchas JD, et al. Gastrin-releasing peptide immunoreactivity in intestinal carcinoids. Am J Clin Pathol 82:428, 1984

Boumsell L, Bernard A, Reinherz EL, et al. Surface antigens on malignant Sezary and T-CLL cells correspond to those of mature T cells. Blood 57:526, 1981

Bowen DM, Smith CB, White P, et al. Neurotransmitter-related enzymes and indices of hypoxia in senile dementia and other abiotrophies. Brain 99:459, 1976.

Bowes D, Clark AE, Corrin B. Ultrastructural localisation of lactoferrin and glycoprotein in human bronchial glands. Thorax 36:108, 1981

Bowling MC. Lymph node specimens: achieving technical excellence. Lab Med 10:467, 1979

Boxer ME. Cardiac myxoma: an immunoperoxidase study of histogenesis. Histopathology 8:861, 1984

Boyd JF. Immunohistochemical staining of the Dutcher-Fahey intranuclear inclusion body in a case of Waldenström's macroglobulinemia. J Pathol 132:81, 1980

Boyd JF, McWilliams E. Immunoperoxidase staining of *Legionella pneumophila*. Histopathology 6:191, 1982

Boyer RS, Sun NC, Verity A, et al. Immunoperoxidase staining of the choroid plexus in systemic lupus erythematosus. J Rheumatol 7:645, 1980

Brabon AC, Williams JF, Cardiff RD. A monoclonal antibody to a human breast tumor protein released in response to estrogen. Cancer Res 44:2704, 1984

Bramwell ME, Bhavanandan VP, Wiseman G, et al. Structure and function of the Ca antigen. Br J Cancer 48:177, 1983

Brandtzaeg P. Mucosal and glandular distribution of immunoglobulin components. Immunohistochemistry with cold ethanol-fixation technique. Immunology 26:1101, 1974

Brandtzaeg P. Structural, functional and cellular studies of human J chain. Ric Clin Lab (Suppl 3) 6:15, 1976a

Brandtzaeg P. Studies on J chain and binding site for secretory component in circulating human B cells. II. The cytoplasm. Clin Exp Immunol 25:59, 1976b

Brandtzaeg P. Prolonged incubation time in immunohistochemistry: effects on fluorescence staining of immunoglobulins and epithelial components in ethanol- and formaldehyde-fixed paraffin-embedded tissues. J Histochem Cytochem 29:1302, 1981

Braylan RC, Rappaport H. Tissue immunoglobulins in nodular lymphomas as compared with reactive follicular hyperplasias. Blood 42:579, 1973

Braziel RM, Keneklis T, Donlon JA, et al. Terminal deoxynucleotidyl transferase in non-Hodgkin's lymphoma. Am J Clin Pathol 80:655, 1983

Breathnach SM, Melrose SM, Bhogal B, et al. Immunohistochemical studies of amyloid P component in disorders of cutaneous elastic tissue. Br J Dermatol 107:443, 1982

Brierley JB, Brown AW. The origin of lipid phagocytes in the central nervous system: I. The intrinsic microglia. J Comp Neurol 211:397, 1982

Briggs RC, Montiel MM, Wojtkowiak Z. Nuclear localization of lactoferrin in the human granulocyte: artifact incurred during slide preparation. J Histochem Cytochem 31:1157, 1983

Brisbane JU, Lessell S, Finkel HE, et al. Malignant lymphoma presenting in the orbit: a clinicopathologic study of a rare immunoglobulin-producing variant. Cancer 47:548, 1981

Britton CB, Mesa-Tejada R, Fenoglio CM, et al. A new complication of AIDS: thoracic myelitis caused by herpes simplex virus. Neurology 35:1071, 1985

Bröcker EB, Suter L, Sorg C. HLA-DR antigen expression in primary melanomas of the skin. J Invest Dermatol 82:244, 1984

Brodal A. Anterograde and retrograde degeneration of nerve cells in the central nervous system. In: Haymaker W, Adams RD, eds. Histology and Histopathology of the Nervous System, Vol I. Springfield, Ill., Charles C Thomas, p 276, 1982

Broder S, Edelson R, Lutzner M, et al. The Sezary syndrome. A malignant proliferation of helper T cells. J Clin Invest 58:1297, 1976

Brodsky FM, Parham P, Barnstable CJ, et al. Monoclonal antibodies for analysis of the HLA system. Immunol Rev 47:3, 1979

Broers J, Huysmans A, Moesker O, et al. Small cell lung cancers contain intermediate filaments of the cytokeratin type. Lab Invest 52:113, 1985

Brooks JJ. Immunohistochemistry of soft tissue tumors. Myoglobin as a tumor marker for rhabdomyosarcoma. Cancer 50:1757, 1982

Brooks JJ, Ernst CS. Immunoreactive secretory component of IgA in human tissues and tumors. Am J Clin Pathol 82:660, 1984

Brooks JSJ, Freeman M, Enterline HT. Malignant "Triton" tumors: natural history and immunohistochemistry of nine new cases with literature review. Cancer 55:2543, 1985

Brouet JC, Mason DY, Danon F, et al. Alpha-chain disease: evidence for common clonal origin of intestinal immunoblastic lymphoma and plasmacytic proliferation. Lancet 1:861, 1977

Brown G, Biberfeld P, Christensson B, et al. The distribution of HLA on human lymphoid, bone marrow and peripheral blood cells. Eur J Immunol 9:272, 1979

Brown JP, Nishiyama K, Hellstrom I, et al. Structural characterization of human melanoma-associated antigen with monoclonal antibodies. J Immunol 127:539, 1981a

Brown JP, Woodbury RG, Head CE, et al. Quantitative analysis of melanoma-associated antigen in normal and neoplastic tissues. Proc Natl Acad Sci USA 78:539, 1981b

Brown WR. Neoplastic human colon cells in studies on the translocation of dimeric IgA. Cancer (Suppl 5) 45:1234, 1980

Brubaker DB, Whiteside TL. Localization of human T lymphocytes in tissue sections by a rosetting technique. Am J Pathol 88:323, 1977

Brun A, Jonsson N. Angiosarcomas in hamsters after inoculation of brain tissue from a case of progressive multifocal leukoencephalopathy. Cancer 53:1714, 1984

Bruner JM, Humphreys JH, Armstrong DL. Immunocytochemistry of recurring intracerebral nerve sheath tumor. J Neuropathol Exp Neurol 43:296, 1984

Bryant MG, Buchan AM, Gregor M, et al. Development of intestinal regulatory peptides in the human fetus. Gastroenterology 83:47, 1982

Brynes RK, McKenna RW, Sundberg RD. Bone marrow aspiration and trephine biopsy. An approach to a thorough study. Am J Clin Pathol 70:753, 1978

Buchan AM, Polak JM. The classification of the human gastroenteropancreatic endocrine cells. Invest Cell Pathol 3:51, 1980

Budka H. Hyaline inclusions (pseudopsammoma bodies) in meningiomas: immunocytochemical demonstration of epithel-like secretion of secretory component and immunoglobulins A and M. Acta Neuropathol 56:294, 1982

Budka H, Lassmann H, Popow-Kraupp T. Measles virus antigen in panencephalitis. An immunomorphological study stressing dendritic involvement in SSPE. Acta Neuropathol 56:52, 1982

Budka H, Majdic O, Knapp W. Monoclonal antibodies

raised against hemopoietic cells: crossreactivity with nervous tissues and tumors. J Neuropathol Exp Neurol 43:300, 1984

Budka H, Popow-Kraupp T. Rabies and herpes simplex virus encephalitis. An immunohistological study on site and distribution of viral antigens. Virchows Arch [Pathol Anat] 390:353, 1981

Budka H, Shah KV. Papova viral antigens in PML brains. J Neuropathol Exp Neurol 41:366, 1982

Bulman AS, Heyderman E. Alkaline phosphatase for immunocytochemical labelling: problems with endogenous enzyme activity. J Clin Pathol 34:1349, 1981

Bunn PA Jr, Linnoila I, Minna JD, et al. Small cell lung cancer, endocrine cells of the fetal bronchus, and other neuroendocrine cells express the Leu-7 antigenic determinant present on natural killer cells. Blood 65:764, 1985

Burchiel KJ, Shaw C-M, Kelly WA. A mixed functional microadenoma and ganglioneuroma of the pituitary fossa. Case report. J Neurosurg 58:416, 1983

Burgdorf WH, Duray P, Rosai J. Immunohistochemical identification of lysozyme in cutaneous lesions of alleged histiocytic nature. Am J Clin Pathol 75:162, 1981b

Burgdorf WH, Mukai K, Rosai J. Immunohistochemical identification of factor VIII-related antigen in endothelial cells of cutaneous lesions of alleged vascular nature. Am J Clin Pathol 75:167, 1981a

Burns BF, Warnke RA, Doggett RS, et al. Expression of a T-cell antigen (Leu-1) by B-cell lymphomas. Am J Pathol 113:165, 1983

Burns J. Background staining and sensitivity of the unlabelled antibody-enzyme (PAP) method: comparison with the peroxidase labelled antibody sandwich method using formalin fixed paraffin embedded material. Histochemistry 43:291, 1975

Burns J, Dixon AJ, Woods JC. Immunoperoxidase localisation of fibronectin in glomeruli of formalin fixed paraffin processed renal tissue. Histochemistry 67:73, 1980

Burns J, Hambridge M, Taylor CR. Intracellular immunoglobulins. A comparative study of three standard tissue processing methods using horseradish peroxidase and fluorochrome conjugates. J Clin Pathol 27:548, 1974

Burns JC. Diagnostic methods for herpes simplex infection: a review. Oral Surg 50:346, 1980

Burt A, Goudie RB. Diagnosis of primary thyroid carcinoma by immunohistological demonstration of thyroglobulin. Histopathology 3:279, 1979

Burtin P, Calmettes C, Fondaneche MC. CEA and nonspecific cross-reacting antigen (NCA) in medullary carcinomas of the thyroid. Int J Cancer 23:741, 1979

Busachi CA, Ray MB, Desmet VJ. An immunoperoxidase technique for demonstrating membrane localized HBsAg in paraffin sections of liver biopsies. J Immunol Meth 19:95, 1978

Bussolati G, Alfani V, Weber K, et al. Immunocytochemical detection of actin on fixed and embedded tissues: its potential use in routine pathology. J Histochem Cytochem 28:169, 1980a

Bussolati G, Botta G, Gugliotta P. Actin-rich (myoepithelial) cells in ductal carcinoma-in-situ of the breast. Virchows Arch [B] 34:251, 1980b

Bussolati G, Papotti M, Sapino A. Binding of antibodies against human prealbumin to intestinal and bronchial carcinoids and to pancreatic endocrine tumours. Virchows Arch [B] 45:15, 1984

Butenandt O, Knorr D, Hecker WC, et al. Precocious

puberty in a boy with LCG-producing hepatoma. Case report. Helv Paediatr Acta 35:155, 1980

Cabral GA, Marciano-Cabral F, Fry D, Lumpkin CK, Mercer L, Goplerud D. Expression of herpes simplex virus type 2 antigens in premalignant and malignant human vulvar cells. Am J Obstet Gynecol 143:611, 1982

Caillaud JM, Bellett D. [Immunoperoxidase study of 80 germ cell tumours of the testis in adults.] Nouv Presse Med 10:1057, 1981

Caillaud JM, Bellet D, Arrang JM. Essai de mise un évidence de la beta H.C.G. dans des tumeurs testiculaires germinales de l'adulte par une méthode d'immunopéroxidase indirecte. Ann Anat Pathol 24:193, 1979

Caillaud JM, Benjelloun S, Bosq J, Braham K, Lipinski M. HNK-1–defined antigen detected in paraffin-embedded neuroectoderm tumors and those derived from cells of the amine precursor uptake and decarboxylation system. Cancer Res 44:4432, 1984

Callihan TR, Jaffe ES. Identification of crystalline deposits. Arch Ophthalmol 98:386, 1980

Camilleri JP, Hinglais N, Bruneval P, Bariety J, Tricottet V, Rouchon M, Mancilla-Jimenez R, Corvol P, Menard J. Renin storage and cell differentiation in juxtaglomerular cell tumors: an immunohistochemical and ultrastructural study of three cases. Hum Pathol 15:1069, 1984

Campbell GT, Bhatnagar AS. Simultaneous visualization by light microscopy of two pituitary hormones in a single tissue section using a combination of indirect immunohistochemical methods. J Histochem Cytochem 24:448, 1976

Campbell JA, Bass NM, Kirsch RE. Immunohistological localization of ligandin in human tissues. Cancer 45:503, 1980

Canale DD Jr, Collins RD. Use of bone marrow particle sections in the diagnosis of multiple myeloma. Am J Clin Pathol 61:382, 1974

Candy JM, Oakley AE, Perry EK, et al. Existence in vitro of fibrillary aggregates of substance P, cholecystokinin octapeptide, somatostatin and related molecules. J Physiol (Lond) 32:112P, 1981

Capella C, Cornaggia M, Usellini L, et al. Neoplastic cells containing lysozyme in gastric carcinomas. Pathology 16:87, 1984

Carbone A, Micheau C. Pitfalls in microscopic diagnosis of undifferentiated carcinoma of nasopharyngeal type (lymphoepithelioma). Cancer 50:1344, 1982

Carbone A, Micheau C, Caillaud JM, A cytochemical and immunohistochemical approach to malignant histiocytosis. Cancer 47:2862, 1981

Cardiff RD, Taylor CR, Wellings SR, et al. Monoclonal antibodies in immunoenzyme studies of breast cancer. Ann NY Acad Sci 420:140, 1983

Carlei F, Polak JM, Ceccamea A, et al. Neuronal and glial markers in tumours of neuroblastic origin. Virchows Arch [A] 404:313, 1984

Carlo JR, Ruddy S, Conway AF. Localization of the receptors for activated complement on the visceral epithelial cells by the human renal glomerulus by immunoenzymatic microscopy. Am J Clin Pathol 75:23, 1981

Carmichael GP, Lee YT. Granulocytic sarcoma simulating "nonsecretory" multiple myeloma. Hum Pathol 6:697, 1977

Carr I, Carr J, Trew JA, et al. Lysozyme production by a granuloma in vivo: output in blood and lymph in

relation to ultrastructure and immunochemistry. J Pathol 132:105, 1980

Carrel S, Schreyer M, Schmidt-Kessen A, et al. Reactivity spectrum of 30 monoclonal antimelanoma antibodies to a panel of 28 melanoma and control cell lines. Hybridoma 1:387, 1982

Caselitz J, Löning T, Seifert G. An approach to stain actin in parotid gland cells in paraffin-embedded material. Staining by human anti-actin antibodies using the indirect unlabeled immunoperoxidase technique. Virchows Arch [A] 387:301, 1980

Caselitz J, Löning T, Staquet MJ, et al. Immunocytochemical demonstration of filamentous structures in the parotid gland. Occurrence of keratin and actin in normal and tumoral parotid gland with special respect to the myoepithelial cells. J Cancer Res Clin Oncol 100:59, 1981a

Caselitz J, Seifert G, Jaup T. Presence of carcinoembryonic antigen (CEA) in the normal and inflamed human parotid gland. An immunohistochemical study of 31 cases. J Cancer Res Clin Oncol 100:205, 1981b

Casper S, van Nagell JR Jr, Powell DF, et al. Immunohistochemical localization of tumor markers in epithelial ovarian cancer. Am J Obstet Gynecol 149:154, 1984

Castro A, Buschbaum P, Nadji M, et al. Immunochemical demonstration of human chorionic gonadotrophin (hCG) in tissue of breast carcinoma. Acta Endocrinol 94:511, 1980a

Castro A, Ziegels-Weissman J, Buschbaum P, et al. Immunochemical demonstration of immunoreactive insulin in human breast cancer. Res Commun Chem Pathol Pharmacol 29:171, 1980b

Cebelin MS, Velasco ME, de las Mulas JM, et al. Galactorrhea associated with lymphocytic adenohypophysitis. Case report. Br J Obstet Gynaecol 88:675, 1981

Cevenini R, Donati M, Moroni A, et al. Rapid immunoperoxidase assay for detection of respiratory syncytial virus in nasopharyngeal secretions. J Clin Microbiol 18:947, 1983

Chamness GC, Mercer WD, McGuire WL. Are histochemical methods for estrogen receptor valid? J Histochem Cytochem 28:792, 1980

Chapman CM, Allhoff EP, Proppe KH, et al. Use of monoclonal antibodies for the localization of tissue isoantigens A and B in transitional cell carcinoma of the upper urinary tract. J Histochem Cytochem 31:557, 1983

Charpin C, Andrac L, Monier-Faugere MC, et al. ·Calcitonin, somatostatin and ACTH immunoreactive cells in a case of familial bilateral thyroid medullary carcinoma. Cancer 50:1806, 1982a

Charpin C, Argemi B, Cannoni M, et al. [Immunohistochemical detection of calcitonin, ACTH, beta-MSH, beta-endorphin and somatostatin in medullary carcinoma of the thyroid. Immunoperoxidase study (PAP, ABC) of 10 cases.] Ann Pathol 4:27, 1984

Charpin C, Bhan AK, Zurawski VR Jr, et al. Carcinoembryonic antigen (CEA) and carbohydrate determinant 19-9 (CA 19-9) localization in 121 primary and metastatic ovarian tumors: an immunohistochemical study with the use of monoclonal antibodies. Int J Gynecol Pathol 1:231, 1982b

Charpin C, Hassoun J, Oliver C, et al. Immunohistochemical and immunoelectron-microscopic study of pituitary adenomas associated with Cushing's disease. A report of 13 cases. Am J Pathol 109:1, 1982c

Chase DR, Enzinger FM, Weiss SW, et al. Keratin in

epithelioid sarcoma. An immunohistochemical study. Am J Surg Pathol 8:435, 1984

Chasey D. A simple and rapid immunoperoxidase test for the detection of virus antigens in tissue culture. Vet Rec 106:506, 1980

Chasey D, Woods SB. Detection of immunoperoxidase labelled mycoplasmas in cell culture by light microscopy and electronmicroscopy. J Med Microbiol 17:23, 1984

Chechik BE, Rao J, Greaves MF, et al. Human thymus/leukaemia-associated antigen (a low-molecular weight form of adenosine deaminase) and the phenotype of leukaemic cells. Leuk Res 4:343, 1980

Chechik BE, Schrader WP, Minowada J. An immunomorphologic study of adenosine deaminase distribution in human thymus tissue, normal lymphocytes, and hematopoietic cell lines. J Immunol 126:1003, 1981

Chee DO, Yonemoto RH, Leong SP, et al. Mouse monoclonal antibody to a melanoma-carcinoma–associated antigen synthesized by a human melanoma cell line propagated in serum-free medium. Cancer Res 42:3142, 1982

Childs G, Unabia G. Application of the avidin-biotin-peroxidase complex (ABC) method to the light microscopic localization of pituitary hormones. J Histochem Cytochem 30:713, 1982

Childs GV, Ellison DG. A critique of the contributions of immunoperoxidase cytochemistry to our understanding of pituitary cell function, as illustrated by our current studies of gonadotropes, corticotropes and endogenous pituitary GnRH and TRH. Histochem J 12:405, 1980

Chilosi M, Iannucci AM, Pizzolo G, et al. Immunohistochemical analysis of thymoma. Evidence for medullary origin of epithelial cells. Am J Surg Pathol 8:309, 1984

Cho C, Linscheer WG, Bell R, et al. Colonic lymphoma producing alpha-chain disease protein. Gastroenterology 83:121, 1982

Choi BH, Kim RC. Expression of glial fibrillary acidic protein in immature oligodendroglia. Science 223:407, 1984

Choi BS, Kim RC, Lapham LW. Do radial glia give rise to both astroglial and oligodendroglial cells? Dev Brain Res 8:119, 1983

Choi H-SH, Anderson PJ. Immunohistochemical diagnosis of olfactory neuroblastoma. J Neuropathol Exp Neurol 44:18, 1985

Chowdhury C, Roy S, Mahapatra AK, et al. Medullomyoblastoma: a teratoma. Cancer 55:1495, 1985

Christensen AK, Wisner JR, Orth J. Preliminary observations on the localization of androgen and FSH receptors in the rat seminiferous tubule, studied by autoradiography at the light microscope level. In: The Testis in Normal and Infertile Men. Troen P, Nankin HR (eds). New York, Raven Press, 1977, p 153

Chu A, Eisinger M, Lee JS, et al. Immunoelectron microscopic identification of Langerhans cells using a new antigenic marker. J Invest Dermatol 78:177, 1982

Chu AC, MacDonald DM. Identification in situ of T lymphocytes in the dermal and epidermal infiltrates of mycosis fungoides. Br J Dermatol 100:177, 1979

Cibull ML, Coleman MS, Hutton JJ, et al. Unusual immunofluorescence patterns for terminal deoxynucleotidyl transferase in blast crisis chronic myelogenous leukemia. Am J Clin Pathol 75:363, 1981

Ciocca DR, Adams DJ, Bjercke RJ, et al. Immunohistochemical detection of an estrogen-regulated protein by monoclonal antibodies. Cancer Res 42:4256, 1982

Clark A, Grant AM. Quantitative morphology of endocrine cells in human fetal pancreas. Diabetologia 25:31, 1983

Clark ES, Carney JA. Pancreatic islet cell tumor associated with Cushing's syndrome. Am J Surg Pathol 8:917, 1984

Clarke SM, Merchant DJ, Starling JJ. Monoclonal antibodies against a soluble cytoplasmic antigen in human prostatic epithelial cells. Prostate 3:203, 1982

Claudy AL, Schmitt D, Viac J, et al. Morphological, immunological and immunocytochemical identification of lymphocytes extracted from cutaneous infiltrates. Clin Exp Immunol 23:61, 1976

Clausen PP. Immunohistochemical demonstration of alpha-1-antitrypsin in liver tissue. A methodological investigation. Acta Pathol Microbiol Scand [A] 88:299, 1980

Clausen PP, Jacobsen M, Johansen P, et al. Immunohistochemical demonstration of intracellular immunoglobulin in formalin fixed, paraffin embedded sections, as staining method in diagnostic work. Acta Pathol Microbiol Scand [C] 87:307, 1979

Clausen PP, Lindskov J, Gad I, Kreutzfeldt M, Orholm M, Reinicke V, Larsen HR, Strom P. The diagnostic value of alpha 1-antitrypsin globules in liver cells as a morphological marker of alpha 1-antitrypsin deficiency. Liver 4:353, 1984

Clausen PP, Møller AM, Praetorius Clausen P, et al. Methods for localization of hepatitis B surface antigen in liver tissue. An evaluation of different staining and tissue preparation methods. Acta Pathol Microbiol Immunol Scand [A] 91:329, 1983

Clausen PP, Thomsen P. Demonstration of hepatitis B-surface antigen in liver biopsies. A comparative investigation of immunoperoxidase and orcein staining on identical sections of formalin fixed, paraffin embedded tissue. Acta Pathol Microbiol Scand [A] 86A:383, 1978

Clayton F, Ordóñez NG, Hanssen GM, et al. Immunoperoxidase localization of lactalbumin in malignant breast neoplasms. Arch Pathol Lab Med 106:268, 1982

Clough DG, Coghill GR, Holley MP. Evaluation of the Ca 1 antibody in the diagnosis of invasive breast cancer. J Clin Pathol 37:10, 1984

Cochran AJ, Wen DR, Herschman HR, et al. Detection of S-100 protein as an aid to the identification of melanocytic tumors. Int J Cancer 30:295, 1982

Cochran AJ, Wen DR, Herschman HR. Occult melanoma in lymph nodes detected by antiserum to S-100 protein. Int J Cancer 34:159, 1984

Coffin CM, Mukai K, Dehner LP. Glial differentiation in medulloblastomas: histogenetic insight, glial reaction, or invasion of brain? Am J Surg Pathol 7:555, 1983

Cohen C, Berson SD, Budgeon LR. Alpha-1-antitrypsin deficiency in Southern African hepatocellular carcinoma patients. An immunoperoxidase and histochemical study. Cancer 49:2537, 1982a

Cohen C, Budgeon LR. Commercial immunoperoxidase kits in the study of 13 pancreatic islet-cell tumors. Am J Clin Pathol 78:364, 1982

Cohen C, Shulman G, Budgeon LR. Endocervical and endometrial adenocarcinoma: an immunoperoxidase and histochemical study. Am J Surg Pathol 6:151, 1982b

Cohen C, Shulman G, Budgeon LR. Immunohistochemical ferritin in testicular seminoma. Cancer 54:2190, 1984

Colcher D, Hand PH, Nuti M, et al. Differential binding to human mammary and nonmammary tumors of monoclonal antibodies reactive with carcinoembryonic antigen. Cancer Invest 1:127, 1983

Collings LA, Poulter LW, Janossy G. The demonstration of cell surface antigens on T cells, B cells and accessory cells in paraffin-embedded human tissues. J Immunol Methods 75:227, 1984

Collins RD, Waldron JA, Glick AD. Results of multiparameter studies of T cell lymphoid neoplasms. Am J Clin Pathol (Suppl 4) 72:699, 1979

Conley FK, Jenkins KA. Immunohistological study of the anatomic relationship of toxoplasma antigens to the inflammatory response in the brains of mice chronically infected with *Toxoplasma gondii*. Infect Immun 31:1184, 1981

Coon JS, Weinstein RS. Detection of ABH tissue isoantigens by immunoperoxidase methods in normal and neoplastic urothelium. Comparison with the erythrocyte adherence method. Am J Clin Pathol 76:163, 1981

Coon JS, Weinstein RS, Summers JL. Blood group precursor T-antigen expression in human urinary bladder carcinoma. Am J Clin Pathol 77:692, 1982

Cooney T, Benediktsson H, Mukai K. Immunohistochemical evaluation of a complex endocrinopathy. Am J Surg Pathol 4:491, 1980

Coons AH, Creech HJ, Jones RN. Immunological properties of an antibody containing a fluorescent group. Proc Soc Exp Biol 47:200, 1941

Cooper CW, Peng TC, Obie JF, et al. Calcitonin-like immunoreactivity in rat and human pituitary glands: histochemical, in vitro, and in vivo studies. Endocrinology 107:98, 1980

Cordon-Cardo C, Bander NH, Fradet Y, et al. Immunoanatomic dissection of the human urinary tract by monoclonal antibodies. J Histochem Cytochem 32:1035, 1984

Corson JM, Pinkus GS. Intracellular myoglobin—a specific marker for skeletal muscle differentiation in soft tissue sarcomas. An immunoperoxidase study. Am J Pathol 103:384, 1981

Corson JM, Pinkus GS. Mesothelioma: profile of keratin proteins and carcinoembryonic antigen: an immunoperoxidase study of 20 cases and comparison with pulmonary adenocarcinomas. Am J Pathol 108:80, 1982

Cossman J. Diffuse, aggressive non-Hodgkin's lymphomas. In: Surgical Pathology of Lymph Nodes and Related Organs. Jaffe ES, ed. Philadelphia, WB Saunders, 1985, p 203

Cote RJ, Morrissey DM, Houghton AN, et al. Generation of human monoclonal antibodies reactive with cellular antigens. Proc Natl Acad Sci 80:2026, 1983

Courtoy PJ, Lombart C, Feldmann G, et al. Synchronous increase of four acute phase proteins synthesized by the same hepatocytes during the inflammatory reaction: a combined biochemical and morphologic kinetics study in the rat. Lab Invest 44:105, 1981

Cox CE, VanVickle J, Froome LC, et al. Carcinoembryonic antigen and calcitonin as markers of malignancy in medullary thyroid carcinoma. Surg Forum 30:120, 1979

Cravioto H, Fukaya T, Zimmerman EA, et al. Immunohistochemical and electron-microscopic studies of functional and non-functional pituitary adenomas including one TSH-secreting tumor in a thyrotoxic patient. Acta Neuropathol (Berl) 53:281, 1981

Crifò S, Russo M. IgA transport mechanism through the human nasal mucosa: an immunoenzymatic ultrastructural study. Acta Otolaryngol 89:214, 1980

Croghan GA, Papsidero LD, Valenzuela LA, et al. Tissue distribution of an epithelial and tumor-associated antigen recognized by monoclonal antibody F36/22. Cancer Res 43:4980, 1983

Croghan GA, Wingate MB, Gamarra M, et al. Reactivity of monoclonal antibody F36/22 with human ovarian adenocarcinomas. Cancer Res 44:1954, 1984

Crum CP, Braun LA, Shah KV, et al. Vulvar intraepithelial neoplasia: correlation of nuclear DNA content and the presence of a human papilloma virus (HPV) structural antigen. Cancer 49:468, 1982a

Crum CP, Egawa K, Fenoglio CM, et al. Chronic endometritis: the role of immunohistochemistry in the detection of plasma cells. Am J Obstet Gynecol 147:812, 1983

Crum CP, Fenoglio CM. The immunoperoxidase technique: a review of its application to diseases of the female genital tract. Diagn Gynecol Obstet 2:103, 1980

Crum CP, Fu YS, Levine RU, et al. Intraepithelial squamous lesions of the vulva: biologic and histologic criteria for the distinction of condylomas from vulvar intraepithelial neoplasia. Am J Obstet Gynecol 144:77, 1982b

Crum CP, Mitao M, Winkler B, et al. Localizing chlamydial infection in cervical biopsies with the immunoperoxidase technique. Int J Gynecol Pathol 3:191, 1984

Culling CFA. Handbook of Histopathological and Histochemical Techniques, 3rd ed. London, Butterworths, 1974

Culling CFA. Histopathological and Histochemical Techniques. London, Butterworths, 1974

Curran RC, Gregory J. Demonstration of immunoglobulin in cryostat and paraffin sections of human tonsil by immunofluorescence and immunoperoxidase techniques. J Clin Pathol 31:974, 1978

Curran RC, Gregory J. Effects of fixation and processing on immunohistochemical demonstration of immunoglobulin in paraffin sections of tonsil and bone marrow. J Clin Pathol 33:1047, 1980

Curran RC, Gregory J, Jones EL. The distribution of immunoglobulin and other plasma proteins in human reactive lymph nodes. J Pathol 136:307, 1982

Custer RP. Pitfalls in the diagnosis of lymphoma and leukemia from the pathologist's point of view. In: Proceedings of the Second National Cancer Conference, vol 1. American Cancer Society, 1954, p 554

Cuttitta F, Rosen S, Gazdar AF, et al. Monoclonal antibodies that demonstrate specificity for several types of human lung cancer. Proc Natl Acad Sci USA 78:4595, 1978

Czernielewski JM, Schmitt D, Faure MR, et al. Functional and phenotypic analysis of isolated human Langerhans cells and indeterminate cells. Br J Dermatol 108:129, 1983

Daar AS, Fabre JW. The membrane antigens of human colorectal cancer cells: demonstration with monoclonal antibodies of heterogeneity within and between tumours and of anomalous expression of HLA-DR. Eur J Cancer Clin Oncol 19:209, 1983

Dahl D. Immunohistochemical differences between neurofilaments in perikarya, dendrites and axons. Immunofluorescence study with antisera raised to neurofilament polypeptides (200K, 150K, 70K) isolated by anion exchange chromatography. Exp Cell Res 149:397, 1983

Dahl D. The vimentin-GFA protein transition in rat neuroglia cytoskeleton occurs at the time of myelination. J Neurosci Res 6:741, 1981

Dahl D, Bignami A, Weber K, et al. Filament proteins in rat optic nerves undergoing wallerian degeneration:

localization of vimentin, the fibroblastic 100-Å filament protein, in normal and reactive astrocytes. Exp Neurol 73:495, 1981a

Dahl D, Chi NH, Miles LE, et al. Glial fibrillary acidic (GFA) protein in Schwann cells: fact or artifact? J Histochem Cytochem 30:912, 1982

Dahl D, Grossi M, Bignami A. Masking of epitopes in tissue sections. A study of glial fibrillary acidic (GFA) protein with antisera and monoclonal antibodies. Histochemistry 81:525, 1984

Dahl D, Rueger DC, Bignami A, et al. Vimentin, the 57,000 molecular weight protein of fibroblast filaments, is the major cytoskeletal component in immature glia. Eur J Cell Biol 24:191, 1981b

Daimaru Y, Hashimoto H, Enjoji M. Malignant "triton" tumors: a clinicopathologic and immunohistochemical study of nine cases. Hum Pathol 15:768, 1984

Dairaku M, Sueishi K, Tanaka K, et al. Immunohistological analysis of surfactant-apoprotein in the bronchiolo-alveolar carcinoma. Virchows Arch [A] 400:223, 1983

Dalakas MC, Fujihara S, Askanas V, et al. Nature of amyloid deposits in hypernephroma. Immunocytochemical studies in 2 cases associated with amyloid polyneuropathy. Am J Pathol 116:447, 1984

Danilovs JA, Hofman FM, Taylor CR, et al. Expression of HLA-DR antigens in human fetal pancreas tissue. Diabetes 31:23, 1982

Davis RL. Pathologic tumor type and response to treatment. In: Natl Cancer Inst Monograph No 46. Modern Concepts in Brain Tumor Therapy: Laboratory and Clinical Investigations. p 83, 1977

Davis RL, Erlich SS. Neuroepithelial tumors of the central nervous system. In: The Clinical Neurosciences. Section III. Neuropathology. Rosenberg RN, ed. New York, Churchill Livingstone, p 85, 1983

Davison PF, Jones RN. Filament proteins in central, cranial, and peripheral mammalian nerves. J Cell Biol 88:67, 1981

Davydova AA, Shubladze AK, Zakharova NA, et al. [Comparative results from the use of the direct immunoperoxidase and immunofluorescence methods to diagnose chronic herpetic infection.] Vopr Virusol 1:100, 1980

Daya-Grosjean L, Azzarone B, Maunoury R, et al. SV40 immortalization of adult human mesenchymal cells from neuroretina. Biological, functional and molecular characterization. Int J Cancer 33:319, 1984

Dayal Y, Doos WG, O'Brien MJ, et al. Psammomatous somatostatinomas of the duodenum. Am J Surg Pathol 7:653, 1983

Dayal Y, O'Brian DS, DeLellis RA, et al. Carcinoid tumors in gastrointestinal and extraintestinal sites. A comparative study of polypeptide hormonal profiles. Regul Pept (Suppl 1)1:22, 1980

De Armond SJ, Eng LF, Rubinstein LJ. The application of glial fibrillary acidic (GFA) protein immunohistochemistry in neurooncology. Pathol Res Pract 168:374, 1980

Dearnaley DP, Sloane JP, Ormerod MG, et al. Increased detection of mammary carcinoma cells in marrow smears using antisera to epithelial membrane antigen. Br J Cancer 44:85, 1981

De Boer WG, Ma J, Rees JW, et al. Inappropriate mucin production in gall bladder metaplasia and neoplasia—an immunohistological study. Histopathology 5:295, 1981

DeBoni U, Crapper McLachlan DR. Controlled induction of paired helical filaments of the Alzheimer type

in cultured human neurons, by glutamate and aspartate. J Neurol Sci 68:105, 1985

Debus E, Moll R, Franke WW, et al. Immunohistochemical distinction of human carcinomas by cytokeratin typing with monoclonal antibodies. Am J Pathol 114:121, 1984

Deck JHN, Eng LF, Bigbee J, et al. The role of glial fibrillary acidic protein in the diagnosis of central nervous system tumors. Acta Neuropathol (Berl) 42:183, 1978

Deck JHN, Rubinstein LJ. Glial fibrillary acidic protein in stromal cells of some capillary hemangioblastomas: significance and possible implications of an immunoperoxidase study. Acta Neuropathol (Berl) 54:173, 1981

Deftos LJ, Bone HG 3rd, Parthemore JG. Immunohistological studies of medullary thyroid carcinoma and C cell hyperplasia. J Clin Endocrinol Metab 51:857, 1980

De Ikonicoff LK. [Immunohistochemistry of the basal plate of the full-term human placenta: X cell characterization with anti-hCS and anti-hCG sera labeled with peroxidase.] C R Acad Sci [D] 288:97, 1979

De Leij L, Poppema S, Nulend JK, et al. Immunoperoxidase staining on frozen tissue sections as a first screening assay in the preparation of monoclonal antibodies directed against small cell carcinoma of the lung. Eur J Cancer Clin Oncol 20:123, 1984

DeLellis RA, Sternberger LA, Mann RB, et al. Immunoperoxidase technics in diagnostic pathology. Report of a workshop sponsored by the National Cancer Institute. Am J Clin Pathol 71:483, 1979

DeLellis RA, Wolfe HJ. The polypeptide hormone-producing neuroendocrine cells and their tumors: an immunohistochemical analysis. Methods Achiev Exp Pathol 10:190, 1981

Dell'Orto P, Viale G, Colombi R, et al. Immunohistochemical localization of human immunoglobulins and lysozyme in epoxy-embedded lymph nodes: effect of different fixatives and of proteolytic digestion. J Histochem Cytochem 30:630, 1982

del Poggetto CB, Virtanen I, Lehto V-P, et al. Expression of intermediate filaments in ovarian and uterine tumors. Int J Gynecol Pathol 1:359, 1983

Del Rio-Hortega P. Microglia. In: Penfield W, ed. Cytology and Cellular Pathology of the Nervous System. vol 2. New York, Paul B. Hoeber. p 483, 1932

Delsol G, Al Saati T, Caveriviere P, et al. [Immunoperoxidase study of normal and pathologic lymphoid tissue. Value of monoclonal antibodies.] Ann Pathol 4:165, 1984a

Delsol G, Gatter KC, Stein H, et al. Human lymphoid cells express epithelial membrane antigen. Implications for diagnosis of human neoplasms. Lancet 2:1124, 1984b

Delsol G, Pradere M, Voigt JJ, et al. Warthin-Finkeldey-like cells in benign and malignant lymphoid proliferations. Histopathology 6:451, 1982

Demaree RS Jr, Hillyer GV. Immunoperoxidase localization of _Fasciola hepatica_ worm tegument antigens by electron microscopy. Int J Parasitol 12:179, 1982

Deng J-S, Beutner EH. Effect of formaldehyde, glutaraldehyde and sucrose on the tissue antigenicity. Int Arch Allergy 47:562, 1974

DeSchryver-Kecskemeti K, Kyriakos M, et al. Pulmonary oat cell carcinomas. Expression of plasma membrane antigen correlated with presence of cytoplasmic neurosecretory granules. Lab Invest 41:432, 1979

De Waele M, De Mey J, Moeremans M, et al. Cytochemical profile of immunoregulatory T-lymphocyte subsets defined by monoclonal antibodies. J Histochem Cytochem 31:471, 1983

Dhillon AP, Rode J, Leathem A. Neurone specific enolase: an aid to the diagnosis of melanoma and neuroblastoma. Histopathology 6:81, 1982b

Dhillon AP, Rode J, Leathem A, et al. Somatostatin: a paracrine contribution to hypothyroidism in Hashimoto's thyroiditis. J Clin Pathol 35:764, 1982a

Dickson DW, Hart MN, Menezes A, et al. Medulloblastoma with glial and rhabdomyoblastic differentiation. A myoglobin and glial fibrillary acidic protein immunohistochemical study. J Neuropathol Exp Neurol 42:639, 1983

Dictor M. Ovarian malignant mixed mesodermal tumor: the occurrence of hyaline droplets containing alpha$_1$-antitrypsin. Hum Pathol 13:930, 1982

Dietel M. Discrimination between benign, borderline, and malignant epithelial ovarian tumors using tumor markers: an immunohistochemical study. Cancer Detect Prev 6:255, 1983

Dietel M, Lehmann E, Kaspar M, et al. Distribution pattern of PTH in human parathyroid adenomas. An immunohistochemical study. Horm Metab Res 12:640, 1980

Dighiero G, Bodega E, Mayzner R, et al. Individual cell-by-cell quantitation of lymphocyte surface membrane Ig in normal and CLL lymphocytes and during ontogeny of mouse B lymphocytes by immunoperoxidase assay. Blood 55:93, 1980

Dighiero G, Mayzner R, Roisin JP, et al. Automated recognition of B and T lymphocytes by immunoperoxidase on the hemalog D system and its applications. Blood Cells 8:447, 1982

DiPersio LP, Weiss MA, Michael JG, et al. Evaluation of the peroxidase-antiperoxidase method for demonstrating cell membrane β2-microglobulin. Am J Clin Pathol 77:700, 1982

Dippold WG, Lloyd KO, Li LTC, et al. Cell surface antigens of human malignant melanoma: definition of six antigenic systems with mouse monoclonal antibodies. Proc Natl Acad Sci USA 77:6114, 1980

DiStefano HS, Marucci AA, Dougherty RM. Immunohistochemical demonstration of avian leukosis virus antigens in paraffin embedded tissue. Proc Soc Exp Bio Med 142:1111, 1973

Dix RD, Waitzman DM, Follansbee S, et al. Herpes simplex virus type 2 encephalitis in two homosexual men with persistent lymphadenopathy. Ann Neurol 17:203, 1985

Dixon AJ, Burns J, Dunnill MS, et al. Distribution of fibronectin in normal and diseased human kidneys. J Clin Pathol 33:1021, 1980

Dixon RG, Eng LF. Processing techniques for the demonstration of myelin basic protein in paraffin-embedded optic nerve: an immunoperoxidase study of the developing albino rat. J Histochem Cytochem 30:270, 1982

Dobersen MJ, Gascon P, Trost S, et al. Murine monoclonal antibodies to the myelin-associated glycoprotein react with large granular lymphocytes of human blood. Proc Natl Acad Sci 82:552, 1985

Doggett RS, Wood GS, Horning S, et al. The immunologic characterization of 95 nodal and extranodal diffuse large cell lymphomas in 89 patients. Am J Pathol 115:245, 1984

Dohan FC Jr, Kornblith PL, Wellum GR, et al. S-100 protein and 2′, 3′-cyclic nucleotide 3′-phosphohydrolase in human brain tumors. Acta Neuropathol (Berl) 40:123, 1977

Donohue JP, Garrett RA, Baehner RL, et al. The multiple manifestations of neuroblastoma. J Urol 111:260, 1974

Dormeyer HH, Arnold W, Schönborn H, et al. The significance of serologic, histologic, and immunohistologic findings in the prognosis of 88 asymptomatic carriers of hepatitis B surface antigen. J Infect Dis 144:33, 1981

Dorreen MS, Habeshaw JA, Stansfeld AG, et al. Characteristics of Sternberg-Reed and related cells in Hodgkin's disease: an immunohistological study. Br J Cancer 49:465, 1984

Dragosics B, Bauer P, Radaszkiewicz T. Primary gastrointestinal non-Hodgkin's lymphomas. A retrospective clinicopathologic study of 150 cases. Cancer 55:1060, 1985

Drenckhahn D, Steffens R, Gröschel-Stewart U. Immunocytochemical localization of myosin in the brush border region of the intestinal epithelium. Cell Tissue Res 205:163, 1980

Druguet M, Pepys MB. Enumeration of lymphocyte populations in whole peripheral blood with alkaline phosphatase-labelled reagents. A method for routine clinical use. Clin Exp Immunol 29:162, 1977

Dubois MP. Immunocytochemistry of polypeptide hormones: a review. Acta Histochem (Suppl) 22:141, 1980

Ducatelle R, Coussement W, Hoorens J. Demonstration of canine distemper viral antigen in paraffin sections, using an unlabeled antibody-enzyme method. Am J Vet Res 41:1860, 1980

Ducatman BS, Wick MR, Morgan TW, et al. Malignant histiocytosis: a clinical, histologic, and immunohistochemical study of 20 cases. Hum Pathol 15:368, 1984

Dudek RW, Childs GV, Boyne AF. Quick-freezing and freeze-drying in preparation for high quality morphology and immunocytochemistry at the ultrastructural level: application to pancreatic beta cell. J Histochem Cytochem 30:129, 1982

Dudley AW Jr. Cerebrospinal blood vessels: normal and diseased. In: Haymaker W, Adams RD, eds. Histology and Histopathology of the Nervous System, vol 1. Springfield, Ill., Charles C Thomas, p 714, 1982

Duello TM, Halmi NS. Ultrastructural-immunocytochemical localization of growth hormone and prolactin in human pituitaries. J Clin Endocrinol Metab 49:189, 1979

Duffy PE, Graf L, Rapport MM. Immunocytochemical diagnosis of brain tumor biopsies. Trans Am Neurol Assoc 103:108, 1978

Duffy PE, Huan Y-Y, Rapport MM, et al. Glial fibrillary acidic protein in giant cell tumors of brain and other gliomas. A possible relationship to malignancy, differentiation, and pleomorphism of glia. Acta Neuropathol (Berl) 52:51, 1980

Dura WT, Gladkowska-Dura MJ. Application of immunoperoxidase technique to electron microscopy. Acta Med Pol 21:319, 1980

Dyck RF, Lockwood CM, Kershaw M, et al. Amyloid P–component is a constituent of normal human glomerular basement membrane. J Exp Med 152:1162, 1980

Dyson JL, Walker PG, Singer A. Human papillomavirus infection of the uterine cervix: histological appearances in 28 cases identified by immunohistochemical techniques. J Clin Pathol 37:126, 1984

Eckert H. [Immunohistochemical findings in intrathoracic tumors. II. Demonstration of alpha$_1$-antitrypsin in tumor tissue.] Z Erkr Atmungsorgane 161:319, 1983

Edelson R. Cutaneous T-cell lymphoma. J Dermatol Surg Oncol 6:358, 1980a

Edelson R. Cutaneous T cell lymphoma: mycosis fungoides, Sézary syndrome, and other variants. J Am Acad Dermatol 2:89, 1980b

Edelson RL, Smith RW, Frank MM, et al. Identification of subpopulations of mononuclear cells in cutaneous infiltrates. 1. Differentiation between B cells, T cells, and histiocytes. J Invest Dermatol 61:82, 1973

Edwards GA, Zawadzki ZA. Extraosseous lesions in plasma cell myeloma: a report of six cases. Am J Med 43:194, 1967

Eikelenboom P, Stam FC. Immunoglobulins and complement factors in senile plaques. An immunoperoxidase study. Acta Neuropathol 57:239, 1982

Eikelenboom P, Stam FC. An immunohistochemical study on cerebral vascular and senile plaque amyloid in Alzheimer's dementia. Virchows Arch [B] 47:17, 1984

Eishi Y, Hatakeyama S, Takemura T, et al. Demonstration of various antigens on paraffin sections of formalin-fixed tissues: trypsin-treated, indirect peroxidase-labelled antibody technique. Bull Tokyo Med Dent Univ 28:27, 1981

Elema JD, Atmosoerodjo-Briggs JE. Langerhans cells and macrophages in eosinophilic granuloma. An enzyme-histochemical, enzyme-cytochemical, and ultrastructural study. Cancer 54:2174, 1984

El Etreby MF, Mahrous AT. Immunocytochemical technique for detection of prolactin (PRL) and growth hormone (GH) in hyperplastic and neoplastic lesions of dog prostate and mammary gland. Histochemistry 64:279, 1979

Elias JM. Principles and Techniques of Diagnostic Histopathology: Development in Immunohistochemistry and Enzyme Histochemistry. Park Ridge, N.J., Noyes Press, 1982

Elliott PR, Forsey T, Darougar S, et al. Chlamydiae and inflammatory bowel disease. Gut 22:25, 1981

Ellis DW, Leffers S, Davies JS, et al. Multiple immunoperoxidase markers in benign hyperplasia and adenocarcinoma of the prostate. Am J Clin Pathol 81:279, 1984

Ellis IO, Robins RA, Elston CW, et al. A monoclonal antibody, NCRC-11, raised to human breast carcinoma. 1. Production and immunohistological characterization. Histopathology 8:501, 1984

Elovaara I, Paetau A, Lehto V-P, et al. Immunocytochemical studies of Alzheimer neuronal perikarya with intermediate filament antisera. J Neurol Sci 62:315, 1983

Eng LF. Localization of specific brain antigens. In: Boese A, ed. Search for the Cause of Multiple Sclerosis and Other Chronic Diseases of the Central Nervous System. Basel, Verlag Chemie, p 15, 1980

Eng LF, Rubinstein LJ. Contribution of immunohistochemistry to diagnostic problems of human cerebral tumors. J Histochem Cytochem 26:513, 1978

Engleman EG, Warnke R, Fox RI, et al. Studies of a human T lymphocyte antigen recognized by a monoclonal antibody. Proc Natl Acad Sci USA 78:1791, 1981

Engvall E, Miyashita M, Ruosiahti E. Monoclonal antibodies in analysis of oncoplacental protein SP1 in vivo and in vitro. Cancer Res 42:2028, 1982

Epenetos AA, Bobrow LG, Adams TE, et al. A monoclonal antibody that detects HLA–D region antigen in routinely fixed, wax embedded sections of normal and neoplastic lymphoid tissues. J Clin Pathol 38:12, 1985

Epenetos AA, Canti G, Taylor-Papadimitriou J, et al. Use of two epithelium-specific monoclonal antibodies for diagnosis of malignancy in serous effusions. Lancet 2:1004, 1982

Epenetos AA, Travers P, Gatter KC, et al. An immunohistological study of testicular germ cell tumours using two different monoclonal antibodies against placental alkaline phosphatase. Br J Cancer 49:11, 1984

Epstein AL, Marder RJ, Winter JN, et al. Two new monoclonal antibodies (LN-1, LN-2) reactive in B5 formalin-fixed, paraffin-embedded tissues with follicular center and mantle zone human B lymphocytes and derived tumors. J Immunol 133:1028, 1984

Epstein JI, White CL III, Mendelsohn G. Factor VIII–related antigen and glial fibrillary acidic protein immunoreactivity in the differential diagnosis of central nervous system hemangioblastomas. Am J Clin Pathol 81:285, 1984

Erber WN, Pinching AJ, Mason DY. Immunocytochemical detection of T and B cell populations in routine blood smears. Lancet 1:1042, 1984

Ernst C, Thurin J, Atkinson B, et al. Monoclonal antibody localization of A and B isoantigens in normal and malignant fixed human tissues. Am J Pathol 117:451, 1984

Eross KJ, Pangalis GA, Staatz CG, et al. Demonstration of cell surface antigens and their antibodies by the peroxidase-antiperoxidase method. Transplantation 25:331, 1978

Esiri MM. Poliomyelitis: immunoglobulin-containing cells in the central nervous system in acute and convalescent phases of the human disease. Clin Exp Immunol 40:42, 1980

Esiri MM. Herpes simplex encephalitis. An immunohistological study of the distribution of viral antigen within the brain. J Neurol Sci 54:209, 1982

Esiri MM, Adams CB, Burke C, et al. Pituitary adenomas: immunohistology and ultrastructural analysis of 118 tumors. Acta Neuropathol 62:1, 1983

Esiri MM, Booss J. Comparison of methods to identify microglial cells and microphages in the human central nervous system. J Clin Pathol 37:150, 1984

Esiri MM, Oppenheimer DR, Brownell B, Distribution of measles antigen and immunoglobulin-containing cells in the CNS in subacute sclerosing panencephalitis (SSPE) and atypical measles encephalitis. J Neurol Sci 53:29, 1982

Esiri MM, Taylor CR, Mason DY. Application of an immunoperoxidase method to a study of the central nervous system: preliminary findings in a study of human formalin-fixed material. Neuropathol Appl Neurobiol 2:233, 1976

Espinoza CG, Azar HA. Immunohistochemical localization of keratin-type proteins in epithelial neoplasms. Correlation with electron microscopic findings. Am J Clin Pathol 78:500, 1982

Espinoza CG, Balis JU, Saba SR, et al. Ultrastructural and immunohistochemical studies of bronchiolo-alveolar carcinoma. Cancer 54:2182, 1984a

Espinoza CG, Pillarisetti SG, Azar HA. Immunohistochemistry of hepatocellular carcinoma associated with cirrhosis. Ann Clin Lab Sci 14:467, 1984b

Eto H, Hashimoto K, Kobayashi H, et al. Differential staining of cytoid bodies and skin-limited amyloids with monoclonal anti-keratin antibodies. Am J Pathol 116:473, 1984

Ettinger DS, Rosenshein NB, Parmley TH, et al. Tumor cell origin of histaminase activity in ascites fluid from patients with ovarian carcinoma. Cancer 45:2568, 1980

Facer P, Bishop AE, Polak JM. Immunocytochemistry: its applications and drawbacks for the study of gut neuroendocrinology. Invest Cell Pathol 3:13, 1980

Fagraeus A. Plasma cellular reaction and its relation to formation of antibodies in vitro. J Immunol 58:1, 1948

Falini B, De Solas I, Halverson C, et al. Double labeled–antigen method for demonstration of intracellular antigens in paraffin-embedded tissues. J Histochem Cytochem 30:21, 1982a

Falini B, De Solas I, Levine AM, et al. Emergence of B-immunoblastic sarcoma in patients with multiple myeloma: a clinicopathologic study of 10 cases. Blood 59:923, 1982b

Falini B, Martelli MF, Tarallo F, et al. Immunohistological analysis of human bone marrow trephine biopsies using monoclonal antibodies. Br J Haematol 56:365, 1984

Falini B, Tabilio A, Zuccaccia M, et al. Protein A-peroxidase conjugates for two-stage immunoenzyme staining of intracellular antigens in paraffin-embedded tissues. J Immunol Methods 39:111, 1980

Falini B, Taylor CR. New developments in immunoperoxidase techniques and their application. Arch Pathol Lab Med 107:105, 1983

Falkmer S. Immunocytochemical studies of the evolution of islet hormones. J Histochem Cytochem 27:1281, 1979

Farley AL, O'Brien T, Moyer D, et al. The detection of estrogen receptors in gynecologic tumors using immunoperoxidase and the dextran–coated charcoal assay. Cancer 49:2153, 1982

Faulk WP, Hsi BL, Stevens PJ. Transferrin and transferrin receptors in carcinoma of the breast. Lancet 2:390, 1980

Favre L, Rogers LM, Cobb CA, et al. Gigantism associated with a pituitary tumour secreting growth hormone and prolactin and cured by transsphenoidal hypophysectomy. Acta Endocrinol 91:193, 1979

Fedoroff S, Whit R, Neal J, et al. Astrocyte cell lineage. II. Mouse fibrous astrocytes and reactive astrocytes in cultures have vimentin- and GFP-containing intermediate filaments. Dev Brain Res 7:303, 1983

Feller AC, Parwaresch MR. Simultaneous enzyme-immunocytochemical detection of antigens in monocellular specimens with monoclonal antibodies. J Immunol Methods 63:273, 1983

Fenoglio CM, Crum CP, Pascal RR, et al. Carcinoembryonic antigen in gynecologic patients. Diagn Gynecol Obstet 31:291, 1981

Fenoglio CM, Hayata T, Crum CP, et al. The expression of human chorionic gonadotropin in the female genital tract: localization by the immunoperoxidase technique. Diagn Gynecol Obstet 4:97, 1982a

Fenoglio CM, Tlamsa G, Habif DV. Pituitary-containing benign cystic teratoma of the ovary in a patient with metastatic breast cancer: a case report. Diagn Histopathol 5:143, 1982b

Ferenczy A, Braun L, Shah KV. Human papillomavirus (HPV) in condylomatous lesions of cervix. Am J Surg Pathol 5:661, 1981

Ferguson AM, Fox H. A study of the Ca antigen in epithelial tumours of the ovary. J Clin Pathol 37:6, 1984a

Ferguson AM, Fox H. The expression of Ca antigen in normal, hyperplastic and neoplastic endometrium. Br J Obstet Gynaecol 91:1042, 1984b

Feurle GE, Linke RP, Kuhn E, et al. Clinical value of immunohistochemistry with AF-antibody in the diagnosis of familial amyloid neuropathy. J Neurol 231:237, 1984

Fields KL, Raine CS. Ultrastructure and immunocytochemistry of rat Schwann cells and fibroblasts in vitro. J Neuroimmunol 2:155, 1982

Fields PA, Larkin LH. Purification and immunohistochemical localization of relaxin in the human term placenta. J Clin Endocrinol Metab 52:79, 1981

Finan PJ, Grant RM, de Mattos C, et al. Immunohistochemical techniques in the early screening of monoclonal antibodies to human colonic epithelium. Br J Cancer 46:9, 1982

Fink B, Loepfe E, Wyler R. Demonstration of viral antigen in cryostat sections by a new immunoperoxidase procedure eliminating endogenous peroxidase activity. J Histochem Cytochem 27:686, 1979

Finstad CL, Cordon-Cordo C, Bauder NH, et al. Specificity analysis of mouse monoclonal antibodies detecting cell surface antigens of human renal cancer. Proc Natl Acad Sci USA 82:2955, 1985

Fischer EG, Morris JH, Kettyle WM. Intrasellar gangliocytoma and syndromes of pituitary hypersecretion. Case report. J Neurosurg 59:1071, 1983

Fishman WH. Perspectives on alkaline phosphatase isoenzymes. Am J Med 56:617, 1974

Flanigan RC, King CT, Clark TD, et al. Immunohistochemical demonstration of blood group antigens in neoplastic and normal human urothelium: a comparison with standard red cell adherence. J Urol 130:499, 1983

Fleischer I, Caselitz J, Löning T, et al. Histological and immunocytochemical examinations of the stromal reaction in carcinomas of the parotid gland. Analysis of 52 cases. J Cancer Res Clin Oncol 96:193, 1980

Folberg R, Donoso LA, Herlyn MF, et al. Antigens in ocular and cutaneous melanomas. Am J Ophthalmol 96:394, 1983

Fontana A. Astrocytes and lymphocytes: intercellular communication by growth factors. J Neurosci Res 8:443, 1982

Fontana A, Fierz W. The endothelium-astrocyte immune control system of the brain. Springer Sem Immunopathol 8:57, 1985

Fontana A, Fierz W, Wekerle H. Astrocytes present myelin basic protein to encephalitogenic T-cell lines. Nature 307:273, 1984

Fontana A, Weber E, Grob PJ, et al. Dual effect of glia maturation factor on astrocytes—differentiation and release of interleukin 1–like factors. J Neuroimmunol 5:261, 1983

Forni M, Hofman FM, Parker JW, et al. B- and T-lymphocytes in Hodgkin's disease. An immunohistochemical study utilizing heterologous and monoclonal antibodies. Cancer 55:728, 1985

Forni M, Meyer PR, Levy NB, et al. An immunohistochemical study of hemoglobin A, hemoglobin F, muramidase and transferrin in erythroid hyperplasia and neoplasia. Am J Clin Pathol 80:145, 1983

Foster NL, Chase TN, Mansi L, et al. Cortical abnormalities in Alzheimer' disease. Ann Neurol 16:649, 1984

Foucar K, Rydell RE. Richter's syndrome in chronic lymphocytic leukemia. Cancer 46:118, 1980

Fox B, Shousha S, James KR, et al. Immunohistological study of human lungs by immunoperoxidase technique. J Clin Pathol 35:144, 1982

Frable WJ. Thin-Needle Aspiration Biopsy. Major Problems in Pathology, vol 14. Philadelphia, WB Saunders, 1983

Fradet Y, Cordon-Cordo C, Thomsen T, et al. Cell surface antigens of human bladder cancer defined by mouse monoclonal antibodies. Proc Natl Acad Sci USA 81:224, 1984

Frankel AE, Rouse RV, Wang MC, et al. Monoclonal antibodies to a human prostate antigen. Cancer Res 42:3714, 1982

Franko MC, Masters CL, Gibbs CJ Jr, et al. Monoclonal antibodies to central nervous system antigens. J Neuroimmunol 1:391, 1981

Franssila KO, Harach HR, Wasenius VM. Mucoepidermoid carcinoma of the thyroid. Histopathology 8:847, 1984

Fray RE, Husain OA, To AC, et al. The value of immunohistochemical markers in the diagnosis of cervical neoplasia. Br J Obstet Gynaecol 91:1037, 1984

Frelinger JG, Hood L, Hill S, et al. Mouse epidermal Ia molecules have a bone marrow origin. Nature 282:324, 1979

Frenkel JK. Toxoplasmosis. In: Marcial-Rojas RA, ed. Pathology of Protozoal and Helminthic Diseases, with Clinical Correlation. p 254, Baltimore, Williams & Wilkins, 1971.

Friede RL, Gliofibroma. A peculiar neoplasia of collagen forming glia-like cells. J Neuropathol Exp Neurol 37:300, 1978

Friedman CJ, Mills SE. Immunoperoxidase staining for CEA in ulcerative colitis. J Clin Gastroenterol 5:453, 1983

Fritz P, Müller J, Wegner G, et al. [Enzyme histochemical demonstration of immunoglobulins in joint capsules in chronic polyarthritis and active inflammatory arthritis.] J Rheumatol 39:331, 1980

Fu SM, Chiorazzi N, Wang CY, et al. Ia bearing T cells in man. Their identification and role in the generation of allogenic helper activity. J Exp Med 148:1423, 1978

Fu YS, Braun L, Shah KV, et al. Histologic, nuclear DNA, and human papillomavirus studies of cervical condylomas. Cancer 52:1705, 1983

Fuchs E, Hanukoglu I. Unraveling the structure of the intermediate filaments. Cell 34:332, 1983

Fujihara S. Differentiation of amyloid fibril proteins in tissue sections. Two simple and reliable histological methods applied to fifty-one cases of systemic amyloidosis. Acta Pathol Jpn 32:771, 1982

Fujihara S, Balow JE, Costa JC, et al. Identification and classification of amyloid in formalin-fixed, paraffin-embedded tissue sections by the unlabeled immunoperoxidase method. Lab Invest 43:358, 1980

Fujihara S, Glenner GG. Primary localized amyloidosis of the genitourinary tract: immunohistochemical study on eleven cases. Lab Invest 44:55, 1981

Fujii S. Development of pancreatic endocrine cells in the rat fetus. Arch Histol Jpn 42:467, 1979

Fujimoto, S, Kimoto K, Inokuchi H, et al. G-cell population and serum gastrin response to cimetidine-OXO test meal in relation to histopathological alterations in resected stomachs from patients with peptic ulcer disease. Gastroenterol Jpn 15:101, 1980

Fujita S, Kitamura T. Origin of brain macrophages and the nature of the microglia. Prog Neuropathol 3:1, 1976

Fujita S, Tsuchihashi Y, Kitamura T. Absence of hematogenous cells in the normal brain tissue as revealed by leucocyte-specific immunofluorescent staining. J Neuropathol Exp Neurol 37:615, 1978

Fujita S, Tsuchihashi Y, Kitamura T. Origin, morphology and function of the microglia. Prog Clin Biol Res 59A:141, 1981

Fulthorpe JJ, Hudgson P. Immunocytochemical localization of immunoglobulins in the inflammatory lesions of polymyositis. J Neuroimmunol 2:145, 1982

Furcht LT, Smith D, Wendelschafer-Crabb G, et al. Fibronectin presence in native collagen fibrils of human fibroblasts: immunoperoxidase and immunoferritin localization. J Histochem Cytochem 28:1319, 1980

Furomoto M. Cellular localization of AFP, hCG and its free subunits, and SP1 in embryonal carcinoma of the testis and ovary. Pathol Res Pract 173:12, 1981

Gabbiani G, Kapanci Y, Barazzone P, et al. Immunochemical identification of intermediate-sized filaments in human neoplastic cells: a diagnostic aid for the surgical pathologist. Am J Pathol 104:206, 1981

Gabbiani G, Kocher O. Cytocontractile and cytoskeletal elements in pathologic processes: pathogenetic role and diagnostic value. Arch Pathol Lab Med 107:622, 1983

Gambarelli D, Hassoun J, Choux M, et al. Complex cerebral tumor with evidence of neuronal, glial and Schwann cell differentiation: a histologic, immunocytochemical and ultrastructural study. Cancer 49:1420, 1982

Gambetti P, Autillio-Gambetti L, Papasozomenos SC. Bodian's silver method stains neurofilament polypeptides. Science 213:1521, 1981

Gambetti P, Autilio-Gambetti L, Perry G, et al. Antibodies to neurofibrillary tangles of Alzheimer's disease raised from human and animal neurofilament fractions. Lab Invest 49:430, 1983a

Gambetti P, Roessmann U, Velasco ME. Immunofluorescence technique for rapid diagnosis of glial tumors. Am J Surg Pathol 4:277, 1980

Gambetti P, Shecket G, Ghetti B, et al. Neurofibrillary changes in human brain: an immunocytochemical study with a neurofilament antiserum. J Neuropathol Exp Neurol 42:69, 1983b

Gamliel H, Polliack A. Scanning immunoelectron microscopy markers. Isr J Med Sci 15:639, 1979

Ganjei P, Nadji M, Penneys NS, et al. Immunoreactive prekeratin in Brenner tumors of the ovary. Int J Gynecol Pathol 1:353, 1983

Ganser AL, Kirschner DA, Willinger M. Ganglioside localization on myelinated nerve fibres by cholera toxin binding. J Neurocytol 12:921, 1983

Garancis JC, Miller LS, Tomita JT, et al. Immunoperoxidase localization of estrogen receptors in human breast carcinoma. Cancer Detect Prev 6:235, 1983

Garaud JC, Eloy R, Moody AJ, et al. Glucagon- and glicentin-immunoreactive cells in the human digestive tract. Cell Tissue Res 213:121, 1980

Gardner MB, Lund JK, Cardiff RD. Prevalence and distribution of murine mammary tumor virus antigen detectable by immunocytochemistry in spontaneous breast tumors of wild mice. J Natl Cancer Inst 64:1251, 1980

Garrigues HJ, Tilgen W, Hellström I, et al. Detection of a human melanoma-associated antigen, p97, in histological sections of primary human melanomas. Int J Cancer 29:511, 1982

Garson JA, Beverley PCL, Coakham HB, et al. Monoclonal antibodies against human T lymphocytes label Purkinje neurones of many species. Nature 298:375, 1982

Gatter KC, Alcock C, Heryet A, et al. The differential diagnosis of routinely processed anaplastic tumors using monoclonal antibodies. Am J Clin Pathol 82:33, 1984a

Gatter KC, Alcock C, Heryet A, et al. Clinical importance of analysing malignant tumours of uncertain origin with immunohistological techniques. Lancet 1:1302, 1985

Gatter KC, Pulford KA, Vanstapel MJ, et al. An immunohistological study of benign and malignant skin tumours: epithelial aspects. Histopathology 8:209, 1984b

Geddie WR, Bedard YC, Strawbridge HT. Medullary carcinoma of the thyroid in fine-needle aspiration biopsies. Am J Clin Pathol 82:552, 1984

Gerber MA, Shah KV, Thung SN, et al. Immunohistochemical demonstration of common antigen of polyomaviruses in routine histologic tissue sections of animals and man. Am J Clin Pathol 73:795, 1980

Gerdes J, Stein H. Complement (C3) receptors on dendritic reticulum cells of normal and malignant lymphoid tissue. Clin Exp Immunol 48:348, 1982

Ghandour MS, Langley OK, Vincendon G, et al. Double labeling immunohistochemical technique provides evidence of the specificity of glial cell markers. J Histochem Cytochem 27:1634, 1979

Ghandour MS, Langley OK, Vincendon G, et al. Immunochemical and immunohistochemical study of carbonic anhydrase II in adult rat cerebellum: a marker for oligodendrocytes. Neuroscience 5:559, 1980a

Ghandour MS, Vincendon G, Gombos G, et al. Carbonic anhydrase and oligodendroglia in developing rat cerebellum: a biochemical and immunohistological study. Dev Bio 77:73, 1980b

Ghazizadeh M, Kagawa S, Izumi K, et al. Immunohistochemical localization of T antigenlike substance in benign hyperplasia and adenocarcinoma of the prostate. J Urol 132:1127, 1984a

Ghazizadeh M, Kagawa S, Izumi K, et al. Immunohistochemical detection of carcinoembryonic antigen in benign hyperplasia and adenocarcinoma of the prostate with monoclonal antibody. J Urol 131:501, 1984b

Ghazizadeh M, Kagawa S, Maebayashi K, et al. Prostatic origin of metastases: immunoperoxidase localization of prostate-specific antigen. Urol Int 39:9, 1984c

Gheuens J, Noppe M, Karcher D, et al. Immunochemical determination and immunocytological localization of brain-specific protein α-albumin (GFA) in isolated astrocytes. Neurochem Res 5:757, 1980

Ghosh AK, Mason DY, Spriggs AI. Immunocytochemical staining with monoclonal antibodies in cytologically "negative" serous effusions from patients with malignant disease. J Clin Pathol 36:1150, 1983a

Ghosh AK, Spriggs AI, Taylor-Papadimitriou J, Mason DY. Immunocytochemical staining of cells in plueral and peritoneal effusions with a panel of monoclonal antibodies. J Clin Pathol 36:1154, 1983b

Ghosh L, Ghosh B, Das Gupta TK. Immunocytological localization of estrogen in human mammary carcinoma cells by horseradish–anti-horseradish peroxidase complex. J Surg Oncol 10:221, 1978

Gibson WC, Peng TC, Croker BP. C-cell nodules in adult human thyroid. A common autopsy finding. Am J Clin Pathol 75:347, 1981

Gibson, WG, Peng TC, Croker BP. Age-associated C-cell hyperplasia in the human thyroid. Am J Pathol 106:388, 1982

Giddings J, Griffin RL, Maciver AG. Demonstration of immunoproteins in araldite-embedded tissues. J Clin Pathol 35:111, 1982

Giddings JC, Brookes LR, Piovella F, et al. Immunohistological comparison of platelet factor 4 (PF4), fibronectin (Fn) and factor VIII related antigen (VIII:Ag) in human platelet granules. Br J Haematol 52:79, 1982

Gillis TP, Buchanan TM. Production and partial characterization of monoclonal antibodies to Mycobacterium leprae. Infect Immun 37:172, 1982

Giorno R. Characterization of mononuclear cells in cytocentrifuge and imprint preparations using monoclonal antibodies and an avidin-biotin immunoperoxidase staining system. J Histochem Cytochem 31:1326, 1983

Giraldo AA, Ruby SG, Humes JJ. Blood group antigens in urothelium in transitional cell carcinoma. Ann Clin Lab Sci 13:307, 1983

Gleason TH, Hammar SP. Plasmacytoma of the colon: case report with lambda light chain, demonstrated by immunoperoxidase studies. Cancer 50:130, 1982

Glenner GG, Wong CW. Alzheimer's disease: initial report of the purification and characterization of a novel cerebrovascular amyloid protein. Biochem Biophys Res Commun 120:885, 1984

Glynn, AA, Parkman R. Studies with an antibody to rat lysozyme. Immunology 7:l724, 1964

Gold DV. Immunoperoxidase localization of colonic mucoprotein antigen in neoplastic tissues. Cancer Res 41:767, 1981

Goldschneider I, Gregorie KE, Barton RW, et al. Demonstration of terminal deoxynucleotidyl transferase in thymocytes by immunofluorescence. Proc Natl Acad Sci USA 74:734, 1977

Gomes MA, Staquet MJ, Thivolet J. Staining of colloid bodies by keratin antisera in lichen planus. Am J Dermatopathol 3:341, 1981

Goodman, ZD, Ishak KG, Langloss JM, et al. Combined hepatocellular-cholangiocarcinoma. A histologic and immunohistochemical study. Cancer 55:124, 1985

Gooi JH, Burns GF, Cawley JC. Hairy-cell leukaemia: an immunoperoxidase study of paraffin-embedded tissues. J Clin Pathol 32:1244, 1979

Gorin NC, Najman A, Parrot G, et al. [Non-secretory plasma cell leukemia with intracytoplasmic kappa light chains.] Sem Hop Paris 00:1581, 1979

Goslin R, O'Brien MJ, Steele G, et al. Correlation of plasma CEA and CEA tissue staining in poorly differentiated colorectal cancer. Am J Med 71:246, 1981

Gould SF, Lopez RL, Speers WC. Malignant struma ovarii. A case report and literature review. J Reprod Med 28:415, 1983

Gould VE, Memoli VA, Dardi LE, et al. Nesidiodysplasia and nesidioblastosis of infancy: structural and functional correlations with the syndrome of hyperinsulinemic hypoglycemia. Pediatr Pathol 1:7, 1983

Gourdin MF, Farcet JP, Reyes F. The ultrastructural localization of immunoglobulins in human B cells of immunoproliferative diseases. Blood 59:1132, 1982

Gourdin MF, Reyes F, Laurent G, et al. Immunoelectron microscopy and immunocytochemistry in pathology, with special reference to immunoglobulin-producing cells. Isr J Med Sci 15:693, 1979

Goust J-M, Mangum M, Powers JM. An immunologic assessment of brain-associated IgG in senile cerebral amyloidosis. J Neuropathol Exp Neurol 43:481, 1984

Govindarajan S, Lim B, Peters RL. Immunohistochemical localization of the delta antigen associated with hepatitis B virus in liver biopsy sections embedded in Araldite. Histopathology 8:1984

Gown, AM, Vogel AM. Monoclonal antibodies to intermediate filament proteins of human cells: unique and cross-reacting antiibodies. J Cell Biol 95:414, 1982

Gown AM, Vogel AM. Monoclonal antibodies to human intermediate filament proteins. II. Distribution of filament proteins in normal human tissues. Am J Pathol 114:309, 1984

Grafe MR, Forno LS, Eng LF. Immunocytochemical studies of substance P and met-enkephalin in the basal ganglia and substantia nigra in Huntington's, Parkinson's and Alzheimer's diseases. J Neuropathol Exp Neurol 44:47, 1985

Graham BS, Snell JD Jr. Herpes simplex virus infection of the adult lower respiratory tract. Medicine 62:384, 1983

Graham DI, Thomas DGT, Brown I. Nervous system antigens. Histopathology 7:1, 1983.

Graham DY, Estes MK. Comparison of methods for immunocytochemical detection of rotavirus infections. Infect Immun 26:686, 1979

Grampag et al. Hypoglycemia in infancy caused by beta cell nesidioblastosis. M J Dis Child 128:226, 1974

Graus F, Cordon-Cardo C, Posner JB. Neuronal antinuclear antibody in sensory neuronopathy from lung cancer. Neurology 35:538, 1985

Gray A, Downing R, Hill R, et al. Demonstration of carcinoembryonic antigen in bone marrow from patients with carcinoma. J Clin Pathol 37:1090, 1984

Greaves MF, Janossy G. Antisera to human T lymphocytes. In: Bloom BR, David JR, eds. In Vitro Methods in Cell-Mediated and Tumor Immunity, vol 2. New York, Academic Press, p 89, 1976

Greenberger JS, Campos-Neto A, Parkma R, et al. Immunologic detection of intracellular and cell surface lysozyme with human and experimental leukemic leukocytes. Clin Immunol Immunopathol 8:318, 1977

Greenlee JE, Brashear HR. Antibodies to cerebellar Purkinje cells in patients with paraneoplastic cerebellar degeneration and ovarian carcinoma. Ann Neurol 14:609, 1983

Griffiths DF, Jasani B, Newman GR, et al. Glandular duodenal carcinoid—a somatostatin-rich tumour with neuroendocrine associations. J Clin Pathol 37:163, 1984

Grimaud JA, Druguet M, Peyrol S, et al. Collagen immunotyping in human liver: light and electron microscope study. J Histochem Cytochem 28:1145, 1980

Grogan TM, Hicks MJ, Jolley CS, et al. Identification of two major B cell forms of nodular mixed lymphoma. Lab Invest 51:504, 1984

Groopman JE, Golde DW. The histiocytic disorders: pathophysiologic analysis. Ann Intern Med 94:95, 1981

Gross DS, Longer JD. Developmental correlation between hypothalamic somatostatin and hypophysial growth hormone. Cell Tissue Res 202:251, 1979

Grube D. Immunoperoxidase methods: increased efficiency using fluorescence microscopy for 3,3-diaminobenzidine (DAB)–stained semithin sections. Histochemistry 70:19, 1980

Grube D, Aebert H. [Specificity control in the immunohistochemistry of enteral peptide hormones.] Acta Histochem (Suppl) 24:277, 1981

Grundke-Iqbal I, Iqbal K, Tung YC, et al. Alzheimer-paired helical filaments: immunochemical identification of polypeptides. Acta Neuropathol (Berl) 62:259, 1984

Grundke-Iqbal I, Iqbal K, Tung YC, et al. Alzheimer-paired helical filaments: cross-reacting polypeptides normally present in brain. Acta Neuropathol 66:52, 1985

Grundke-Iqbal I, Johnson AB, Terry RD, et al. Alz-

heimer neurofibrillary tangles: antiserum and immunohistological staining. Ann Neurol 6:532, 1979

Gu J, de Mey J, Moeremans M, et al. Sequential use of the PAP and immunogold staining method for the light microscopical double staining of tissue antigens. Regul Pept 1:365, 1981

Guarda LG, Ordóñez NG, Smith JL Jr, et al. Immunoperoxidase localization of factor VIII in angiosarcomas. Arch Pathol Lab Med 106:515, 1982

Guarda LG, Silva EG, Ordóñez NG, et al. Factor VIII in Kaposi's sarcoma. Am J Clin Pathol 76:197, 1981

Guesdon JL, Ternynck T, Avrameas S. The use of avidin-biotin interaction in immunoenzymatic techniques. J Histochem Cytochem 27:1131, 1979

Gullotta F, Dickopf KE. Is progressive multifocal leukoencephalopathy exclusively due to Papova viruses? Pathologica 74:763, 1982

Gunby P. Herpes simplex virus type 2: a not-so-simple problem. Arch Int Med 141:835, 1981

Gupta JW, Gupta PK, Shah KV, et al. Distribution of human papillomavirus antigen in cervicovaginal smears and cervical tissues. Int J Gynecol Pathol 2:160, 1983

Gusterson B, Mitchell D, Warburton M, et al. Immunohistochemical localization of keratin in human lung tumors. Virchows Arch [A] 394:269, 1982

Gutman GA, Weissman IL. Lymphoid tissue architecture. Experimental analysis of the origin and distribution of T cells and B cells. Immunology 23:465, 1972

Guy J, Leclerc R, Vaudry H, et al. Localisation immunocytochimique de l'ACTH, de la gamma-endorphine et du précurseur commun de ces peptides dans l'hypophyse humaine. Union Med Can 109:483, 1980

Haberland C. Primary systemic amyloidosis. Cerebral involvement and senile plaque formation. J Neuropathol Exp Neurol 23:135, 1964

Haghighi P, Kharazmi A, Gerami C, et al. Primary upper small-intestinal lymphoma and alpha-chain disease. Report of 10 cases emphasizing pathological aspects. Am J Surg Pathol 2:147, 1978

Haglid K, Carlsson C-A, Stavrou D. An immunological study of human brain tumors concerning the brain specific proteins S-100 and 14.3.2. Acta Neuropathol 24:187, 1973

Haglund C, Roberts PJ, Nordling S, et al. Expression of laminin in pancreatic neoplasms and in chronic pancreatitis. Am J Surg Pathol 8:669, 1984

Hall CL, Lampert PW. Immunohistochemistry as an aid in the diagnosis of Hirschsprung's disease. Am J Clin Pathol 83:177, 1981

Hall CL, Lampert PW. Immunochemistry as an aid in the diagnosis of Hirschsprung's disease. J Neuropathol Exp Neurol 43:311, 1984

Halmi NS. Immunostaining of growth hormone and prolactin in paraffin-embedded and stored or previously stained materials. J Histochem Cytochem 26:486, 1978

Halmi NS. Occurrence of both growth hormone–and prolactin-immunoreactive material in the cells of human somatotropic pituitary adenomas containing mammotropic elements. Virchows Arch [A] 398:19, 1982

Halmi NS, Parsons JA, Erlandson SL, et al. Prolactin and growth hormone cells in the human hypophysis: a study with immunoenzyme histochemistry and differential staining. Cell Tissue Res 158:497, 1975

Halper JP, Knowles DM, Want CY. Ia antigen expression

by human malignant lymphomas: correlation with conventional lymphoid markers. Blood 55:373, 1980

Halter, SA, Fraker LD, Parmenter M, et al. Carcinoembryonic antigen expression and patient survival in carcinoma of the breast. Oncology 41:297, 1984

Halverson C, Falini B, Taylor CR, et al. Detection of terminal transferase in paraffin sections with the immunoperoxidase techniques. Am J Pathol 105:241, 1981

Hamada Y, Yamamura M, Hioki K, et al. Immunohistochemical study of carcinoembryonic antigen in patients with colorectal cancer. Correlation with plasma carcinoembryonic antigen levels. Cancer 55:136, 1985

Hand PH, Nuti M, Colchi D, et al. Definition of antigenic heterogeneity and modulation among human mammary carcinoma cell populations using monoclonal antibodies to tumor associated antigens. Cancer Res 43:726, 1983

Hanker JS, Yates PE, Metz CB, et al. A new specific sensitive and non-carcinogenic reagent for the demonstration of horseradish peroxidase. Histochem J 9:789, 1977

Hanna W, Ryder DI, Mobbs BG. Cellular localization of estrogen binding sites in human breast cancer. Am J Clin Pathol 77:391, 1982

Hansen BL, Hansen GN, Vestergaard BF. Immunoelectron microscopic localization of herpes simplex virus antigens in infected cells using the unlabeled antibody–enzyme method. J Histochem Cytochem 27:1455, 1979

Hara H, Yamane T, Yamashita K. Extramedullary plasmacytoma of the gastrointestinal tract in a renal transplant recipient. Acta Pathol Jpn 29:661, 1979

Harach HR, Skinner M, Gibbs AR. Biological markers in human lung carcinoma: an immunopathological study of six antigens. Thorax 38:937, 1983

Hardy TJ, Myerowitz RL, Bender BL. Diffuse parenchymal amyloidosis of lungs and breast. Its association with diffuse plasmacytosis and kappa-chain gammopathy. Arch Pathol Lab Med 103:583, 1979

Harper JR, Bumol TF, Reisfeld RA. Serological and biochemical analyses of monoclonal antibodies to human melanoma-associated antigens. Hybridoma 1:423, 1982

Harris NL, Data RE. The distribution of neoplastic and normal B-lymphoid cells in modular lymphomas: use of an immunoperoxidase technique on frozen sections. Hum Pathol 13:610, 1982

Harris NL, Pilch BZ, Bhan AK, et al. Immunohistologic diagnosis of orbital lymphoid infiltrates. Am J Surg Pathol 8:83, 1984

Harris NL, Poppema S, Data RE. Demonstration of immunoglobulin in malignant lymphomas. Use of an immunoperoxidase technic on frozen sections. Am J Clin Pathol 78:14, 1982

Harrist TJ, Bhan AK, Murphy GF, et al. Lymphomatoid papulosis and lymphomatoid granulomatosis: T cell subset populations, refined light microscopic morphology and direct immunofluorescence observations. Clin Res 29:597A, 1981

Harrist TJ, Bhan AK, Murphy GF, et al. Histiocytosis-X: in situ characterization of cutaneous infiltrates with monoclonal antibodies. Am J Clin Pathol 79:294, 1983

Harrowe D, Taylor CR. Immunoperoxidase staining for carcinoembryonic antigen in colonic carcinoma, osteosarcoma, and chordoma. J Surg Oncol 16:1, 1981

Hasleton PS, Shah S, Buckley CH. Ampullary carcinoma associated with multiple duodenal villous adenomas. Am J Gastroenterol 73:418, 1980

Hasselbacher P. Extracellular aggregates of immunoglobulin in synovial fluid from rheumatoid arthritis. J Rheumatol 6:374, 1979

Hasselbacher P, Nacht JL, Labosky DA, et al. Antigen-induced arthritis: an immunohistologic study of articular tissue and synovial fluid using the horseradish peroxidase technique. J Rheumatol 7:596, 1980

Hassoun J, Charpin C, Jaquet P, et al. [Immunocytochemical similarities between basophilic and chromophobe pituitary adenomas. Light and electron microscopic study of 13 cases.] Ann Endocrinol 40:559, 1979

Hassoun J, Monges G, Giraud P, et al. Immunohistochemical study of pheochromocytomas. An investigation of methionine-enkephalin, vasoactive intestinal peptide, somatostatin, corticotropin, beta-endorphin, and calcitonin in 16 tumors. Am J Pathol 114:56, 1984

Haugen OA, Taylor CR. Immunohistochemical studies of ovarian and testicular teratomas with antiserum to glial fibrillary acidic protein. Acta Pathol Microbiol Immunol Scand (A) 92:9, 1984

Hauser SL, Bhan AK, Gilles FH, et al. Immunohistochemical staining of human brain with monoclonal antibodies that identify lymphocytes, monocytes, and the Ia antigen. J Neuroimmunol 5:197, 1983

Hautzer NW, Wittkuhn JF, McCaughey WT. Trypsin digestion in immunoperoxidase staining. J Histochem Cytochem 28:52, 1980

Hayata T, Fenoglio CM, Crum CP, et al. The simultaneous expression of human chorionic gonadotropin and carcinoembryonic antigen in the female genital tract. Diagn Gynecol Obstet 3:309, 1981

Haynes BF, Metzgar RS, Minna JD, et al. Phenotypic characterization of cutaneous T-cell lymphoma. Blood 304:1319, 1981

Heald J, Buckley CH, Fox H. An immunohistochemical study of the distribution of CEA in epithelial tumours of the ovary. J Clin Pathol 32:910, 1979

Heaney-Kieras J, Bystryn JC. Identification and purification of a Mr 75,000 cell surface human melanoma-associated antigen. Cancer Res 42:2310, 1982

Hecht T, Forman SJ, Bross KJ, et al. Immunoenzymatical staining for terminal deoxynucleotidyl transferase. N Engl J Med 304:848, 1981

Hedin A, Hammarström S, Larsson A. Specificities and binding properties of eight monoclonal antibodies against carcinoembryonic antigen. Mol Immunol 19:1641, 1982

Hedman K. Intracellular localization of fibronectin using immunoperoxidase cytochemistry in light and electron microscopy. J Histochem Cytochem 28:1233, 1980

Heggeness MH, Ash JF. Use of the avidin-biotin complex for the localization of actin and myosin with fluorescence microscopy. J Cell Biol 73:783, 1977

Hehlmann R, Baumgarten A, Schreiber MA, et al. [Cross-reaction of human breast cancers with the envelope glycoprotein gp 52 of the mouse mamma tumorvirus (MMTV).] Verh Dtsch Ges Pathol 65:275, 1981

Heidl G. Demonstration of carcinoembryonic antigen (CEA) by means of the immunoperoxidase technique in paraffin-embedded specimens of tumour tissues. Exp Pathol 21:79, 1982

Heitz PU. Immunocytochemistry—theory and application. Acta Histochem (Suppl) 25:17, 1982

Heitz PU, Wegmann W. Identification of neoplastic Paneth cells in an adenocarcinoma of the stomach using lysozyme as a marker, and electron microscopy. Virchows Arch [A] 386:107, 1980

Hellström I, Brown JP, Hellström KE. Workshop on monoclonal antibodies to human melanoma-associated antigens: findings of the Seattle group. Hybridoma 1:399, 1982

Herbert A, Gallagher PJ. Interpretation of pleural biopsy specimens and aspirates with the immunoperoxidase technique. Thorax 37:822, 1982

Herlyn D, Atkinson B, Koprowski H. Monoclonal antibodies derived from immunosuppressed mice grafted with human melanoma. J Immunol Methods 57:155, 1983

Herlyn M, Steplewski Z, Atkinson BF, et al. Comparative study of the binding characteristics of monoclonal antimelanoma antibodies. Hybridoma 1:403, 1982

Herlyn M, Steplewski Z, Herlyn D, et al. Colorectal carcinoma-specific antigen: detection by means of monoclonal antibodies. Proc Natl Acad Sci USA 76:1438, 1979

Herpers MJHM, Budka H. Glial fibrillary acidic protein (GFAP) in oligodendroglial tumors: gliofibrillary oligodendroglioma and transitional oligoastrocytoma as subtypes of oligodendroglioma. Acta Neuropathol (Berl) 64:265, 1984

Herpers MJHM, Budka H, McCormick D. Production of glial fibrillary acidic protein (GFAP) by neoplastic cells: adaptation to the microenvironment. Acta Neuropathol (Berl) 64:333, 1984

Herrera GA, Pinto de Moraes H. Neurogenic sarcomas in patients with neurofibromatosis (von Recklinghausen's disease). Light, electron microscopy and immunohistochemistry study. Virchows Arch [A] 403:361, 1984

Herrick MK, Rubinstein LJ. The cytological differentiating potential of pineal parenchymal neoplasms (true pinealomas). A clinicopathological study of 28 tumours. Brain 102:289, 1979

Herva E, Ryhänen P, Blanco G, et al. Acid alpha-naphthyl acetate esterase (ANAE) activity and DNA synthesis of lymph node cells in Hodgkin's disease. Scand J Haematol 23:277, 1979

Heyderman E. Immunoperoxidase technique in histopathology: applications, methods, and controls. J Clin Pathol 32:971, 1979

Heyderman E. The role of immunocytochemistry in tumour pathology: a review. J R Soc Med 73:655, 1980

Heyderman E, Gibbons AR, Rosen SW. Immunoperoxidase localisation of human placental lactogen: a marker for the placental origin of the giant cells in "syncytial endometritis" of pregnancy. J Clin Pathol 34:303, 1981

Heyderman E, Graham RM, Chapman DV, et al. Epithelial markers in primary skin cancer: an immunoperoxidase study of the distribution of epithelial membrane antigen (EMA) and carcinoembryonic antigen (CEA) in 65 primary skin carcinomas. Histopathology 8:423, 1984

Heyderman E, Monaghan P. Immunoperoxidase reactions in resin embedded sections. Invest Cell Pathol 2:119, 1979

Heyderman E, Neville MA. A shorter immunoperoxidase technique for the demonstration of carcinoembryonic antigen and other cell products. J Clin Pathol 30:138, 1977

Heyderman E, Steele K, Ormerod MG. A new antigen on the epithelial membrane: its immunoperoxidase localization in normal and neoplastic tissue. J Clin Pathol 32:35, 1979

Heyworth MF. Influence of two different fixatives on the identification of plasma cells in human rectal mucosa. J Histochem Cytochem 9:1018,1980

Higgins PJ, Correa P, Cuello C, et al. Fetal antigens in the precursor stages of gastric cancer. Oncology 41:73, 1984

Hilkens J, Buijs F, Hilgers J, et al. Monoclonal antibodies against human milk–fat globule membranes detecting differentiation antigens of the mammary gland and its tumors. Int J Cancer 34:197, 1984

Hind CR, Tennent GA, Evans DJ, et al. Demonstration of amyloid A (AA) protein and amyloid P component (AP) in deposits of systemic amyloidosis associated with renal adenocarcinoma. J Pathol 139:159, 1983

Hinton DR, Halliday WC. Primary rhabdomyosarcoma of the cerebellum—a light, electron microscopic, and immunohistochemical study. J Neuropathol Exp Neurol 43:439, 1984

Hirsh M-R, Wietzerbin J, Pierres M, et al. Expression of Ia antigens by cultured astrocytes treated with gamma-interferon. Neurosci Lett 41:199, 1983

Ho AD, Helmstädter V, Hunstein W. Immunocytochemical method for the detection of terminal deoxynucleotidyl transferase in acute leukemia. Klin Wochenschr 60:451, 1982

Hockey MS, Stokes HJ, Thompson H, et al. Carcinoembryonic antigen (CEA) expression and heterogeneity in primary and autologous metastatic gastric tumours demonstrated by a monoclonal antibody. Br J Cancer 49:129, 1984

Hoefler H, Kerl H, Rauch HJ, et al. New immunocytochemical observations with diagnostic significance in cutaneous neuroendocrine carcinoma. Am J Dermatopathol 6:525, 1984

Hofer JF, Schwarzmeier JD, Marosi L, et al. [Clinical and laboratory chemical examination in the diagnostic demarcation of chronic lymphatic leukemia.] Acta Med Austriaca 6:222, 1979

Hoffmann-Fezer G, Löhrs U, Rodt HV, et al. Immunohistochemical identification of T- and B-lymphocytes delineated by the unlabelled antibody enzyme method. III. Topographical and quantitative distribution of T- and B-cells in human palatine tonsils. Cell Tissue Res 216:361, 1981

Hoffmann-Fezer G, Rodt H, Eulitz M, et al. Immunohistochemical identification of T- and B-lymphocytes delineated by the unlabeled antibody enzyme method. I. Anatomical distribution of theta-positive and Ig-positive cells in lymphoid organs of mice. J Immunol Methods 1:261, 1976

Höfler H, Denk H. Immunocytochemical demonstration of cytokeratin in gastrointestinal carcinoids and their probable precursor cells. Virchows Arch [A] 403:235, 1984

Höfler H, Denk H, Walter GF. Immunohistochemical demonstration of cytokeratins in endocrine cells of the human pituitary gland and in pituitary adenomas. Virchows Arch [A] 404:359, 1984

Hofman FM, Billing RJ, Parker JW, et al. Cytoplasmic as opposed to surface Ia antigens expressed on human peripheral blood lymphocytes and monocytes. Clin Exp Immunol 49:355, 1982

Hofman FM, Danilovs JA, Husmann L, et al. Ontogeny of B cell markers in human fetal liver. J Immunol 133:1197, 1984a

Hofman FM, Danilovs JA, Taylor CR. HLA-DR (Ia)-positive dendritic-like cells in human fetal nonlymphoid tissues. Transplantation 37:590, 1984b

Hofman FM, Yanagihara E, Byrne B, et al. Analysis of B cell antigens in normal reactive lymphoid tissue using four B cell monoclonal antibodies. Blood 4:775, 1983

Holck S. Plasma cell granuloma of the thyroid. Cancer 48:830, 1981

Holden CA, Hay RJ, MacDonald DM. The antigenicity of trichophyton rubrum: in situ studies by an immunoperoxidase technique in light and electron microscopy. Acta Derm Venereol 61:207, 1981

Holden CA, Staughton RC, Campbell MA, et al. Differential loss of T lymphocyte markers in advanced cutaneous T cell lymphoma. J Am Acad Dermatol 6:507, 1982

Holden J, Churg A. Immunohistochemical staining for keratin and carcinoembryonic antigen in the diagnosis of malignant mesothelioma. Am J Surg Pathol 8:277, 1984

Holmberg V, Wahren B, Esposti PL. Carcinoembryonic antigen in cytological specimens of urothelial carcinoma. Cytometry 5:437, 1984

Holt JM, Robb-Smith AHT. Multiple myeloma: development of plasma cell sarcoma during apparently successful chemotherapy. J Clin Pathol 26:649, 1973

Holthöfer H, Miettinen A, Paasivuo R, et al. Cellular origin and differentiation of renal carcinomas. A fluorescence microscopic study with kidney-specific antibodies, antiintermediate filament antibodies, and lectins. Lab Invest 49:317, 1983

Holubar K, Wolff K, Konrad K, et al. Ultrastructural localization of immunoglobulins in bullous pemphigoid skin. J Invest Dermatol 64:220, 1975

Hølund B, Clemmensen I, Junker P, et al. Fibronectin in experimental granulation tissue. Acta Pathol Microbiol Immunol Scand [A] 90:159, 1982

Hood IC, Qizilbash AH, Young JE, et al. Needle aspiration cytology of a benign and a malignant schwannoma. Acta Cytol 28:157, 1984

Horie Y, Gomyoda M, Kishimoto Y, et al. Plasma carcinoembryonic antigen and acinar cell carcinoma of the pancreas. Cancer 53:1137, 1984

Horne CHW, Reid IN, Milne GD. Prognostic significance of inappropriate production of pregnancy proteins by breast cancer. Lancet 2:279, 1976

Horning SJ, Doggett RS, Warnke RA, et al. Clinical relevance of immunologic phenotype in diffuse large cell lymphoma. Blood 63:1209, 1984

Horoupian DS, Lax F, Suzuki K. Extracerebral leptomeningeal astrocytoma mimicking a meningioma. Arch Pathol Lab Med 103:676, 1979

Horten B, Price RW, Jimenez D. Multifocal varicella-zoster virus leukoencephalopathy temporally remote from herpes zoster. Ann Neurol 9:251, 1981

Horvath E, Kovacs K. Gonadotropin adenomas of the human pituitary: sex-related fine-structural dichotomy. A histologic, immunocytochemical, and electron-microscopic study of 30 tumors. Am J Pathol 117:429, 1984

Horvath E, Kovacs K, Singer W, et al. Acidophil stem cell adenoma of the human pituitary: clinicopathologic analysis of 15 cases. Cancer 47:761, 1981

Houghton AN, Brooks H, Cote RJ, et al. Detection of cell surface and intracellular antigens by human monoclonal antibodies. J Exp Med 158:53, 1983

Houghton AN, Eisinger M, Albino AP, et al. Surface antigens of melanocytes and melanomas. J Exp Med 156:1755, 1982

Houthoff HJ, Poppema S, Ebels EJ, et al. Intracranial malignant lymphomas. A morphologic and immunocytologic study of twenty cases. Acta Neuropathol 44:203, 1978

Howard DR, Batsakis JG. Cytostructural localization of a tumor-associated antigen. Science 210:201, 1980

Howard DR, Batsakis JG. Peanut agglutinin: a new marker for tissue histiocytes. Am J Clin Pathol 77:401, 1982

Howard DR, Taylor CR. A method for distinguishing benign from malignant breast lesions utilizing antibody present in normal human sera. Cancer 43:2279, 1979

Howard DR, Taylor CR. An antitumor antibody in normal human serum: reaction of anti-T with breast carcinoma cells. Oncology 37:142, 1980

Hsu HC, Lin WS, Tsai MJ. Hepatitis-B surface antigen and hepatocellular carcinoma in Taiwan. With special reference to types and localization of HBsAg in the tumor cells. Cancer 52:1825, 1983

Hsu SM, Hsu PL. Demonstration of IgA and secretory component in human hepatocytes. Gut 21:985, 1980

Hsu SM, Hsu PL, Nayak RN. Warthin's tumor: an immunohistochemical study of its lymphoid stroma. Hum Pathol 12:251, 1981a

Hsu SM, Jaffe ES. Leu M1 and peanut agglutinin stain the neoplastic cells of Hodgkin's disease. Am J Clin Pathol 82:29, 1984

Hsu SM, Raine L. Versatility of biotin-labeled lectins and avidin-biotin-peroxidase complex for localization of carbohydrate in tissue sections. J Histochem Cytochem 30:157, 1982

Hsu SM, Raine L, Fanger H. Use of avidin-biotin-peroxidase complex (ABC) in immunoperoxidase techniques: a comparison of ABC and unlabeled antibody (PAP) procedure. J Histochem Cytochem 29:577, 1981b

Hsu SM, Raine L, Fanger H. A comparative study of the peroxidase-antiperoxidase method and an avidin-biotin complex method for studying polypeptide hormones with radioimmunoassay antibodies. Am J Clin Pathol 75:734, 1981c

Hsu SM, Raine L, Fanger H. The use of antiavidin antibody and avidin-biotin-peroxidase complex in immunoperoxidase technics. Am J Clin Pathol 75:816, 1981d

Hsu SM, Raine L, Martin HF. Spironolactone bodies. An immunoperoxidase study with biochemical correlation. Am J Clin Pathol 75:92, 1980

Hsu SM, Ree HJ. Self-sandwich method. An improved immunoperoxidase technic for the detection of small amounts of antigens. Am J Clin Pathol 74:32, 1980

Hsu SM, Yang K, Jaffe ES. Phenotypic expression of Hodgkin's and Reed-Sternberg cells in Hodgkin's disease. Am J Pathol 118:209, 1985

Huang S-N. Immunohistochemical demonstration of hepatitis B core and surface antigens in paraffin section. Lab Invest 33:88, 1975

Huang SN, Neurath AR. Immunohistologic demonstration of hepatitis B viral antigens in liver with reference to its significance in liver injury. Lab Invest 40:1, 1979

Huber H, Gattringer C. [Immunopathology of lymphatic systemic diseases.] Wien Klin Wochenschr 95:319, 1983

Huber H, Gattringer C, Knapp W, et al. Immunopathology of non-Hodgkin lymphomas. Klin Wochenschr 62:1001, 1984

Hui PK, Lawton JW. Immunoperoxidase detection of T and B cells in blood compared with conventional methods. J Clin Pathol 37:1343, 1984

Hullin DA, Brown K, Kynoch PAM, et al. Purification, radioimmunoassay, and distribution of human brain 14-3-2 protein (nervous-system specific enolase) in human tissues. Biochim Biophy Acta 628:98, 1980

Humphrey DM, Aufdemorte TB, Mattox DE. Immunoperoxidase characterization of pharyngeal plasmacytoma. Arch Otolaryngol 108:362, 1982a

Humphrey DM, Cortez EA, Spiva DA. Immunohistologic studies of cytoplasmic immunoglobulins in rheumatic diseases including two patients with monoclonal patterns and subsequent lymphoma. Cancer 49:2049, 1982b

Huntrakoon M, Lin F, Heitz PU, et al. Thymic carcinoid tumor with Cushing's syndrome. Report of a case with electron microscopic and immunoperoxidase studies for neuron-specific enolase and corticotropin. Arch Pathol Lab Med 108:551, 1984

Hurlimann J, Gloor E. Adenocarcinoma in situ and invasive adenocarcinoma of the uterine cervix. An immunohistologic study with antibodies specific for several epithelial markers. Cancer 54:103,1984

Huszar M, Halkin H, Herczeg E, et al. Use of antibodies to intermediate filaments in the diagnosis of metastatic amelanotic malignant melanoma. Hum Pathol 14:1006, 1983

Ibelgaufts H, Jones KW. Papovavirus-related RNA sequences in human neurogenic tumours. Acta Neuropathol (Berl) 56:118, 1982

Iglesias JR, Richardson EP Jr, Collia F, et al. Prenatal intramedullary gliofibroma. A light and electron microscope study. Acta Neuropathol (Berl) 62:230, 1984

Ilardi CF, Ying YY, Ackerman LV, et al. Hepatitis B surface antigen and hepatocellular carcinoma in the People's Republic of China. Cancer 46:1612, 1980

Imada Y, Nonomura I, Hayashi S, et al. Immunoperoxidase technique for identification of *Mycoplasma gallisepticum* and *M. synoviae*. Natl Inst Anim Health Q 19:40, 1979

Imam A, Drushella MM, Taylor CR, et al. Generation and immunohistologic characterization of human monoclonal antibodies to mammary carcinoma cells. Cancer Res 45:263, 1985a

Imam A, Mitchell MS, Modlin RL, et al. Human monoclonal antibodies that distinguish cutaneous malignant melanomas from benign nevi in fixed tissue sections. J Invest Dermatol, in press, 1985b

Imam A, Tayor CR, Tökés ZA. Immunohistochemical study of the expression of human milk fat globule membrane glycoprotein 70. Cancer Res 44:2016, 1984

Imam A, Tökés ZA. Immunoperoxidase localization of a glycoprotein on plasma membrane of secretory epithelium from human breast. J Histochem Cytochem 29:581, 1981

Inaba N, Renk T, Daume E, et al. Ectopic production of placenta-"specific" tissue proteins (PP5 and PP11) by malignant breast tumors. Arch Gynecol 231:87, 1981

Inaba N, Renk T, Wurster K, et al. Ectopic synthesis of pregnancy specific beta 1-glycoprotein (SP1) and placental specific tissue proteins (PP5, PP10, PP11, PP12) in nontrophoblastic malignant tumours. Possible markers in oncology. Klin Wochenschr 58:789, 1980

Inokuchi H, Kawai K, Takeuchi Y, et al. Identification of EC cells in the human intestine: a comparative study between immunohistochemical and silver impregnation techniques. Histochemistry 79:9, 1983

Inoue A, Aozasa K, Tsujimoto M, et al. Immunohistological study on malignant fibrous histiocytoma. Acta Pathol Jpn 34:759, 1984

Inoue M, Ueda G, Yamasaki M, et al. A follicular adenoma arising from the thyroid tissue of a benign cystic teratoma during pregnancy—light microscopical, ultrastructural and endocrinological studies. Nippon Sanka Fujinka Gakkai Zasshi 32:953, 1980

Inoue M, Ueda G, Yamasaki M, et al. Immunohistochemical demonstration of peptide hormones in endometrial carcinomas. Cancer 54:2127, 1984

Inoue T, Kanayama Y, Ohe A, et al. Immunopathologic studies of pneumonitis in systemic lupus erythematosus. Ann Intern Med 91:30, 1979

Ioachim HL, Lerner CW, Tapper ML. The lymphoid lesions associated with the acquired immunodeficiency syndrome. Am J Surg Pathol 7:543, 1983

Ioannidis C, Papamichail M, Agnanti N, et al. The detection of glucocorticoid receptors in breast cancer by immunocytochemical and biochemical methods. Int J Cancer 29:147, 1982

Iqbal K, Zaidi T, Thompson CH, et al. Alzheimer paired helical filaments: bulk isolation, solubility, and protein composition. Acta Neuropathol (Berl) 672:167, 1984

Irie T, Watanabe H, Kawaoi A, et al. Alpha-fetoprotein (AFP), human chorionic gonadotropin (HCG), and carcinoembryonic antigen (CEA) demonstrated in the immature glands of mediastinal teratocarcinoma: a case report. Cancer 50:1160, 1982

Isaacson C, Paterson AC, Berson SD. Hepatitis B surface antigen and hepatocellular carcinoma in Southern Africa. Virchows Arch [A] 385:61, 1979

Isaacson P. Immunochemical demonstration of J chain: a marker of B-cell malignancy. J Clin Pathol 32:802, 1979a

Isaacson P. Middle East lymphoma and alpha-chain disease. An immunohistochemical study. Am J Surg Pathol 3:431, 1979b

Isaacson P. Immunoperoxidase study of the secretory immunoglobulin system and lysozyme in normal and diseased gastric mucosa. Gut 23:578, 1982a

Isaacson P. Immunoperoxidase study of the secretory immunoglobulin system in colonic neoplasia. J Clin Pathol 35:14, 1982b

Isaacson P, Jones DB, Sworn MJ, et al. Malignant histiocytosis of the intestine: report of three cases with immunological and cytochemical analysis. J Clin Pathol 35:510, 1982

Isaacson P, Le Vann HP. The demonstration of carcinoembryonic antigen in colorectal carcinoma and colonic polyps using an immunoperoxidase technique. Cancer 38:1348, 1976

Isaacson P, Wright DH. Anomalous staining patterns in immunohistologic studies of malignant lymphoma. J Histochem Cytochem 27:1197, 1979

Isaacson P, Wright DH, Judd MA, et al. Primary gastrointestinal lymphomas. A classification of 66 cases. Cancer 43:1805, 1979

Isaacson P, Wright DH, Judd MA, et al. The nature of the immunoglobulin-containing cells in malignant lymphoma: an immunoperoxidase study. J Histochem Cytochem 28:761, 1980

Ishiguro Y, Kato K, Ito T, et al. Nervous system–specific enolase in serum as a marker for neuroblastoma. Pediatrics 72:696, 1983a

Ishiguro Y, Kato K, Ito T, et al. Determination of three enolase isoenzymes and S-100 protein in various tumors in children. Cancer Res 43:6080, 1983b

Ishiguro Y, Kato K, Shimizu A, et al. High levels of immunoreactive nervous system–specific enolase in sera of patients with neuroblastoma. Clin Chim Acta 121:173, 1982

Ishii T, Haga S. Immuno-electron-microscopic localization of complements in amyloid fibrils of senile plaques. Acta Neuropathol 63:296, 1984

Isobe K, Isobe Y, Sakurami T. Cytochemical demonstration of transferrin in the mitochondria of immature human erythroid cells. Acta Haematol 65:2, 1981

Isobe T, Ichimori K, Nakajima T, et al. The alpha subunit of S100 protein is present in tumor cells of human malignant melanoma, but not in schwannoma. Brain Res 294:381, 1984

Ito S, Iwanaga T, Yamada Y, et al. Immunohistological demonstration of ACTH-like immunoreactivity in the foetal adrenal medulla in the 23rd week of gestation. Acta Endocrinol 97:412, 1981

Itoh G, Miura S, Suzuki I. Immunohistochemical detection of Fc receptor. I. Light microscopic demonstration of Fc receptor by using soluble immune complexes of peroxidase-antiperoxidase immunoglobulin G. J Histochem Cytochem 25:252, 1977

Itoyama Y, Sternberger NH, Kies MW, et al. Immunocytochemical method to identify myelin basic protein in oligodendroglia and myelin sheaths of the human nervous system. Ann Neurol 7:157, 1980a

Itoyama Y, Sternberger NH, Webster H deF, et al. Immunocytochemical observations on the distribution of myelin-associated glycoprotein and myelin basic protein in multiple sclerosis lesions. Ann Neurol 7:167, 1980b

Itoyama Y, Webster H deF, Sternberger NH, et al. Distribution of papovavirus, myelin-associated glycoprotein, and myelin basic protein in progressive multifocal leukoencephalopathy lesions. Ann Neurol 11:396, 1982

Jabłońska S. [Human papillomavirus and oncogenesis.] Z Hautkr 57:551, 1982

Jacobs M, Choo QL, Thomas C. Vimentin and 70K neurofilament protein co-exist in embryonic neurones from spinal ganglia. J Neurochem 38:969, 1982

Jacobsen GK, Jacobsen M. Possible liver cell differentiation in testicular germ cell tumours. Histopathology 7:537, 1983a

Jacobsen GK, Jacobsen M. Immunohistochemical demonstration of hemoglobin F (HbF) in testicular germ cell tumors. Oncodev Biol Med 4:C45, 1983b

Jacobsen GK, Jacobsen M, Clausen PP. Distribution of tumor-associated antigens in the various histologic components of germ cell tumors of the testis. Am J Surg Pathol 5:257, 1981

Jacobsen GK, Nørgaard-Pedersen B. Placental alkaline phosphatase in testicular germ cell tumours and in carcinoma-in-situ of the testis. An immunohistochemical study. Acta Pathol Microbiol Immunol Scand [A] 92:323, 1984

Jacobsen M, Clausen PP, Smidth S. The effect of fixation and trypsinization on the immunohistochemical demonstration of intracellular immunoglobulin in paraffin-embedded material. Acta Pathol Microbiol Scand [A] 88A:369, 1980

Jäger G. A simple test for the terminal deoxynucleotidyl transferase using the peroxidase-antiperoxidase technique. Blut 42:259, 1981

Jäger G, Dörmer P. Quantitation of the Pap reaction on single cells by absorption cytophotometry. J Immunol Methods 44:55, 1981

Jäger G, Lau B. Normal mononuclear blood cells in diffusion chambers: occurrence of cALLA and TdT. Adv Exp Med Biol 145:371, 1982

Jahnke U, Fischer EH, Alvord EC Jr. Sequence homology between certain viral proteins and proteins related to encephalomyelitis and neuritis. Science 229:282, 1985

Janossy G, Montano L, Selby WS, et al. T cell subset abnormalities in tissue lesions developing during autoimmune disorders, viral infection, and graft-vs.-host disease. J Clin Immunol 2:42S, 1982

Janossy G, Pizzolo G, Thomas JA. Differentiation of human thymocytes. In: Aiuti F, Wigzell H, eds. Thymus Hormones and T Lymphocytes, p 15, 1980a

Janossy G, Thomas JA, Bollum FJ, et al. The human thymic microenvironment: an immunohistologic study. J Immunol 125:202, 1980b

Janossy G, Thomas JA, Habeshaw JA. Immunofluorescence analysis of normal and malignant lymphoid tissues with selected combination of antisera. J Histochem Cytochem 28:1207, 1980c

Janossy G, Thomas JA, Pizzolo G, et al. Immuno-histological diagnosis of lymphoproliferative diseases by selected combinations of antisera and monoclonal antibodies. Br J Cancer 42:224, 1980d

Janossy G, Tidman N, Papageorgiou ES, et al. Distribution of T lymphocyte subsets in the human bone marrow and thymus: an analysis with monoclonal antibodies. J Immunol 126:1608, 1981

Janossy G, Tidman N, Selby WS, et al. Human T lymphocytes of inducer and suppressor type occupy different microenvironments. Nature 288:81, 1980e

Janunger KG, Lindgren J, Sipponen P, et al. Carcinoembryonic antigen (CEA) in the gastric mucosa after partial gastrectomy. Scand J Gastroenterol 14:555, 1979

Jardon-Jeghers C, Reznik M. [Immunohistochemical study in 16 cases of primary lymphoma of the central nervous system.] J Neurol Sci 53:331, 1982

Jautzke G, Altenaehr E. Immunohistochemical demonstration of carcinoembryonic antigen (CEA) and its correlation with grading and staging on tissue sections of urinary bladder carcinomas. Cancer 50:2052, 1982

Javadpour N. Tumor markers in urologic cancer. Urology 16:127, 1980a

Javadpour N. Radioimmunoassay and immunoperoxidase of pregnancy-specific beta$_1$-glycoprotein in sera and tumor cells of patients with certain testicular germ cell tumors. J Urol 123:514, 1980b

Javadpour N, Utz M, Soares T. Immunocytochemical discordance in localization of pregnancy-specific beta$_1$-glycoprotein, alpha-fetoprotein and human chorionic gonadotropin in testicular cancers. J Urol 124:615, 1980

Jennette JC, Wilkman AS, Bagnell CR. Insulin receptor autoantibody-induced pancreatic islet beta (B) cell hyperplasia. Arch Pathol Lab Med 106:218, 1982

Jenson AB, Lancaster WD, Hartmann DP, et al. Frequency and distribution of papillomavirus structural antigens in verrucae, multiple papillomas, and condylomata of the oral cavity. Am J Pathol 107:212, 1982a

Jenson AB, Sommer S, Payling-Wright C, et al. Human papillomavirus. Frequency and distribution in plantar and common warts. Lab Invest 47:491, 1982b

Jessen KR, Mirsky R. Glial cells in the enteric nervous system contain glial fibrillary acidic protein. Nature 286:736, 1980

Jessen KR, Thorpe R, Mirsky R. Molecular identity, distribution and heterogeneity of glial fibrillary acidic protein: an immunoblotting and immunohistochemical study of Schwann cells, satellite cells, enteric glia and astrocytes. J Neurocytol 13:187, 1984

Jha RS, Wickenden C, Anderson MC, et al. Monoclonal antibodies for the histopathological diagnosis of cervical neoplasia. Br J Obstet Gynaecol 91:483, 1984

Jöbsis AC. Prostate. In: Filipe MI, Lake BD, eds. Histochemistry in Pathology, p 263. Edinburgh, Churchill Livingston, 1983

Jöbsis AC, De Vriies GP, Meijer AE, et al. The immunohistochemical detection of prostatic acid phosphatase: its possibilities and limitations in tumour histochemistry. Histochem J 13:961, 1981

Johansen P, Jensen MK. Enzymecytochemistry and immunohistochemistry in monoclonal gammopathy and reactive plasmacytosis. Acta Pathol Microbiol Scand [A] 88A:377, 1980

Johnson GD, Holborow EJ, Dorling J. Immunofluorescence and immunoenzyme techniques. In: Weir DM, ed. Handbook of Experimental Immunology, vol 1. Immunochemistry, p 15. Blackwell Scientific, Oxford, 1978

Johnson KP, Swoveland PT, Emmons RW. Diagnosis of rabies by immunofluorescence in trypsin-treated histologic sections. J Am Med Assoc 244:41, 1980

Johnson RT, Olson LC, Buescher EL. Herpes simplex virus infections of the nervous system: problems in laboratory diagnosis. Arch Neurol 18:260, 1968

Jolivet J, Beauregard H, Somma M, et al. ACTH-secreting medullary carcinoma of the thyroid: monitoring of clinical course with calcitonin and cortisol assays and immunohistochemical studies. Cancer 46:2667, 1980

Jong AS, van Vark M, Albus-Lutter CE, et al. Myosin and myoglobin as tumor markers in the diagnosis of rhabdomyosarcoma. A comparative study. Am J Surg Pathol 8:521, 1984

Jordon RE. Immunohistopathology of the skin. In: Rose NR, Friedman H, eds. Manual of Clinical Immunology, 2nd ed, p 895. Washington DC, American Society for Microbiology, 1980

Jos J, Labbe F, Geny B, et al. Immunoelectron-microscopic localization of immunoglobulin A and secretory component in jejunal mucosa from children with coeliac disease. Scand J Immunol 9:441, 1979

Joseph SA, Sternberger LA. The unlabeled antibody method. Contrasting color staining of beta-lipotropin and ACTH-associated hypothalamic peptides without antibody removal. J Histochem Cytochem 27:1430, 1979

Jothy S, Knaack J, Onerheim RM, et al. Renal involvement in malignant histiocytosis. An immunoperoxidase marker study. Am J Clin Pathol 76:183, 1981

Judd MA. One micrometre paraffin sections: an aid to interpretation of immunoperoxidase staining of immunoglobulins. J Microsc 120:201, 1980.

Judd MA, Britten KJ. Tissue preparation for the demonstration of surface antigen by immunoperoxidase techniques. Histochem J 14:747, 1982

Jurco S 3rd, Nadji M, Harvey DG, et al. Hemangioblastomas: histogenesis of the stromal cell studied by immunocytochemistry. Hum Pathol 13:13, 1982

Justice DL, Rhodes RH, Tokes ZA. Immunohistochemical demonstration of proteinase inhibitor alpha-1-antichymotrypsin in the human central nervous system. Fed Proc Fed Am Soc Exp Biol 44:743, 1985

Kabawat SE, Bast RC Jr, Bhan AK, et al. Tissue distribution of a coelomic epithelium-related antigen recognized by the monoclonal antibody OC125. Int J Gynecol Pathol 2:275, 1983

Kadin M. Ia-like (HLA-DR) antigens in the diagnosis of lymphoma and undifferentiated tumors. Arch Pathol Lab Med 104:503, 1980

Kadin ME. The Reed-Sternberg cell: biological and clinical significance. In: Bennett JM, ed. Controversies in the Management of Lymphomas, Boston, Martinus Nijhoff, 1983

Kageoka T, Nakashima K, Miwa S. Simultaneous demonstration of peroxidase and lysozyme activities in leukemic cells. Am J Clin Pathol 67:481, 1977

Kahn HJ, Baumal R, Marks A. The value of immunohistochemical studies using antibody to S100 protein in dermatopathology. Int J Dermatol 23:38, 1984a

Kahn HJ, Hanna W, Yeger H, et al. Immunohistochemical localization of prekeratin filaments in benign and malignant cells in effusions. Comparison with intermediate filament distribution by electron microscopy. Am J Pathol 109:206, 1982

Kahn HJ, Huang SN, Hanna WM, et al. Immunohistochemical localization of epidermal and Mallory body cytokeratin in undifferentiated epithelial tumors. Comparison with ultrastructural features. Am J Clin Pathol 81:184, 1984b

Kahn HJ, Marks A, Thom H, et al. Role of antibody to S100 protein in diagnostic pathology. Am J Clin Pathol 79:341, 1983

Kallioinen M, Autio-Harmainen H, Dammert K, et al. Discontinuity of the basement membrane in fibrosing basocellular carcinomas and basosquamous carcinomas of the skin: an immunohistochemical study with human laminin and type IV collagen antibodies. J Invest Dermatol 82:248, 1984

Kalyan-Raman UP, Cancilla PA, Case MJ. Solitary, primary malignant astrocytoma of the spinal leptomeninges. J Neuropathol Exp Neurol 42:517, 1983

Kalyan-Raman UP, Kalyan-Raman K. Cerebral amyloid angiopathy causing intracranial hemorrhage. Ann Neurol 16:321, 1984

Kalyan-Raman UP, Taraska JJ, Fierer JA, et al. Malignant fibrous histiocytoma of the meninges. Histological, ultrastructural, and immunocytochemical studies. J Neurosurg 55:957, 1981

Kameda Y, Harada T, Ito K, et al. Immunohistochemical study of the medullary thyroid carcinoma with reference to C-thyroglobulin reaction of tumor cells. Cancer 44:2071, 1979

Kameda Y, Ikeda A. Immunohistochemical study of the C-cell complex of dog thyroid glands with reference to the reactions of calcitonin, C-thyroglobulin and 19S thyroglobulin. Cell Tissue Res 208:405, 1980

Kameda Y, Shigemoto H, Ikeda A. Development and cytodifferentiation of C cell complexes in dog fetal thyroids. An immunohistochemical study using anti-calcitonin, anti-C-thyroglobulin and anti-19S thyroglobulin antisera. Cell Tissue Res 206:403, 1980

Kameya T, Bessho T, Tsumuraya M, et al. Production of gastrin releasing peptide by medullary carcinoma of the thyroid. An immunohistochemical study. Virchows Arch [A] 401:99, 1983

Kami K, Igarashi J, Mitsui T. Immunohistological demonstration of lysozyme in human leukocytes, salivary corpuscles and nasal discharge cells after blockade of myeloperoxidase activity. Okajimas Folia Anat Jpn 58:195, 1981

Kanitakis J, Schmitt D, Thivolet J. Immunohistologic study of cellular populations of histiocytofibromas ("dermatofibromas"). J Cutan Pathol 11:88, 1984

Kapadia SB, Dekker A, Cheng VS, et al. Malignant lymphoma of the thyroid gland: a clinicopathologic study. Head Neck Surg 4:270, 1982

Kaplan C, Blanc WA, Elias J. Identification of erythrocytes in intervillous thrombi: a study using immunoperoxidase identification of hemoglobins. Hum Pathol 13:554, 1982

Kaplan C, Hawley R. Dysgerminoma with giant cells. A case report with immunoperoxidase. Diagn Gynecol Obstet 3:325, 1981

Kariniemi AL, Forsman L, Wahlström T, et al. Expression of differentiation antigens in mammary and extramammary Paget's disease. Br J Dermatol 110:203, 1984a

Kariniemi AL, Forsman L, Wahlström T, et al. Expression of differentiation antigens in benign sweat gland tumours. Br J Dermatol 111:175, 1984b

Kariniemi AL, Forsman L, Wahlström T, et al. Expression of differentiation antigens in mammary Paget's disease. Br J Dermatol 110:203, 1984c

Karle H, Hansen NE, Killmann S-A. Intracellular lysozyme in mature neutrophils and blast cells in acute leukemia. Blood 44:247, 1974

Kasai M, Saxton RE, Holmes EC, et al. Membrane antigens detected on human lung carcinoma cells by hybridoma monoclonal antibody. J Surg Res 30:403, 1981

Kasajima T, Shinzawa H, Matsuda M, et al. Watery diarrhea, hypokalemia and achlorhydria syndrome. Acta Pathol Jpn 30:639, 1980

Kasurinen J, Syrjänen KJ. Stainability of the peptide hormones in gastrointestinal apudomas as demonstrated by immunoperoxidase kits. Scand J Gastroenterol 19:167, 1984

Katano M, Irie K, Irie RF. Immunotherapy of human melanoma with a human monoclonal antibody. In: Proceedings AACR, Abstract 893, 1983

Katayama I, Shimizu M, Miura M, et al. Histochemical demonstration of endogenous estrogen in breast carcinomas: biochemical and clinical correlation. Virchows Arch [A] 402:353, 1984

Katayama Y, Shimoyama N, Yagihashi S, et al. Primary cerebral malignant lymphoma with macroglobulinemia and carcinoma of the colon. Acta Pathol Jpn 31:335, 1981

Kato K, Ishiguro Y, Suzuki F, et al. Distribution of nervous system-specific forms of enolase in peripheral tissues. Brain Res 237:441, 1982

Katz RL, Raval P, Brooks TE, et al. Role of immunocytochemistry in diagnosis of prostatic neoplasia by fine-needle aspiration biopsy. Diagnos Cytopathol 1:28, 1985

Kawakami K, Takahashi KP, Yamagata K. Localization of terminal deoxynucleotidyl transferase (TdT) in rat thymus using immunoperoxidase methods. Histochemistry 73:377, 1981

Kawaoi A, Okano T, Nemoto N, et al. Simultaneous detection of thyroglobulin (Tg), thyroxine (T4), and triiodothyronine (T3) in nontoxic thyroid tumors by the immunoperoxidase method. Am J Pathol 108:39, 1982

Käyhkö K. Optimal fixation conditions for the immunoperoxidase identification of human J chain from tissue sections. Histochemistry 70:23, 1980

Kazimiera J, Gajl-Peczalska KJ, Kersey JH. The value of combined cell suspension and tissue frozen section study in surface marker evaluation of non-Hodgkin's malignant lymphomas. Lab Invest 40:254, 1979

Keifer J, Zaino R, Ballard JO. Erythroleukemic infiltration of a lymph node: use of hemoglobin immunohistochemical techniques in diagnosis. Hum Pathol 15:1090, 1984

Kelly JK, Taylor TV, Milford-Ward A. Alpha-1-antitrypsin Pi S phenotype and liver cell inclusion bodies in alcoholic hepatitis. J Clin Pathol 32:706, 1979

Kemény E, Iványi B, Németh A, et al. Application of the immunoperoxidase technique to formalin fixed, paraffin embedded kidney biopsies. Zentralbl Allg Pathol 128:119, 1983

Kemshead JT, Coakham HB. The use of monoclonal antibodies for the diagnosis of intracranial malignancies and the small round cell tumours of childhood. J Pathol 141:249, 1983

Kendall PA, Polak JM, Pearse AGE. Carbodiimide fixation for immunohistochemistry. Experientia 27:1104, 1971

Kenney RM, Michaels IA, Flomenbaum NE, et al. Poisoning with N-3-pyridylmethyl-N'-p-nitrophenylurea (Vacor). Immunoperoxidase demonstration of beta-cell destruction. Arch Pathol Lab Med 105:367, 1981

Kepes JJ. Meningiomas: Biology, Pathology, and Differential Diagnosis. New York, Masson, 1982

Kepes JJ, Fulling KH, Garcia JH. The clinical significance of "adenoid" formations of neoplastic astrocytes, imitating metastatic carcinoma, in gliosarcomas. A review of five cases. Clin Neuropathol 1:139, 1982

Kepes JJ, Rengachary SS, Lee SH. Astrocytes in hemangioblastomas of the central nervous system and their relationship to stromal cells. Acta Neuropathol (Berl) 47:99, 1979a

Kepes JJ, Rubinstein LJ, Chian H. The role of astrocytes in the formation of cartilage in gliomas: an immunohistochemical study of four cases. Am J Pathol 117:471, 1984

Kepes JJ, Rubinstein LJ, Eng LF. Pleomorphic xanthoastrocytoma: a distinctive meningocerebral glioma of young subjects with relatively favorable prognosis. A study of 12 cases. Cancer 44:1839, 1979b

Kerdel FA, Morgan EW, Holden CA, et al. Demonstration of alpha-1-antitrypsin and alpha-1-antichymotrypsin in cutaneous histiocytic infiltrates and a comparison with intracellular lysozyme. J Am Acad Dermatol 7:177, 1982

Keshgegian AA, Kline TS. Immunoperoxidase demonstration of prostatic acid phosphatase in aspiration biopsy cytology (ABC). Am J Clin Pathol 82:586, 1984

Kew MC, Ray MB, Desmet VJ, et al. Hepatitis-B surface antigen in tumour tissue and non-tumorous liver in black patients with hepatocellular carinoma. Br J Cancer 41:399, 1980

Kierszenbaum AL, Feldman M, Lea O, et al. Localization of androgen-binding protein in proliferating Sertoli cells in culture. Proc Natl Acad Sci USA 77:5322, 1980

Kilpi A, Bergroth V, Konttinen YT, et al. Lymphocyte infiltrations of the gastric mucosa in Sjögren's syndrome. An immunoperoxidase study using monoclonal antibodies in the avidin-biotin-peroxidase method. Arthritis Rheum 26:1196, 1983

Kim SU, Moretto G, Shin DH. Isolation and culture of adult human oligodendroglia. J Neuropathol Exp Neurol 43:329, 1984

Kindblom LG. Factor VIII related antigen and mast cells. Acta Pathol Microbiol Immunol Scand [A] 90:437, 1982

Kindblom LG, Seidal T, Karlsson K. Immuno-histochemical localization of myoglobin in human muscle tissue and embryonal and alveolar rhabdomyosarcoma. Acta Pathol Microbiol Immunol Scand [A] 90:167, 1982

King CT, Clark TD, Lovett J, et al. A comparison of clinical course with blood group antigen testing by specific red cell adherence and immunoperoxidase in ureteral and renal pelvic tumors. J Urol 130:871, 1983

King WJ, DeSombre ER, Jensen EV, et al. Comparison of immunocytochemical and steroid-binding assays for estrogen receptor in human breast tumors. Cancer Res 45:293, 1985

Kingston D, Pearson JR, Penna FJ. Plasma cell counts on human jejunal biopsy specimens examined by immunofluorescence and immunoperoxidase techniques: a comparative study. J Clin Pathol 35:381, 1981

Kini SR, Miller JM, Hamburger JI, et al. Cytopathologic features of medullary carcinoma of the thyroid. Arch Pathol Lab Med 108:156, 1984

Kirshenbaum G, Rhone DP. Solitary extramedullary plasmacytoma of the breast with serum monoclonal protein: a case report and review of the literature. Am J Clin Pathol 83:230, 1985

Kitamura T, Miyake T, Fujita S. Genesis of resting microglia in the gray matter of mouse hippocampus. J Comp Neurol 226:421, 1984

Kittas C, Aroni K, Kotsis L, et al. Distribution of lysozyme, alpha 1-antichymotrypsin and alpha 1-antitrypsin in adenocarcinomas of the stomach and large intestine. An immunohistochemical study. Virchows Arch [A] 398:139, 1982

Kjeldsberg CR, Kim H. Polykaryocytes resembling Warthin-Finkeldey giant cells in reactive and neoplastic lymphoid disorders. Hum Pathol 12:267, 1981

Klavins JV. Tumor markers of pancreatic carcinoma. Cancer (Suppl 6) 47:1597, 1981

Klempa I, Helmstädter V, Feurle G, et al. [Endocrine tumors of the gastrointestinal and pancreatic systems. Multiple endocrine adenoma from another viewpoint.] Chirurg 51:321, 1980

Klockars M, Pettersson T, Riska H, et al. Pleural fluid lysozyme in human disease. Arch Intern Med 139:73, 1979

Knapp RH, Fritz SR, Reiman HM. Primary embryonal carcinoma and choriocarcinoma of the mediastinum. A case report. Arch Pathol Lab Med 106:507, 1982

Knowles DM II. Non-Hodgkin's lymphomas. II. Current immunologic concepts. In: Fenoglio CM, Wolff M, eds. Progress in Surgical Pathology, p 107. New York, Masson, 1980.

Knowles DM, Winchester RJ, Kunkel HG. A comparison of peroxidase- and fluorochrome-conjugated antisera for the demonstration of surface and intracellular antigens. Clin Immunol Immunopathol 7:410, 1977

Koh S-J, Vargas GF, Caces JN, et al. Malignant "histiocytic" lymphoma in childhood. Cancer 74:417, 1980

Kohama MT, Cardenas JM, Seto JT. Immunoelectron microscopic study of the detection of the glycoproteins of influenza and Sendai viruses in infected cells by the immunoperoxidase method. J Virol Methods 3:293, 1981

Kojima M, Mori N. Immunohistological analysis of malignant lymphoma of B cell origin. Acta Pathol Jpn 32 (Suppl 1):155, 1982

Kojima O, Ikeda E, Uehara Y, et al. Correlation between carcinoembryonic antigen in gastric cancer tissue and survival of patients with gastric cancer. Gann 75:230, 1984a

Kojima O, Tanioku T, Kitagawa N, et al. Comparative study of CEA staining in gastric and colorectal cancer tissues. Gastroenterol Jpn 19:18, 1984b

Kojiro M, Kawano Y, Isomura T, et al. Distribution of albumin- and/or alpha-fetoprotein-positive cells in hepatocellular carcinoma. Lab Invest 44:221, 1981

Konttinen YT, Reitamo S. Effect of fixation on the antigenicity of human lactoferrin in paraffin-embedded tissues and cytocentrifuged cell smears. Histochemistry 62:55, 1979

Kornstein MJ, Bonner H, Cohen R, et al. Leu M1 and S-100 in Hodgkin's disease and non-Hodgkin's lymphoma. Lab Invest 52:36A, 1985

Kovacs K, Horvath E. Pathology of pituitary adenomas. Bull Los Angeles Neurol Soc 42:92, 1977

Kovacs K, Horvath E, Ezrin C, et al. Adenoma of the human pituitary producing growth hormone and thyrotropin. A histologic, immunocytologic, and fine-structural study. Virchows Arch [A] 395:59, 1982

Kovacs K, Horvath E, Killinger DW, et al. Growth hormone-producing pituitary adenoma with giant secretory granules. Acta Neuropathol 46:239, 1977

Kovacs K, Horvath E, Rewcastle NB, et al. Gonadotroph cell adenoma of the pituitary in a woman with long-standing hypogonadism. Arch Gynecol 229:57, 1980a

Kovacs K, Horvath E, Ryan N. Immunocytology of the human pituitary. In: DeLellis RA, ed. Diagnostic Immunohistochemistry, p 17. Monographs in Diagnostic Pathology. New York, Masson, 1981

Kovacs K, Horvath E, Ryan N, et al. Null cell adenoma of the human pituitary. Virchows Arch [A] 387:165, 1980b

Kovacs K, Ryan N, Horvath E, et al. Pituitary adenomas in old age. J Gerontol 35:16, 1980c

Krajs GJ, et al. Somatostatinoma syndrome. N Engl J Med 301:285, 1979

Kramer SA, Wold LE, Gilchrist GS, et al. Yolk sac carcinoma: an immunohistochemical and clinicopathologic review. J Urol 131:315, 1984

Kreth HW, Dunker R, Rodt H, et al. Immunohistochemical identification of T-lymphocytes in the central nervous system of patients with multiple sclerosis and subacute sclerosing panencephalitis. J Neuroimmunol 2:177, 1982

Krugliak L, Meyer PR, Taylor CR. The distribution of lysozyme, alpha-1-antitrypsin, alpha-1-antichymotrypsin in normal hematopoietic cells and in myeloid leukemias: an immunoperoxidase study on cytocentrifuge preparations, smears and paraffin sections. Am J Hematol, 21:99, 1986.

Kuhajda FP, Bohn H, Mendelsohn G. Pregnancy-specific beta-1 glycoprotein (SP-1) in breast carcinoma. Pathologic and clinical considerations. Cancer 54:1392, 1984

Kuhajda FP, Offutt LE, Mendelsohn G. The distribution of carcinoembryonic antigen in breast carcinoma. Diagnostic and prognostic implications. Cancer 52:1257, 1983a

Kuhajda FP, Sun TT, Mendelsohn G. Polypoid squamous carcinoma of the esophagus. A case report with immunostaining for keratin. Am J Surg Pathol 7:495, 1983b

Kuhlmann WD, Kuhlmann M. Immunohistological localization of alpha 1-fetoprotein in normal and diseased liver. Acta Histochem 25:63, 1982

Kuhlmann WD, Peschke P. Advances in ultrastructural postembedment localization of antigens in Epon sections with paroxidase-labelled antibodies. Histochemistry 75:151, 1982

Kumanishi T, Hirano A. An immunoperoxidase study on herpes simplex virus encephalitis. J Neuropathol Exp Neurol 37:790, 1978

Kumanishi T, In S. SSPE: immunohistochemical demonstration of measles virus antigen(s) in paraffin sections. Acta Neuropathol (Berl) 48:161, 1979

Kumpulainen T. Immunohistochemical localization of human carbonic anhydrase isoenzyme C. Histochemistry 62:271, 1979

Kumpulainen T, Dahl D, Korhonen LK, et al. Immunolabeling of carbonic anhydrase isoenzyme C and glial fibrillary acidic protein in paraffin-embedded tissue sections of human brain and retina. J Histochem Cytochem 31:879. 1983

Kumpulainen T, Nyström SHM. Immunohistochemical localization of carbonic anhydrase isoenzyme C in human brain. Brain Res 220:220, 1981

Kung, PC, Berger CL, Goldstein G, et al. Cutaneous T cell lymphoma: characterization by monoclonal antibodies. Blood 57:261, 1981

Kung PC, Goldstein G, Reinherz EK, et al. Monoclonal antibodies defining distinctive human T cell surface antigens. Science 206:347, 1979

Kuriyama M, Loor R, Wang MC, et al. Prostatic acid phosphatase and prostate-specific antigen in prostate cancer. Int Adv Surg Oncol 5:29, 1982

Kurman RJ, Andrade D, Goebelsmann U, et al. An immunohistological study of steroid localization in Sertoli-Leydig tumors of the ovary and testis. Cancer 42:1772, 1978

Kurman RJ, Goebelsmann U, Taylor CR. Steroid localization in granulosa-theca tumors of the ovary. Cancer 43:2377, 1979

Kurman RJ, Goebelsmann U, Taylor CR. Steroid hormones in functional ovarian tumours. In: DeLellis RA, ed. Monographs in Diagnostic Pathology, p 137. New York, Masson, 1981a

Kurman RJ, Jenson AB, Lancaster WD. Papillomavirus infection of the cervix. II. Relationship to intraepithelial neoplasia based on the presence of specific viral structural proteins. Am J Surg Pathol 7:39, 1983

Kurman RJ, Scardino PT. Alpha-fetoprotein and human chorionic gonadotropin in ovarian and testicular germ cell tumors. In: DeLellis RA, ed. Diagnostic Immunohistochemistry, p 277. Monographs in Diagnostic Pathology. New York, Masson, 1981

Kurman RJ, Shah KH, Lancaster WD, et al. Immunoperoxidase localization of papillomavirus antigens in cervical dysplasia and vulvar condylomas. Am J Obstet Gynecol 140:931, 1981b

Kurman RJ. Contributions of immunocytochemistry to gynaecological pathology. Clin Obstet Gynaecol 11:5, 1984

Kurucz J, Charbonneau R, Kurucz A, et al. Quantitative clinicopathologic study of senile dementia. J Am Geriatr Soc 29:158, 1981

Kutteh WH, Mestecky J, Preud'homme JL, et al. J-chain and immunoglobulin synthesis in human lymphoid cells. Fed Proc 39:1152, 1980

Kuwano H, Hashimoto H, Enjoji M. Atypical fibroxanthoma distinguishable from spindle cell carcinoma in sarcoma-like skin lesions. A clinicopathologic and immunohistochemical study of 21 cases. Cancer 55:172, 1985

Kyritsis AP, Tsokos M, Triche TJ, et al. Retinoblastoma—origin from a primitive neuroectodermal cell? Nature 307:471, 1984

Kyrkou KA, Iatridis SG, Athanassiadou PP, et al. Detection of benign or malignant origin of ascites with combined indirect immunoperoxidase assays of carcinoembryonic antigen and lysozyme. Acta Cytol 29:57, 1985

Lack EE, Jenson AB, Smith HG, et al. Immunoperoxidase localization of human papillomavirus in laryngeal papillomas. Intervirology 14:148, 1980

Lajtha LG. Cellular mechanisms of red cell production. Scand J Haematol 2:26, 1965

Lake BD. Lysosomal enzyme deficiencies. In: Adams JH, Corsellis JAN, Duchen LW, eds. Greenfield's Neuropathology, 4th ed, p 491. New York, John Wiley & Sons, 1984

Lampert IA, Pizzolo G, Thomas A, et al. Immunohistochemical characterisation of cells involved in dermatopathic lymphadenopathy. J Pathol 131:145, 1980

Landaas TO, Godal T, Marton PF, et al. Cell-associated immunoglobulin in human non-Hodgkin lymphomas. A comparative study of surface immunoglobulin on cells in suspension and cytoplasmic immunoglobulin by immunohistochemistry. Acta Pathol Microbiol Scand [A] 89:91, 1981

Landolt AM. Pituitary adenomas. Clinico-morphologic correlations. J Histochem Cytochem 27:1395, 1979

Landolt AM, Minder H. Immunohistochemical examination of the paraadenomatous "normal" pituitary. An evaluation of prolactin cell hyperplasia. Virchows Arch [A] 403:181, 1984

Langley OK, Ghandour MS. An immunocytochemical investigation of non-neuronal enolase in cerebellum: a new astrocyte marker. Histochem J 13:137, 1981

Langley OK, Ghandour MS, et al. Carbonic anhydrase: an ultrastructural study in rat cerebellum. Histochem J 12:473, 1980

Lansdorp PM, Astaldi GCB, Oostehof F, et al. Immunoperoxidase procedures to detect monoclonal antibodies against cell surface antigens. Quantitation of binding and staining of individual cells. J Immunol Methods 39:393, 1980

Larsson LI. Pathology of gastrointestinal endocrine cells. Scand J Gastroenterol (Suppl 53) 14:1, 1979

Larsson LI. Immunocytochemical characterization of ACTH-like immunoreactivity in cerebral nerves and in endocrine cells of the pituitary and gastrointestinal tract by using region-specific antisera. J Histochem Cytochem 28:133, 1980

Larsson LI, Golterman N, DeMagistris L, et al. Somatostatin cell processes as pathway for paracrine secretion. Science 205:1393, 1979

Lascano EF, Patitó JA, Salama AA, et al. Immunostaining of carcinoembryonic antigen in colorectal adenocarcinomas and polyps. Media 39:369, 1979

Lass JH, Jenson AB, Papale JJ, et al. Papillomavirus in human conjunctival papillomas. Am J Ophthalmol 95:364, 1983

Lauder I, Holland D, Mason DY, et al. Identification of large cell undifferentiated tumours in lymph nodes using leucocyte common and keratin antibodies. Histopathology 8:259, 1984

Laurent G, Delsol G, Reyes F, et al. Detection of J chain in lymphomas and related disorders. Clin Exp Immunol 44:620, 1981

Laurent G, Gourdin M, Reyes F. Immunoperoxidase detection of immunoglobulins in cells of immunoproliferative diseases. A comparison between conjugate and nonconjugate (PAP) procedures. Am J Clin Pathol 74:265, 1980

Laurent G, Gourdin MF, Reyes F. Detection of surface immunoglobulins of human lymphoid cells: a comparative study of live and fixed cells using a direct immunoperoxidase procedure. J Clin Pathol 35:139, 1982

Lauriola L, Michetti F, Stolfi VM, et al. Detection by S-100 immunolabelling of interdigitating reticulum cells in human thymomas. Virchows Arch [B] 45:187, 1984

Laverson S, McKeever PE, Kornblith PL, et al. Diagnosis of glioma on frozen section by immunofluorescence for glial fibrillary acidic protein. Lancet 1:674, 1981

Lavker RM, Sun TT. Heterogeneity in epidermal basal keratinocytes: morphological and functional correlations. Science 215:1239, 1982

Lawrence EC, Broder S, Jaffe ES, et al. Evolution of a lymphoma with helper T-cell characteristics in Sezary syndrome. Blood 52:481, 1978

Lazarides E. Intermediate filaments—chemical heterogeneity in differentiation. Cell 23:649, 1981

Le Bouton AV, Masse JP. A random arrangement of albumin-containing hepatocytes seen with histo-immunologic methods. I. Verification of the artifact. Anat Rec 197:183, 1980

Le Doussal V, Zangerle PF, Collette J, et al. Immunohistochemical detection of alphalactalbumin in breast lesions. Eur J Cancer Clin Oncol 20:1069, 1984

Leader M, Jass JR. Increased alpha-fetoprotein concentration in association with ileal adenocarcinoma complicating Crohn's disease. J Clin Pathol 37:293, 1984

Leathem A, Atkins N. Fixation and immunohistochemistry of lymphoid tissue. J Clin Pathol 33:1010, 1980

Lechago J, Sun NC, Weinstein WM. Simultaneous visualization of two antigens in the same tissue section by combining immunoperoxidase with immunofluorescence techniques. J Histochem Cytochem 27:1221, 1979

Leduque P, Paulin C, Chayvialle JA, et al. Immunocytological evidence of motilin- and secretin-containing cells in the human fetal gastro-entero-pancreatic system. Cell Tissue Res 218:519, 1981

Lee AK, DeLellis RA, Rosen PP, et al. Alpha-lactalbumin as an immunohistochemical marker for metastatic breast carcinomas. Am J Surg Pathol 8:93, 1984

Lee CL, Li CY, Jou YH, et al. Immunochemical characterization of prostatic acid phosphatase with monoclonal antibodies. Ann NY Acad Sci 390:52, 1982

Lee JC, Olszewski J. Increased cerebrovascular permeability after repeated electroshocks. Neurology (NY) 11:515, 1961

Lee JN, Wahlström T, Ouyang PC, et al. Immunohistochemical evidence of prolactin in trophoblastic tumors. Gynecol Oncol 11:299, 1981

Lee P, Lam KW, Li CY, et al. A simple immunohistochemical method for the detection of prostatic acid phosphatase. Arch Pathol Lab Med 105:205, 1981

Lehto V-P, Miettinen M, Dahl D, et al. Bronchial carcinoid cells contain neural-type intermediate filaments. Cancer 545:624, 1984

Lehto V-P, Stenman S, Miettinen M., et al. Expression of a neural type of intermediate filament as a distinguishing feature between oat cell carcinoma and other lung cancers. Am J Pathol 110:113, 1983

Lehy T, Peranzi G, Cristina ML. Correlative immunocytochemical and electron microscopic studies: identification of (entero) glucagon-somatostatin- and pancreatic polypeptide-like–containing cells in the human colon. Histochemistry 71:67, 1981

Lehy T, Grès L, Ferreira de Castro E. Quantitation of gastrin and somatostatin cell populations in the antral mucosa of the rat. Comparative distribution and evolution through different life stages. Cell Tissue Res 198:325, 1979

Lennert K. Malignant lymphomas other than Hodgkin's disease. In: Uehlinger E, ed. Handbuch der speziellen pathologischen Anatomie und Histologie, p 263. Berlin, Springer-Verlag, 1978

Lennert K, Stein H, Kaiserling E. New criteria for the classification of malignant lymphomata. Br J Cancer 31 (suppl 31):29, 1975

Levine AM, Lichtenstein AK, Gresik MV, et al. Clinical and immunologic spectrum of plasmacytoid lymphocytic lymphoma without serum monoclonal IgM. Br J Haematol 46:225, 1980

Levine AM, Taylor CR, Schneider DR, et al. Immunoblastic sarcoma of T-cell versus B-cell origin: I. Clinical features. Blood 58:52, 1981

Levy N, Nelson J, Meyer P, Lukes RF, Parker JW. Reactive lymphoid hyperplasia with single class (monoclonal) surface immunoglobulin. Am J Clin Pathol 80:300, 1983

Levy R, Warnke R, Dorfman RF, et al. The monoclonality of human B cell lymphomas. J Exp Med 145:1014, 1977

Li CY, Lam WK, Yam LT. Immunohistochemical diagnosis of prostatic cancer with metastasis. Cancer 46:706, 1980

Li JY, Dubois MP, Dubois PM. Ultrastructural localization of immunoreactive corticotropin, beta-lipotropin, alpha- and beta-endorphin in cells of the human fetal anterior pituitary. Cell Tissue Res 204:37, 1979

Lillehoj HS, Choe BK, Rose NR. Monoclonal antibodies to human prostatic acid phosphatase: probes for antigenic study. Proc Natl Acad Sci USA 79:5061, 1982

Lillie RD, Fullmer HM. Histopathologic Technic and Practical Histochemistry. New York, McGraw-Hill, 1976

Lillie RD, Pizzolato P. Histochemical use of borohydride as aldehyde blocking reagent. Stain Technol 13:16, 1976

Linch DC, Jones HM, Berliner N, et al. Hodgkin-cell leukemia of B-cell origin. Lancet 1:78, 1985

Lindenberg R, Haymaker W. Tissue reactions in the gray matter of the central nervous system. In: Haymaker W, Adams RD, eds. Histology and Histopathology of the Nervous System, vol I, p 973. Springfield, Ill., Charles C Thomas, 1982

Lindop GB, Fleming S. Renin in renal cell carcinoma—an immunocytochemical study using an antibody to pure human renin. J Clin Pathol 37:27, 1984

Ling EA, Kaur C, Wong WC. Light and electron microscopic demonstration of non-specific esterase in amoeboid microglial cells in the corpus callosum in postnatal rats: a cytochemical link to monocytes. J Ant 135:385, 1982

Linke RP. Monoclonal antibodies against amyloid fibril protein AA. Production, specificity, and use for immunohistochemical localization and classification of AA-type amyloidosis. J Histochem Cytochem 32:322, 1984

Linke RP, Nathrath WB. [Classification of amyloidoses at biopsy by the immunoperoxidase method.] MMW 122:1772, 1980

Linke RP, Nathrath WB. Immunochemical typing of amyloid from tissue biopsies. Acta Neuropathol 56:285, 1982

Linnemann CC Jr, First MR, Alvira MM, et al. Herpesvirus hominis type 2 meningoencephalitis following renal transplantation. Am J Med 61:703, 1976

Lipinski M, Braham K, Caillaud JM, et al. HNK-1 antibody detects an antigen expressed on neuroectodermal cells. J Exp Med 158:1775, 1983

Livni N, Abramowitz A, Londner M, et al. Immunoperoxidase method of identification of Leishmania in routinely prepared histological sections. Virchows Arch [A] 401:147, 1983

Livni N, Laufer A, Levo Y. Demonstration of amyloid in murine and human secondary amyloidosis by the immunoperoxidase technique. J Pathol 132:343, 1980

Ljungberg O, Ericsson UB, Bondeson L, et al. A compound follicular-parafollicular cell carcinoma of the thyroid: a new tumor entity? Cancer 52:1053, 1983

Llena J, Hirano A. Fine structure of an intracerebral benign hemangioendothelioma. J Neuropathol Exp Neurol 42:355, 1983

Lloyd JM, O'Dowd T, Driver M, et al. Demonstration of an epitope of the transferrin receptor in human cervical epithelium—a potentially useful cell marker. J Clin Pathol 37:131, 1984a

Lloyd JM, O'Dowd T, Driver M, et al. Immunohistochemical detection of Ca antigen in normal dysplastic and neoplastic squamous epithelia of the human uterine cervix. J Clin Pathol 37:14,1984b

Lloyd RV, Caceres V, Warner TF, et al. Islet cell adenomatosis: a report of two cases and review of the literature. Arch Pathol Lab Med 105:198, 1981

Lloyd RV, Shapiro B, Sisson JC, et al. An immunohistochemical study of pheochromocytomas. Arch Pathol Lab Med 108:541, 1984

Lloyd RV, Wilson BS. Specific endocrine tissue marker defined by a monoclonal antibody. Science 222:628, 1983

Lobo A, Carr I, Malcolm D. The EM immunocytochemical demonstration of lysozyme in macrophage giant cells in sarcoidosis. Experentia 34:1088, 1978

Löhler J. Immunohistochemical demonstration of viral antigens in paraffin-embedded autopsy specimens of virally infected central nervous system. Acta Neuropathol (Suppl) 7:139, 1981

Löhler J. Virusinfektionen des Zentralnervensystems. Nachweis virales Antigen in paraffin-eingebettetem Autopsiematerial mit Hilfe der PAP-Technik (Sternberger). Acta Histochem [Suppl] 25:107, 1982

Lojek MA, Fer MF, Kasselberg AG, et al. Cushing's syndrome with small cell carcinoma of the uterine cervix. Acta Pathol Microbiol Scand [A] 88:175, 1980

Loke YW, Day S. Monoclonal antibody to human cytotrophoblast. Am J Reprod Immunol 5:106, 1984

Long TT 3rd, Barton TK, Draffin R, et al. Conservative management of the Zollinger-Ellison syndrome. Ectopic gastrin production by an ovarian cystadenoma. J Am Med Assoc 243:1837, 1980

Löning T, Burkhardt A. Dyskeratosis in human and experimental oral precancer and cancer. An immunohistochemical and ultrastructural study in men, mice and rats. Arch Oral Biol 27:361, 1982

Loor R, Shimano T, Manzo ML, et al. Purification and characterization of human pancreas-specific antigen. Biochim Biophys Acta 668:222, 1981

Loosli H, Hurlimann J. Immunohistological study of malignant diffuse mesotheliomas of the pleura. Histopathology 8:793, 1984

Lowenthal A, Flament-Durand J, Karcher D, et al. Glial cells identified by anti-α-albumin (anti-GFA) in human pineal gland. J Neurochem 38:863, 1982

Lozano de Arce EA, Bedrossian CWM, Bedrossian UK, Reitmeyer W, Burgeois PL. Detection of herpes virus cervicovaginitis by a sequential Papanicolaou-immunoperoxidase technique. Diagnos Cytopathol 1:23, 1985

Lukes RJ, Collins RD. New approaches to the classification of the lymphomata. Br J Cancer (Suppl 2) 31:1, 1975

Lukes RJ, Parker JW, Taylor CR, et al. Immunologic approach to non-Hodgkin's lymphoma and related leukemias. An analysis of the results of multiparameter studies of 425 cases. Semin Hematol 15:322, 1978

Lukes RJ, Tindle B. An approach to bone marrow evaluation by pathologists. In: Proceedings of the VIII

World Congress of Anatomic and Clinical Pathology, Munich, September 1972. Amsterdam, Excerpta Medica, p 86, 1972

Lutzner M, Edelson R, Schein P, et al. Cutaneous T-cell lymphomas: the Sezary syndrome, mycosis fungoides, and related disorders. Ann Intern Med 83:534, 1975

Lutzner M, Kuffer R, Blanchet-Bardon C, et al. Different papillomaviruses as the cause of oral warts. Arch Dermatol 118:393, 1982

Ma BI, Joseph BS, Walsh MJ, et al. Multiple sclerosis serum and cerebrospinal fluid immunoglobulin binding to Fc receptors of oligodendrocytes. Ann Neurol 9:371, 1981

Ma J, De Boer WG, Nayman J. The presence of oncofoetal antigens in large bowel carcinoma. Aust NZ J Surg 52:30, 1982

Ma J, Handley CJ, de Boer WG. An ovarian tumour specific mucin antigen—immunohistological and biochemical studies. Pathology 15:385, 1983

Maciejewski W, Braun-Falco O, Scherer R. Immunoelectron-microscopical localization of in vivo–bound complement C3 in bullous pemphigoid with the use of the peroxidase-antiperoxidase multistep technique. Arch Dermatol Res 266:205, 1979

MacIver AG, Giddings J, Mepham BL. Demonstration of extracellular immunoproteins in formalin-fixed renal biopsy specimens. Kidney Int 16:632, 1979

MacIver AG, Mepham BL. Immunoperoxidase technique and controls. J Clin Pathol 33:1218, 1980

MacIver AG, Mepham BL. Immunoperoxidase techniques in human renal biopsy. Histopathology 6:249, 1982

Mackie RM, Campbell I, Turbitt ML. Use of NK1 C3 monoclonal antibody in the assessment of benign and malignant melanocytic lesions. J Clin Pathol 37:367, 1984

MacLean GD, Seehafer J, Shaw AR, et al. Antigenic heterogeneity of human colorectal cancer cell lines analyzed by a panel of monoclonal antibodies. I. Heterogeneous expression of Ia-like and HLA-like antigenic determinants. J Natl Cancer Inst 69:357, 1982

MacPherson BR, Kottmeyer ME. Detection of anti-lymphocyte antibodies using immunoperoxidase antiglobulin technic. Am J Clin Pathol 68:347, 1977

Madri JA, Barwick KW. An immunohistochemical study of nasopharyngeal neoplasms using keratin antibodies: epithelial versus nonepithelial neoplasms. Am J Surg Pathol 6:142, 1982

Mahan DE, Bruce AW, Manley PN et al. Immunohistochemical evaluation of prostatic carcinoma before and after radiotherapy. J Urol 124:488, 1980

Malik NJ, Daymon ME. Improved double immunoenzyme labeling using alkaline phosphatase and horseradish peroxidase. J Clin Pathol 35:1092, 1982

Mallory FB. Principles of Pathologic Histology. Philadelphia, WB Saunders, 1923

Mambo NC, Irwin SM. Anaplastic small cell neoplasms of the thyroid: an immunoperoxidase study. Hum Pathol 15:55, 1984

Mandache E, Moldoveanu E, Móta G, et al. Multivalent hybrid antibody with double specificity as a tool for locating cell surface antigens by electron microscopy. J Immunol Meth 35:33, 1980

Manley PN, Mahan DE, Bruce AW, et al. Prostate-specific acid phosphatase. In: DeLellis RA, ed. Diagnostic Immunohistochemistry, p. 313. Masson Monographs in Diagnostic Pathology, Masson Publishing, 1981

Mann DMA, Tinkler AM, Yates PO. Neurological disease and herpes simplex virus. An immunohistochemical study. J Neurochem 38:24, 1983

Mann G. Physiologic Histology. Oxford, Oxford University Press, 1902

Mannoji H, Takeshita I, Fukui M, et al. Glial fibrillary acidic protein in medulloblastoma. Acta Neuropathol (Berl) 55:63, 1981

Manz HJ, Phillips TM, McCullough DC. Herpes simplex type 2 encephalitis concurrent with known cerebral metastases. Acta Neuropathol (Berl) 47:237, 1979

Marangos PJ, Schmechel D, Zis AP, et al. The existence and neurobiological significance of neuronal and glial forms of the glycolytic enzyme enolase. Biol Psychiatry 14:563, 1979

Marcollet M, Morin J, Lecher P. Comparison between two chromogenic substrates for revealing an immunoperoxidase reaction of human metaphase chromosomes. Stain Technol 55:35, 1980

Mariani-Costantini R, Barbanti P, Colnaghi MI, et al. Reactivity of a monoclonal antibody with tissues and tumors from the human breast. Immunohistochemical localization of a new antigen and clinicopathologic correlations. Am J Pathol 115:47, 1984

Mariuzzi GM, Beltrami CA, Di Loreto C, et al. Human papillomavirus in cervical condylomata. An immunohistochemical study. Ric Clin Lab 13:255, 1983

Marks SM, Baltimore D, McCaffrey R. Terminal transferase as a predictor of initial responsiveness to vincristine and prednisone in blastic chronic myelogenous leukemia. A co-operative study. N Engl J Med 198:812, 1978

Marmar JL, Gisser S, Praiss DE, et al. The identification of functioning plasma cells in cervical tissue by an immunoperoxidase technique. Int J Fertil 26:25, 1981

Marsden HB, Kumar S, Kahn J, et al. A study of glial fibrillary acidic protein (GFAP) in childhood brain tumours. Int J Cancer 31:439, 1983

Marsh WL Jr, Stevenson DR, Long HJ III. Primary leptomeningeal presentation of T-cell lymphoma. Report of a patient and review of the literature. Cancer 51:1125, 1983

Marshall PE, Landis DMD, Zalneraitis EL. Immunocytochemical studies of substance P and leucine-enkephalin in Huntington's disease. Brain Res 289:11, 1983

Marshall RJ, Herbert A, Braye SG, et al. Use of antibodies to carcinoembryonic antigen and human milk fat globule to distinguish carcinoma, mesothelioma, and reactive mesothelium. J Clin Pathol 37:1215, 1984

Martelli MF, Falini B, Tabilio A, et al. Topographical localization of intracellular immunoglobulins in hairy cells by immunoelectron microscopy. Acta Haematol 64:251, 1980

Martelli MF, Falini B, Tabilio A, et al. Multiple myeloma and related conditions: an immunoperoxidase study of paraffin-embedded bone marrow biopsies. Haematologica 67:1, 1982

Martin JF, Kittas C, Triger DR. Giant cell arteritis of coronary arteries causing myocardial infarction. Br Heart J 43:487, 1980

Martin SE, Zhang HZ, Magyarosy E, et al. Immunologic methods in cytology: definitive diagnosis of non-Hodgkin's lymphomas using immunologic markers for T- and B-cells. Am J Clin Pathol 82:666, 1984

Martinez AJ. Acanthamoebiasis and immunosuppression. Case report. J Neuropathol Exp Neurol 41:548, 1982

Martinez AJ, Lee A, Moossy J, et al. Pituitary adenomas: clinicopathological and immunohistochemical study. Ann Neurol 7:24, 1980

Martinez D, Barthe D. Heterogeneous pituitary adenomas: a light microscopic, immunohistochemical and electron microscopic study. Virchows Arch [A] 394: 221, 1982

Mason DY. Intracellular lysozyme and lactoferrin in myeloproliferative disorders. J Clin Pathol 30:541, 1977

Mason DY, Abdulaziz Z, Falini B, et al. Single and double immunoenzymatic techniques for labeling tissue sections with monoclonal antibodies. Ann NY Acad Sci 420:127, 1983

Mason DY, Bell JI, Christensson B, et al. An immunohistological study of human lymphoma. Clin Exp Immunol 40:235, 1980a

Mason DY, Biberfeld P. Technical aspects of lymphoma immunohistology. J Histochem Cytochem 28:731, 1980

Mason DY, Cordell JL, Abdulaziz Z, et al. Preparation of PAP complexes for immunohistological labeling of monoclonal antibodies. J Histochem Cytochem 30: 1114, 1982

Mason DY, Farrel C, Taylor CR. The detection of intracellular antigens in human leucocytes by immunoperoxidase staining. Br J Haematol 31:361, 1975

Mason DY, Leonard RCF, Laurent G, et al. Immunoperoxidase staining of surface and intercellular immunoglobulin in human neoplastic lymphoid cells. J Clin Pathol 33:609, 1980b

Mason DY, Sammons R. Alkaline phosphatase and peroxidase for double immunoenzymatic labelling of cellular constituents. J Clin Pathol 31:454, 1978

Mason DY, Stein H. Reactive and neoplastic human lymphoid cells producing J chain in the absence of immunoglobulin: evidence for the existence of 'J chain disease'? Clin Exp Immunol 46:305, 1981

Mason DY, Stein H, Naiem M, et al. Immunohistological analysis of human lymphoid tissue by double immunoenzymatic labelling. J Cancer Res Clin Oncol 101:13, 1981

Mason DY, Taylor CR. The distribution of muramidase (lysozyme) in human tissues. J Clin Pathol 28:124, 1975

Mason DY, Taylor CR. Distribution of transferrin, ferritin, and lactoferrin in human tissues. J Clin Pathol 31:316, 1978

Mason TE, Phifer RF, Spicer SS, et al. An immunoglobulin-enzyme bridge method for localizing tissue antigens. J Histochem Cytochem 17:573, 1969

Mather EL, Koshland ME. The role of J chain in B cell activation. In Sercarz EE, Herzenberg LA, Fox DF, eds. Immune System: Genetics and Regulation, p 727. Symposium of Molecular and Cell Biology, vol 6. New York, Academic Press, 1977

Mathew RC, Gupta SK, Katayama I, et al. Macrophage specific antigen is expressed by resting microglia in the CNS but not by Langerhans cells in the skin. J Pathol 141:435, 1983

Mathews T, Moossy J. Gliomas containing bone and cartilage. J Neuropathol Exp Neurol 33:456, 1974

Matsuba I, Tanese T, Abe M. Human pancreatic islet cell clones secreting insulin, glucagon and somatostatin: immunocytochemical and functional studies. Arch Histol Jpn 45:111, 1982

Matsumoto H, Kikuchi S, Chiba S, et al. [A comparative study on clinical signs and computed tomography in spinocerebellar degenerations.] Rinsho Shinkeigaku 19:27, 1979

Matsuta M. Immunohistochemical and electron microscope studies on Hashimoto's thyroiditis. Acta Pathol Jpn 32:41, 1982

Mattes MJ, Cordon-Cardo C, Lewis JL Jr, et al. Cell surface antigens of human ovarian and endometrial carcinoma defined by mouse monoclonal antibodies. Proc Natl Acad Sci USA 81:568, 1984

Matthews JB. Influence of clearing agent on immunohistochemical staining of paraffin-embedded tissue. J Clin Pathol 34:103, 1981

Matthews JB. The immunoglobulin nature of Russell bodies. Br J Exp Pathol 64:331, 1983

Matthews JB, Basu MK. Oral tonsils: an immunoperoxidase study. Int Arch Allergy Appl Immunol 69:21, 1982

Maurer R, Taylor CR, Parker JW, et al. Immunoblastic sarcoma: morphologic criteria and the distinction of B and T cell types. Oncology 39:42, 1982

Maurer R, Taylor CR, Schmucki O, et al. Extratesticular gonadal stromal tumor in the pelvis: a case report with immunoperoxidase findings. Cancer 44:985, 1980

Maurer R, Taylor CR, Terry R, et al. Non-Hodgkin lymphomas of the thyroid: a clinico-pathological review of 29 cases applying the Lukes-Collins classification and an immunoperoxidase method. Virchows Arch (A) 383:293, 1979

Maxwell A, Ward HA, Nairn RC. Freezing in an isopentane-liquid nitrogen mixture and storage in 2-octanol: technical improvements for immunofluorescence. Stain Technol 41:305, 1966

Mazauric T, Mitchell KF, Letchworth GJ 3rd, et al. Monoclonal antibody-defined human lung cell surface protein antigens. Cancer Res 42:150, 1982

Mazoujian G, Pinkus GS, Haagensen DE Jr. Extramammary Paget's disease—evidence for an apocrine origin. An immunoperoxidase study of gross cystic disease fluid protein-15, carcinoembryonic antigen, and keratin proteins. Am J Surg Pathol 8:43, 1984

McAlpine RG, Javadpour N, Vafier JA, et al. Avidin-biotin technique is more sensitive than lectin assay for detecting the Thomsen-Friedenreich antigen (T-antigen) in transitional cell carcinoma of the bladder. J Surg Oncol 27:255, 1984

McArdle JP, Roff BT, Muller HK, et al. The basal lamina in basal cell carcinoma, Bowen's disease, squamous cell carcinoma and keratoacanthoma: an immunoperoxidase study using an antibody to type IV collagen. Pathology 16:67, 1984

McCallister JA, Boxer LA, Baehner RL. The use and limitation of labeled staphylococcal protein A for study of antineutrophil antibodies. Blood 54:1330, 1979

McComb DJ, Bayley TA, Horvath E, et al. Monomorphous plurihormonal adenoma of the human pituitary: a histologic, immunocytologic and ultrastructural study. Cancer 53:1538, 1984

McComb RD, Jones TR, Pizzo SV, et al. Specificity and sensitivity of immunohistochemical detection of factor VIII/von Willebrand factor antigen in formalin-fixed paraffin-embedded tissue. J Histochem Cytochem 30:371, 1982a

McComb RD, Jones TR, Pizzo SV, et al. Localization of factor VIII/von Willebrand factor and glial fibrillary acidic protein in the hemangioblastoma: implications for stromal cell histogenesis. Acta Neuropathol 56:207, 1982b

McDicken IW, Rainey M. The immunohistological demonstration of carcinoembryonic antigen in intra-epithelial and invasive squamous carcinoma of the cervix. Histopathology 7:475, 1983

McDougall JK, Crum CP, Fenoglio CM, et al. Herpes virus–specific RNA and protein in carcinoma of the uterine cervix. Proc Natl Acad Sci USA 79:3853, 1982

McGee JO, Woods JC, Ashall F, et al. A new marker for human cancer cells. II. Immunohistochemical detection of the Ca antigen in human tissues with the Ca1 antibody. Lancet 2:7, 1982

McLaren KM, Holloway L, Pepper DS. Human platelet factor 4 and tissue mast cells. Thromb Res 19:293, 1980

McMillan EM, Brubaker DB, Peters S, et al. Demonstration of cells bearing the OKT6 determinant in human tonsil and lymph node. Cancer Immunol Immunother 15:221, 1983

McMillan EM, Martin D, Wasik R, et al. Demonstration in situ of "T" cells and "T" cell subsets in lichen planus using monoclonal antibodies. J Cutan Pathol 8:228, 1981

McMillan EM, Wasik R, Jackson I, et al. OKT 9 reactive cells in mycosis fungoides. J Cutan Pathol 9:55, 1982

Meier C, Vandevelde M, Steck A, et al. Demyelinating polyneuropathy associated with monoclonal IgM-paraproteinaemia—histological, ultrastructural and immunocytochemical studies. J Neurol Sci 63:353, 1984

Meijer CJ, Albeda F, Van der Valk P, et al. Immunohistochemical studies of the spleen in hairy-cell leukemia. Am J Pathol 115:266, 1984

Meinke GC, Spiegelberg HL. Antigenic studies of J chain. J Immunol 112:1401, 1974

Meisels A, Roy M, Fortier M, et al. Human papillomavirus infection of the cervix: the atypical condyloma. Acta Cytol 25:7, 1981

Meissner K, Löning T, Heckmayr M, et al. Predominant cutaneous infiltration of OKT6- and OKT8-positive cells in a case of Sézary syndrome. Arch Dermatol Res 275:168, 1983

Meister P, Huhn D, Nathrath W. Malignant histiocytosis. Immunohistochemical characterization on paraffin embedded tissue. Virchows Arch (A) 385:233, 1980

Meister P, Nathrath W. Immunohistochemical markers of histiocytic tumors. Hum Pathol 11:300, 1980

Melmed C, Frail D, Duncan I, et al. Peripheral neuropathy with IgM kappa monoclonal immunoglobulin directed against myelin-associated glycoprotein. Neurology (NY) 33:1397, 1983

Mendell JR, Sahenk Z, Whitaker JN, et al. Polyneuropathy and IgM monoclonal gammopathy: studies on the pathogenetic role of anti-myelin–associated glycoprotein antibody. Ann Neurol 17:243, 1985

Mendelsohn G. Histaminase localization in medullary thyroid carcinoma and small cell lung carcinoma. In: Delellis RA, ed. Diagnostic Immunohistochemistry, p 299. Masson Monographs in Diagnostic Pathology, Masson Publications, 1981

Mendelsohn G, Baylin SB, Bigner SH, et al. Anaplastic variants of medullary thyroid carcinoma: a light-microscopic and immunohistochemical study. Am J Surg Pathol 4:333, 1980a

Mendelsohn G, Baylin SB, Eggleston JC. Relationship of metastatic medullary thyroid carcinoma to calcitonin content of pheochromocytomas: an immunohistochemical study. Cancer 45:498, 1980b

Mendelsohn G, Eggleston JC, Mann RB. Relationship of lysozyme (muramidase) to histiocytic differentiation in malignant histiocytosis. An immunohistochemical study. Cancer 45:273, 1980c

Meneses ACO, Kepes JJ, Sternberger NH. Astrocytic differentiation of neoplastic oligodendrocytes. J Neuropathol Exp Neurol 41:368, 1982

Mepham BL, Frater W, Mitchell BS. The use of proteolytic enzymes to improve immunoglobulin staining by the PAP technique. Histochem J 11:345, 1979

Mercer WD, Lippman ME, Wahl TM, et al. The use of immunocytochemical techniques for the detection of steroid hormones in breast cancer cells. Cancer (Suppl 12) 46:2859, 1980

Merkel KH, Zimmer M. Herpes simplex encephalitis. A modified indirect immunoperoxidase technique for rapid diagnosis in paraffin-embedded tissue. Arch Pathol Lab Med 105:351, 1981

Merkel KH, Zimmer M. The immunoperoxidase method for rapid diagnosis of herpes simplex encephalitis (HSE) using touch preparations. Am J Clin Pathol 77:605, 1982

Merrill JE, Kutsunai S, Mohlstrom C, et al. Proliferation of astroglia and oligodendroglia in response to human T cell-derived factors. Science 224:1428, 1984

Merson AG. [Cytoplasmic immunoglobulins in lymph node cells in angioimmunoblastic lymphadenopathies.] Arkh Patol 42:30, 1980

Merson AG, Rudens IuF. [Immunohistochemical study of intracellular immunoglobulins in the lymph nodes of malignant lymphomas.] Vopr Onkol 27:39, 1981

Merz PA, Somerville RA, Wisniewski HM, et al. Scrapie-associated fibrils in Creutzfeldt-Jakob disease. Nature 306:474, 1983

Mesa-Tejada R, Keydar I, Ramanarayanan M, et al. Immunohistochemical evidence of RNA virus related components in human breast cancer. Ann Clin Lab Sci 9:202, 1979

Mestecky J, Preud'homme JL, Crago SS, et al. Presence of J chain in human lymphoid cells. Clin Exp Immunol 39:371, 1980

Metz K, Leder LD. Myeloma with immunohistochemically different cell populations: implication for the validity of immunohistochemical assessment of lymphoma cell monoclonality. Klin Wochenschr 58:409, 1980

Metzgar RS, Gaillard MT, Levine SJ, et al. Antigens of human pancreatic adenocarcinoma cells defined by murine monoclonal antibodies. Cancer Res 42:601, 1982

Meuris S, Soumenkoff G, Malengreau A, et al. Immunoenzymatic localization of prolactin-like immunoreactivity in decidual cells of the endometrium from pregnant and nonpregnant women. J Histochem Cytochem 28:1347, 1980

Meyer MP, Amortegui AJ. Rapid detection of herpes simplex virus using a combination of human fibroblast cell cultures and peroxidase-antiperoxidase staining. Am J Clin Pathol 81:43, 1984

Meyer PR, Ormerod LD, Osborn KG, et al. An immunologic evaluation of lymph nodes from monkey and man with acquired immune deficiency syndrome and related conditions. Hematol Oncol 3:199, 1985

Miettinen M. Chordoma. Antibodies to epithelial membrane antigen and carcinoembryonic antigen in differential diagnosis. Arch Pathol Lab Med 108:891, 1984

Miettinen M, Foidart JM, Ekblom P. Immunohistochemical demonstration of laminin, the major glycoprotein of basement membranes, as an aid in the diagnosis of soft tissue tumors. Am J Clin Pathol 79:306, 1983a

Miettinen M, Lehto VP, Badley RA, et al. Expression of intermediate filaments in soft-tissue sarcomas. Int J Cancer 30:541, 1982a

Miettinen M, Lehto VP, Dahl D, et al. Differential diagnosis of chordoma, chondroid, and ependymal tumors as aided by anti-intermediate filament antibodies. Am J Pathol 112:160, 1983b

Miettinen M, Lehto VP, Virtanen I. Neuroendocrine carcinoma of the skin (Merkel cell carcinoma): ultrastructural and immunohistochemical demonstration of neurofilaments. Ultrastruct Pathol 4:219, 1983c

Miettinen M, Lehto VP, Virtanen I. Monophasic synovial sarcoma of spindle cell type: epithelial differentiation as revealed by ultrastructural features, content of prekeratin and binding of peanut agglutinin. Virchows Arch [B] 44:187, 1983d

Miettinen M, Lehto VP, Virtanen I. Expression of intermediate filaments in normal ovaries and ovarian epithelial, sex cord–stromal, and germinal tumors. Int J Gynecol Pathol 2:64, 1983e

Miettinen M, Lehto VP, Virtanen I. Nasopharyngeal lymphoepithelioma. Histological diagnosis as aided by immunohistochemical demonstration of keratin. Virchows Arch [B] 40:163, 1982b

Miettinen M, Lehtonen E, Lehtola H, et al. Histogenesis of granular cell tumour—an immunohistochemical and ultrastructural study. J Pathol 142:221, 1984

Miettinen M, Virtanen I. Synovial sarcoma—a misnomer. Am J Pathol 117:18, 1984

Millar DA, Williams ED. A step-wedge standard for the quantification of immunoperoxidase techniques. Histochem J 14:609, 1982

Miller CA, Benzer S. Monoclonal antibody cross-reactions between Drosophila and human brain. Proc Natl Acad Sci 80:7641, 1983

Miller EP, Hogg RM. Long-term storage of fresh tissue at −20° C embedded for cryotomy. Med Lab Sci 37:93, 1980

Miller JM, Kini SR. Needle Biopsy of the Thyroid: Current Concepts. New York, Praeger, 1983

Miller ML, Tubbs RR, Fishleder AJ, et al. Immunoregulatory Leu-7+ and T8+ lymphocytes in B-cell follicular lymphomas. Hum Pathol 15:810, 1984

Miller RA, Coleman CN, Fawcett HD, et al. Sézary syndrome: a model for migration of T lymphocytes to skin. N Engl J Med 303:89, 1980

Mills BG, Singer FR, Weiner LP, et al. Cell cultures from bone affected by Paget's disease. Arthritis Rheum 23:1115, 1980

Mills BG, Singer FR, Weiner LP, et al. Immunohistological demonstration of respiratory syncytial virus antigens in Paget disease of bone. Proc Natl Acad Sci USA 78:1209, 1981

Minna JD, Cuttitta R, Rosen S, et al. Methods for production of monoclonal antibodies with specificity for human lung cancer cells. In Vitro 17:1058, 1981

Mirecka J. Anti-steroid antibodies and their application for immunohistochemical localization of sex hormones. Acta Histochem [Suppl] 22:245, 1980

Mitao M, Reumann W, Winkler B, et al. Chlamydial cervicitis and cervical intraepithelial neoplasia: an immunohistochemical analysis. Gynecol Oncol 19:90, 1984

Mitchell DP, Gusterson BA. Simultaneous demonstration of keratin and mucin. J Histochem Cytochem 30:707, 1982

Mitchell KF, Fuhrer JP, Steplewski Z, et al. Structural characteristics of the melanoma-specific antigen detected by monoclonal antibody 691 15 Nu-4-B. Mol Immunol 18:207, 1981

Mitchell WM, Halter SA, Schuffman SS, et al. Molecular and morphological evidence for type B retrovirus (oncornavirus) expression in human mammary carcinoma. An overview using scanning electron microscopy, immunoperoxidase staining, and transmission election microscopy. Scan Electron Microsc (3):1, 1980

Miwa M, Senoue I, Watanabe H, et al. Serum CEA levels

in gastrointestinal diseases. Tokai J Exp Clin Med 5:151, 1980

Miyake T, Tsuchihashi Y, Kitamura T, et al. Immuno-histochemical studies of blood monocytes infiltrating into the neonatal rat brain. Acta Neuropathol (Berl) 62:291, 1984

Modlin RL, Hofman FM, Horwitz DA, et al. In situ identification of cells in human leprosy granulomas with monoclonal antibodies to interleukin 2 and its receptor. J Immunol 132:3085, 1984a

Modlin RL, Rowden G, Taylor CR, et al. Comparison of S-100 and OKT6 antisera in human skin. J Invest Dermatol 83:206, 1984b

Modlin RL, Vaccaro SA, Gottlieb B, et al. Granuloma annulare. Identification of cells in the cutaneous infiltrate by immunoparoxidase techniques. Arch Pathol Lab Med 108:379, 1984c

Mogollon R, Penneys N, Albores-Saavedra J, et al. Malignant schwannoma presenting as a skin mass. Confirmation by the demonstration of myelin basic protein within tumor cells. Cancer 53:1190, 1984

Mohabeer J, Buckley CH, Fox H. An immunohistochemical study of the incidence and significance of human chorionic gonadotrophin synthesis by epithelial ovarian neoplasms. Gynecol Oncol 16:78, 1983

Moir DJ, Ghosh AK, Abdulaziz Z, et al. Immunoenzymatic staining of haematological samples with monoclonal antibodies. Br J Haematol 55:395, 1983

Møller M, Ingild A, Bock E. Immunohistochemical demonstration of S-100 protein and GFA protein in interstitial cells of rat pineal gland. Brain Res 140:1, 1978

Möller P. Peanut lectin: a useful tool for detecting Hodgkin cells in paraffin sections. Virchows Arch [A] 396:313, 1982

Möller P, Achsätter H, Butzengeiger M, et al. The distribution of fibronectin in lymph nodes infiltrated by Hodgkin's disease. An immunoperoxidase study on paraffin sections. Virchows Arch [A] 400:319, 1983

Monier JC, Dardenne M, Pleau JM, et al. Characterization of facteur thymique serique (FTS) in the thymus. I. Fixation of anti-FTS antibodies on thymic reticulo-epithelial cells. Clin Exp Immunol 42:470, 1980

Montero C. Immunocytochemical methods and their achievements in pathology. Methods Achiev Exp Pathol 10:1, 1981

Morell A, Maurer W, Skvaril F, et al. Differentiation between benign and malignant monoclonal gammopathies by discriminant analysis on serum and bone marrow parameters. Acta Haematol 60:129, 1978

Morgan AC, Galloway DR, Reisfeld RA. Production and characterization of monoclonal antibody to a melanoma-specific glycoprotein. Hybridoma 1:27, 1981

Morgan DA, Caillaud JM, Bellet D, et al. Gonadotrophin-producing seminoma: a distinct category of germ cell neoplasm. Clin Radiol 33:149, 1982

Morgello S, Block G, Price RW, et al. Case #3, Diagnostic slide session. Proceedings of American Association of Neuropathologists, San Diego, California, 16 June, 1984

Mori H, Soeda O, Kamano T, et al. Choriocarcinomatous change with immunocytochemically HCG-positive cells in the gastric carcinoma of the males. Virchows Arch [A] 396:141, 1982

Mori N, Abe M, Kojima M. Study of malignant lymphomas from the aspect of immunoglobulin production. Acta Pathol Jpn 29:705, 1979

Morin C, Braun L, Casas-Cordero M, et al. Confirmation of the papillomavirus etiology of condylomatous cervix lesions by the peroxidase-antiperoxidase technique. J Natl Cancer Inst 66:831, 1981

Morinaga S, Ojima M, Sasano N. Human chorionic gonadotrophin and alpha-fetoprotein in testicular germ cell tumors. An immunohistochemical study in comparison with tissue concentrations. Cancer 52:1281, 1983

Morise K. [Immunohistochemical studies on gastric tissues with intestinal metaplasia and cancer.] Nippon Shokakibyo Gakkai Zasshi 79:18, 1982

Mornaghi R, Rubinstein P, Franklin EC. Familial renal amyloidosis: case reports and genetic studies. Am J Med 73:609, 1982

Morris JA, Bird CC. Ultrastructural and immunohistological study of immunoblastic sarcoma developing in child with immunoblastic lymphadenopathy. Cancer 44:171, 1979

Morrison JH, Rogers J, Scherr S, et al. Somatostatin immunoreactivity in neuritic plaques of Alzheimer's patients. Nature 314:90, 1985

Morton JA, Fleming KA, Trowell JM, et al. Mallory bodies—immunohistochemical detection by antisera to unique non-prekeratin components. Gut 21:727, 1980

Moseley RC, Corey L, Benjamin D, et al. Comparison of viral isolation, direct immunofluorescence, and indirect immunoperoxidase techniques for detection of genital herpes simplex virus infection. J Clin Microbiol 13:913, 1981

Moskowitz LB, Gregarios JB, Hensley GT, et al. Cytomegalovirus-induced demyelination associated with acquired immune deficiency syndrome. Arch Pathol Lab Med 108:873, 1984b

Moskowitz LB, Hensley GT, Chan JC, et al. The neuropathology of acquired immune deficiency syndrome. Arch Pathol Lab Med 108:867, 1984a

Mostofi FK, Price EB Jr. Tumors of the male genital system. Atlas of Tumor Pathology. Fascicle 7, series 2. Washington, DC. Armed Forces Institute of Pathology. 1973

Motoi M, Stein H, Lennert K. Demonstration of lysozyme, alpha 1-antichymotrypsin, alpha 1-antitrypsin, albumin, and transferrin with the immunoperoxidase method in lymph node cells. Virchows Arch (B) 35:73, 1980

Motoi M, Yoshino T, Hayashi K, et al. Immunohistochemical studies on human brain tumors using anti-Leu 7 monoclonal antibody in paraffin-embedded specimens. Acta Neuropathol (Berl) 66:75, 1985

Mounts P, Shah KV, Kashima H. Viral etiology of juvenile- and adult-onset squamous papilloma of the larynx. Proc Natl Acad Sci USA 79:5425, 1982

Mshana RN, Humber DP, Harboe M, et al. Demonstration of mycobacterial antigens in nerve biopsies from leprosy patients using peroxidase-antiperoxidase immunoenzyme technique. Clin Immunol Immunopathol 29:359, 1983

Muehleck SD, McKenna RW, Gale PF, et al. Terminal deoxynucleotidyl transferase (TdT)-positive cells in bone marrow in the absence of hematologic malignancy. Am J Clin Pathol 79:277, 1983

Mukai K. Functional pathology of pancreatic islets: immunocytochemical exploration. Pathol Annu 18:87, 1983

Mukai K, Grotting JC, Greider MH, et al. Retrospective study of 77 pancreatic endocrine tumors using the immunoperoxidase method. Am J Surg Pathol 6:387, 1982

Mukai K, Rosai J, Bergdorf WH. Localization of factor VIII-related antigen in vascular endothelial cells using an immunoperoxidase method. Am J Surg Pathol 4:273, 1980a

Mukai K, Rosai J, Hallaway BE. Localization of myoglobin in normal and neoplastic human skeletal muscle cells using an immunoperoxidase method. Am J Surg Pathol 3:373, 1979

Mukai K, Schollmeyer JV, Rosai J. Immunohistochemical localization of actin: applications in surgical pathology. Am J Surg Pathol 5:91, 1981

Mukai K, Varela-Duran J, Nochomovitz LE. The rhabdomyoblast in mixed müllerian tumors of the uterus and ovary. An immunohistochemical study of myoglobin in 25 cases. Am J Clin Pathol 74:101, 1980b

Mukai M. Immunohistochemical localization of S-100 protein and peripheral nerve myelin proteins (P2 protein, P0 protein) in granular cell tumors. Am J Pathol 112:139, 1983

Müller-Mennelink HK, Kaiserling E. Different reticulum cells of the lymph node: microecological concept of lymphoid tissue organization. In: Bosman F, van den Tweel J, Taylor CR, eds. Malignant Lymphomas, the Pathophysiology of the Lymphocyte and its Neoplasms, p 57. Leiden, Leiden University Press, 1980

Mulshine JL, Cuttitta F, Bibro M, et al. Monoclonal antibodies that distinguish non–small cell from small cell lung cancer. J Immunol 131:497, 1983

Munoz-Garcia D, Ludwin SK. Classic and generalized variants of Pick's disease: a clinicopathological, ultrastructural, and immunocytochemical comparative study. Ann Neurol 16:467, 1984

Murabe Y, Sano Y. Morphological studies on neuroglia. VII. Distribution of "brain macrophages" in brains of neonatal and adult rats, as determined by means of immunohistochemistry. Cell Tissue Res 229:85, 1983

Murao T, Toda K, Tomiyama Y. Papillary and solid neoplasm of pancreas in a child. Report of a case in which acinar differentiation was demonstrated by immunohistochemistry and electron microscopy. Acta Pathol Jpn 33:565, 1983

Murphy GF, Flynn TC, Rice RH, et al. Involucrin expression in normal and neoplastic human skin: a marker for ketatinocyte differentiation. J Invest Dermatol 82:453, 1984

Murray N, Steck AJ. Indication of a possible role in a demyelinating neuropathy for an antigen shared between myelin NK cells. Lancet 1:711, 1984

Mussini JM, Hauw JJ, Escourolle R. Immunofluorescence studies of intracytoplasmic immunoglobulin binding lymphoid cells (CILC) in the central nervous system. Report of 32 cases including 19 multiple sclerosis. Acta Neuropathol (Berl) 40:227, 1977

Myers FJ, Cardiff RD, Taylor CR, et al. Hairy cell leukemia has a B-cell genotype. Hematol Oncol 2:745, 1984

Myerson D, Hackman RC, Nelson JA, et al. Widespread presence of histologically occult cytomegalovirus. Hum Pathol 15:430, 1984

Nadji M. The potential value of immunoperoxidase techniques in diagnostic cytology. Acta Cytol 24:442, 1980

Nadji M, Morales AR. Immunohistochemistry of prostatic acid phosphatase. Ann NY Acad Sci 390:133, 1982

Nadji M, Morales AR, Girtanner RE, et al. Paget's disease of the skin. A unifying concept of histogenesis. Cancer 50:2203, 1982

Nadji M, Morales AR, Ziegles-Weissman J, Penneys NS. Kaposi's sarcoma: immunohistologic evidence for an endothelial origin. Arch Pathol Lab Med 105:274, 1981

Nadji M, Tabei SZ, Castro A, et al. Prostatic origin of tumors. An immunoperoxidase study. Am J Clin Pathol 73:735, 1980

Nadler LM, Korsmeyer SJ, Anderson KC, et al. B cell origin of non–T cell acute lymphoblastic leukemia. A model for discrete stages of neoplastic and normal pre–B cell differentiation. J Clin Invest 74:332, 1984

Naganuma H, Inoue H, Misumi S, et al. Intracranial germ-cell tumors. Immunohistochemical study of three autopsy cases. J Neurosurg 61:931, 1984

Nagashima K, Yasui D, Kimura J, et al. Induction of brain tumors by a newly isolated JC virus (Tokyo-1 strain). Am J Pathol 116:455, 1984

Nagle RB, Clark VA, McDaniel KM, et al. Immunohistochemical demonstration of keratins in human ovarian neoplasms. A comparison of methods. J Histochem Cytochem 31:1010, 1983a

Nagle RB, McDaniel KM, Clark VA, et al. The use of antikeratin antibodies in the diagnosis of human neoplasms. Am J Clin Pathol 79:458, 1983b

Nahmias AJ, Whitley RJ, Visintine AN, et al. Collaborative Antiviral Study Group. Herpes simplex virus encephalitis: laboratory evaluations and their diagnostic significance. J Infect Dis 145:829, 1982

Naiem M, Gerdes J, Abdulaziz Z, et al. Production of monoclonal antibodies for the immunohistological analysis of human lymphoma. In: Knapp W, ed. Leukemia Markers, p 117. New York, Academic Press, 1981

Naiem M, Gerdes J, Abdulaziz Z, et al. The value of immunohistological screening in the production of monoclonal antibodies. J Immunol Methods 50:145, 1982

Naiem M, Gerdes J, Abdulaziz Z, et al. Production of a monoclonal antibody reactive with human dendritic reticulum cells and its use in the immunohistological analysis of lymphoid tissue. J Clin Pathol 36:167, 1983

Nakagawa Y, Okada M, Tanimoto K, et al. [Primary endodermal sinus tumor of the fourth ventricle.] No Shinkei Geka 8:1177, 1980

Nakagawara A, Ikeda K, Hayashida Y, et al. Immunocytochemical identification of human chorionic gonadotropin- and alpha-fetoprotein–producing cells of hepatoblastoma associated with precocious puberty. Virchows Arch [A] 398:45, 1982

Nakajima T, Kameya T, Tsumuraya M, et al. Enolase distribution in human brain tumors, retinoblastomas and pituitary adenomas. Brain Res 308:215, 1984

Nakajima T, Watanabe S, Sato Y, et al. An immunoperoxidase study of S-100 protein distribution in normal and neoplastic tissues. Am J Surg Pathol 6:715, 1982a

Nakajima T, Watanabe S, Sato Y, et al. Immunohistochemical demonstration of S100 protein in malignant melanoma and pigmented nevus, and its diagnostic application. Cancer 50:912, 1982b

Nakakuma K, Tashiro S, Uemura K, et al. Alpha-fetoprotein and human chorionic gonadotropin in embryonal carcinoma of the ovary: an 8–year survival case. Cancer 52:1470, 1983

Nakamura Y, Becker LE, Marks A. S100 protein in human chordoma and human and rabbit notochord. Arch Pathol Lab Med 107:118, 1983a

Nakamura Y, Becker LE, Marks A. Distribution of immunoreactive S-100 protein in pediatric brain tumors. J Neuropathol Exp Neurol 42:136, 1983b

Nakamura Y, Sato T, Nishimura G, et al. Malignant teratoma in the brain: an immunohistochemical study. Cancer 55:103, 1985

Nakane PK, Hartman AL. Immunocytochemical localization of intracellular antigens with SEM. Histochem J 12:435, 1980

Nakatsu H, Kobayashi I, Onishi Y, et al. ABO (H) blood group antigens and carcinoembryonic antigens as indicators of malignant potential in patients with transitional cell carcinoma of the bladder. J Urol 131:252, 1984

Nakazato Y, Ishizeki J, Takahasi K, et al. Localization of S-100 protein and glial fibrillary acidic protein-related antigen in pleomorphic adenoma of the salivary glands. Lab Invest 46:621, 1982a

Nakazato Y, Ishizeki J, Takahasi K, et al. Immunohistochemical localization of S-100 protein in granular cell myoblastoma. Cancer 49:1624, 1982b

Namba K, Jaffe ES, Braylan RC, et al. Alkaline phosphatase-positive malignant lymphoma: a subtype of B-cell lymphomas. Am J Clin Pathol 68:535, 1968

Nap M, Keuning H, Burtin P, et al. CEA and NCA in benign and malignant breast tumors. Am J Clin Pathol 82:526, 1984

Nardelli E, Pizzighella S, Tridente G, et al. Peripheral neuropathy associated with immunoglobulin disorders: an immunological and ultrastructural study. Acta Neuropathol [Suppl] 7:258, 1981

Nardelli J, Bara J, Rosa J, et al. Intestinal metaplasia and carcinomas of the human stomach: an immunohistological study. J Histochem Cytochem 31:366, 1983

Naritoku WY. The immunocytochemical study of tissue and tumor-associated antigens of the prostate and a relationship of immunostaining patterns and the Gleason classification system. Ph.D. Dissertation, University of Southern California, 1982

Naritoku WY, Taylor CR. A comparative study of the use of monoclonal antibodies using three different immunohistochemical methods: an evaluation of monoclonal and polyclonal antibodies against human prostatic acid phosphatase. J Histochem Cytochem 30:253, 1982

Naruse K, Inagami T, Celio MR, et al. Immunohistochemical evidence that angiotensins I and II are formed by intracellular mechanism in juxtaglomerular cells. Hypertension 4:70, 1982

Nash JR. Macrophages in human tumours: an immunohistochemical study. J Pathol 136:72, 1982

Natali PG, Bigotti A, Cavaliere R, et al. Phenotyping of lesions of melanocyte origin with monoclonal antibodies to melanoma-associated antigens and to HLA antigens. J Natl Cancer Inst 73:13, 1984

Natali PG, Cordiali-Fei P, Cavaliere R, et al. Ia-like antigens on freshly explanted human melanoma. Clin Immunopathol 19:250, 1981a

Natali PG, De Martino C, Pellegrino MA, et al. Analysis of the expression of Ia-like antigens in murine fetal and adult tissues with the monoclonal antibody 10-2.16. Scand J Immunol 13:541, 1981b

Natali PG, De Martino C, Quaranta V, et al. Expression of Ia-like antigens in normal human nonlymphoid tissues. Transplanation 31:75, 1981c

Natali PG, Giacomini P, Russo C, et al. Antigenic profile of human melanoma cells. Analysis with monoclonal antibodies to histocompatibility antigens and to melanoma-associated antigens. J Cutan Pathol 10:225, 1983

Nathrath WB, Heidenkummer P, Björklund V. Distribution of tissue polypeptide antigen (TPA) in normal human tissues: immunohistochemical study on unfixed, methanol-, ethanol-, and formalin-fixed tissues. J Histochem Cytochem 33:99, 1985

Nathrath WB, Meister P. Lysozyme (muramidase) and alpha 1-anti-chymotrypsin as immunohistochemical tumour markers. Acta Histochem (Suppl) 25:69, 1982

Nathrath WB, Wilson PD, Trejdosiewicz LK. Immunohistochemical demonstration of epithelial and uro-

thelial antigens at the light- and electron microscope levels. Acta Histochem (Suppl) 25:73, 1982

Neal DE, Marsh C, Bennett MK, et al. Epidermal–growth-factor receptors in human bladder cancer: comparison of invasive and superficial tumours. Lancet 1:366, 1985

Neffen EL, Monti JA, Naves AE. [Carcinoembryonic antigen in the differential diagnosis of colonic polypoid lesions.] Allergol Immunopathol 8:651, 1980

Negishi Y, Mutai Y, Akiya K, et al. Tumor-associated antigen in ovarian carcinoma. Nippon Sanka Fujinka Gakkai Zasshi 36:126, 1984

Neiman RS. Erythroblastic transformation in myeloproliferative disorders. Confirmation by an immunohistologic technique. Cancer 46:1636, 1980

Nelson WG, Battifora H, Santana H, et al. Specific keratins as molecular markers for neoplasms with a stratified epithelial origin. Cancer Res 44:1600, 1984

Nemes Z, Thomázy V, Szeifert G. Follicular centre cell lymphoma with alpha heavy chain disease. A histopathological and immunohistological study. Virchows Arch [A] 394:119, 1981

Nemes Z, Thomázy V, Szeifert G. Sensitivity and specificity of immunohistological methods on freeze-dried paraffin sections. J Immunol Methods 49:53, 1982

Nemoto N, Kawaoi A, Shikata T. Occurrence of alpha-fetoprotien–containing hepatocytes in human embryos and fetuses: an immunohistochemical study using the light and ultrastructural immunoperoxidase methods. J Histochem Cytochem 30:1022, 1982

Neuwelt EA, Smith RG. Presence of lymphocyte membrane surface markers on "small cells" in a pineal germinoma. Ann Neurol 6:133, 1979

Newell DG, Bohane C, Payne S, et al. The intracellular localization of immunoglobulin in human lymphoid cells and haematopoietic cell lines by immunoperoxidase electron microscopy. J Immunol Methods 37:275, 1980

Newell DG, Hannam-Harris A, Karpas A, et al. The differential ultrastructural localization of immunoglobulin heavy and light chains in human haematopoietic cell lines. Br J Haematol 50:445, 1982

Nielsen HO, Halken S, Lorentzen M. Quantitative studies of the gastrin-producing cells of the human antrum. A methodological study. Acta Pathol Microbiol Sand [A] 88:255, 1980a

Nielsen HO, Jensen KB, Christiansen LA. The antral gastrin-producing cells in duodenal ulcer patients. A density study before and during treatment with cimetidine. Acta Pathol Microbiol Scand [A] 88A:383, 1980b

Nielsen HO, Teglbjaerg PS, Hage E. Gastrin and enteroglucagon cells in human antra, with special reference to intestinal metaplasia. Scand J Gastroenterol (Suppl) 54:101, 1979

Nielsen K, Paulsen SM, Johansen P. Carcinoembryonic antigen-like antigen in granular cell myoblastomas. An immunohistochemical study. Virchows Arch [A] 401:159, 1983

Nielsen K, Teglbjaerg PS. Carcino-embryonic antigen (CEA) in gastric adenocarcinomas. Morphologic patterns and their relationship to a histogenic classification. Acta Pathol Microbiol Immunol Scand [A] 90:393, 1982

Nieuwenhuijzen Kruseman AC, Bosman FT, van Bergen Henegouw JC, et al. Medullary differentiation of anaplastic thyroid carcinoma. Am J Clin Pathol 77:541, 1982

Nijhuis-Heddes JM, Lindeman J, Otto AJ, et al. Distribution of immunoglobulin-containing cells in the bronchial mucosa of patients with chronic respiratory disease. Eur J Respir Dis 63:249, 1982

Nilsson P, Berqquist NR, Grundy MS. A technique for preparing defined conjugates of horseradish peroxidase and immunoglobulin. J Immunol Methods 41:81, 1981

Nishida H. [Immunohistochemical localization of carcinoembryonic antigen (CEA) in gastric cancer —a comparative study between tissue CEA and plasma CEA.] Nippon Geka Gakkai Zasshi 84:328, 1983

Nishiyama RH, Thompson NW, Lloyd R, et al. Secretory diarrhea with islet cell hyperplasia and increased immunohistochemical reactivity to serotonin. Surgery 96:1038, 1984

Nishiyama T, Hayashi I, Inoue I, et al. Distribution of histaminase in human tumor tissues. An immunohistochemical study. Oncodev Biol Med 4:197, 1983

Norenberg MD, Martinez-Hernandez A. Fine structural localization of glutamine synthetase in astrocytes of rat brain. Brain Res 161:303, 1979

Nørgaard-Pedersen B, Lundborg CJ, Baursen AM, et al. Infantile vaginal tumour with alpha-fetoprotein synthesis. Acta Pathol Microbiol Scand [A] 87A:223, 1979

Notani GW, Parsons JA, Erlandsen SL. Versatility of *Staphylococcus aureus* protein A in immunocytochemistry. Use in unlabeled antibody enzyme system and fluorescent methods. J Histochem Cytochem 27:1438, 1979

Nusbickel FR. The construction of a closed-chambered incubator for use in such techniques as enzyme and immunoperoxidase histochemistry. J Microsc 118:447, 1980

Nuti M, Teramoto YA, Mariani-Costantini R, et al. A monoclonal antibody (B72.3) defines patients of distribution of a novel tumor-associated antigen in human mammary carcinoma cell populations. Int J Cancer 29:539, 1982

Nygren H, Hansson HA, Lange S. Studies on the conjugation of horseradish peroxidase to immunoglobulin G via glutaraldehyde. Med Biol 57:187, 1979

Obata N, Kodama S, Hando T. et al. [Cellular localization of alpha-fetoprotein (AFP), human chorionic gonadotropin (HCG), and carcinoembryonic antigen (CEA) in malignant germ cell tumors of the ovary using immunoperoxidase technique.] Nippon Sanka Fujinka Gakkai Zasshi 32:757, 1980

Oberley TD, Mosher DF, Mills MD. Localization of fibronectin within the renal glomerulus and its production by cultured glomerular cells. Am J Pathol 96:651, 1979

O'Briain DS, Dayal Y. The pathology of the gastrointestinal endocrine cells. In: DeLellis RA, ed. Diagnostic Immunohistochemistry, p 75. Masson Monographs in Diagnostic Pathology, Sternberg SS, series ed. New York, Masson Publishing, 1981

O'Briain DS, Dayal Y, DeLellis RA, et al. Rectal carcinoids as tumors of the hindgut endocrine cells: a morphological and immunohistochemical analysis. Am J Surg Pathol 6:131, 1982

O'Brien MJ, Kirkham SE, Burke B, et al. CEA, ZGM and EMA localization in cells of pleural and peritoneal effusion: a preliminary study. Invest Cell Pathol 3:251, 1980

O'Brien MJ, Zamcheck N, Burke B, et al. Immunocytochemical localization of carcinoembryonic antigen in benign and malignant colorectal tissues. Assessment of diagnostic value. Am J Clin Pathol 75:283, 1981

Oehmichen M. Inflammatory cells in the central nervous system: an integrating concept based on recent research in pathology, immunology, and forensic medicine. Prog Neuropathol 5:277, 1983

Oehmichen M, Huber H. Reactive microglia with membrane features of mononuclear phagocytes. J Neuropathol Exp Neurol 35:30, 1976

Oehmichen M, Torvik A. The origin of reactive cells in retrograde and Wallerian degeneration. Experiments with intravenous injection of ³H-DFP–labeled microphages. Cell Tissue Res 173:343, 1976

Oehmichen M, Wiethölter H, Greaves MF. Immunological analysis of human microglia: lack of monocytic and lymphoid membrane differentiation antigens. J Neuropathol Exp Neurol 38:99, 1979

Ogawa H, Kami K, Suzuki T, et al. An immunohistochemical study of lysozyme in the human nasal mucosa. Keio J Med 28:73, 1979

Ogawa H, Sato Y, Takeshita I, et al. Transient expression of glial fibrillary acidic protein in developing oligodendrocytes in vitro. Dev Brain Res 18:133, 1985

Oguchi H, Homma T, Kawa S, et al. A pancreatic oncofetal antigen (POA): its characterization and application for enzyme immunoassay. Cancer Detect Prev 7:51, 1984

O'Hara CM, Gardner WA Jr, Bennett BD. Immunoperoxidase staining of *Trichomonas vaginalis* in cytologic material. Acta Cytol 24:448, 1980

Okada S, Ohtsuki H, Midorikawa O, et al. Bronchial plasmacytoma identified by immunoperoxidase technique on paraffin-embedded section. Acta Pathol Jpn 32:149, 1982

Okamura A, Ohkawa J, Fujisawa H, et al. Clinicopathological study on the relationship between serum-CEA and tissue-CEA of resected lung cancer cases. Acta Pathol Jpn 34:1209, 1984

Okamura S, Crane F, Jamal N, et al. Single-cell immunofluorescence assay for terminal transferase: Human leukaemic and non-leukaemic cells. Br J Cancer 41:159, 1980

Okon E, Felder B, Epstein A, et al. Monoclonal antibodies reactive with B-lymphocytes and histiocytes in paraffin sections. Cancer 56:95, 1985.

Okoye MI, Mueller WF Jr, Chang CY, et al. Testicular gonadal stromal (Sertoli cell) tumor. Urology 25:184, 1985

Okudaira Y, Ohtsuru Y, Matsui Y, et al. [Immunohistochemical demonstration of carcinoembryonic antigen and ultrastructural features of endometrial adenocarcinoma.] Nippon Sanka Fujinka Gakkai Zasshi 36:173, 1984

Olding LB, Thurin J, Svalander C, et al. Expression of gastrointestinal carcinoma-associated antigen (GICA) detected in human fetal tissues by monoclonal antibody NS-19-9. Int J Cancer 34:187, 1984

Olson LC, Buescher EL, Artenstein MS, et al. Herpesvirus infections of the human central nervous system. N Engl J Med 277:1271, 1967

Omata M, Liew CT, Ashcavai M, et al. Nonimmunologic binding of horseradish peroxidase to hepatitis B surface antigen. A possible source of error in immunohistochemistry. Am J Clin Pathol 73:626, 1980

Oommen KJ, Johnson PC, Ray CG. Herpes simplex type 2 virus encephalitis presenting as psychosis. Am J Med 73:445, 1982

Ordóñez NG, Ayala AG, von Eschenbach AC, et al. Immunoperoxidase localization of prostatic acid phosphatase in prostatic carcinoma with sarcomatoid changes. Urology 19:210, 1982

Ordóñez NG, Ibañez ML, Samaan NA, et al. Immuno-peroxidase study of uncommon parathyroid tumors. Report of two cases of nonfunctioning parathyroid carcinoma and one intrathyroid parathyroid tumor-producing amyloid. Am J Surg Pathol 7:535, 1983

Ordóñez NG, Manning JT Jr. Comparison of alpha-1-antitrypsin and alpha-1-antichymotrypsin in hepato-cellular carcinoma: an immunoperoxidase study. Am J Gastroenterol 79:959, 1984

Orell SR, Dowling KD. Oncofetal antigens as tumor markers in the cytologic diagnosis of effusions. Acta Cytol 27:625, 1983

Ormerod MG, Sloane JP. Breast tumours. In: Filipe MS, Lake BD, eds. Histochemistry in Pathology. Edinburgh, Churchill Livingstone, 1983

Orntoft TF, Mors NP, Eriksen G, et al. Comparative immunoperoxidase demonstration of T-antigens in human colorectal carcinomas and morphologically abnormal mucosa. Cancer Res 45:447, 1985

Osamura RY, Akatsuka A, Watanabe K. Localization of anterior pituitary hormones on Epon sections by peroxidase-labeled antibody method—light and electron microscopic observations. Acta Histochem Cytochem 11:399, 1978

Osamura RY, Watanabe K, Nakai Y, et al. Adrenocor-ticotropic hormone cells and immunoreactive beta-endorphin cells in the human pituitary gland: normal and pathologic conditions studied by the peroxidase-labeled antibody method. Am J Pathol 99:105, 1980

Osborn M, Ludwig-Festl M, Weber K, et al. Expression of glial and vimentin type intermediate filaments in cultures derived from human glial material. Differentiation 19:161, 1981

Osborn M, Weber K. Intermediate filaments: cell-type–specific markers in differentiation and pathology. Cell 31:303, 1982

Osborn M, Weber K. Biology of disease: tumor diagnosis by intermediate filament typing: a novel tool for surgical pathology. Lab Invest 48:372, 1983

O'Sullivan MJ, Gnemmi E, Morris D, et al. Comparison of two methods of preparing enzyme-antibody con-jugates: application of these conjugates for enzyme immunoassay. Anal Biochem 100:100, 1979

Osung OA, Toh BH, Gray A, et al. Immunoperoxidase EM localisation of cytoplasmic actin in cultured fibro-blasts. J Immunol Methods 34:303, 1980

Otto HF, Gebbers JO, Bettmann I. [Malignant lympho-mas of the intestinal tract. Histological and immuno-histological findings in 22 intestinal lymphomas.] Schweiz Med Wochenschr 110:1043, 1980

Paasivuo R, Saksela E. Non-specific binding of mouse immunoglobulins by swollen-bodied astrocytes—a po-tential source of confusion in human brain immuno-histochemistry. Acta Neuropathol (Berl) 59:103, 1983

Packer RJ, Sutton LN, Rorke LB, et al. Prognostic importance of cellular differentiation in medulloblas-toma of childhood. J Neurosurg 61:296, 1984a

Packer RJ, Sutton LN, Rorke LB, et al. Intracranial embryonal cell carcinoma. Cancer 54:520, 1984b

Palmer JO, Kasselberg AG, Netsky MG. Differentiation of medulloblastoma. Studies including immunohisto-chemical localization of glial fibrillary acidic protein. J Neurosurg 55:161, 1981

Pallesen G, Beverleyt PC, Lane EB, et al. Nature of non-B, non-T lymphomas: an immunohistological study on frozen tissues using monoclonal antibodies. J Clin Pathol 37:911, 1984a

Pallesen G, Kerndrup G, Ellegaard J. Further evidence for the B-cell nature of hairy cells. A study using

immunostaining of splenic tissue with a wide panel of monoclonal antibodies. Blut 49:395, 1984b

Palutke M, Schnitzer B, Mirchandani I, et al. Monoclonal lymphoid populations in lymph nodes with reactive hyperplasia. Lab Invest 44:50A, 1981

Pangalis GA, Nathwani BN, Rappaport H. Detection of cytoplasmic immunoglobulin in well-differentiated lymphoproliferative diseases by the immunoperoxi-dase method. Cancer 45:1334, 1980

Pangalis GA, Rappaport H. Common clonal origin of lymphoplasmacytic proliferation and immunoblastic lymphoma in intestinal alpha-chain disease. Lancet 2:880, 1977

Panitch HS. Antimyelin antibodies in patients with pe-ripheral neuropathy and benign monoclonal gammopathy. J Neuropathol Exp Neurol 41:372, 1982

Papadimitriou CS, Papacharalampous NX, Kittas C. Pri-mary gastrointestinal malignant lymphomas. A mor-phologic and immunohistochemical study. Cancer 55:870, 1985

Papadimitriou CS, Stein H, Papacharalampous NX. Presence of an alpha 1-antichymotrypsin and alpha 1-antitrypsin in haematopoietic and lymphoid tissue cells as revealed by the immunoperoxidase method. Pathol Res Pract 169:287, 1980

Papasozomenos SC. Glial fibrillary acidic (GFA) protein-containing cells in the human pineal gland. J Neuro-pathol Exp Neurol 42:391, 1983

Papasozomenos S, Shapiro S. Pineal astrocytoma: report of a case, confined to the epiphysis, with immunocy-tochemical and electron microscopic studies. Cancer 47:99, 1981

Papotti M, Eusebi V, Gugliotta P, et al. Immunohisto-chemical analysis of benign and malignant papillary lesions of the breast. Am J Surg Pathol 7:451, 1983

Paradinas FJ, Boxer G, Bagshawe KD. Distribution of the Ca (Oxford) antigen in lung neoplasms and non-neoplastic lung tissues. J Clin Pathol 37:1, 1984

Paradis IL, Merrall EJ, Krell JM, et al. Lymphocyte enumeration: a comparison between a modified avi-din-biotin-immunoperoxidase system and flow cytom-etry. J Histochem Cytochem 32:358, 1984

Parham D, Whitaker JN, Berard CW. Cellular distribu-tion of cathepsin D in childhood tumors. Arch Pathol Lab Med 109:250, 1985

Parwaresch MR, Radzun HJ, Hansmann ML, et al. Monoclonal antibody Ki-M4 specifically recognizes hu-man dendritic reticulum cells (follicular dendritic cells) and their possible precursor in blood. Blood 62:585, 1983

Pascal RR, Slovin SF. Tumor-directed antibody and carcinoembryonic antigen in the glomeruli of a patient with gastric carcinoma. Hum Pathol 11:679, 1980

Pasmantier MW, Azar HA. Extraskeletal spread in mul-tiple plasma cell myeloma: a review of 57 autopsied cases. Cancer 23:167, 1969

Pasquier B, Pasquier D, Tanous AM, et al. Le diagnostic des tumeurs nerveuses centrales par un marqueur de la protéine gliofibrillaire acide. Étude préliminaire d'une série de 33 cas. Sem Hop Paris 56:1720, 1980

Pasquier B, Pasquier D, Tanous AM, et al. Détection de la protéine gliofibrillaire acide au sein des tumeurs nerveuses centrales. Applications d'une méthode im-munoperoxydasique sur coupes incluses en paraffine ou en épon. Arch Anat Cytol Pathol 29:90, 1981

Pattengale PK, Taylor CR, Engvall E, et al. Direct tissue visualization of normal cross-reacting antigen in neo-plastic granulocytes. Am J Clin Pathol 73:351, 1980

Paull WK, King JC. A rinsing and incubation chamber

used for immunocytochemistry of vibratome sections. Histochemistry 78:413, 1983

Payne SV, Wright DH, Jones KJ, et al. Macrophage origin of Reed-Sternberg cells: an immunohistochemical study. J Clin Pathol 35:159, 1982

Pearse AGE. Histochemistry, Theoretical and Applied. Edinburgh, Churchill Livingston, 1968

Pearse AGE. Neuroendocrine tumours and hyperplasia. In: Filipe MI, Lake BD, eds. Histochemistry in Pathology, p 274. Edinburgh, Churchill Livingston, 1983

Pearson J. Neurotransmitter immunocytochemistry in the study of human development, anatomy, and pathology. Prog Neuropathol 5:41, 1983

Pearson RCA, Sofroniew MV, Cuello AC, et al. Persistence of cholinergic neurons in the basal nucleus in a brain with senile dementia of the Alzheimer's type demonstrated by immunohistochemical staining for choline acetyltransferase. Brain Res 289:375, 1983

Pedersen JS, Walker M, Toh BH, et al. Flow microfluorometry detects IgM autoantibody to oligodendrocytes in multiple sclerosis. J Neuroimmunol 5:251, 1983

Pelletier G, Puviani R, Bosler O, et al. Immunocytochemical detection of peptides in osmicated and plastic-embedded tissue. An electron microscopic study. J Histochem Cytochem 29:759, 1981

Pelletier G, Robert F, Hardy J. Identification of human anterior pituitary cells by immunoelectron microscopy. J Clin Endocrinol Metab 46:534, 1978

Pelliniemi LJ, Dym M, Karnovsky MJ. Peroxidase histochemistry using diaminobenzidine tetrahydrochloride stored as a frozen solution. J Histochem Cytochem 28:191, 1980

Penneys NS, Nadji M, McKinney EC. Carcinoembryonic antigen present in human eccrine sweat. J Am Acad Dermatol 4:401, 1981

Penneys NS, Nadji M, Morales A. Carcinoembryonic antigen in benign sweat gland tumors. Arch Dermatol 118:225, 1982a

Penneys NS, Nadji M, Ziegels-Weissman J, et al. Carcinoembryonic antigen in sweat-gland carcinomas. Cancer 50:1608, 1982b

Pepys EO, Pepys MB. Enumeration in whole peripheral blood of lymphocytes bearing receptors for Fc(gamma) and C3b using alkaline phosphatase-labelled reagents. J Immunol Methods 32:305, 1980

Perkkiö M. Immunohistochemical study of intestinal biopsies from children with atopic eczema due to food allergy. Allergy 35:573, 1980

Perkkiö M, Savilahti E. Time of appearance of immunoglobulin-containing cells in the mucosa of the neonatal intestine. Pediatr Res 14:953, 1980

Permanetter W, Nathrath WB, Löhrs U. Immunohistochemical analysis of thyroglobulin and keratin in benign and malignant thyroid tumours. Virchows Arch [A] 398:221, 1982

Perry EK, Oakley AE, Candy JM, et al. Properties and possible significance of substance P and insulin fibrils. Neurosci Lett 25:321, 1981

Perry EK, Perry RH. Neurotransmitter and neuropeptide systems in Alzheimer-type dementia. Exp Brain Res [Suppl] 5:140, 1982

Perry EK, Tomlinson BE, Blessed G, et al. Correlation of cholinergic abnormalities with senile plaques and mental test scores in senile dementia. Br Med J [Clin Res] 2:1457, 1978

Pertschuk LP, Tobin EH, Tanapat P, et al. Histochemical analysis of steroid hormone receptors in breast and prostatic carcinoma. J Histochem Cytochem 28:799, 1980

Peschke P, Wurster K, Rapp W. Neue Möglichkeiten und Aufgaben der Bildanalysetechnik im Bereich der Immunoenzymhistologie. Microsc Acta [Suppl] 4:66, 1980

Phifer RF, Spicer SS. Immunohistochemical and histologic demonstration of thyrotropic cells of the human adenohypophysis. J Clin Endocrinol Metab 36:1210, 1973

Phillips LL, Autilio-Gambetti L, Lasek RJ. Bodian's silver method reveals molecular variation in the evolution of neurofilament proteins. Brain Res 278:219, 1983

Pierce DA, Stern R, Jaffe R, et al. Immunoblastic sarcoma with features of Sjögren's syndrome and systemic lupus erythematosus in a patient with immunoblastic lymphadenopathy. Arthritis Rheum 22:911, 1979

Pileri S, Gobbi M, Rivano MT, et al. Immunohistological study of transferrin receptor expression in non-Hodgkin's lymphoma. Br J Haematol 58:501, 1984

Pileri S, Martinelli G, Serra L, et al. Endodermal sinus tumor arising in the endometrium. Obstet Gynecol 56:391, 1980a

Pileri S, Serra L, Martinelli G. The use of pronase enhances sensitivity of the PAP method in the detection of intracytoplasmic immunoglobulins. Basic Appl Histochem 24:203, 1980b

Pilkington GJ, Lantos PL. The role of glutamine synthetase in the diagnosis of cerebral tumours. Neuropathol Appl Neurobiol 8:227, 1982

Pilotti S, Rilke F, Shah KV, et al. Immunohistochemical and ultrastructural evidence of papilloma virus infection associated with in situ and microinvasive squamous cell carcinoma of the vulva. Am J Surg Pathol 8:751, 1984

Pinkus GS. Diagnostic immunocytochemistry of paraffin-embedded tissues. Hum Pathol 13:411, 1982

Pinkus GS, Said JW. Profile of intracytoplasmic lysozyme in normal tissues, myeloproliferative disorders, hairy cell leukemia, and other pathologic processes. Am J Pathol 89:351, 1977

Pinkus GS, Said JW. Intracellular hemoglobin—specific marker of erythroid cells in paraffin sections. An immunoperoxidase study of normal, megaloblastic, and dysplastic erythropoiesis, including erythroleukemia and other myeloproliferative disorders. Am J Pathol 102:308, 1981

Pinkus GS, Said JW. Hodgkin's disease, lymphocyte predominance type, nodular—a distinct entity? Unique staining profile for L&H variants of Reed-Sternberg cells defined by monoclonal antibodies to leukocyte common antigen, granulocyte-specific antigen, and B-cell–specific antigen. Am J Pathol 118:1, 1985

Piris J, Thomas ND. A quantitative study of the influence of fixation on immunoperoxidase staining of rectal mucosal plasma cells. J Clin Pathol 33:361, 1980

Piscioli F, Bondi A, Scappini P, et al. 'True' sarcomatoid carcinoma of the renal pelvis. First case report with immunocytochemical study. Eur Urol 10:350, 1984

Pixley SKR, de Vellis J. Transition between immature radial glia and mature astrocytes studied with a monoclonal antibody to vimentin. Dev Brain Res 15:201, 1984

Pizzolo G, Sloane J, Beverley P, et al. Differential diagnosis of malignant lymphoma and nonlymphoid tumors using monoclonal anti-leucocyte antibody. Cancer 46:2640, 1980

Pollen JJ, Dreilinger A. Immunohistochemical identification of prostatic acid phosphatase and prostate specific antigen in female periurethral glands. Urology 23:303, 1984

Ponder BA, Wilkinson MM. Inhibition of endogenous tissue alkaline phosphatase with the use of alkaline phosphatase conjugates in immunohistochemistry. J Histochem Cytochem 29:981, 1981

Popov VL, Prozorovskiĭ SV, Tartakovskiĭ IS, et al. [Ultrastructural localization of type-specific antigen of legionella pneumophila.] Biull Eksp Biol Med 93:63, 1982

Poppema S. The diversity of the immunohistological staining pattern of Sternberg-Reed cells. J Histochem Cytochem 28:788, 1980

Poppema S, Bhan AK, Reinherz EL, et al. Distribution of T cell subsets in human lymph nodes. J Exp Med 153:30, 1981

Poppema S, Bhan AK, Reinherz EL, et al. In situ immunologic characterization of cellular constituents in lymph nodes and spleens involved by Hodgkin's disease. Blood 59:226, 1982

Poppema S, De Jong B, Atmosoerodjo J, et al. Morphologic, immunologic, enzymehistochemical and chromosomal analysis of a cell line derived from Hodgkin's disease. Evidence for a B-cell origin of Sternberg-Reed cells. Cancer 55:683, 1985

Poppema S, Elema JD, Halie MR. The localization of Hodgkin's disease in lymph nodes. A study with immunohistological, enzyme histochemical and rosetting techniques on frozen section. Int J Cancer 24:532, 1979a

Poppema S, Kaiserling E, Lennert K. Nodular paragranuloma and progressively transformed germinal centers. Ultrastructural and immunohistologic findings. Virchows Arch [B] 31:211, 1979b

Poppema S, Kaiserling E, Lennert K. Hodgkin's disease with lymphocyte predominance, nodular type, and progressively transformed germinal centers. Histopathology 3:295, 1979c

Poppema S, Visser L, De Leij L. Reactivity of presumed anti-natural killer cell antibody Leu 7 with intrafollicular T lymphocytes. Clin Exp Immunol 54:834, 1983

Porstmann B, Porstmann T, Nugel E. Comparison of chromogens for the determination of horseradish peroxidase as a marker in enzyme immunoassay. J Clin Chem Clin Biochem 19:435, 1981

Poulsen HS, Ozzello L, King WJ, et al. The use of monoclonal antibodies to estrogen receptors (ER) for immunoperoxidase detection of ER in paraffin sections of human breast cancer tissue. J Histochem Cytochem 33:87, 1985

Powers JM, Schlaepfer WW, Willingham MC, et al. An immunoperoxidase study of senile cerebral amyloidosis with pathogenetic considerations. J Neuropathol Exp Neurol 40:592, 1981

Press MF, Greene GL. An immunocytochemical method for demonstrating estrogen receptor in human uterus using monoclonal antibodies to human estrophilin. Lab Invest 50:480, 1984

Press MF, Nousek-Goebl N, King WJ, et al. Immunohistochemical assessment of estrogen receptor distribution in the human endometrium throughout the menstrual cycle. Lab Invest 51:495, 1984

Price RA, Lee PA, Albright AL, et al. Treatment of sexual precocity by removal of a luteinizing hormone–releasing hormone secreting hamartoma. J Am Med Assoc 251:2247, 1984

Primus FJ, Clark CA, Goldenberg DM. Immunohistochemical detection of carcinoembryonic antigen. In: DeLellis RA, ed. Diagnostic Immunohistochemistry, p

263. Masson Monographs in Diagnostic Pathology, Sternberg SS, series ed., 1981

Prineas JW, Kwon EE, Sternberger NH, et al. The distribution of myelin-associated glycoprotein and myelin basic protein in actively demyelinating multiple sclerosis lesions. J Neuroimmunol 6:251, 1984

Probst A, Anderton BH, Ulrich J, et al. Pick's disease: an immunocytochemical study of neuronal changes. Monoclonal antibodies show that Pick bodies share antigenic determinants with neurofibrillary tangles and neurofilaments. Acta Neuropathol (Berl) 60:175, 1983

Pukel CS, Lloyd KO, Travassos LR, et al. GD3, a prominent ganglioside of human melanoma. J Exp Med 155:1133, 1982

Purnell DM, Heatfield BM, Trump BF. Immunocytochemical evaluation of human prostatic carcinomas for carcinoembryonic antigen, nonspecific cross-reacting antigen, beta-chorionic gonadotrophin, and prostate-specific antigen. Cancer Res 44:285, 1984

Purnell DM, Hillman EA, Heatfield BM, et al. Immunoreactive prolactin in epithelial cells of normal and cancerous human breast and prostate detected by the unlabeled antibody peroxidase-antiperoxidase method. Cancer Res 42:2317, 1982

Quick CA, Watts SL, Krzyzek RA, et al. Relationship between condylomata and laryngeal papillomata. Clinical and molecular virological evidence. Ann Otol Rhinol Laryngol 89:467, 1980

Rachlin J, Wollmann R, Dohrmann G. SV40 viral DNA in human CNS tumors. J Neuropathol Exp Neurol 43:301, 1984

Racklin B, Bearman R, Sheibani K, et al. The demonstration of terminal deoxynucleotidyl transferase on frozen tissue sections and smears by the avidin-biotin complex (ABC) method. Leuk Res 7:431, 1983

Radaszkiewicz T, Dragosics B, Abdelfattahgad M, et al. Effect of protease pretreatment on immunomorphologic demonstration of hepatitis-B–surface antigen in conventional paraffin-embedded liver biopsy material: quantitative evaluation. J Immunol Method 29:27, 1979

Raff M, Abney ER, Miller RH. Two glial cell lineages diverge prenatally in rat optic nerve. Dev Biol 106:53, 1984

Raff MC, Miller RH, Noble M. A glial progenitor cell that develops in vitro into an astrocyte or an oligodendrocyte, depending on culture medium. Nature 303:390, 1983

Rahier J, Wallon J, Henquin JC. Abundance of somatostatin cells in the human neonatal pancreas. Diabetologia 18:251, 1980

Rahman AF, Longenecker BM. A monoclonal antibody specific for the Thomsen Freidenreich cryptic T antigen. J Immunol 129:2021, 1982

Ramaekers FCS, Puts JJG, Moesker O, et al. Intermediate filaments in malignant melanomas. Identification and use as marker in surgical pathology. J Clin Invest 71:635, 1983

Ramanarayanan M, Francis P, Spiegelman S, et al. Preparation of horseradish peroxidase (PO) conjugates of several human and viral proteins and their use in immunohistochemistry by the enzyme-labeled antigen method. J Histochem Cytochem 29:892, 1981

Rambaud JC, Modigliani R, Phuoc BKN, et al. Nonsecretory alpha-chain disease in intestinal lymphoma. N Engl J Med 303:53, 1980

Rambaud JC, Piel JL, Galian A, et al. Rémission complète clinique, histologique et immunologique d'un cas de maladie des chaines alpha traité par antibiothérapie orale. Gastroenterol Clin Biol 2:49, 1978

Ranscht B, Clapshaw PA, Price J, et al. Development of oligodendrocytes and Schwann cells studied with a monoclonal antibody against galactocerebroside. Proc Natl Acad Sci 79:2709, 1982

Rao PE, Talle MA, Kung PC, et al. Five epitopes of a differentiation antigen on human inducer T cells distinguished by monoclonal antibodies. Cell Immunol 80:310, 1983

Rapp W, Wurster K. Gastric marker proteins. Purification and immunohistological demonstration of the chief cell esterase. Virchows Arch [A] 390:151, 1981

Rappaport H, Thomas LB. Mycosis fungoides: the pathology of extracutaneous involvement. Cancer 34:1198, 1974

Rasool CG, Abraham C, Anderton BH, et al. Alzheimer's disease: immunoreactivity of neurofibrillary tangles with anti-neurofilament and anti-paired helical filament antibodies. Brain Res 310:249, 1984

Rasool CG, Selkoe DJ. Sharing of specific antigens by degenerating neurons in Pick's disease and Alzheimer's disease. N Engl J Med 312:700, 1985

Rathlev T, Hocko JM, Franks GF, et al. Glucose oxidase immunoenzyme methodology as a substitute for fluorescence microscopy in the clinical laboratory. Clin Chem 27:1513, 1981

Raux H, Labbe F, Fondaneche MC, et al. A study of gastrointestinal cancer-associated antigen (GICA) in human fetal organs. Int J Cancer 32:315, 1983

Ravazzola M, Siperstein A, Moody AJ, et al. Glicentin immunoreactive cells: their relationship to glucagon-producing cells. Endocrinology 105:499, 1979

Rebel A, Basle M. [Paget's bone disease and virus.] Ann Pathol 1:21, 1981

Ree HJ, Crowley JP, Leone LA. Macrophage-histiocyte lysozyme activity in relation to the clinical presentation of Hodgkin's disease. An immunohistochemical study. Cancer 47:1988, 1981a

Ree HJ, Rege VB, Knisley RE, et al. Malignant lymphoma of Waldeyer's ring following gastrointestinal lymphoma. Cancer 46:1528, 1980

Ree HJ, Song JY, Leone LA, et al. Occurrence and patterns of muramidase containing cells in Hodgkin's disease, non-Hodgkin's lymphomas, and reactive hyperplasia. Hum Pathol 12:49, 1981b

Reid R, Crum CP, Herschman BR, et al. Genital warts and cervical cancer. III. Subclinical papillomaviral infection and cervical neoplasia are linked by a spectrum of continuous morphologic and biologic change. Lab Invest 48:A70, 1983

Reid R, Fu YS, Herschman BR, et al. Genital warts and cervical cancer. VI. The relationship between aneuploid and polyploid cervical lesions. Am J Obstet Gynecol 150:189, 1984

Reik L Jr. Disseminated vasculomyelinopathy: an immune complex disease. Ann Neurol 7:291, 1979

Reinecke M, Schlüter P, Yanaihara N, et al. VIP immunoreactivity in enteric nerves and endocrine cells of the vertebrate gut. Peptides (Suppl 2)2:149, 1981

Reinherz EL, Kung PC, Goldstein G, et al. Separation of functional subsets of human T cells by a monoclonal antibody. Proc Natl Acad Sci USA 76:4061, 1979

Reinherz EL, Kung PC, Goldstein G, et al. Discrete stages of human intrathymic differentiation: analysis of normal thymocytes and leukemic lymphoblasts of T cell lineage. Proc Natl Acad Sci USA 77:1588, 1980a

Reinherz EL, Kung PC, Goldstein G, et al. A monoclonal antibody reactive with the human cytotoxic/suppressor T cell subset previously defined by a heteroantiserum termed TH2. J Immunol 124:1301, 1980b

Reinherz EL, Schlossman SF. The characterization and function of human immunoregulatory T lymphocyte subsets. Pharmacol Rev 34:17, 1982

Reintoft I, Hägerstrand IE. Does the Z gene variant of alpha-1-antitrypsin predispose to hepatic carcinoma? Hum Pathol 10:419, 1979

Reisfeld RA. Monoclonal antibody to human malignant melanoma. Nature 298:325, 1982

Reitamo S. Lysozyme antigenicity and tissue fixation. Histochemistry 55:197, 1978

Reitamo S, Konttinen YT, Segerberg-Konttinen M. Distribution of lactoferrin in human salivary glands. Histochemistry 66:285, 1980a

Reitamo S, Ranki A, Konttinen YT, et al. Immunoperoxidase identification of intracellular immunoglobulins from cell smears. Am J Clin Pathol 73:248, 1980b

Reitamo S, Reitamo JJ, Konttinen YT, et al. Lysozyme in neoplastic Paneth cells of a jejunal adenocarcinoma. Acta Pathol Microbiol Scand [A] 89:165, 1981

Rhodes RH. Development of the optic nerve. In: Jakobiec FA, ed. Ocular Anatomy, Embryology, and Teratology, p 601. Philadelphia, Harper & Row, 1982

Rhodes RH. Ultrastructure of Müller cells in the developing human retina. Graefes Arch Clin Exp Ophthalmol 221:171, 1984

Rhodes RH, Davis RL, Berne TV, et al. Disseminated toxoplasmosis with brain involvement in a renal allograft recipient. Bull Los Angeles Neurol Soc 42:16, 1977

Rhodes RH, Dusseau JJ, Boyd AS Jr, et al. Intrasellar neural-adenohypophyseal choristoma: a morphological and immunocytochemical study. J Neuropathol Exp Neurol 41:267, 1982

Rhodes RH, Novak R, Beattie JF, et al. Immunoperoxidase demonstration of herpes simplex virus type 1 in the brain of a psychotic patient without history of encephalitis. Clin Neuropathol 3:59, 1984

Rijntjes NVM, Van de Putte LBA, Van der Pol M, et al. Cryosectioning of undecalcified tissues for immunofluorescence. J Immunol Methods 30:263, 1979

Risdall RJ, Sibley RK, McKenna RW, et al. Malignant histiocytosis. A light- and electron-microscopic and histochemical study. Am J Surg Pathol 4:439, 1980

Robb JA. A new enzyme immunoelectron tissue stain. Diagn Med, Oct Spec Issue:87, 1981

Robb-Smith AHT, Taylor CR. Lymph Node Biopsy. London, Miller Heyden Ltd; New York, Oxford University Press, 1981

Roberts DA. A rapid staining method giving sharp nuclear definition in frozen sections. J Med Lab Tech 23:110, 1966

Roberts GW, Crow TJ, Polak JM. Location of neuronal tangles in somatostatin neurones in Alzheimer's disease. Nature 314:92, 1985

Robertson AJ, McIntosh W, Lamont P, et al. Malignant granular cell tumour (myoblastoma) of the vulva: report of a case and review of the literature. Histopathology 5:69, 1981

Robinson G, Dawson I. Immunochemical studies of the endocrine cells of the gastrointestinal tract. I. The use and value of peroxidase-conjugated antibody techniques for the localization of gastrin-containing cells in human pyloric antrum. Histochem J 7:321, 1975

Robinson G, Dawson I. A formalin fixative for immunochemical and ultrastructural studies on gastrointestinal endocrine cells. J Clin Pathol 32:40, 1979

Rodning CB, Erlandsen SL, Coulter HD, et al. Immunohistochemical localization of IgA antigens in sections embedded in epoxy resin. J Histochem Cytochem 28:199, 1980a

Rodning CB, Erlandsen SL, Wilson ID. Immunohistochemical identification of immunoglobulin A on ultrathin tissue sections. Am J Anat 157:221, 1980b

Roessmann U, Velasco ME, Gambetti P, et al. Neuronal and astrocytic differentiation in human neuroepithelial neoplasms. An immunohistochemical study. J Neuropathol Exp Neurol 42:113, 1983a

Roessmann U, Velasco ME, Gambetti P, et al. Vimentin intermediate filaments are increased in human neoplastic astrocytes. J Neuropathol Exp Neurol 42:309, 1983b

Roessmann U, Velasco ME, Sindely SD, et al. Glial fibrillary acidic protein (GFAP) in ependymal cells during development. An immunocytochemical study. Brain Res 200:13, 1980

Romas NA, Veenema RJ, Hsu KC, et al. Bone marrow acid phosphatase in prostate cancer: an assessment by immunoassay and biochemical methods. Trans Am Assoc Genitourin Surg 71:26, 1979

Romet-Lemonne JL, Barin F, Goudeau A, et al. [Hepatitis B virus and hepatoma: evidence for a cytoplasmic tumor antigen in transformed hepatocytes.] C R Seances Acad Sci [III] 294:9, 1982

Rorke LB. The cerebellar medulloblastoma and its relationship to primitive neuroectodermal tumors. J Neuropathol Exp Neurol 42:1, 1983

Rosai J, Pinkus GS. Immunohistochemical demonstration of epithelial differentiation in adamantinoma of the tibia. Am J Surg Pathol 6:427, 1982

Rosekrans PC, Meijer CJ, Cornelisse CJ, et al. Use of morphometry and immunohistochemistry of small intestinal biopsy specimens in the diagnosis of food allergy. J Clin Pathol 33:125, 1980a

Rosekrans PC, Meijer CJ, Polanco I, et al. Long-term morphological and immunohistochemical observations on biopsy specimens of small intestine from children with gluten-sensitive enteropathy. J Clin Pathol 34:138, 1981

Rosekrans PC, Meijer CJ, van der Wal AM, et al. Immunoglobulin containing cells in inflammatory bowel disease of the colon: a morphometric and immunohistochemical study. Gut 21:941, 1980b

Rosekrans PC, Meijer CJ, van der Wal AM, Lindeman J. Allergic proctitis, a clinical and immunopathological entity. Gut 21:1017, 1980c

Rosenberg SA, et al. National Cancer Institute sponsored study of classification of non-Hodgkin's lymphomas: Summary and description of a working formulation for clinical usage. Cancer 49:2112, 1982

Rossiello R, Carriero MV, Giordano GG. Distribution of ferritin, transferrin and lactoferrin in breast carcinoma tissue. J Clin Pathol 37:51, 1984

Roth A, Le Pelletier O, Cukier J. [Prognostic value of extraembryonic components in testicular dysgerminoma (seminoma excluded).] Presse Med 12:2863, 1983

Rouget P, Penit C. Terminal deoxynucleotidyl transferase during the development of chicken thymus. Cell Differ 9:329, 1980

Rowden G. Expression of Ia antigens on Langerhans cells in mice, guinea pigs, and man. J Invest Dermatol 75:22, 1980

Rowden G. The Langerhans cell. CRC Crit Rev Immunol 3:95, 1981

Rowe DJ, Beverley PC. Characterisation of breast cancer infiltrates using monoclonal antibodies to human leucocyte antigens. Br J Cancer 49:149, 1984

Rowe IF, Jensson O, Lewis PD, et al. Immunohistochemical demonstration of amyloid P component in cerebro-vascular amyloidosis. Neuropathol Appl Neurobiol 10:53, 1984

Royds JA, Parson MA, Taylor CB, et al. Enolase isoenzyme distribution in the human brain and its tumours. J Pathol 137:37, 1982

Rubel LR, Ishak KG, Benjamin SB, et al. Alpha 1-antitrypsin deficiency and hepatocellular carcinoma. Association with cirrhosis, copper storage, and Mallory bodies. Arch Pathol Lab Med 106:678, 1982

Rubinstein LJ, Brucher J-M. Focal ependymal differentiation in choroid plexus papillomas: an immunoperoxidase study. Acta Neuropathol (Berl) 53:29, 1981

Ruppenthal M. Changes of the central nervous system in herpes zoster. Acta Neuropathol (Berl) 52:59, 1980.

Russell DS, Rubinstein LJ. Pathology of Tumours of the Nervous System, 4th ed. Baltimore, Williams and Wilkins, 1977

Ruttman E, Klöppel G, Bommer G, et al. Pancreatic glucagonoma with and without syndrome. Virchows Arch [A] 388:51, 1980

Rygaard-Olsen C, Boedker A, Emus HC, et al. Extramedullary plasmacytoma of the small intestine: a case report studied with electron microscopy and immunoperoxidase technique. Cancer 50:573, 1982

Saad MR, Ordóñez NG, Guido JJ, et al. The prognostic value of calcitonin immunostaining in medullary carcinoma of the thyroid. J Clin Endocrinol Metab 59:850, 1984

Sadun AA, Schaechter JD. Tracing axons in the human brain: a method utilizing light and TEM techniques. J Electron Microsc Tech 2:175, 1985

Said JW. Immunohistological localization of keratin proteins in tumor diagnosis. Hum Pathol 14:1017, 1983

Said JW, Nash G, Banks-Schlegel S, et al. Keratin in human lung tumors. Patterns of localization of different-molecular-weight keratin proteins. Am J Pathol 113:27, 1983

Said JW, Sassoon AF, Shintaku IP, et al. Involucrin in squamous and basal cell carcinomas of the skin: an immunohistochemical study. J Invest Dermatol 82:449, 1984

Saigo PE, Brigati DJ, Sternberg SS, et al. Primary gastric choriocarcinoma. An immunohistological study. Am J Surg Pathol 5:333, 1981

St. George JA, Cardiff RD, Young LJ, et al. Immunocytochemical distribution of mouse mammary tumor virus antigens in BALB/cfC3H mammary epithelium. J Natl Cancer Inst 63:813, 1979

Sainte-Marie G. A paraffin embedding technique for studies employing immunofluorescence. J Histochem Cytochem 10:250, 1962

Saito H, Saito S, Sano T, et al. Immunoreactive somatostatin in catecholamine-producing extra-adrenal paraganglioma. Cancer 50:560, 1982

Saksela O, Wahlström T, Lehtovirta P, et al. Presence of alpha 2-macroglobulin in normal but not in malignant human syncytiotrophoblasts. Cancer Res 41:2507, 1981

Samoszuk MK, Epstein AL, Said J, et al. Sensitivity and specificity of immunostaining in the diagnosis of mantle zone lymphoma. Am J Clin Pathol (in press), 1986

Sandhaus L, Strom RL, Mukai K. Primary embryonal-choriocarcinoma of the mediastinum in a woman. A case report with immunohistochemical study. Am J Clin Pathol 75:573, 1981

Sandhaus LM, Gajl-Peczalska KJ, Brunning RD. Immunophenotyping of leukaemia: an immunoperoxidase method using air-dried smears. Br J Haematol 56:131, 1984

Sappino AP, Ellison ML, Gusterson BA. Immunohisto-chemical localisation of keratin in small cell carcinoma of the lung: correlation with response to combination chemotherapy. Eur J Cancer Clin Oncol 19:1365, 1983

Sarno EN, Vieira LM, Alvariz FG. [Identification of hepatitis B antigens in hepatic tissue in various forms of acute hepatitis.] Arg Gastroenterol 21:68, 1984

Sasaki R, Bollum FJ, Takaku F, et al. Detection of terminal deoxynucleotidyl transferase (TdT)-positive leukemia cells by an immunoperoxidase staining. Jpn J Med 23:114, 1984

Sassen A, Vander Plaetse F. Detection and spontaneous alteration of lymphocyte antigens on slide smears. Med Microbiol Immunol 168:129, 1980

Sato A, Spicer SS. Ultrastructural visualization of galac-tose in the glycoprotein of gastric surface cells with a peanut lectin conjugate. Histochem J 14:125, 1982

Sato A, Spicer SS, Tashian RE. Ultrastructural localiza-tion of carbonic anhydrase in gastric parietal cells with the immunoglobulin-enzyme bridge method. Histo-chem J 12:651, 1980

Sato S, Tanaka M, Miyatani N, et al. Shared antigen between the myelin-associated glycoprotein (MAG) and a cell line from human T cell leukemia (HSB-2). J Neuroimmunol 7:287, 1985

Sato Y, Kim SU, Ghetti B. Induction of neurofibrillary tangles in cultured mouse neurons by maytanprine. J Neurol Sci 68:191, 1985

Saurat JH, Chavaz P, Carraux P, et al. A human mon-oclonal antibody reacting with Merkel cells: immuno-fluorescence, immunoperoxidase, and immunoelec-tron microscopy. J Invest Dermatol 81:249, 1983

Schachner M. Cell type–specific neural cell surface an-tigens. Fed Proc Fed Am Soc Exp Biol 38:2363, 1979

Schaumburg-Lever G, Gavris V, Lever WF, et al. Cell-surface carbohydrates in proliferative epidermal le-sions. Distribution of A, B, and H blood group anti-gens in benign and malignant lesions. Am J Derma-topathol 6:583, 1984

Schechter J. Electron microscopic studies of human pituitary tumors. I. Chromophobic adenomas. Am J Anat 138:371, 1973

Scheithauer BW, Kovacs K, Randall RV, et al. Hypotha-lamic neuronal hamartoma and adenohypophyseal neuronal choristoma: their association with growth hormone adenoma of the pituitary gland. J Neuro-pathol Exp Neurol 42:648, 1983

Scheithauer BW, Rubinstein LJ, Herman MM. Leukoen-cephalopathy in Waldenstrom's macroglobulinemia. Immunohistochemical and electron microscopic ob-servations. J Neuropathol Exp Neurol 43:408, 1984

Schienle HW, Stein N, Müller-Ruchholtz W. Neutrophil granulocytic cell antigen defined by a monoclonal antibody—its distribution within normal haemic and non-haemic tissue. J Clin Pathol 35:959, 1982

Schlegel R, Banks-Schlegel S, McLeod JA, et al. Immu-noperoxidase localization of keratin in human neo-plasms: a preliminary survey. Am J Pathol 101:41, 1980a

Schlegel R, Banks-Schlegel S, Pinkus GS. Immunohis-tochemical localization of keratin in normal human tissues. Lab Invest 42:91, 1980b

Schlom J, Wunderlich D, Teramoto YA. Generation of human monoclonal antibodies reactive with human mammary carcinoma cells. Proc Natl Acad Sci USA 77:6841, 1980.

Schmidt GM, Bross KJ, Blume KG, et al. Detection of platelet-directed immunoglobulin G in sera using the peroxidase–anti-peroxidase (PAP) slide technique. Blood 55:299, 1980.

Schmidt NJ, Dennis J, Devlin V, et al. Comparison of direct immunofluorescence and direct immunoperox-idase procedures for detection of herpes simplex virus antigen in lesion specimens. J Clin Microbiol 18:445, 1983

Schmiegel WH, Becker WM, Arndt R, et al. Pancreatic oncofetal antigen in pancreatic juices. Partial chemical characterization and diagnostic application of a pan-creatic cancer-associated antigen. Scand J Gastroen-terol 16:1033, 1981

Schneider DR, Taylor CR, Parker JW, et al. Immuno-blastic sarcoma of T- and B-cell types: morphologic description and comparison. Hum Pathol 16:885, 1985

Schnitzer J, Franke WW, Schachner M. Immunocyto-chemical demonstration of vimentin in astrocytes and ependymal cells of developing and adult mouse ner-vous system. J Cell Biol 90:435, 1981

Schober R, Itoyama Y, Sternberger NH, et al. Immu-nocytochemical study of P_0 glycoprotein, P_1 and P_2 basic proteins, and myelin-associated glycoprotein (MAG) in lesions of idiopathic polyneuritis. Neuro-pathol Appl Neurobiol 7:421, 1981

Schrell U, Sofroniew MV. Use of serial 1–2 micrometer paraffin sections in neuropeptide immunocytochem-istry for sequential analysis of different substances contained within the same neurons. J Histochem Cy-tochem 30:512, 1982

Schrieber JR, Reid R, Ross GT. A receptor-like testos-terone binding protein in ovaries from immature female rats. Endocrinology 98:1206, 1976

Schröder R. Later changes in brain death. Signs of partial recirculation. Acta Neuropathol (Berl) 62:15, 1983

Schron DS, Gipson T, Mendelsohn G. The histogenesis of small cell carcinoma of the prostate. An immuno-histochemical study. Cancer 53:2478, 1984

Schuller-Petrovic S, Gebhart W, Lassman H, et al. A shared antigenic determinant between natural killer cells and nervous tissue. Nature 306:179, 1983

Schumacher HR, Thomas WJ, Strong M, et al. Acute lymphoblastic leukemia—hand mirror variant—viral immune interrelationship as demonstrated by ultra-structural studies. Am J Hematol 10:399, 1981

Schwechheimer K, Kartenbeck J, Moll R, et al. Vimentin filament-desmosome cytoskeleton of diverse types of human meningiomas: a distinctive diagnostic feature. Lab Invest 51:584, 1984

Schwerer B, Lassmann H, Bernheimer H. Antisera against ganglioside G_{M2}: immunochemical and immu-nohistological studies. Neuropathol Appl Neurobiol 8:217, 1982

Scott DL, Morris CJ, Blake AE, et al. Distribution of fibronectin in the rectal mucosa. J Clin Pathol 34:749, 1981b

Scott DL, Wainwright AC, Walton KW, et al. Significance of fibronectin in rheumatoid arthritis and osteoar-throsis. Ann Rheum Dis 40:142, 1981a

Scott H, Solheim GB, Brandtzaeg P, et al. HLA-DR–like antigens in the epithelium of the human small intes-tine. Scand J Immunol 12:82, 1980

Scurry J, de Boer WG. Carcinoembryonic antigen in skin and related tumours as determined by immuno-histological techniques. Pathology 15:379, 1983

Searle RF, Billington WD, Whyte A, et al. Detection of human and murine trophoblast–specific antigens and an assessment of their species specificity. Placenta 2:93, 1981

Seddon JM, Corwin JM, Weiter JJ, et al. Solitary extramedullary plasmacytoma of the palpebral conjunctiva. Br J Ophthalmol 66:450, 1982

Sehested M, Hirsch FR, Hou-Jensen K. Immunoperoxidase staining for carcinoembryonic antigen in small cell carcinoma of the lung. Eur J Cancer Clin Oncol 17:1125, 1981

Sehested M, Hou-Jensen K. Factor VIII related antigen as an endothelial cell marker in benign and malignant diseases. Virchows Arch [A] 391:217, 1981

Seifert G, Caselitz J. Tumor markers in parotid gland carcinomas: immunohistochemical investigations. Cancer Detect Prev 6:119, 1983

Selby WS, Janossy G, Goldstein G, et al. T lymphocyte subsets in human intestinal mucosa: the distribution and relationship to MHC-derived antigens. Clin Exp Immunol 44:453, 1981a

Selby WS, Janossy G, Jewell DP. Immunohistological characterisation of intraepithelial lymphocytes of the human gastrointestinal tract. Gut 22:169, 1981b

Selby WS, Janossy G, Mason DY, et al. Expression of HLA-DR antigens by colonic epithelium in inflammatory bowel disease. Clin Exp Immunol 53:614, 1983

Seligmann M. Summing up immunologic markers in malignant lymphomas. Adv Exp Med Biol 114:635, 1979

Sens MA, Garvin AJ, Drew S, et al. Skeletal muscle differentiation in Wilms' tumor. Antibody identification and explant culture. Arch Pathol Lab Med 108:58, 1984

Seo IS, Binkley WB, Warner TF, et al. A combined morphologic and immunologic approach to the diagnosis of gastrointestinal lymphomas: I. Malignant lymphoma of the stomach (a clinicopathologic study of 22 cases). Cancer 49:493, 1982

Seppälä M, Wahlström T, Lehtovirta P, et al. Immunohistochemical demonstration of luteinizing hormone–releasing factor-like material in human syncytiotrophoblast and trophoblastic tumours. Clin Endocrinol 12:441, 1980

Serebrin R, Robertson DM. Ganglioneuroma arising in the pituitary fossa: a twenty year follow-up. J Neurol Neurosurg Psychiatry 47:97, 1984

Sero SF, et al. International histological classification of tumors (benign). Histologic typing of ovarian tumors. World Health Organization, Geneva, 1973

Sethi P, Lipton HL. The growth of four human and animal enteroviruses in the central nervous systems of mice. J Neuropathol Exp Neurol 40:258, 1981

Seymour GJ, Greaves MF, Janossy G. Identification of cells expressing T and p28,33 (Ia-like) antigens in sections of human lymphoid tissue. Clin Exp Immunol 39:66, 1980

Shabana AH, Ivany L, Kramer IR. Expression of the CA1 determinant by carcinomas and by non-malignant epithelial cells in oral lesions. Br J Cancer 48:527, 1983

Shah LC, Ogbimi AO, Johnson PM. A cell membrane antigen expressed by both human breast carcinoma cells and normal human trophoblast. Placenta 1:299, 1980

Sharkey RM, Primus FJ, Goldenberg DM. Comparison of the sensitivity of the indirect, antibody-conjugated and the triple-bridge immunoperoxidase methods for immunohistochemical detection of carcinoembryonic antigen. Histochemistry 66:35, 1980

Sharp G, Osborn M, Weber K. Occurrence of two different intermediate filament proteins in the same filament in situ within a human glioma cell line. An immunoelectron microscopical study. Exp Cell Res 141:385, 1982

Shaw G, Osborn M, Weber K. An immunofluorescence microscopical study of the neurofilament triplet proteins, vimentin and glial fibrillary acidic protein within the adult rat brain. Eur J Cell Biol 26:68, 1981

Shaw GM, Harper ME, Hahn BH, et al. HTLV-III infection in brains of children and adults with AIDS encephalopathy. Science 227:177, 1985

Shaw ST Jr, Roche PC, Schmer G, et al. Immunohistochemical identification of mast cells in paraffin- and epon-embedded tissues using platelet factor 41. J Histochem Cytochem 30:185, 1982

Sheffield WD, Strandberg JD, Braun L, et al. Simian virus 40–associated fatal interstitial pneumonia and renal tubular necrosis in a rhesus monkey. J Invest Dis 142:618, 1980

Sheibani K, Tubbs RR, Gephardt GN, et al. Comparison of alternative chromogens for renal immunohistochemistry. Lab Invest 42:150, 1980

Sheibani K, Tubbs RR, Gephardt GN, et al. Comparison of alternative chromogens for renal immunohistochemistry. Human Pathol 12:349, 1981

Sheibani K, Tubbs RR, Velasco ME, et al. Immunocytochemical identification of human chorionic gonadotropin (hCG): comparative study of diaminobenzidine (DAB) and 3-amino-9-ethylcarbazole (AEC), a nonhazardous chromogen. Lab Invest 40:284, 1979

Sheppard MN, Corrin B, Bennett MH, et al. Immunocytochemical localization of neuron specific enolase in small cell carcinomas and carcinoid tumours of the lung. Histopathology 8:171, 1984

Sheppard MN, Johnson NF, Cole GA, et al. Neuron specific enolase (NSE) immunostaining detection of endocrine cell hyperplasia in adult rats exposed to asbestos. Histochemistry 74:505, 1982

Sherry SH, Guay AT, Lee AK, et al. Concurrent production of adrenocorticotropin and prolactin from two distinct cell lines in a single pituitary adenoma: a detailed immunohistochemical analysis. J Clin Endocrinol Metab 55:947, 1982

Shevchuk MM, Fenoglio CM, Richart RM. Histogenesis of Brenner tumors, II: histochemistry and CEA. Cancer 46:2617, 1980

Shevchuk MM, Fenoglio CM, Richart RM. Carcinoembryonic antigen localization in benign and malignant transitional epithelium. Cancer 47:899, 1981

Shevchuk MM, Romas NA, Ng PY, et al. Acid phosphatase localization in prostatic carcinoma. A comparison of monoclonal antibody to heteroantisera. Cancer 52:1642, 1983

Shi SR, Bhan AK, Pilch BZ, et al. Keratin antibody localization in head and neck tissues and neoplasms. J Laryngol Otol 98:1241, 1984a

Shi SR, Goodman ML, Bhan AK, et al. Immunohistochemical study of nasopharyngeal carcinoma using monoclonal keratin antibodies. Am J Pathol 117:53, 1984b

Shimada H, Aoyama C, Chiba T, et al. Prognostic subgroups for undifferentiated neuroblastoma: immunohistochemical study with anti–S-100 protein antibody. Hum Pathol 16:471, 1985

Shimano T, Loor RM, Papsidero LD, et al. Isolation, characterization and clinical evaluation of a pancreas cancer-associated antigen. Cancer (Suppl 6) 47:1602, 1981

Shimatani N, Arakawa S, Ohno S, et al. [Immunohistochemical study of testicular tumor on cellular localization of HCG beta-subunit, alpha-fetoprotein and beta 1-pregnancy specific glycoprotein.] Nippon Hinyokika Gakkai Zasshi 71:1438, 1980

Shimizu M, Wajima O, Miura M, et al. PAP immunoperoxidase method demonstrating endogenous estrogen in breast carcinomas. Cancer 52:486, 1983

Shimizu YK, Shikata T, Beninger PR, et al. Detection of hepatitis A antigen in human liver. Infect Immun 36:320, 1982

Shimokawara I, Imamura M, Yamanaka N, et al. Identification of lymphocyte subpopulations in human breast cancer tissue and its significance: an immunoperoxidase study with anti-human T- and B-cell sera. Cancer 49:1456, 1982

Shioda Y, Nagura H, Tsutsumi Y, et al. Distribution of Leu 7 (HNK-1) antigen in human digestive organs: an immunohistochemical study with monoclonal antibody. Histochem J 16:843, 1984.

Shirahama T, Skinner M, Westermark P, et al. Senile cerebral amyloid: prealbumin as a common constituent in the neuritic plaque, in the neurofibrillary tangle, and in the microangiopathic lesion. Am J Pathol 107:41, 1982

Shirai T, Itoh T, Yoshiki T, et al. Immunofluorescent demonstration of alpha-fetoprotein and other plasma proteins in yolk. Cancer 38:1661, 1976

Shousha S, Miller GC. A histochemical and immunohistological study of a testicular malignant teratoma containing embryonic and extraembryonic elements in various stages of development. Histopathology 8:125, 1984

Shuangshoti S, Samranvej P, Netsky MG. Phagocytic astrocytes and neurons in old encephalomalacia. J Neuropathol Exp Neurol 38:235, 1979

Shuangshoti S, Samranvej P, Netsky MG. Solitary primary intracranial extracerebral glioma. Case report. J Neurosurg 61:777, 1984

Siegal GP, Barsky SH, Terranova VP, et al. Stages of neoplastic transformation of human breast tissue as monitored by dissolution of basement membrane components. An immunoperoxidase study. Invasion Metastasis 1:54, 1981

Siegal GP, Taylor LL 3rd, Nelson KG, et al. Characterization of a pure heterologous sarcoma of the uterus: rhabdomyosarcoma of the corpus. Int J Gynecol Pathol 2:303, 1983

Sikora K. The characterization of gliomas using human monoclonal antibodies. Minireview on cancer research. Exp Cell Biol 52:189, 1984

Sikora K, Wright R. Human monoclonal antibodies to lung cancer antigens. Br J Cancer 43:696, 1981

Silva EG, Kott MM, Ordóñez NG. Endocrine carcinoma intermediate cell type of the uterine cervix. Cancer 54:1705, 1984a

Silva EG, Ordóñez NG, Lechago J. Immunohistochemical studies in endocrine carcinoma of the skin. Am J Clin Pathol 81:558, 1984b

Simpson HW, Candlish W, Liddle C, et al. A critical investigation of the Oxford tumour marker Ca1 in the histological diagnosis of breast cancer and precancer. Histopathology 8:481, 1984

Simpson S, Vinik AI, Marangos PJ, et al. Immunohistochemical localization of neuron-specific enolase in gastroenteropancreatic neuroendocrine tumors. Correlation with tissue and serum levels of neuron-specific enolase. Cancer 54:1364, 1984

Sindelar WF, Dresdale AR, Hadley NA. Demonstration of tissue-specific antigens shared by normal pancreas and pancreatic neoplasms. Experientia 39:87, 1983

Singer S, Boddington MM, Hudson EA. Immunocytochemical reaction of Ca1 and HMFG2 monoclonal antibodies with cells from serous effusions. J Clin Pathol 38:180, 1985

Singh G, Katyal SL, Ordóñez NG, et al. Type II pneumocytes in pulmonary tumors. Implications for histogenesis. Arch Pathol Lab Med 108:44, 1984

Singh G, Katyal SL, Torikata C. Carcinoma of type II pneumocytes: immunodiagnosis of a subtype of "bronchioloalveolar carcinomas." Am J Pathol 102:195, 1981

Sisson SP, Vernier RL. Methods for immunoelectron microscopy: localization of antigens in rat kidney. J Histochem Cytochem 28:441, 1980

Skinner JM, Manousos ON, Economidou J, et al. Alpha-chain disease with localized plasmacytoma of the intestine. Clin Exp Immunol 25:112, 1976

Skinner JM, Whitehead R. Carcinoplacental alkaline phosphatase in malignant and premalignant conditions of the human digestive tract. Virchows Arch [A] 394:109, 1981

Skinner JM, Whitehead R. Tumor markers in carcinoma and premalignant states of the stomach in humans. Eur J Cancer Clin Oncol 18:227, 1982

Slager UT, Kaufman RL, Cohen KL, et al. Primary lymphoma of the spinal cord. J Neuropathol Exp Neurol 41:437, 1982

Slemmon JR, Salvaterra PM, Saito K. Preparation and characterization of peroxidase: antiperoxidase-Fab complex. J Histochem Cytochem 28:10, 1980

Sloane JP, Hughes F, Ormerod MG. An assessment of the value of epithelial membrane antigen and other epithelial markers in solving diagnostic problems in tumour histopathology. Histochem J 15:645, 1983

Sloane JP, Ormerod MG, Imrie SF, et al. The use of antisera to epithelial membrane antigen in detecting micrometastases in histological sections. Br J Cancer 42:392, 1980

Sloane JP, Ormerod MG. Distribution of epithelial membrane antigen in normal and neoplastic tissues and its value in diagnostic tumor pathology. Cancer 47:1786, 1981

Slocombe GW, Berry CL, Swettenham KV. The variability of blood group antigens in gastric carcinoma as demonstrated by the immunoperoxidase technique. Virchows Arch [A] 387:289, 1980

Smart Y, Millard PR. The localisation of intracellular immunoglobulin and alpha-1-antitrypsin by immunoelectron staining of post-osmicated, resin-embedded tissue. J Immunol Methods 56:97, 1983

Smith MT, Ludwig CL, Godfrey AD, et al. Grading of oligodendrogliomas. Cancer 52:2107, 1983a

Smith MT, Redick JA, Baron J. Quantitative immunohistochemistry: a comparison of microdensitometric analysis of unlabeled antibody peroxidase-antiperoxidase staining and of microfluorometric analysis of indirect fluorescent antibody staining for nicotinamide adenosine dinucleotide phosphate (NADPH)-cytochrome c (P-450) reductase in rat liver. J Histochem Cytochem 31:1183, 1983b

Smith TW, Davidson RI. Medullomyoblastoma: a histologic, immunohistochemical, and ultrastructural study. Cancer 54:323, 1984

Soeur M, Monseu G, Ketelbant P, et al. Intramedullary ependymoma producing collagen. A clinical and pathological study. Acta Neuropathol (Berl) 47:159, 1979

Soffer D, Siegal T. Solitary dural plasmacytoma with conspicuous cytoplasmic inclusions. Cancer 49:250, 1982

Sofroniew MV, Schrell U. Long-term storage and regular repeated use of diluted antisera in glass staining jars for increased sensitivity, reproducibility, and convenience of single- and two-color light microscopic immunocytochemistry. J Histochem Cytochem 30:504, 1982

Sofroniew MV, Weindl A, Schrell U, et al. Immunohistochemistry of vasopressin, oxytocin and neurophysin in the hypothalamus and extrahypothalamic regions of the human and primate brain. Acta Histochem (Suppl) 24:79, 1981

Spiers AS, Halpern R, Ross SC, et al. Meningeal myelomatosis. Arch Intern Med 140:256, 1980

Springall DR, Lackie P, Levene MN, et al. Immunostaining of neuron-specific enolase is a valuable aid to the cytological diagnosis of neuroendocrine tumours of the lung. J Pathol 143:259, 1984

Springer GF, Taylor CR, Howard DR, et al. Tn, a carcinoma-associated antigen, reacts with anti-Tn of normal human sera. Cancer 55:561, 1985

Stachura I, Mendelow H. Endodermal sinus tumor originating in the region of the pineal gland: ultrastructural and immunohistochemical study. Cancer 45:2131, 1980

Stam FC, van Alphen HA, Boorsma DM. Meningioma with conspicuous plasma cell components. A histopathological and immunohistochemical study. Acta Neuropathol (Berl) 49:241, 1980

Stass SA, Dean L, Peiper SC, et al. Determination of terminal deoxynucleotidyl transferase on bone marrow smears by immunoperoxidase. Am J Clin Pathol 77:174, 1982

Stass SA, Schumacher HR, Keneklis TP, et al. Terminal deoxynucleotidyl transferase immunofluorescence of bone marrow smears. Experience in 156 cases. Am J Clin Pathol 72:898, 1979

Steck AJ, Murray N, Meier C, et al. Demyelinating neuropathy and monoclonal IgM antibody to myelin-associated glycoprotein. Neurology 33:19, 1983a

Steck AJ, Murray N, Vandevelde M, et al. Human monoclonal antibodies to myelin-associated glycoprotein: comparison of specificity and use for immunocytochemical localization of the antigen. J Neuroimmunol 5: 145, 1983b

Stefaneanu L, Simionescu L, Aman E, Tasca C. Immunohistochemical demonstration of thyroglobulin in thyroid pathology. Endocrinologie 22: 55, 1984

Stefansson K, Molnar ML, Marton LS, Molnar GK, Mihovilovic M, Tripathi RC, Richman DP. Myelin-associated glycoprotein in human retina. Nature 307:548, 1984

Stefansson K, Wollman R. Distribution of glial fibrillary acid protein in central nervous system lesions of tuberculous sclerosis. Acta Neuropathol (Berl) 52:135, 1980

Stefansson K, Wollmann R. Distribution of the neuronal specific protein, 14-3-2, in central nervous system lesions of tuberous sclerosis. Acta Neuropathol (Berl) 53:113, 1981

Stefansson K, Wollmann RL. S-100 protein in granular cell tumors (granular cell myoblastomas). Cancer 49:1834, 1982

Stefansson K, Wollmann R, Jerkovic M. S-100 protein in soft-tissue tumors derived from Schwann cells and melanocytes. Am J Pathol 106:261, 1982a

Stefansson K, Wollmann RL, Moore BW, Arnason BG. S-100 protein in human chondrocytes. Nature 295:63, 1982b

Stegehuis F, de Vries GP, Jöbsis AC, Meijer AE. Comparative investigation of the mixed aggregation immunocytochemical technique and the indirect perox-

idase technique for the detection of prostate specific acid phosphatase in paraffin or paraplast sections. Histochemistry 62:45, 1979

Stein H, Bonk A, Tolksdorf G, et al. Immunohistologic analysis of the organization of normal lymphoid tissue and non-Hodgkin's lymphomas. J Histochem Cytochem 28:746, 1980

Stein H, Gatter KC, Heryet A, et al. Freeze-dried paraffin-embedded human tissue for antigen labelling with monoclonal antibodies. Lancet 2:71, 1984

Stein H, Gerdes J, Schwab U, et al. Identification of Hodgkin and Sternberg-Reed cells as a unique cell type derived from a newly detected small-cell population. Int J Cancer 30:445, 1982

Stein H, Gerdes J, Tolksdorf G, et al. Human membrane-bound C3 receptors. I. Serological and immunohistological demonstration of C3 receptors. Scand J Immunol 13:67, 1981a

Stein H, Mason DY, Gerdes J, et al. Immunohistology of B cell lymphomas. In: Knapp W et al, eds. Leukemia Markers, p 99. New York, Academic Press, 1981b

Steinman RM, Kaplan G, Witmer MD, et al. Identification of a novel cell type in peripheral lymphoid organs of mice. V. Purification of spleen dendritic cells, new surface markers, and maintenance in vitro. J Exp Med 149:1, 1979

Steinman G, Mertelsmann R, deHarven E, et al. Ultrastructural demonstration of terminal deoxynucleotidyl transferase (TdT). Blood 57:368, 1981

Stenman S, von Smitten K, Vaheri A. Fibronectin and atherosclerosis. Acta Med Scand [Suppl] 642:165, 1980

Sternberger LA. Immunocytochemistry. Englewood Cliffs, NJ, Prentice-Hall, 1974

Sternberger LA. Immunocytochemistry, 2nd ed. New York, John Wiley and Sons, 1979a

Sternberger LA. The labeled antibody method. Hormone receptor, Golgi-like and dual color immunocytochemistry. J Histochem Cytochem 27:1658, 1979b

Sternberger LA, Hardy PH Jr, Cuculis JJ, et al. The unlabeled antibody enzyme method of immunohistochemistry. Preparation and properties of soluble antigen-antibody complex (horseradish peroxidase-antihorseradish peroxidase) and its use in the identification of spirochetes. J Histochem Cytochem 18:315, 1970

Sternberger LA, Joseph SA. The unlabeled antibody method. Contrasting color staining of paired pituitary hormones without antibody removal. J Histochem Cytochem 27:1424, 1979

Stiller D, Katenkamp D. Histochemistry of amyloid: general considerations, light microscopical and ultrastructural examinations. Exp Pathol [Suppl] 1:3, 1975

Stjernholm MR, Freudenbourg JC, Mooney HS, et al. Medullary carcinoma of the thyroid before age 2 years. J Clin Endocrinol Metab 51:252, 1980

Stone JL, Zavala G, Bailery OT. Mixed malignant mesenchymal tumor of the cerebellar vermis. Cancer 44:2165, 1979

Storch W. [Immunohistochemical localization of actin and myosin in liver, kidney, stomach, heart and skeletal muscle: a reference to a cytoplasmic actin fibrillar network in liver cells.] Acta Histochem 68:208, 1981

Straus W. Inhibition of peroxidase by methanol and by methanol-nitroferricyanide for use in immunoperoxidase procedures. J Histochem Cytochem 19:682, 1971

Straus W. Phenylhydrazine as inhibitor of horseradish peroxidase for use in immunoperoxidase procedures. J Histochem Cytochem 20:949, 1972

Straus W. Use of peroxidase inhibitors for immunoperoxidase procedures. In: Feldman et al, eds. First

International Symposium on Immunoenzymatic Techniques. p 117. Amsterdam, North Holland Publishing Co, 1976

Straus W. Staining patterns for the anti-horseradish peroxidase antibody reaction in proplasma cells developing in the medulla of rat popliteal lymph nodes during the secondary response. J Histochem Cytochem 29:525, 1981

Streefkerk JG. Inhibition of erythrocyte pseudoperoxidase activity by treatment with hydrogen peroxide following methanol. J Histochem Cytochem 29:829, 1972

Strefling AM, Knapp AM, Mansbridge JN. Histologic distribution of staining by a monoclonal antibody (psi-3) in psoriasis and occurrence of psi-3 antigen in other cutaneous diseases. J Invest Dermatol 84:100, 1985

Streilein JW, Bergstresser PR. Ia antigens and epidermal Langerhans cells. Transplantation 30:319, 1980

Stromeyer FW, Ishak KG, Gerber MA, et al. Ground-glass cells in hepatocellular carcinoma. Am J Clin Pathol 74:254, 1980

Stuart AE, Volsen SG, Zola H. The reactivity of Reed-Sternberg cells with monoclonal antisera at thin section and ultrastructural levels. J Pathol 141:71, 1983

Stuhlmiller GM, Borowitz MJ, Croker BP, et al. Multiple assay characterization of murine monoclonal antimelanoma antibodies. Hybridoma 1:447, 1982

Suffin SC, Muck KB, Young JC, et al. Improvement of the glucose oxidase immunoenzyme technic. Use of tetrazolium whose formazan is stable without heavy metal chelation. Am J Clin Pathol 71:492, 1979

Sugano I, Nagao K, Matsuzaki O, et al. Immunohistochemical studies on myoepithelial changes in breast tumors. Acta Pathol Jpn 31:35, 1981

Sugimoto M, Bollum FJ. Terminal deoxynucleotidyl transferase (TdT) in chick embryo lymphoid tissues. J Immunol 122:392, 1979

Sumiyoshi H, Taniyama K, Ito H, et al. Secretory component and immunoglobulin in human gastric carcinoma: an immunohistochemical study. Gann 75:166, 1984

Sun NC, Edgington TD, Carpentier CL, et al. Immunohistochemical localization of carcinoembryonic antigen (CEA), CEA-S and nonspecific cross-reacting antigen (NCA) in carcinomas of lung. Cancer 52:1732, 1983

Sun NC, Fishkin BG, Nies KM, et al. Lymphoplasmacytic myeloma: an immunological, immunohistochemical and electron microscopic study. Cancer 43:2268, 1979

Sun TT, Eichner R, Nelson WG, et al. Keratin expression during normal epidermal differentiation. Curr Probl Dermatol 11:277, 1983

SundarRaj N, Martin J, Hrinya N. Development and characterization of monoclonal antibodies to human type III procollagen. Biochem Biophys Res Commun 106:48, 1982

Sunderland CA, Davies JO, Stirrat GM. Immunohistology of normal and ovarian cancer tissue with a monoclonal antibody to placental alkaline phosphatase. Cancer Res 44:4496, 1984

Sunderland CA, Redman CW, Stirrat GM. Monoclonal antibodies to human syncytiotrophoblast. Immunology 43:541, 1981

Sutton AL, Smithwick EM, Seligman SJ, et al. Fatal disseminated herpesvirus hominis type 2 infection in an adult with associated thymic dysplasia. Am J Med 56:545, 1974

Suzumura A, Silberberg DH. Expression of H-2 antigen on oligodendrocytes is induced by soluble factors from concanavalin A activated T cells. Brain Res 336:171, 1985

Sweeney EC, Barry-Walsh C, Robinson A. Sertoli-Leydig cell tumor of the ovary with heterologous elements and carcinoid: an immunohistochemical and ultrastructural study. Ultrastruct Pathol 5:185, 1983

Swenson PD, Escobar MR, Silverman JF. Hepatitis B virus surface and core antigens in the liver of primary hepatocellular carcinoma cases in Virginia. Acta Biol Acad Sci Hung 31:321, 1980

Swerdlow SH, Murray LJ. Natural killer (Leu 7+) cells in reactive lymphoid tissues and malignant lymphomas. Am J Clin Pathol 81:459, 1984

Syrjänen K, Happonen RP, Syrjänen S, et al. Human papillomavirus (HPV) antigens and local immunologic reactivity in oral squamous cell tumors and hyperplasias. Scand J Dent Res 92:358, 1984

Syrjänen K, Syrjänen S, Lamberg M, et al. Morphological and immunohistochemical evidence suggesting human papillomavirus (HPV) involvement in oral squamous cell carcinogenesis. Int J Oral Surg 12:418, 1983a

Syrjänen K, Väyrynen M, Castién O, et al. Morphological and immunohistochemical evidence of human papilloma virus (HPV) involvement in the dysplastic lesions of the uterine cervix. Int J Gynaecol Obstet 21:261, 1983b

Syrjänen KJ, Pyrhönen S. Demonstration of human papilloma virus antigen in the condylomatous lesions of the uterine cervix by immunoperoxidase technique. Gynecol Obstet Invest 14:90, 1982a

Syrjänen KJ, Pyrhönen S. Immunoperoxidase demonstration of human papilloma virus (HPV) in dysplastic lesions of the uterine cervix. Arch Gynecol 233:53, 1982b

Syrjänen KJ. The pattern of human lymph node involvement by the non-Hodgkin lymphomas of B-cell lineage. Neoplasma 26:589, 1979

Syrjänen KJ. Non-Hodgkin malignant lymphomas of B-cell lineage with special reference to their lymph node involvement pattern. Arch Geschwulstforsch 50:66, 1980

Szymendera JJ, Zborzil J, Sikorowa L, et al. Value of five tumor markers (AFP, CEA, hCG, hPL and SP1) in diagnosis and staging of testicular germ cell tumors. Oncology 38:222, 1981

Tabei SZ. Immunohistologic demonstration of Toxoplasma gondii. N Engl J Med 307:1404, 1982

Tabilio A, Falini B, Mecucci C, et al. Light chain plasmacytoid lymphocytic lymphoma. Postgrad Med J 57:588, 1981

Tabuchi K, Kawakami Y, Nishimoto A. Immunohistochemical demonstration of IgG in meningioma. Acta Neurochir (Wien) 55:201, 1981

Tabuchi K, Moriya Y, Furuta T, et al. S-100 protein in human glial tumours qualitative and quantitative studies. Acta Neurochir (Wein) 65:239, 1982

Tabuchi K, Nishimoto A, Kirsch WM. Localization of SV40 T antigen in mitotic cells by an immunoperoxidase method. Experientia 36:1053, 1980

Tahara E, Ito H, Shimamoto F, et al. Lysozyme in human gastric carcinoma: a retrospective immunohistochemical study. Histopathology 6:409, 1982

Takahashi H, Takahashi K, Tanno K, et al. Pagetoid reticulosis (Woringer-Kolopp disease). An ultrastructural and immunocytological study. Acta Pathol Jpn 32:513, 1982

Takahashi K, Isobe T, Ohtsuki Y, et al. Immunohistochemical study on the distribution of α and β subunits of S-100 protein in human neoplasm and normal tissues. Virchows Arch [Cell Pathol] 45:385, 1984

Takahashi K, Yamaguchi H, Ishizeki J, et al. Immunohistochemical and immunoelectron microscopic localization of S-100 protein in the interdigitating reticulum cells of the human lymph node. Virchows Arch [B] 37:125, 1981

Takamiya H, Batsford SR, Tokunaga J, et al. Immuno-histological staining of antigens on semithin sections of specimens embedded in plastic CGMA-Quetol 523. J Immunol Methods 30:277, 1979

Takamiya H, Batsford S, Vogt A. An approach to postembedding staining of protein (immunoglobulin) antigen embedded in plastic prerequisites and limita-tions. J Histochem Cytochem 28:1041, 1980

Takeda A, Ishizuka T, Goto T, et al. Polyembryoma of ovary producing alpha-fetoprotein and HCG: immu-noperoxidase and electron microscopic study. Cancer 49:1818, 1982

Takeuchi T, Kuriyama M, Fujihiro S, et al. Evaluation of serum prostate-specific antigen in urologic cancers. J Surg Oncol 24:157, 1983

Talerman A, Lindeman J, Kievit-Tyson PA, et al. Dem-onstration of calcitonin and carcinoembryonic antigen (CEA) in medullary carcinoma of the thyroid (MCT) by immunoperoxidase technique. Histopathology 3:503, 1979

Tanaka M, Kaneda T, Hirota Y, et al. Terminal deoxy-nucleotidyl transferase in the blastic phase of chronic myelogenous leukemia: An indicator of response to vincristine and prednisone therapy. Am J Hematol 9:287, 1980

Tanaka M, Tanaka H, Ishikawa E. Immunohistochemi-cal demonstration of surface antigen of human lym-phocytes with monoclonal antibody in acetone-fixed paraffin-embedded sections. J Histochem Cytochem 32:452, 1984

Tanimura A, Nakamura Y, Hachisuka H, et al. Heman-gioblastoma of the central nervous system: nature of the stromal cells as studied by the immunoperoxidase technique. Hum Pathol 15:866, 1984

Taratuto AL, Molina HA, Diez B, et al. Primary rhab-domyosarcoma of brain and cerebellum. Report of four Acta Neuropathol (Berl) 66:98, 1985

Taratuto AL, Monges J, Lylyk P, et al. Superficial cerebral astrocytoma attached to dura: report of six cases in infants. Cancer 54:2505, 1984

Tarkkanen A, Tervo T, Tervo K, et al. Substance P immunoreactivity in normal human retina and in retinoblastoma. Ophthalmic Res 15:300, 1983

Tascos NA, Parr J, Gonata NK. Immunocytochemical study of the glial fibrillary acidic protein in human neoplasms of the central nervous system. Hum Pathol 13:454, 1982

Tate DY, Carlton GT, Nesbit ME, et al. Detection of platelet associated IgG in immune thrombocytopenia: a new assay employing protein A and peroxidase anti-peroxidase (PROA-PAP). Am J Hematol 9:349, 1980

Tatsumi E, Kimura K, Takiuchi Y, et al. T lymphocytes expressing human Ia-like antigens in infectious mono-nucleosis (IM). Blood 56:383, 1980

Tavares de Castro J, San Miguel JF, Soler J, et al. Method for the simultaneous labelling of terminal deoxynucleotidyl transferase (TdT) and membrane antigens. J Clin Pathol 37:628, 1984

Taxy JB, Mendelsohn G, Gupta PK. Carcinoid tumors of the rectum. Silver reactions, fluorescence, and ser-otonin content of the cytoplasmic granules. Am J Clin Pathol 74:791, 1980

Taylor CR. The nature of Reed-Sternberg cells and other malignant cells. Lancet 2:802, 1974

Taylor CR. An immunohistological study of follicular lymphoma, reticulum cell sarcoma and Hodgkin's dis-ease. Eur J Cancer 12:61, 1976

Taylor CR. Immunohistological approach to tumor di-agnosis. Oncology 35:189, 1978a

Taylor CR. Immunoperoxidase techniques: theoretical and practical aspects. Arch Pathol Lab Med 102:113, 1978b

Taylor CR. Classification of lymphomas: "new thinking" on old thoughts. Arch Pathol Lab Med 102:549, 1978c

Taylor CR. Immunocytochemical methods in the study of lymphoma and related conditions. J Histochem Cytochem 26:495, 1978d

Taylor CR. Immunohistologic studies of lymphomas: new methodology yields new information and poses new problems. J Histochem Cytochem 27:1189, 1979a

Taylor CR. Results of multiparameter studies of B-cell lymphomas. Am J Clin Pathol (Suppl 4) 72:687, 1979b

Taylor CR. A practical approach to immunohistologic studies of lymphoreticular neoplasia. J Histochem Cytochem 27:118, 1979c

Taylor CR. Changing concepts in classification of lym-phoma. In: Bosman F, van den Tweel J, Taylor CR, eds. Malignant Lymphomas, the Pathophysiology of the Lymphocyte and its Neoplasms, p 175. Leiden, Leiden University Press, 1980a

Taylor CR. Inter-relations of B cell neoplasms. In: Bosman F, van den Tweel J, Taylor CR, eds. Malig-nant Lymphomas, the Pathophysiology of the Lym-phocyte and its Neoplasms, p 399. Leiden, Leiden University Press, 1980b

Taylor CR. Immunohistologic studies of lymphoma: past, present and future. J Histochem Cytochem 28:777, 1980c

Taylor CR. Pathobiology of lymphocyte transformation. In: Ioachim HL, ed. Pathobiology Annuals, p 65. New York, Raven Press, 1982a

Taylor CR. Advances in the classification of lymphomas using histologic and diagnostic criteria. In: Steckel RJ, Kagan AR, eds. Recent Advances in Cancer Diagnosis, p 2. New York, Grune & Stratton, 1982b

Taylor CR. Immunoenzyme techniques and their appli-cation to diagnostic studies. Ann NY Acad Sci 420:115, 1983a

Taylor CR. The enigma of Hodgkin's disease and the Reed-Sternberg cell. In: Bennett JM, ed. Controver-sies in the Management of Lymphomas, II. p 91. Cancer Treatment and Research, McGuire WL, series ed. Boston, Martinus Nijhoff, 1983b

Taylor CR, Burns J. The demonstration of plasma cells and other immunoglobulin containing cells in for-malin-fixed, paraffin-embedded tissues using peroxi-dase labelled antibody. J Clin Pathol 27:14, 1974

Taylor CR, Cooper CL, Kurman RJ, et al. Detection of estrogen receptor in breast and endometrial carci-noma by the immunoperoxidase technique. Cancer 47:2634, 1981

Taylor CR, Kledzik G. Immunohistologic techniques in surgical pathology—a spectrum of "new" special stains. Human Pathol 12:590, 1981

Taylor CR, Kurman RJ, Warner NE. The potential value of immunohistological techniques in the classification of ovarian and testicular tumors. Human Pathol 9:417, 1978a

Taylor CR, Lukes RJ, Parker JW. Advances in the classification of lymphomas using histologic and di-agnostic criteria. In: Steckel RJ, Kagan Ar, eds. Recent Advances in Cancer Diagnosis, p 2. New York, Grune & Stratton, 1982

Taylor CR, Mason DY. Immunohistological detection of intracellular immunoglobulin in formalin-paraffin sec-tions from multiple myeloma using the immunoper-oxidase technique. Clin Exp Immunol 18:417, 1974

Taylor CR, Parker JW. Immuno-methods in diagnostic hematopathology. In: Jasmin G, Cantin M, eds. Methods and Achievements in Experimental Pathology, vol 10. p 37. New York, Karger, 1981

Taylor CR, Russell R, Chandor SB. An immunohistological study of multiple myeloma and related conditions using immunoperoxidase methods. Am J Clin Pathol 70:612, 1978b

Taylor CR, Russell R, Lukes RJ, et al. An immunohistological study of the immunoglobulin content of primary central nervous system lymphomas. Cancer 41:2197, 1978c

Taylor CR, Sherrod AE, Imam A, et al. Immunohistochemical methods: a more precise approach to the diagnosis of malignant disease. In: Directions in Oncology, vol 1, No 9. New Canaan, Nassau, Conn, 1985

Taylor CR, Skinner JM. Evidence for significant hematopoiesis in the human thymus. Blood 47:305, 1976

Taylor CR, Warner NE. Immunohistologic technique in the diagnosis of ovarian and testicular neoplasia. In: Filipe MI, Lake BD, eds. Histochemistry in Pathology. Edinburgh, Churchill Livingstone, 1982

Teitelman G, Joh TH, Reis DJ. Linkage of the brain-skin-gut axis: islet cells originate from dopaminergic precursors. Peptids (Suppl 2) 2:157, 1981

Temple S, Raff MC. Differentiation of a bipotential glial progenitor cell in single cell microculture. Nature 313:223, 1985

Tenovuo O, Rinne UK, Viljanen MK. Substance P immunoreactivity in the post-mortem parkinsonian brain. Brain Res 303:113, 1984

Teramoto YA, Meriani R, Wunderlich D, et al. The immunohistochemical reactivity of a human monoclonal antibody with tissue sections of human mammary tumors. Cancer 50:241, 1982

Terenghi G, Polak JM, Ballesta J, et al. Immunocytochemistry of neuronal and glial markers in retinoblastoma. Virchows Arch [A] 404:61, 1984

Terry RD, Gonata NK, Weiss M. Ultrastructural studies in Alzheimer's presenile dementia. Am J Pathol 44:269, 1964

Terry RD, Katzman R. Senile dementia of the Alzheimer type. Ann Neurol 14:497, 1983

Tetu B, Totovic V, Bechtelsheimer H, et al. [Renin-secreting renal tumor. Apropos of a case with an ultrastructural and immunohistochemical study.] Ann Pathol 4:55, 1984

Theodoropoulos G, Nakopoulou L, Repanti M, et al. Detection of hepatitis B surface antigen in fixed tissues of patients with cirrhosis and hepatoma. Virchows Arch [A] 382:293, 1979

Thivolet J, Viac J, Staquet MJ, et al. [Study of normal and pathological keratinization using anti-keratin polypeptide sera.] Ann Dermatol Venereol 107:357, 1980

Thomas JA, Iliescu V, Crawford DH, et al. Expression of HLA-DR antigens in nasopharyngeal carcinoma: an immunohistological analysis of the tumour cells and infiltrating lymphocytes. Int J Cancer 33:813, 1982

Thomas JA, Janossy G, Eden OB, et al. Nuclear terminal deoxynucleotidyl transferase in leukaemic infiltrates of testicular tissue. Br J Cancer 45:709, 1984

Thomas P, Said JW, Nash G, et al. Profiles of keratin proteins in basal and squamous cell carcinomas of the skin. An immunohistochemical study. Lab Invest 50:36, 1982

Thompson JJ, Herlyn MF, Elder DE, et al. Use of monoclonal antibodies in detection of melanoma associated antigen in intact human tumors. Am J Pathol 107:357, 1982

Thomsen P, Clausen PP. Occurrence of hepatitis B-surface antigen in a consecutive material of 1539 liver biopsies. Acta Pathol Microbiol Immunol Scand [A] 91:71, 1983

Thung SN, Gerber MA. Immunohistochemical study of delta antigen in an American metropolitan population. Liver 3:392, 1983

Tilgen W, Hellström I, Engstner M, et al. Localization of melanoma-associated antigen p97 in cultured human melanoma, as visualized by light and electron microscopy. J Invest Dermatol 80:459, 1983

Tinelli M, Legnani F, Santi G, et al. [Observation about the use of different types of enzymes in immunohistological diagnosis of autoimmune diseases. Comparative study with indirect immunofluorescence technique.] Ann Sclavo 21:561, 1979

Tischler AS, Dichter MA, Biales B, et al. Neuroendocrine neoplasms and their cells of origin. N Engl J Med 296:919, 1977

Toccanier MF, Exquis B, Groebli Y. Granulome plasmocytaire du poumon. Neuf observations avec etude immunohistochimique. Ann Pathol 2:21, 1982

Togo S, Hirayama R, Hirokawa K. Distribution of immunoglobulin-containing cells and localization of secretory component in gastric mucosa bearing carcinoma. Bull Tokyo Med Dent Univ 28:61, 1981

Tokunaga O, Tanimura A, Morimatsu M, et al. Measles giant cell pneumonia in childhood leukemia in remission. Acta Pathol Jpn 30:483, 1980

Tolson ND, Boothroyd B, Hopkins CR. Cell surface labelling with gold colloid particulates: the use of avidin and staphylococcal protein A–coated gold in conjunction with biotin and Fc-bearing ligands. J Microscop 123:215, 1981

Tomita T, Kimmel JR, Friesen SR, et al. Pancreatic polypeptide cell hyperplasia with and without watery diarrhea syndrome. J Surg Oncol 14:11, 1980

Tomlinson BE. The aging brain. In: Smith WT, Cavanagh JB, eds. Recent Advances in Neuropathology, vol I, p 129. Edinburgh, Churchill Livingstone, 1979

Torack RM, Gebel HM. Immunopathology of brain aging and senile dementia of the Alzheimer type. In: Cervos-Navarro J, Sarkander H-I, eds. Brain Aging: Neuropathology and Neuropharmacology, p 373. New York, Raven Press, 1983

Totović V, Kron I. [Diagnosis of congenital deficiency of alpha 1-antitrypsin by the immune peroxidase technique.] Leber Magen Darm 10:91, 1980

Tougard C, Tixier-Vidal A, Avrameas S. Comparison between peroxidase-conjugated antigen or antibody and peroxidase–anti:peroxidase complex in a post-embedding procedure. J Histochem Cytochem 27:1630, 1979

Trachtenberg MC. Glial endocytosis of protein in the traumatized brain. J Neurosci Res 9:413, 1983

Tramu G, Beauvillain JC, Mazzuca M, et al. [Pituitary adenomas with cells containing beta MSH, alpha and beta endorphins and without ACTH.] Ann Endocrinol 40:561, 1979

Traugott U, Scheinberg LC, Raine CS. On the presence of Ia-positive endothelial cells and astrocytes in multiple sclerosis lesions and its relevance to antigen presentation. J Neuroimmunol 8:1, 1985

Treilhou-Lahille F, Cressent M, Taboulet J, et al. Demonstration immunohistochimique des cellules a calcitonine de la thyroide foetale de souris. C R Acad Sci [D] 289:421, 1979

Triarhou LC, de Cerro M, Herndon RM. Ultrastructural evidence for phagocytosis by oliodendroglia. Neurosci Lett 53:185, 1985

Triche TJ, Askin FB. Neuroblastoma and the differential diagnosis of small-, round-, blue-cell tumors. Hum Pathol 14:569, 1983

Trojanowski JQ, Hickey WF. Human teratomas express differentiated neural antigens: an immunohistochemical study with anti-neurofilament, anti-glial filament, and anti-myelin basic protein monoclonal antibodies. Am J Pathol 115:383, 1984

Trojanowski JQ, Kleinman GM, Proppe KH. Malignant tumors of nerve sheath origin. Cancer 46:1202, 1980

Trojanowski JQ, Lee V, Pillsbury N, et al. Neuronal origin of human esthesioneuroblastoma demonstrated with anti-neurofilament monoclonal antibodies. N Engl J Med 307:159, 1982

Trojanowski JQ, Lee V, Schlaepfer WW. An immuno-histochemical study of human central and peripheral nervous system tumors, using monoclonal antibodies against neurofilaments and glial filaments. Hum Pathol 15:248, 1984

Trojanowski JQ, Obrocka MA, Lee VM. A comparison of eight different chromogen protocols for the demonstration of immunoreactive neurofilaments or glial filaments in rat cerebellum using the peroxidase-antiperoxidase method and monoclonal antibodies. J Histochem Cytochem 31:1217, 1983

Trost TH, Galosi A, Enderer K. Intercellular immune complexes in a case of bullous pemphigoid. Dermatologica 164:149, 1980a

Trost TH, Steigleder GK, Bodeux E. Immuno-electron microscopical investigations with a new tracer: peroxidase-labeled protein A: application for detection of pemphigus and bullous pemphigoid antibodies. J Invest Dermatol 75:328, 1980b

Trost TH, Weil HP, Noack M, et al. A new immunoenzyme tracer for localization of antibodies in immunohistology: peroxidase-labeled protein A. J Cutan Pathol 7:227, 1980c

Tsai CC, Blank WF, Roodman ST. IgG Fc receptors in surface membrane of human glial tumors. J Neuropathol Exp Neurol 41:367, 1982

Tschen JA, Migliore PJ, McGavran MH. Multiple myeloma with cutaneous involvement. Arch Dermatol 116:1394, 1980

Tsokos M, Linnoila RI, Chandra RS, et al. Neuron-specific enolase in the diagnosis of neuroblastoma and other small, round-cell tumors in children. Hum Pathol 15:575, 1984

Tsuchihashi Y, Kitamura T, Fujita S. Immunofluorescence studies of the monocytes in the injured rat brain. Acta Neuropathol (Berl) 53:213, 1981

Tsunoda R, Yaginuma Y, Kojima M. Immunocytological studies on the constituent cells of the secondary nodules in human tonsils. Acta Pathol Jpn 30:33, 1980

Tsuto T, Okamura H, Fukui K, et al. An immunohistochemical investigation of vasoactive intestinal polypeptide in the colon of patients with Hirschsprung's disease. Neurosci Lett 34:57, 1982

Tsutsumi Y. Leu 7 immunoreactivity as histochemical marker for paraffin-embedded neuroendocrine tumors. Acta Histochem Cytochem 17:15, 1984

Tsutsumi Y, Nagura H, Watanabe K. Immunohistochemical observations of carcinoembryonic antigen (CEA) and CEA-related substances in normal and neoplastic pancreas. Pitfalls and caveats in CEA immunohistochemistry. Am J Clin Pathol 82:535, 1984

Tsutsumi Y, Osamura RY, Watanabe K, et al. Simulta-

neous immunohistochemical localization of gastrin releasing peptide (GRP) and calcitonin (CT) in human bronchial endocrine-type cells. Virchows Arch [A] 400:163, 1983

Tubbs RR, Fishleder A, Weiss RA, et al. Immunohistologic cellular phenotypes of lymphoproliferative disorders. Comprehensive evaluation of 564 cases including 257 non-Hodgkin's lymphomas classified by the International Working Formulation. Am J Pathol 113:207, 1983

Tubbs RR, Gephardt G, Valenzuela R, et al. An approach to immunomicroscopy of renal disease with immunoperoxidase and periodic acid-Schiff counterstain (IMPAS stain). Am J Clin Pathol 73:240, 1980a

Tubbs RR, Savage RA, Crabtree RH, et al. Expression of monocytic-histiocytic cytochemical markers in epithelial neoplasia. Am J Clin Pathol 72:789, 1977b

Tubbs RR, Sheibani K. Chromogens for immunohistochemistry. Arch Pathol Lab Med 106:205, 1982

Tubbs RR, Sheibani K. Immunohistology of lymphoproliferative disorders. Sem Diag Pathol 1:272, 1984

Tubbs RR, Sheibani K, Hawk WA. Giant cell myocarditis. Arch Pathol Lab Med 104:245, 1980b

Tubbs RR, Sheibani K, Savage R, et al. Muramidase, an immunohistochemical marker of malignant histiocytosis. Hum Pathol 10:483, 1977a

Tubbs RR, Sheibani K, Sebek BA, et al. Immunohistochemistry versus immunofluorescence for non-Hodgkin's lymphomas. Am J Clin Pathol 73:144, 1980c

Tubbs RR, Sheibani K, Weiss RA, et al. Immunohistochemistry of fresh-frozen lymphoid tissue with the direct immunoperoxidase technic. Am J Clin Pathol 75:172, 1981a

Tubbs RR, Sheibani K, Weiss RA, et al. Tissue immunomicroscopic evaluation of monoclonality of B-cell lymphomas: comparison with cell suspension studies. Am J Clin Pathol 76:24, 1981b

Tubbs RR, Velasco ME, Benjamin SP. Immunocytochemical identification of human chorionic gonadotropin. Comparative study of diaminobenzidine and 3-amino, 9-ethylcarbazole, a nonhazardous chromogen. Arch Pathol Lab Med 103:534, 1979

Turner RR, Colby TV, Doggett RS. Well-differentiated lymphocytic lymphoma. A study of 47 patients with primary manifestation in the lung. Cancer 54:2088, 1984

Uchida T, Shikata T, Shimizu SI, et al. Gonadotropin and alkaline phosphatase–producing occult gastric carcinoma with widespread metastasis of generalized bone. Cancer 48:140, 1981

Uchino J, Hata Y, Sasaki F, et al. Alphafetoprotein in congenital biliary atresia and neonatal hepatitis. Jpn J Surg 11:449, 1981

Ueda G, Inoue Y, Yamasaki M, et al. Immunohistochemical demonstration of tumor antigen TA-4 in gynecologic tumors. Int J Gynecol Pathol 3:291, 1984a

Ueda G, Yamasaki M, Inoue M, et al. Immunohistochemical demonstration of peptide hormones in cervical adenocarcinomas with argyrophil cells. Int J Gynecol Pathol 2:373, 1984b

Ueda GT, Yamasaki M, Inoue M, et al. Immunohistological demonstration of calcitonin in endometrial carcinomas with and without argyrophil cells. Nippon Sanka Fujinka Gakkai Zasshi 32:960, 1980

Ulich TR, Cheng L, Glover H, et al. A colonic adenocarcinoma with argentaffin cells. An immunoperoxidase study demonstrating the presence of numerous neuroendocrine products. Cancer 51:1483, 1983

Underwood JC, Dangerfield VJM. Immunohistochemical identification of adult and fetal haemopoiesis in the spleen in lymphoma, leukaemia and myeloproliferative disease. J Pathol 134:71, 1981

Underwood JC, Sher E, Reed M, et al. Biochemical assessment of histochemical methods for oestrogen receptor localisation. J Clin Pathol 35:401, 1982

Unsworth DJ, Scott DL, Almond TJ, et al. Studies on reticulin. I: serological and immunohistological investigations of the occurrences of collagen type III, fibronectin and the non-collagenous glycoprotein of Pras and Glynn in reticulin. Br J Exp Pathol 63:154, 1982

Urbanski SJ, Bilbao JM, Horvath EA, et al. Intrasellar solitary plasmacytoma terminating in multiple myeloma: a report of a case including electron microscopical study. Surg Neurol 14:233, 1980

Urbanski SJ, Kovacs R, McComb DJ, et al. Argyrophil granules in the human pituitary. Acta Histochem 70:69, 1982

Vaalasti A, Linnoila I, Hervonen A. Immunohistochemical demonstraton of VIP, [Met5]- and [Leu5]-enkephalin immunoreactive nerve fibres in the human prostate and seminal vesicles. Histochemistry 66:89, 1980

Vacca LL, Hewett D, Woodson G. A comparison of methods using diaminobenzidine (DAB) to localize peroxidases in erythrocytes, neutrophils, and peroxidase-antiperoxidase complex. Stain Technol 53:331, 1978

Vafier JA, Javadpour N, Worsham GF, et al. Double blind comparison of T-antigen and ABO(H) cell surface antigens in bladder cancer. Urology 23:348, 1984

Valdiserri RO, Yunis EJ. Sacrococcygeal teratomas: a review of 68 cases. Cancer 48:217, 1981

Valentino KL, Jones EG. Morphological and immunocytochemical identification of macrophages in the developing corpus callosum. Anat Embryol (Berl) 163:157, 1981

Valkova B, Ormerod MG, Moncrieff D, et al. Epithelial membrane antigen in cells from the uterine cervix: immunocytochemical staining of cervical smears. J Clin Pathol 37:984, 1984

Valnes K, Brandtzaeg P. Unlabeled antibody peroxidase-antiperoxidase method combined with direct immunofluorescence. J Histochem Cytochem 29:703, 1981

Valnes K, Brandtzaeg P. Comparison of paired immunofluorescence and paired immunoenzyme staining methods based on primary antisera from the same species. J Histochem Cytochem 30:518, 1982

Valnes K, Brandtzaeg P. Paired indirect immunoenzyme staining with primary antibodies from the same species. Application of horseradish peroxidase and alkaline phosphatase as sequential labels. Histochem J 16:477, 1984

Van Alstyne D, Smyrnis EM, et al. Differentiation of glioblasts from adult brain. Neurosci Lett 40:327, 1983

Van Bogaert LJ, Quinones JA, et al. Difficulties involved in diaminobenzidine histochemistry of endogenous peroxidase. Acta Histochem 67:180, 1980

Van Camp B, Reynaerts P, Naets JP, et al. Transient IgA-lambda paraproteinemia during treatment of acute myelomonoblastic leukemia. Blood 55:21, 1980

Vanden Heule B, Taylor CR, Terry R, et al. Presentation of malignant lymphoma in the rectum. Cancer 49:2602, 1982

Van den Oord JJ, De Wolf-Peeters C, Tricot G, et al. A subpopulation of lymph node B-CLL cells expresses the common acute lymphoblastic leukemia antigen. Anticancer Res 4:379, 1984

van den Tweel JG. The T-cell derived neoplasms: an overview. In: Bosman F, van den Tweel J, Taylor CR, eds. Malignant Lymphomas, the Pathophysiology of the Lymphocyte and its Neoplasms. Leiden, Leiden University Press, 1980

van den Tweel JG, Taylor CR, Parker JW, et al. Immunoglobulin inclusions in non-Hodgkin lymphomas. Am J Clin Pathol 69:306, 1978

van den Tweel JG, Taylor CR, McClure J, et al. Detection of thymosin in thymic epithelial cells by an immunoperoxidase method. Adv Exp Med Biol 114:511, 1979

van der Meulen JD, Houthoff HJ, Ebels EJ. Glial fibrillary acidic protein in human gliomas. Neuropathol Appl Neurobiol 4:177, 1978

Van der Valk P, te Velde J. Jansen J, et al. Malignant lymphoma of true histiocytic origin: Histiocytic sarcoma. A morphological, ultrastructural, immunological, cytochemical and clinical study of 10 cases. Virchows Arch [A] 391:249, 1981

Van der Valk P, van der Loo EM, Jansen J, et al. Analysis of lymphoid and dendritic cells in human lymph node, tonsil and spleen. A study using monoclonal and heterologous antibodies. Virchows Arch [B] 45:169, 1984

Vandesande F, Dierickx K, Goossens N. Immunocytochemical localization of the posterior lobe hormones and of their carrier proteins. J Histochem Cytochem 28:469, 1980

van Duinen SG, Mauw BJ, de Graaff-Reitsma CB, et al. Methods in laboratory investigation. Immunoelectron microscopic methods for demonstration of antigens on normal human melanocytes and other epidermal cells. Lab Invest 50:733, 1984a

van Duinen SG, Ruiter DJ, Hageman P, et al. Immunohistochemical and histochemical tools in the diagnosis of amelanotic melanoma. Cancer 53:1566, 1984b

Van Ewijk W, Jenkinson EJ, Owen JJ. Detection of Thy-1, T-200, Lyt-1 and Lyt-2 bearing cells in the developing lymphoid organs of the mouse embryo in vivo and in vitro. Eur J Immunol 12:262, 1982a

Van Ewijk W, Jenkinson EJ, van Soest PL, et al. Detection of MHC, Thy-1, Lyt-1, and Lyt-2 antigens in the developing mouse thymus. Adv Exp Med Biol 149:241, 1982b

Van Heerde P, Feltkamp CA, Feltkamp-Vroom TM, et al. Non-Hodgkin's lymphoma. Immunohistochemical and electron microscopical findings in relation to light-microscopy. A study of 74 cases. Cancer 46:2210, 1980

van Muijen GN, Ruiter DJ, van Leewen C, et al. Cytokeratin and neurofilament in lung carcinomas. Am J Pathol 116:363, 1984

Van Nagell JR Jr, Donaldson ES, Gay EC, et al. Carcinoembryonic antigen in carcinoma of the uterine cervix. 2. Tissue localization and correlation with plasma antigen concentration. Cancer 44:944, 1979

Van Rooijen N. Six methods for separate detection of two different antigens in the same tissue section. J Histochem Cytochem 28:716, 1980

Vecchio FM, Fabiano A, Orsini G, et al. Alpha-1-antitrypsin MZ phenotype and cryptogenic chronic liver disease in adults. Digestion 27:100, 1983

Velasco ME, Dahl D, Roessmann U, et al. Immunohistochemical localization of glial fibrillary acidic protein in human glial neoplasms. Cancer 45:484, 1980

Veltri RW, Maxim PE, Boehlecke JM. A human tumour-associated membrane antigen from squamous-cell carcinoma of the lung. Br J Cancer 41:705, 1980

Venter JC, Eddy B, Hall LM, et al. Monoclonal antibodies detect the conservation of muscarinic cholinergic receptor structure from *Drosophila* to human brain and detect possible structural homology with α_1-adrenergic receptors. Proc Natl Acad Sci 81:272, 1984

Vernon SE. Herpetic tracheobronchitis: immunohistologic demonstration of herpes simplex virus antigen. Hum Pathol 13:683, 1982

Vernon SE, Lewin KJ. Immunoperoxidase and immunofluorescence in lymph node biopsies: a comparative study. Am J Surg Pathol 4:357, 1980

Viac J, Reano A, Brochier J, et al. Reactivity pattern of a monoclonal antikeratin antibody (KL1). J Invest Dermatol 81:351, 1983

Viac J, Reano A, Thivolet J. Cytokeratins in human basal and squamous cell carcinomas: biochemical, immunohistological findings and comparisons with normal epithelia. J Cutan Pathol 9:377, 1982

Viale G, Dell'Orto P, Moro E, et al. Vasoactive intestinal polypeptide-, somatostatin-, and calcitonin-producing adrenal pheochromocytoma associated with the watery diarrhea (WDHH) syndrome. First case report with immunohistochemical findings. Cancer 55:1099, 1985

Vieira LM, Sarno EN, Ruzany F, et al. [Glomerular immunopathology: comparative study with immunofluorescence and immunoperoxidase.] Rev Bras Pesqui Med Biol 12:377, 1979

Vilpo JA, Klemi P, Lassila O, et al. Cytological and functional characterization of three cases of malignant histiocytosis. Cancer 46:1795, 1980

Vimadalal SD, Said JW, Voyles H III. Gastric lymphoreticular neoplasms: an immunologic study of 36 cases. Am J Clin Pathol 80:792, 1983

Vinores SA, Bonnin JM, Rubinstein LJ, et al. Immunohistochemical demonstration of neuron-specific enolase in neoplasms of the CNS and other tissues. Arch Pathol Lab Med 108: 536, 1984

Von Gumberz C, Seifert G. Immunoglobulin-containing plasma cells in chronic parotitis and malignant lymphomas of the parotid gland. Comparing immunocytochemical observations of frequency and localization. Virchows Arch [A] 389:79, 1980.

von Hanwehr RI, Hofman FM, Taylor CR, et al. Mononuclear lymphoid populations infiltrating the microenvironment of primary CNS tumors. Characterization of cell subsets with monoclonal antibodies. J. Neurosurg 60:1138, 1984

Vuitch MF, Mendelsohn G. Relationship of ectopic ACTH production to tumor differentiation: a morphologic and immunohistochemical study of prostatic carcinoma with Cushing's syndrome. Cancer 47:296, 1981

Wachner R, Wittekind C, von Kleist S. Localization of CEA, beta-HCG, Sp1, and keratin in the tissue of lung carcinomas. An immunohistochemical study. Virchows Arch [A] 402:415, 1984a

Wachner R, Wittekind C, von Kleist S. Immunohistological localization of beta-HCG in breast carcinomas. Eur J Cancer Clin Oncol 20:679, 1984b

Wachsmuth ED. The localization of enzymes in tissue sections by immunohistochemistry. Conventional antibody and mixed aggregation techniques. Histochem J 8:253, 1976

Wachsmuth ED. A quantitative approach to efficiency and sensitivity: enzyme histochemistry, immunofluorescence and PAP-technique in tissue sections. Acta Histochem (Suppl) 25:47, 1982

Wagener C, Hain F, Breuer H, et al. Immunohistochemical demonstration of carcinoembryonic antigen in normal, transitional and inflamed colonic mucosa. Oncodev Biol Med 2:331, 1981a

Wagener C, Menzel B, Breuer H, et al. Immunohisto-

chemical localisation of alpha-fetoprotein (AFP) in germ cell tumours: evidence for AFP production by tissues different from endodermal sinus tumour. Oncology 38:236, 1981b

Wagener C, Petzold P, Köhler W, et al. Binding of five monoclonal anti-CEA antibodies with different epitope specificities to various carcinoma tissues. Int J Cancer 33:469, 1984

Wahlström T, Huhtaniemi I, Hovatta O, et al. Localization of luteinizing hormone, follicle-stimulating hormone, prolactin, and their receptors in human and rat testis using immunohistochemistry and radioreceptor assay. J Clin Endocrinol Metab 57:825, 1983

Wahlström T, Lindgren J, Korhonen M, et al. Distinction between endocervical and endometrial adenocarcinoma with immunoperoxidase staining of carcinoembryonic antigen in routine histological tissue specimens. Lancet 2:1159, 1979

Wahlström T, Lindgren J, Korhonen M, et al. [Differential diagnosis of adenocarcinoma of the uterus and cervix using CEA immunohistochemical staining.] Duodecim 96:804, 1980

Wahlström T, Seppälä M. Immunological evidence for the occurrence of luteinizing hormone-releasing factor and the alpha-subunit of glycoprotein hormones in carcinoid tumors. J Clin Endocrinol Metab 53:209, 1981

Wahlström T, Stenman UH, Lundovist C, et al. The use of monoclonal antibodies against human chorionic gonadotropin for immunoperoxidase staining of normal placenta, pituitary gland, and pituitary adenomas. J Histochem Cytochem 29:864, 1981a

Walhlström T, Teisner B, Lee JN, et al. Placenta-associated plasma protein-A (PAPP-A, SP4) in trophoblastic tumours. Acta Pathol Microbiol Scand [A] 89A:65, 1981b

Walker AN, Mills SE, Fechner RE, et al. 'Endometrial' adenocarcinoma of the prostatic urethra arising in a villous polyp. A light microscopic and immunoperoxidase study. Arch Pathol Lab Med 106:624, 1981

Walker DM. Identification of subpopulations of lymphocytes and macrophages in the infiltrate of lichen planus lesions of skin and oral mucosa. Br J Dermatol 94:529, 1976

Walker RA. The demonstration of alpha lactalbumin in human breast carcinomas. J Pathol 129:37, 1979

Walker RA. Demonstration of carcinoembryonic antigen in human breast carcinomas by the immunoperoxidase technique. J Clin Pathol 33:356, 1980

Walker RA. Biological markers in human breast carcinoma. J Pathol 137:109, 1982

Walker RA, Cove DH, Howell A. Histological detection of oestrogen receptor in human breast carcinomas. Lancet 1:171, 1980

Walts AE, Said JW, Banks-Schlegel S. Keratin and carcinoembryonic antigen in exfoliated mesothelial and malignant cells: an immunoperoxidase study. Am J Clin Pathol 80:671, 1983

Walts AE, Said JW, Shintaku IP, et al. Keratins of different molecular weight in exfoliated mesothelial and adenocarcinoma cells—an aid to cell identification. Am J Clin Pathol 81:442, 1984

Wang E, Cairncross JG, Liem RKH. Identification of glial filament protein and vimentin in the same intermediate filament system in human glioma cells. Proc Natl Acad Sci 81:2102, 1984a

Wang GP, Grundke-Iqbal I, Kascsak RJ, et al. Alzheimer neurofibrillary tangles: monoclonal antibodies to inherent antigen(s). Acta Neuropathol (Berl) 62:268, 1984b

Wang WL, Wang BY, Zang JS, Liu WB, et al. HBcAg

in hepatocellular carcinoma and its surrounding tissue. Chin Med J 93:835, 1980

Ware JL, Paulson DF, Parks SF, et al. Production of monoclonal antibody alpha pro 3 recognizing a human prostatic carcinoma antigen. Cancer Res 42:1215, 1982

Warhol MJ, Pinkus GS, Banks-Schlegel SP. Localization of keratin proteins in the human epidermis by a postembedding immunoperoxidase technique. J Histochem Cytochem 31:517, 1983

Warhol MJ, Pinkus GS, Said JW. The ultrastructural localization of Leu-M1 in Reed-Sternberg cells and normal myeloid cells. Lab Invest 52:73A, 1985

Warhol MJ, Rice RH, Pinkus GS, et al. Evaluation of squamous epithelium in adenoacanthoma and adenosquamous carcinoma of the endometrium: immunoperoxidase analysis of involucrin and keratin localization. Int J Gynecol Pathol 3:82, 1984

Warner TFCS, Lloyd RV, Hafez GF, et al. Immunocytochemistry of neurotropic melanoma. Cancer 53:254, 1984

Warnke R, Levy R. Detection of T and B cell antigens hybridoma monoclonal antibodies: a biotin-avidin-horseradish peroxidase method. J Histochem Cytochem 28:771, 1980

Warnke R, Levy R. Tissue section immunologic methods in lymphomas. In: DeLellis RA, ed. Diagnostic Immunohistochemistry, p 203. Masson Monographs in Diagnostic Pathology, Sternberg SS, series ed. New York, Masson, 1981

Warnke R, Miller R, Grogan T, et al. Immunologic phenotype in 30 patients with diffuse large-cell lymphoma. N Engl J Med 303:293, 1980

Warren WH, Memoli VA, Gould VE. Immunohistochemical and ultrastructural analysis of bronchopulmonary neuroendocrine neoplasms. I. Carcinoids. Ultrastruct Pathol 6:15, 1984

Watanabe S, Nakajima T, Shimosato Y, et al. Malignant histiocytosis and Letterer-Siwe disease. Cancer 51:1412, 1983

Watanabe S, Shimosato Y, Sato Y, et al. Immunologic characterization of Reed-Sternberg cells and other cell components in lymph nodes with Hodgkin's disease. Acta Pathol Jpn 34:241, 1984

Watanabe S, Shimosato Y, Shimoyama M, et al. Adult T cell lymphoma with hypergammaglobulinemia. Cancer 46:2472, 1980

Watts G, Leathem AJ. A non-immunoglobulin link reagent for use in the unlabelled antibody method (PAP) of immunohistochemistry. Med Lab Sci 37:359, 1980

Wear DJ, Margileth AM, Hadfield TL, et al. Cat scratch disease: a bacterial infection. Science 221:1403, 1983

Webb KS, Paulson DF, Parks SF, et al. Characterization of prostate-tissue-directed monoclonal antibody, alpha-Pro 13. Cancer Immunol Immunother 17-7, 1984

Wechsler LR, Gross RA, Miller DC. Meningeal gliomatosis with "negative" CSF cytology: the value of GFAP staining. Neurology (NY) 34:1611, 1984

Weindl A, Sofroniew MV. Immunohistochemical localization of hypothalamic peptide hormones in neural target areas. In: Ferring Symposium on Brain and Pituitary Peptides, p 97. Munich, 1979. Basel, Karger, WL300 F392b

Weir EE, Pretlow TG, Pitts A, et al. Destruction of endogenous peroxidase activity in order to locate cellular antigens by peroxidase-labeled antibodies. J Histochem Cytochem 22:51, 1974

Weiss LM, Crabtree GS, Rouse RV, et al. Morphologic and immunologic characterization of 50 peripheral T-cell lymphomas. Am J Pathol 118:316, 1985

Weiss RA, Guillet GY, Freedberg IM, et al. The use of monoclonal antibody to keratin in human epidermal disease: alterations in immunohistochemical staining pattern. J Invest Dermatol 81:224, 1983

Weiss SW, Langloss JM, Enzinger FM. Value of S-100 protein in the diagnosis of soft tissue tumors with particular reference to benign and malignant Schwann cell tumors. Lab Invest 49:299, 1983

Wells CA, Heryet A, Brochier J, et al. The immunocytochemical detection of axillary micrometastases in breast cancer. Br J Cancer 50:193, 1984

Wells CA, Taylor SM, Cuello AC. Argentaffin and argyrophill reactions and sertotonin content of endocrine tumours. J Clin Pathol 38:49, 1985

Wen DR, Bhuta S, Herschman HR, et al. S100 protein: a marker for melanocytic tumors. Ann NY Acad Sci 420:261, 1983

Westergaard E, Hertz MM, Bolwig TG. Increased permeability to horseradish peroxidase across cerebral vessels, evoked by electrically induced seizures in the rat. Acta Neuropathol 41:73, 1978

Westermark P, Shirahama T, Skinner M, et al. Immunohistochemical evidence for the lack of amyloid P component in some intracerebral amyloids. Lab Invest 46:457, 1982

Westermark P, Shirahama T, Skinner M, et al. Amyloid P-component (protein AP) in localized amyloidosis as revealed by an immunocytochemical method. Histochemistry 71:171, 1981

Western H, Bainton DF. Association of alkaline phosphatase-positive reticulum cells in bone marrow with granulocyte precursors. J Exp Med 150:919, 1981

Weston PD, Devries JA, Wrigglesworth R. Conjugation of enzymes to immunoglobulins using dimaleimides. Biochim Biophys Acta 612:40, 1980

Wahley K. Biosynthesis of the complement components and the regulatory proteins of the alternative complement pathway by human peripheral blood monocytes. J Exp Med 151:501, 1980

Wheeler GE, Eiferman RA. Immunohistochemical identification of the AA protein in lattice dystrophy. Exp Eye Res 36:181, 1983

Whitaker JN. The distribution of myelin basic protein in central nervous system lesions of multiple sclerosis and acute experimental allergic encephalomyelitis. Ann Neurol 3:291, 1978

Whitaker D, Sterrett GF, Shilkin KB. Detection of tissue CEA-like substance as an aid in the differential diagnosis of malignant mesothelioma. Pathology 14:255, 1982

Whitaker JN, Terry LC, Whetsell WO Jr. Immunocytochemical localization of cathepsin D in rat neural tissue. Brain Res 216:109, 1981

Whitley RJ, Soong S-J, Hirsch MS, et al. (NIAID Collaborative Antiviral Study Group). Herpes simplex encephalitis: vidarabine therapy and diagnostic problems. N Engl J Med 304:313, 1981

Whyte A, Loke YW. Antigens of the human trophoblast plasma membrane. Clin Exp Immunol 37:359, 1979

Wick MR, Perrone TL, Burke BA. Sarcomatoid transitional cell carcinomas of the renal pelvis. An ultrastructural and immunohistochemical study. Arch Pathol Lab Med 109:55, 1985

Wick MR, Scheithauer BW, Kovacs K. Neuron-specific enolase in neuroendocrine tumors of the thymus, bronchus, and skin. Am J Clin Path 79:703, 1983.

Wiernik PH, Serpick AA. Granulocytic sarcoma (chloroma). Blood 35:361, 1970

Wijesinha SS, Steer HW. Studies of the immunoglobulin-producing cells of the human intestine: the defunctioned bowel. Gut 1982 23:211, 1982

Wilander E, Grimelius L, Portela-Gomes G, et al. Substance P and enteroglucagon-like immunoreactivity in argentaffin and argyrophil midgut carcinoid tumours. Scand J Gastroenterol [Suppl] 14:19, 1979

Wiley EL, Mendelsohn G, Droller MJ. Immunoperoxidase detection of carcinoembryonic antigen and blood group substances in papillary transitional cell carcinoma of the bladder. J Urol 128:276, 1982

Wiley EL, Mendelsohn G, Eggleston JC. Distribution of carcinoembryonic antigens and blood group substances in adenocarcinoma of the colon. J Lab Invest 44:507, 1981

Wilke H, Harms D. [Alpha-1-fetoprotein in tumour tissue.] Dtsch Med Wochenschr 104:1527, 1979

Wilkerson EH, Wilkerson JA. New developments in surgical pathology. III. Immunocytochemistry. Ala J Med Sci 19:55, 1982

Wilkinson MJ, Howell A, Harris M, et al. The prognostic significance of two epithelial membrane antigens expressed by human mammary carcinomas. Int J Cancer 33:299, 1984

Willis RA. Pathology of Tumours. London, Butterworths, 1948

Wilson AJ. Factor VIII–related antigen staining by immunoperoxidase technic in smaller laboratories: a potential problem. Am J Clin Pathol 81:117, 1984

Wilson BS, Herzig MA, Lloyd RV. Immunoperoxidase staining for Ia-like antigens in paraffin-embedded tissues from human melanoma and lung carcinomas. Am J Pathol 115:102, 1984

Wilson TS, McDowell EM, McIntire KR, et al. Elaboration of human chorionic gonadotropin by lung tumors: an immunocytochemical study. Arch Pathol Lab Med 105:169, 1981

Wiltshaw E. The natural history of extramedullary plasmacytoma and its relation to solitary myeloma of bone and myelomatosis. Medicine 55:217, 1976

Winchester RJ, Kunkel HG. The human Ia system. Adv Immunol 28:221, 1979

Winchester RJ, Wang C-Y, Gibofsky A, et al. Expression of Ia-like antigens on cultured human malignant melanoma cells lines. Proc Natl Acad Sci 75:6235, 1978

Winkler B, Crum CP, Fujii T, et al. Koilocytotic lesions of the cervix. The relationship of mitotic abnormalities to the presence of papillomavirus antigens and nuclear DNA content. Cancer 53:1081, 1984a

Winkler B, Reumann W, Mitao M, et al. Chlamydial endometritis. A histological and immunohistochemical analysis. Am J Surg Pathol 8:771, 1984b

Winkler CF, Goodman GK, Eiferman RA, et al. Orbital metastasis from prostatic carcinoma. Identification by an immunoperoxidase technique. Arch Opthalmol 99:1406, 1981

Wirdnam PK, Milner RD. Quantitation of the B and A cell fractions in human pancreas from early fetal life to puberty. Early Hum Dev 5:299, 1981

Wischik CM, Crowther RA, Stewart M, et al. Subunit structure of paired helical filaments in Alzheimer's disease. J Cell Biol 100:1905, 1985

Wisniewski H, Johnson AB, Raine CS, et al. Senile plaques and cerebral amyloidosis in aged dogs. A histochemical and ultrastructural study. Lab Invest 23:287, 1970

Wisniewski HM, Brown HR, Thormar H. Pathogenesis of viral encephalitis: demonstration of viral antigen(s) in the brain endothelium. Acta Neuropathol (Berl) 60:107, 1983a

Wisniewski HM, Kozlowski PB. Evidence for blood-brain barrier changes in senile dementia of the Alzheimer type (SDAT). Ann NY Acad Sci 396:119, 1982

Wisniewski HM, Lossinsky AS, Moretz RC, et al. Increased blood-brain barrier permeability in scrapie-infected mice. J Neuropathol Exp Neurol 42:615, 1983b

Wisniewski HM, Merz GS, Merz PA, et al. Morphology and biochemistry of neuronal paired helical filaments and amyloid fibers in humans and animals. Prog Neuropathol 5:139, 1983c

Wisniewski HM, Merz PA, Igbal K. Ultrastructure of paired helical filaments of Alzheimer's neurofibrillary tangle. J Neuropathol Exp Neurol 43:643, 1984

Witorsch RJ. The application of immunoperoxidase methodology for the visulization of prolactin binding sites in human prostate tissue. Hum Pathol 10:521, 1979

Witorsch RJ. Evaluation of immunoperoxidase-stained tissue sections with an electrophoresis densitometer. J Histochem Cytochem 30:179, 1982

Wittekind C, Wichmann T, Von Kleist S. Immunohistological localization of AFP and HCG in uniformly classified testis tumors. Anticancer Res 3:327, 1983

Wittekind C, von Kleist S, Sandritter W. [Comparative immunohistological studies of the localization of the carcinoembryonic antigen in benign and malignant breast tissue.] Acta Histochem (Suppl) 25:83, 1982a

Wittekind C, von Kleist S, Sandritter W. [Immunohistological studies for demonstration of carcinoembryonic antigen in benign breast lesions.] Onkologie (Suppl) 5:25, 1982b

Wolfe HJ, Palmer PE. Alpha-antitrypsin: its immunohistochemical localization and significance in diagnostic pathology. In: DeLellis RA, ed. Diagnostic Immunohistochemistry, p 227. Masson Monographs in Diagnostic Pathology, Sternberg SS, series ed, 1981

Wong GHW, Bartlett PF, Clark-Lewis I, et al. Inducible expression of H-2 and Ia antigens on brain cells. Nature 310:688, 1984

Wong GHW, Bartlett PF, Clark-Lewis I, et al. Interferon-γ induces the expression of H-2 and Ia antigens on brain cells. J Neuroimmunol 7:255, 1985

Wong LY, Chan SH, Oon CJ, et al. Immunocytochemical localization of testosterone in human hepatocellular carcinoma. Histochem J 16:687, 1984

Wood GS, Deneau DG, Miller RA, et al. Subtypes of cutaneous T-cell lymphoma defined by expression of Leu-1 and Ia. Blood 59:876, 1982

Wood GS, Warnke R. Suppression of endogenous avidin-binding activity in tissues and its relevance to biotin-avidin detection system. J Histochem Cytochem 29:1196, 1981

Wood GS, Warnke RA. The immunologic phenotyping of bone marrow biopsies and aspirates: frozen section techniques. Blood 59:913, 1982

Wood GW, Gollahon KA, Tilzer SA, et al. The failure of microglia in normal brain to exhibit mononuclear phagocyte markers. J Neuropathol Exp Neurol 38:369, 1979

Wood GW, Travers H. Non-Hodgkin's lymphoma: identification of the monoclonal B lymphocyte component in the presence of polyclonal immunoglobulin. J Histochem Cytochem 30:1015, 1982

Woodard BH, Eisenbarth G, Wallace NR, et al. Adrenocorticotropin production by a mammary carcinoma. Cancer 47:1823, 1981

Woodruff JD, Braun L, Cavlieri R, et al. Immunologic identification of papillomavirus antigen in condyloma tissues from the female genital tract. Obstet Gynecol 56:727, 1980

Woods JC, Spriggs AI, Harris H, et al. A new marker for human cancer cells. 3. Immunocytochemical detection of malignant cells in serous fluids with the Ca1 antibody. Lancet 2:512, 1982

Wowra B, Peiffer, J. An immunoperoxidase study of a

human pituitary adenoma associated with Cushing's syndrome. Pathol Res Pract 178:349, 1984

Wright DH, Isaacson P. Follicular center cell lymphoma of childhood: a report of three cases and a discussion of its relationship to Burkitt's lymphoma. Cancer 47:915, 1981

Wright GL Jr, Beckett ML, Starling JJ, et al. Immuno-histochemical localization of prostate carcinoma–associated antigens. Cancer Res 43:5509, 1983

Wright GM, Lebloud CP. Immunohistochemical localization of procollagens. III. Type I procollagen antigenicity in osteoblasts and prebone (osteoid). J Histochem Cytochem 29:791, 1981

Wright J, Abolfathi A, Penman E, et al. Pancreatic somatostatinoma presenting with hypoglycaemia. Clin Endocrinol 12:603, 1980

Wright JE. Immunoperoxidase in dermatopathology. J Assoc Military Dermatologists 9:46, 1983

Wright JR, Calkins, E. Relationship of amyloid deposits in the human aorta to aortic atherosclerosis. A postmortem study of 100 individuals over 60 years of age. Lab Invest 30:767, 1974

Wright SD, Rao PE, Van Voorhis WC, et al. Identification of the C3bi receptor of human monocytes and macrophages by using monoclonal antibodies. Proc Natl Acad Sci USA 80:5699, 1983

Wurster K, Rapp W. Histological and immunohistological studies on gastric mucosa. I. The presence of CEA in dysplastic surface epithelium. Pathol Res Pract 164:270, 1979

Yachi A, Imai K, Moriya Y, et al. Human gastric cancer-associated antigens and carcinoembryonic antigen detected by monoclonal antibodies. Ann NY Acad Sci 417:158, 1983

Yagihasi S, Shimoyama N, Morita T, et al. Ganglioneuroblastoma containing several kinds of neuronal peptides with watery diarrhea syndrome. Acta Pathol Jpn 32:807, 1982

Yamada G, Takahashi T, Mizuno M, et al. Immunoelectron miocroscopic observation of hepatitis B surface antigen on the surface of liver cells from patients with hepatitis B virus infection. Acta med Okayama 34:175, 1980

Yamamoto M, Takahashi I, Iwamoto T, et al. Endocrine cells in extrahepatic bile duct carcinoma. J Cancer Res Clin Oncol 108:331, 1984

Yamanaka N, Ishii Y, Koshiba H, et al. A study of surface markers in non-Hodgkin's lymphoma by using anti-T and anti-B lymphocyte sera. Cancer 47:311, 1981

Yamasaki M, Tateishi R, Hongo J, et al. Argyrophil small cell carcinomas of the uterine cervix. Int J Gynecol Pathol 3:146, 1984

Yamasaki M, Ueda G, Inoue M, et al. Correlative light and immunohistological study of the HCG-like antigen in the squamous cell carcinoma of the human uterine cervix. Nippon Sanka Fujinka Gakkai Zasshi 33:151, 1981

Yamase HT. Peroxidase-antiperoxidase method for tissue antigens: improved shelf life for reagents. Arch Pathol Lab Med 106:102, 1982

Yasuda N, Kauch T, Uchino H. J chain synthesis in human myeloma cells: light and electron microscopic studies. Clin Exp Immunol 40:573, 1980

Yasuda K, Yamamoto N, Yamashita S. Use of peroxidase-avidin conjugate for the demonstration of intracellular antigen. Experientia 37:306, 1981

Yen S-H, Fields KL. Antibodies to neurofilament, glial filament, and fibroblast intermediate filament proteins bind to different cell types of the nervous system. J Cell Biol 88:115, 1981

Yen S-H, Gaskin F, Fu SM. Neurofibrillary tangles in senile dementia of the Alzheimer type share an antigenic determinant with intermediate filaments of the vimentin class. Am J Pathol 113:373, 1983a

Yen S-H, Horoupian DS, Terry RD. Immunocytochemical comparison of neurofibrillary tangles in senile dementia of Alzheimer type, progressive supranuclear palsy, and postencephalitic Parkinsonism. Ann Neurol 13:172, 1983b

York JC, Taylor CR, Lukes RJ. Monoclonality in giant lymph node hyperplasia. Lab Invest 44:77A, 1981

Yu GS, Kadish AS, Johnson AB, et al. Breast carcinoma-associated antigen. An immunocytochemical study. Am J Clin Pathol 74:453, 1980

Yung WKA, Borit A, Dahl D, et al. Keratin and vimentin in meningiomas. J Neuropathol Exp Neurol 43:299, 1984

Yung WKA, Tepper SJ, Young DF. Diffuse bone marrow metastatis by gilobblastoma: premortem diagnosis by peroxidase-antiperoxidase staining for glial fibrillary acidic protein. Ann Neurol 14:581, 1983

Zafrani ES, Maurice M, Feldmann G. Comparison between conjugate and non-conjugate immunoperoxidase procedures with special reference to intracellular penetration. Application to albumin localization in rat hepatocytes. J Immunol Methods 56:245, 1983

Zakharova NA, Novikova AV, Shakhanina KL, et al. [Comparative study of modifications in the immunoperoxidase and immunofluorescent methods of detecting human tissue immunoglobulins.] Zh Mikrobiol Epidemiol Immunobiol (8):54, 1979

Zaki FG, Keim GR, Takii Y, et al. Hyperplasia of juxtaglomerular cells and renin localization in kidney of normotensive animals given captopril. Electron microscopic and immunohistochemical studies. Ann Clin Lab Sci 12:200, 1982

Zarrabi MH, Stark RS, Kane P, et al. IgM myeloma, a distinct entity in the spectrum of B-cell neoplasia. Am J Clin Pathol 75:1, 1981

Zipser B, McKay R. Monoclonal antibodies distinguish identifiable neurons in the leech. Nature 289:549, 1981

Zülch KJ. Principles of the new World Health Organization (WHO) classification of brain tumors. Neuroradiology 19:59, 1980

Zweibaum A, Hauri HP, Sterchi E, et al. Immunohistological evidence, obtained with monoclonal antibodies, of small intestinal brush border hydrolases in human colon cancers and foetal colons. Int J Cancer 34:591, 1984

Index

Note: Page numbers followed by (t) refer to tables; page numbers in *italics* refer to illustrations; and page numbers followed by (s) refer to source lists.

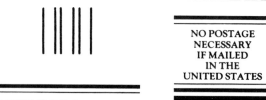

BUSINESS REPLY MAIL
FIRST CLASS   PERMIT NO. 5152   NEW YORK, NEW YORK

POSTAGE WILL BE PAID BY ADDRESSEE

CBS Educational & Professional Publishing
W.B.Saunders Company
Order Fulfillment Department
383 Madison Avenue
New York, NY 10017

NO POSTAGE
NECESSARY
IF MAILED
IN THE
UNITED STATES